Mild Traumatic Brain Injury

Dominic A. Carone, PhD, ABPP-CN earned his undergraduate degree (BA in psychology) at Le Moyne College. He completed his graduate training at Nova Southeastern University, where he earned a PhD in the neuropsychology specialization program. He completed his neuropsychology internship at The University of Oklahoma Health Sciences Center and a neuropsychology fellowship in the Department of Neurology at SUNY Buffalo School of Medicine and Biomedical Sciences.

Dr. Carone is board certified in clinical neuropsychology through the American Board of Professional Psychology. He served as President of the New York State Association of Neuropsychology for 3½ years and of the Central New York Psychological Association (one-year term). He is currently employed as a neuropsychologist and clinical assistant professor at SUNY Upstate Medical University, where he coordinates the Neuropsychology Assessment Program. In that role, he assesses adults and children with a wide variety of acquired and developmental brain disorders including all levels of traumatic brain injury. He also trains undergraduate and graduate psychology students, provides continuing education seminars, conducts research, and serves as a journal reviewer for scientific journals (e.g., editorial board for *The Clinical Neuropsychologist*). He has published numerous journal articles in psychology, neurology, and neuroimaging journals, as well as book chapters. His main research interests include traumatic brain injury and symptom validity testing. He is also the founder and webmaster of the popular medical information website, MedFriendly.com.

Shane S. Bush, PhD, ABPP, ABN is the Director of Long Island Neuropsychology, P.C., a Clinical Assistant Professor in the Department of Psychiatry and Behavioral Science at Stony Brook University School of Medicine, and a neuropsychologist with the VA New York Harbor Healthcare System. He is board certified in neuropsychology and rehabilitation psychology, a fellow of the American Psychological Association and the National Academy of Neuropsychology, and past President of the National Academy of Neuropsychology. He has published 9 books, 2 special journal issues, and numerous articles and book chapters, and has presented at national and international conferences.

Mild Traumatic Brain Injury

Symptom Validity Assessment and Malingering

Dominic A. Carone, PhD, ABPP-CN

Shane S. Bush, PhD, ABPP, ABN

EDITORS

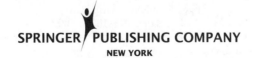

SPRINGER PUBLISHING COMPANY
NEW YORK

Springer Publishing Company, LLC
11 West 42nd Street
New York, NY 10036
www.springerpub.com

Acquisitions Editor: Nancy Hale
Production Editor: Joseph Stubenrauch
Composition: Absolute Service, Inc.

ISBN: 978-0-8261-0915-6
E-book ISBN: 978-0-8261-0916-3

12 13 14 15/ 5 4 3 2 1

The author and the publisher of this Work have made every effort to use sources believed to be reliable to provide information that is accurate and compatible with the standards generally accepted at the time of publication. The author and publisher shall not be liable for any special, consequential, or exemplary damages resulting, in whole or in part, from the readers' use of, or reliance on, the information contained in this book. The publisher has no responsibility for the persistence or accuracy of URLs for external or third-party Internet websites referred to in this publication and does not guarantee that any content on such websites is, or will remain, accurate or appropriate.

Library of Congress Cataloging-in-Publication Data

Mild traumatic brain injury : symptom validity assessment and malingering / Dominic A. Carone, Shane S. Bush, editors.
    p. cm.
  Includes bibliographical references and index.
  ISBN 978-0-8261-0915-6
  1. Brain damage—Diagnosis. 2. Brain—Concussion. I. Carone, Dominic A.
II. Bush, Shane S., 1965-
  RC387.5.M528 2013
  617.4'81044—dc23
                                2012029944

Special discounts on bulk quantities of our books are available to corporations, professional associations, pharmaceutical companies, health care organizations, and other qualifying groups.

If you are interested in a custom book, including chapters from more than one of our titles, we can provide that service as well.

For details, please contact:
Special Sales Department, Springer Publishing Company, LLC
11 West 42nd Street, 15th Floor, New York, NY 10036-8002
Phone: 877-687-7476 or 212-431-4370; Fax: 212-941-7842
Email: sales@springerpub.com

Printed in the United States of America by Bradford & Bigelow.

To Pam, Jessica, and Dominic —Dominic A. Carone

To Dana, Sarah, and Megan —Shane S. Bush

This book is also dedicated to our dear friend and colleague, Dr. Tony M. Wong, who passed away suddenly on April 23, 2011. The content of this book covers topics he cared deeply about, and we are saddened that he did not live to see the finished product.

Contents

Contributors

Bradley N. Axelrod, PhD, ABN
John D. Dingell Veterans Affairs Medical Center, Detroit, MI

Kevin J. Bianchini, PhD, ABN
University of New Orleans and Jefferson Neurobehavioral Group, New Orleans, LA

Kyle Brauer Boone, PhD, ABPP-CN
Center for Forensic Studies, Los Angeles Campus, Alliant International University and Los Angeles Biomedical Institute, Los Angeles, CA

Steven Broglio, PhD, ATC
University of Michigan, Ann Arbor, MI

Jeffrey N. Browndyke, PhD
Duke University Medical Center and Durham Veterans Affairs Medical Center, Durham, NC

Shane S. Bush, PhD, ABPP, ABN
Long Island Neuropsychology, PC, Lake Ronkonkoma, NY
Veterans Affairs New York Harbor Healthcare System, St. Albans, NY
Stony Brook University Medical School, Stony Brook, NY

Dominic A. Carone, PhD, ABPP-CN
State University of New York Upstate Medical University, Syracuse, NY

Michael D. Chafetz, PhD, ABPP-CN
Independent practice, New Orleans, LA

Kelly L. Curtis, MS
University of New Orleans, New Orleans, LA

Bridget M. Doane, PhD
Minneapolis Veterans Affairs Health Care System, Minneapolis, MN

Jacobus Donders, PhD, ABPP-CN/RP
Mary Free Bed Rehabilitation Hospital, Grand Rapids, MI

Christopher J. Graver, PhD, ABPP-CN
Madigan Healthcare System, Tacoma, WA
University of Washington School of Medicine, Seattle, WA

Paul Green, PhD
Private practice, Edmonton, Alberta, Canada

Kevin W. Greve, PhD, ABPP-CN
University of New Orleans and Jefferson Neurobehavioral Group, New Orleans, LA

Leslie M. Guidotti Breting, PhD
NorthShore University HealthSystem, Evanston, IL
University of Chicago Pritzker School of Medicine, Chicago, IL

Thomas J. Guilmette, PhD, ABPP-CN
Providence College and Alpert Medical School of Brown University
Providence, RI

Robert L. Heilbronner, PhD, ABPP-CN
Chicago Neuropsychology Group, Chicago, IL

George K. Henry, PhD, ABPP-CN
Los Angeles Neuropsychology Group, Los Angeles, CA

Grant L. Iverson, PhD
University of British Columbia, Vancouver, British Columbia, Canada

Michael W. Kirkwood, PhD, ABPP-CN
Children's Hospital Colorado, Aurora, CO

Alexis D. Kulick, PhD, ABPP-CN
Greater Los Angeles Veterans Affairs Healthcare System, Los Angeles, CA

Stephen N. Macciocchi, PhD, ABPP-CN
Shepherd Center, Atlanta, GA

Thomas Merten, PhD
Vivantes Netzwerk für Gesundheit, Berlin, Germany

Nathaniel W. Nelson, PhD, ABPP-CN
University of St. Thomas, Graduate School of Professional Psychology
Saint Paul, MN

Christian Schutte, PhD
John D. Dingell Veterans Affairs Medical Center, Detroit, MI

Elisabeth M. S. Sherman, PhD
Faculty of Medicine, University of Calgary, Calgary, Alberta
Copeman Healthcare Centre, Calgary, Alberta, Canada

Daniel J. Slick, PhD
Alberta Children's Hospital, Calgary, Alberta, Canada

Jerry J. Sweet, PhD, ABPP-CN
NorthShore University HealthSystem, Evanston, IL
University of Chicago Pritzker School of Medicine, Chicago, IL

Tara L. Victor, PhD, ABPP-CN
California State University, Dominguez Hills, Carson, CA
University of California, Los Angeles, CA
Greater Los Angeles Veterans Affairs Healthcare System, Los Angeles, CA

Foreword

Deception and its behavioral cousin, mimicry, are all over nature. The source of deception can be ultimate and fixed, such as the bright colorings of butterflies that are actually not poisonous, a defense that evolved over millennia. Deception can be proximately motivated, such as the bird that feigns injury to draw predators away from a nest or the spouse who claims a headache prior to an intimate moment. King David and Ulysses faked insanity to avoid death. Then there is the dangerous emotional mimicry of predatory psychopaths. Yet, because of training and professional culture issues, many psychologists and neuropsychologists are reluctant to fully address prospects for deception in their patients. This is puzzling because psychologists first brought to the world's attention that deception (of both self and other) is common and that most behavior is unconsciously motivated and goal-directed. So if the reader is willing to tentatively presume that deception is a part of evolutionary adaptation, the question becomes how can clinical neuropsychologists help carve nature at its joints? We begin by asking where neuropsychologists should look for deception.

Legendary bank robber Willie Sutton explained his motivation for robbing banks in plain terms: "That's where the money is." The development of clinical constructs and the validation of neuropsychological tests also require choosing a path to places where the "caseness" is. The neuropsychologist seeks the settings where a problem is most likely to be encountered in its clearest and most severe form. Rehabilitation centers, not community mental health clinics, are the place to study recovery from severe traumatic brain injury (TBI). If personality change associated with frontal lobe damage is your interest, a brain cancer treatment center is a better place to search for "frontal caseness" than an anxiety disorder clinic. Contact sports are the ideal venue for studying acute concussion, but courtrooms and law offices definitely aren't. However, legal settings are rife with abnormal illness-seeking behavior, defined as a motivated pursuit of the sick role.

There are several reasons why mild traumatic brain injury (MTBI) is an ideal population for studying feigned deficits. First, MTBI is a self-contained condition that resolves quickly without special treatment, a generally accepted conclusion by fair-minded neuropsychologists. This fact supports the researcher's confidence that false positive diagnosis of faking is made less likely. Second, claims of failure to recover from MTBI are strongly associated with incentives that could motivate exaggerated disability, such as wage loss payments, narcotic drugs, jury awards, work avoidance, and/or reducing criminal culpability. The longer the period of subjective disability, the greater the likelihood you are dealing with abnormal illness-seeking behavior and not dealing with chronic cognitive deficits. Third, the medical records of patients with MTBI are rich in the extra test data needed to objectively define research groups. Examples include the universally used Glasgow Coma Scale, the Revised Trauma Scale (if posttraumatic stress disorder [PTSD] is your interest), and neuroimaging studies. Fourth, there are many important public policy issues associated with persistent MTBI claims, such as the outcome, care, and treatment of combat soldiers with concussion, accident victims, and athletes.

Dominic Carone and Shane Bush's book focuses exclusively on MTBI claims and their association with validity issues. The book's 19 chapters inform on many key issues. Every clinician must know the boundary conditions of malingering caseness, and four chapters clearly inform this issue: Chapter 2 on the limits of clinical judgment, Chapter 3 on ethics, Chapter 4 on differential diagnosis, and Chapter 19 on special populations. Other chapters provide instruction on how neuropsychologists can cope with the counterarguments often raised in response to conclusions that somebody is feigning his or her deficits. Chapter 5 summarizes those counterarguments (providing some comic relief within scholarly limits), and Chapter 6 discusses ways to cope with the counterarguments made by patients caught with their validity scores down. Most of the chapters focus on the specific methods for assessing performance validity (low effort or high effort to look impaired) and symptom validity (over-statement of symptoms). The reader is treated to cutting-edge research into various simulation-detection methods, including freestanding and embedded indicators (Chapters 7, 8, and 9), symptom validity tests (Chapters 10, 16–18), atypical scores on common neuropsychological measures (Chapters 12 and 13), and functional neuroimaging (Chapter 14). The specific medicolegal contexts in which MTBI is assessed are also covered, such as military (Chapter 18), sports (Chapter 17), personal injury, and administratively adjudicated disability (Chapter 16) settings. Chapter 7 is the go-to guide for a novice researcher desiring a crash course on what questions to ask and what variables to define before starting a data collection project.

The content of this book is not monolithic. The discerning reader will appreciate differences of opinion regarding the willingness to attach a malingering label. My philosophy is to always scale your conclusions about effort to the *strongest* statement that the facts allow. Conclusions can range anywhere from "all results valid," to "some findings consistent with questionable effort," and topping out at "clearly faked neurocognitive deficits and symptoms." This book provides plenty of reasonable alternative language for scaling the strength of conclusions without becoming a Tower of Babel.

If after reading this book you are still not convinced that at least *some* persons can and do mimic deficits to fulfill personal needs after an MTBI, you should not be practicing clinical neuropsychology.

Manfred F. Greiffenstein, PhD, ABPP-CN
Psychological Systems
Royal Oak, Michigan

Preface

Neuropsychologists provide clinical and forensic evaluation of persons who have sustained traumatic brain injuries, with mild traumatic brain injuries (i.e., concussions) being, by far, the most common. The assessment of symptom validity (i.e., effort, exaggeration) is typically an essential part of such evaluations or may be the primary goal of the evaluation. As such, symptom validity assessment and mild traumatic brain injury are two of the most popular, researched, and discussed topics in neuropsychology. However, outside of neuropsychology, many health care providers who treat these patients are unaware that such assessment methods exist, and how much the use of such methods can drastically alter case conceptualization, treatment, and proper allocation of resources. Likewise, whereas stories abound in the popular media regarding the short- and long-term effects of concussions, there is rarely a discussion of the importance of symptom validity assessment as it pertains to these cases.

This book is the first specifically devoted to the integration of symptom validity assessment with persons who have sustained mild traumatic brain injuries. The book covers the different types of symptom validity assessment measures and procedures that are employed in the context of mild traumatic brain injury, as well as separate chapters on specific settings and populations (e.g., clinical, forensic, sports, military). It clearly emphasizes the importance of using symptom validity assessment techniques in this population before making conclusions about the cause(s) of symptom persistence. There is a focus on professional and research issues, including providing feedback about symptom validity, ethical issues, and diagnostic schemas. Although the book covers numerous self-report scales and personality inventories, we did not include coverage of the Rorschach test because it is not used routinely (if at all) as a symptom validity measure by neuropsychologists (Sharland & Gfeller, 2007).

This book is intended to be concise and focused while covering the primary issues of importance to practicing neuropsychologists and also retaining relevance for other professions. We recognize that this book attempts to cover a complex and sometimes controversial topic. As such, different chapter authors may have different positions or beliefs on particular issues. We attempted to allow for the presentation of alternate views on specific topics while maintaining a general consistency to the book.

As referring health care providers, courts, disability insurance companies, and athletic teams/leagues increasingly turn to neuropsychologists to address symptom validity concerns in mild traumatic brain injury cases, a comprehensive book discussing these issues will be in high demand. Given the rapid evolution of the knowledge and practices in symptom validity assessment and mild traumatic brain injury over the last 10 to 15 years, this volume provides a timely updated resource for many. We hope that this book assists practitioners in their work with those who present with problems associated with, or attributed to, mild traumatic brain injuries.

REFERENCE

Sharland, M. J., & Gfeller, J. D. (2007). A survey of neuropsychologists' beliefs and practices with respect to the assessment of effort. *Archives of Clinical Neuropsychology*, 22(2), 213–223.

Acknowledgments

We are very grateful to the contributing authors, who are leaders in the field on the topics they cover, for bringing their expertise and experience to bear in their writing. We are also thankful to Springer Publishing, and Nancy Hale in particular, for their understanding of the importance of this topic and their assistance and support throughout the process.

Dominic A. Carone would like to acknowledge the following individuals for providing important background information for use in Chapter 11: Deon Louw, MD, Paul Green, PhD, Jack Richman, MD, and Christopher Stewart-Patterson, MD.

Introduction: Historical Perspectives on Mild Traumatic Brain Injury, Symptom Validity Assessment, and Malingering

1

Dominic A. Carone & Shane S. Bush

"You have to know the past to understand the present."—Dr. Carl Sagan, Cosmos

MILD TRAUMATIC BRAIN INJURY (CONCUSSION)

The Beginnings

In antiquity, head/brain injuries were regarded as serious events that eventually led to death (Feinsod, 1997). Consistent with this view, the first physical evidence of neurosurgery (i.e., trephination) dates back to 10,000 BCE and was likely used to treat skull fractures by removing pieces of bone from the skull (Kshettry, Mindea, & Batjer, 2007). Some of the earliest written accounts of head/brain injuries are presented in three stories from the Holy Bible (King James Version), dating back to between the 12th and 10th centuries BCE (Feinsod, 1997). The three stories included Jael using a mallet to impale tent nails through Sisera's temples (Judges 4:21; 5:25), David embedding a stone in Goliath's forehead with a slingshot (Samuel I 17:49–51), and a woman fracturing Abimelech's skull by striking it with a piece of millstone from above (Judges 9:53–54). Sisera quickly lost consciousness and died from what would today be described as a severe penetrating traumatic brain injury (TBI). Goliath fell face first to the ground but it is unknown if he lost consciousness or suffered a brain injury before David immediately decapitated him with a sword. Abimelech did not lose consciousness and *immediately* called out so he could be slayed by a man rather than a woman. Because we are not told of the size of the millstone piece, the height from which it was dropped on his head, or whether he had any specific symptoms (e.g., altered mental status), it remains technically possible that the story of Abimelech is the first written account of a concussive injury as it would be thought of today. Shapiro and Mintz (1990) have speculated that the injuries to Abimelech and Goliath likely represent examples of cerebral concussion and/or contusion. However, because so many details are lacking, the most that can be said is that Abimelech's head and skull were clearly injured and that Goliath also suffered trauma to the head. Lastly, British rabbi Jonathan Magonet (1992) has stated that there may have been a Hebrew translational problem leading to interpretation that Goliath was struck in the head when he may have actually been struck in the leg, causing him to fall.

Aside from Biblical writings, (which are fictional to some and non-fictional to others) classical Greek writers such as Homer (8th century BCE) and Aristophanes (ca. 446 BCE–386 BCE) are said to have written the first fictional accounts of transient symptoms after mild trauma to the head/brain (Wrightson, 2000). Regarding nonfiction accounts, the ancient Greek physician Hippocrates of Kos (ca. 460 BCE–370 BCE) is said by modern translators to have used the term "concussion" in a general sense to refer to the whole spectrum of head injury (mild to severe) in describing symptoms such as loss of speech and hearing. However, McCrory and Berkovic (2001) posited that because the term concussion was not otherwise known to have been used since the Renaissance (14th–17th century), it is likely that early translators of the Hippocratic writings were applying modern concepts to the injury under consideration.

Very detailed historical accountings of the evolution of the concepts of concussion and mild traumatic brain injury (MTBI) are provided by Wrightson (2000) and McCrory and Berkovic (2001). A brief summary of their accounting is that the Arabic physician Rhazes (CE 865–925) first distinguished concussion as an abnormal transient physiological state rather than a severe or generic description of brain injury. A similar concept was carried forward by the Arabian physicians Albucasis (936–1013) and Avicenna (980–1037) and later by medieval physicians in the 1300s. One such physician, Lanfrancus, hypothesized that concussion symptoms were the result of a transient paralysis of cerebral function caused by brain shaking (or *commotion*).

In 1518, the Italian physician Jacopo Berengario da Carpi suggested that loss of consciousness (LOC) without head wounds or skull fractures was caused by the thrusting of the brain against the skull. The terms "commotio cerebri" and "embranlement" were used to describe shaking of the brain within the skull but were applied to all injury severities. The term concussion (meaning "to shake" in Latin) was used more widely in the 1500s and 1600s, with some specific symptoms (e.g., memory problems, lethargy, vertigo) delineated by several physicians during the era. Between the 1600s and 1700s, the term concussion began to be used to refer to signs (e.g., LOC) after head trauma that were presumed independent of structural brain injury, with some assuming that circulatory failure was the cause (later disproved).

The 19th Century and Beyond

In 1831, John Abernethy was the first to note that chronic postconcussive symptoms were more related to "constitutional weakness" (i.e., psychological factors) than the neurological effects of the injury. In 1863, John Hilton was the first to suggest reassurance and fatigue management as treatments after concussion. In the mid- to late 1800s, Sir John Erichsen wrote that concussion was an impairment of consciousness lasting minutes to hours, followed by a few days of giddiness and confusion. Recovery after concussion was described as complete to incomplete, and the symptoms were considered partly caused by brain damage and partly caused by psychological reactions to disability. These writings begin to lay the foundation for the concern that psychological factors, malingering, litigation, and disability claims are significant confounds that must be considered when assessing postconcussive symptomatology. Consideration of these potential confounds became an increasing problem with the beginning of workers compensation systems in the late 1880s and early 1900s (described in more detail in subsequent sections of this chapter). In the 1930s, a standard surgical text of the day stated that concussive symptoms persisting more than 2 weeks were caused by psychological factors and that disability claims were associated with immorality (Romanis & Mitchiner, 1934).

In the next decade, Denny-Brown and Ritchie (1941) published a seminal paper concluding that LOC after concussion was caused by a direct functional effect on the brainstem neurons without any vascular or pathologic lesion. They noted that concussions without pathological lesions (known as "uncomplicated concussions") could only occur if the head and brain were free to accelerate, which would result in shear-strain injuries that damaged cell bodies and broke axons.

A few decades later, Oppenheimer (1968) published a frequently cited neuro-pathological study which he reported as demonstrating that concussions (in the sense they are discussed today) can cause areas of microscopic brain damage and that if such injuries are repetitive (e.g., boxing), they may result in progressive, cumulative loss of tissue and nervous function. This condition in boxers was first described clinically as "punch drunk" by Martland (1928). These early writings would later influence the modern day discussion of chronic traumatic encephalopathy (CTE), which is a broad term used to refer to repetitive, often subclinical (e.g., asymptomatic), injury to the brain from various contact sports and other causes (Carone & Bush, in press). In cases of single concussive injuries, however, Gennarelli (1986) criticized Oppenheimer's study because the disrupted axons were too small in number and not distributed widely enough to explain all of the clinical phenomena of concussion. He thus concluded that many more axons must be damaged at a functional level without permanent damage (i.e., axotomy) but acknowledged that such permanent damage is possible.

A classic primate study by Ommaya and Gennarelli (1974) showed that microscopic lesions in the brain (especially the temporal lobes) can be found in cases of LOC after concussion—a finding later documented in rats (Foda & Marmarou, 1994). In 2001, Giza and Hovda (2001) published a seminal paper showing that cerebral pathophysiology after concussion can be adversely affected for days in animals and up to weeks in humans. For a detailed review of more recent advances in the biomechanics and neurophysiology of concussion, see McCrea (2008) and Guskiewicz and Mihalik (2011).

Although there was some research documenting objective evidence of brain injury after concussion(s), a very influential study by Livdall, Linderoth, and Norlin (1974) found no objective evidence of brain injury via cognitive tests, behavioral tests, electroencephalography (EEG), and vestibular studies. They concluded that persisting symptoms after concussion were caused by psychiatric and/or psychological factors (e.g., depression, anxiety, motivational) as opposed to brain damage. As Wrightson (2000) noted, these views influenced European neurology for 20 years (and likely still have an influence today), even though the standard psychometric tests used at the time were not those that were later found to be more sensitive to the effects of MTBI. However, as time progressed and neuropsychological test instrumentation and research designs improved (e.g., prospective studies, meta-analyses), a clear pattern began to emerge over the decades demonstrating that cognitive test results were generally at normal levels by 3 months postinjury (Belanger & Vanderploeg, 2005; Binder, 1997; Binder, Rohling & Larrabee, 1997; Dikmen, Machamer, Winn, & Temkin, 1995; Frencham, Fox, & Maybery, 2005; Iverson, 2005; Rohling et al., 2011; Schretlen & Shapiro, 2003).

The debate regarding whether persisting concussive symptoms (i.e., greater than 3 months) are caused by neurological factors, psychological factors, physical pain, the effects of medications, secondary gain, or some combination of these or other factors continues (Bigler, 2008; McCrea, 2008; Ruff & Jamora, 2009; Spencer, Drag, Walker, & Bieliauskas, 2010). The debate persists because of nonspecific nature of "postconcussive" symptoms (Lees-Haley, Fox, & Courtney, 2001) and the absence of objective biomarkers of structural brain injury in the majority of concussion cases despite advances in neuroimaging technology (Hughes et al., 2004; Iverson, Lovell,

Smith, & Franzen, 2000; Jeret et al., 1993; Kurca, Sivák, & Kucera, 2006; Livingston, Loder, Koziol, & Hunt, 1991). However, absence of evidence is not *always* evidence of absence, as revealed by the fact that magnetic resonance imaging (MRI) of the brain has revealed evidence of acute pathology in 30% of cases where no such abnormality was documented on computerized tomography (CT; Bazarian, Blyth, & Cimpello, 2006). Moreover, stronger MRI magnets sometimes show evidence of pathology not shown on weaker MRI magnets (Frayne, Goodyear, Dickhoff, Lauzon, & Sevick, 2003). A further problem is that not all patients go to the emergency room (ER) after a concussion; and, for those who do, brain CT is the standard imaging modality, whereas brain MRI is rarely used in the ER unless there are significant complications (e.g., sudden and unexpected neurological decompensation) that might suggest the presence of intracranial hemorrhage or edema.

One problem with the absence of evidence argument, however, is that it can be taken to the extreme, making brain injury claims unfalsifiable. For example, even if a brain MRI with high magnet strength (e.g., 3.0 Tesla) in the ER showed no evidence of neuropathology after concussion, someone can always argue that more sensitive diagnostics (e.g., an even stronger MRI magnet; brain biopsy; or autopsy, if the patient died from other causes) might have been able to detect brain damage that other methods did not. To take the argument to the most extreme end of the continuum, one can argue that a standard autopsy might have produced a false-negative result regarding the presence of subtle brain damage because an electron scanning microscope (SEM) was not used in the analysis. Overall, although it is true that absence of evidence is not always evidence of absence, there are certainly cases where negative test results accurately reflect that no structural brain damage is present.

Although there have been advances in functional neuroimaging indicating that functional neuronal disruption, as opposed to structural brain damage, is present after concussion, functional neuroimaging modalities remain research instruments at this time, as opposed to clinical tools that can assist in evaluation, management, and decision making with individual patients. In addition, such studies often have significant problems with generalizability to patients with persisting symptoms after a single concussion because of methodological limitations. For example, many of the studies that were performed in the acute to subacute phase of recovery (i.e., from days to 3 months postinjury), included patients with multiple concussions, had small samples sizes, combined patients, with mild and moderate traumatic brain injury (TBI) together, did not list the exclusion criteria, and/or included patients with significant psychiatric comorbidities (Bonne et al., 2003; Chen et al., 2004; Gowda et al., 2006; Hofman et al., 2001; Kant, Smith-Seemiller, Isaac, & Duffy, 1997; Umile, Plotkin, & Sandel, 1998; Varney & Bushnell, 1998). For a more complete review of neuroimaging techniques after MTBI, see Belanger, Vanderploeg, Curtiss, and Warden (2007).

As a result of these limitations and practical constraints involving neuroimaging after MTBI, clinical and forensic health care specialists often find themselves evaluating patients who are reporting persisting symptoms after a known or suspected MTBI without any objective biomarkers of brain injury. This situation poses a potential problem because malingering is most common when the presenting condition is one that has little to no objective evidence of neurological damage (e.g., MTBI, chronic fatigue syndrome, fibromyalgia, somatoform disorders, alleged chemical exposures), particularly if the person is seeking some form of compensation for the condition (Mittenberg, Patton, Canyock, & Condit, 2002). Because many MTBIs occur as a result of motor vehicle collisions or accidents in the workplace or in some other context (e.g., assault) in which a compensation claim can be made (e.g., workers compensation, no-fault insurance, disability application, personal injury litigation), the possibility that poor motivation, exaggeration, and malingering can contribute to persisting symptom reporting is significant. A brief history of malingering in general and its relationship to concussion follows.

MALINGERING

The Beginnings

The word "malingering" comes from the French word "malinger" meaning "poor or weakly" because these are the characteristics feigned or exaggerated by the malingerer (Stedman, 2006). Like concussions, malingering is as old as human existence because illness is a socially acceptable way to avoid obligations and responsibilities. Written documentation of malingering dates back as far as the writings in the Hebrew Bible (I Sam 21:10–15), in which David feigns insanity to escape a king he was afraid of by acting like a madman, drumming on the doors of a gate, and drooling onto his beard. The Greco-Roman physician, Galen of Pergamon (CE 129–199/217) reported two cases of malingering: (a) simulated colic (intermittent pain) to avoid a public meeting; and (b) a feigned knee injury to avoid a long journey (Lund, 1941).

The 19th Century and Beyond

Early books on malingering were brought about by concerns about exaggeration and/or feigning of symptoms in the context of avoiding military service (Bartholow, 1864; Gavin, 1843). For example, in the American Civil War (1861–1865), all symptoms or disability not accompanied by verifiable physical injury were considered malingering unless proven otherwise (Keen, Mitchell, & Morehouse, 1864). Other early books on malingering were written in the context of workers' compensation claims (Collie, 1917; Dawson, 1906; Jones, 1917; McKendrick, 1912; Sherman, 1913). The publications of these books occurred shortly after the introduction of workers' compensation laws in Germany, Britain, and the United States between the mid to late 1800s and early 1900s (Harger, 2010). Only a few years after Germany first introduced workers' compensation laws in 1871 (Employers Liability Law), Rigler (1879) coined the term "compensation neurosis" to describe the increasing compensation claims after German railway accidents (Ackerman, 2010). The term, which was later referred to as "accident neurosis" by Miller (1961a, 1961b), came to refer to patients with compensable injuries who claimed that their injuries were much more severe and disabling than objective medical evidence would support. As such, the cause of the reported symptoms and disability was presumed to be primarily related to psychological factors (e.g., stress) and/or malingering. At the time, workers' compensation was the only practical mechanism that workers had to pursue grievances against their employer for alleged harm, because litigation was almost never successful against employers at the time (Wessely, 2003).

One of the earliest books on malingering was titled *Perjury for Pay: An Exposé of the Methods and Criminal Cunning of the Modern Malingerer*, written by a surgeon for the Missouri Pacific Railway System (King, 1906). The book focused on individuals who exaggerated or feigned various physical injuries and included a specific chapter devoted to malingered TBI. The chapter included one of the first known descriptions of malingering after alleged MTBI. The case was that of a 38-year-old widowed woman who unsuccessfully tried to run her late husband's drug store, forcing the business to close. That business failure was followed by an unsuccessful attempt to sue an engineer for $900 for breach of marriage promise. She claimed to have suffered a MTBI (brief LOC) after a train she was on struck the caboose with considerable force. She demanded a large sum of money from the train company, which failed; and that failure prompted her to file a lawsuit. She reported that she experienced a constant headache, failing memory, sudden right eye dilation, and that she could barely read ordinary newspaper print because of worsening eyesight. Two physicians for the defense examined her and found nothing objectively wrong. However, two of her own physicians reported that her dilating pupil was a sign of a "serious brain lesion." Modern day clinicians will note the uncanny similarities between this woman's reported symptoms, normal findings from the defense physicians, and claims of significant brain injury from her presumably sympathetic treatment providers.

Upon trial, inconsistencies were noted, such as her sister-in-law (who was sitting next to her on the train and not holding anything except for a baby) having not been thrown or much disturbed by the collision. Most telling was the testimony of her landlady who stated that she observed the patient placing drops in her eyes to dilate them before going to the courthouse and begged her not to say anything because such a revelation would hurt her case. When confronted in court, the patient stated that the drops were treatment for her eyes. The judge ordered her to bring the eye drops to court for inspection, but she never did. Dr. King concluded that the woman was malingering, and the jury only awarded her $75.

Between 1880 and the turn of the century, the legal profession in the United States was blossoming, workers' compensation claims flooded the court system, and an increasing percentage of claims were found in favor of the worker (Harger, 2010). Between 1880 and 1900, about 33% of functional nervous diseases were classified as malingering by German doctors; but the percentages dropped dramatically in the next two decades because of concerns of malingering leading to overdiagnosis (Wessely, 2003). In England, however, detecting malingering became a moral, economic, and patriotic duty during World War I (1914–1918) because of the scale of the war effort and the possibility that England might not survive if soldiers attempted to avoid military service to defend the motherland (Wessely, 2003). While objective methods to assess physical malingering came into use around this time (e.g., x-rays, various chemical analyses), physicians also began offering opinions about malingering in the context of alleged psychological war trauma (Cooter, 1998). This advance in the detection of noncredible symptoms was particularly important when considering that soldiers were increasingly presenting with unexplainable signs and symptoms given the nature of their injuries, some of which were invisible (Myers, 1916). By the 1920s, most states in the United States had a workers' compensation system in place (California Department of Insurance [CDI], 2010).

Beginning in the early 1930s, malingering was common in the Soviet Union to obtain certified physician sick notes to escape increased work responsibilities and punishments for missing work (e.g., forced labor, imprisonment) that emerged when the country embarked on a new industrialization program. The presence of malingering further diminished the number of medical dispensations Soviet physicians could issue and changed the traditional doctor–patient relationship from one of mutual trust in which the well-being of the patient is the physician's only concern to one of reciprocal mistrust in which the interests of society take precedence over the individual (Field, 1953). As such, physicians became detective-like gatekeepers for the state (and later for insurance companies) against fraudulent claims in countries in which patients attempted to receive compensation or avoid obligations because of a reported injury. Field reported one physician's recollection that 50% of patients at a railroad clinic were malingering and that 20% of 539 displaced workers later retrospectively admitted to malingering. Some began to view these gatekeeper physicians as "hired guns"—a view that still exists today amongst many injured workers who are evaluated by a health care provider paid for by the insurance company or defense attorneys in civil litigation (although the same charge is made against some health care providers retained by the plaintiff).

The forms malingering take can be dependent on social-cultural factors. For example, because fever was required to obtain a sick note in the Soviet Union, artificial production of fever was the most common form of malingering; simulation of nervous system disease was the least common (Field, 1953).

Between 1917 and 1987, English-language book publications on malingering were virtually nonexistent, with the exception of a book on medicolegal fraud by Collie (1932) and two government publications in 1959 (Bergan; Meltzer). The main reason why the topic was not written about as much was because physicians were fearful of retaliatory actions by patients, either in the form of lawsuits (e.g., for defamation of character) or violence (Hofling, 1965). For example, in 1955, three of four orthopedists who labeled a patient as malinger were shot and two were killed (Parker, 1979).

Between the early 1960s and early 1970s, the U.S. military was involved in combat operations in Vietnam. Many soldiers returned home from Vietnam with genuine posttraumatic stress disorder (PTSD), but the subjective nature of the symptoms, wide availability of the criteria, and the fact that even a delayed onset of the condition was considered compensable by the Veterans Administration all made it prone to malingering (Atkinson, Henderson, Sparr, & Deale, 1982; Bitzer, 1980; Burkett & Whitley, 1998). This increased the need for psychologists and psychiatrists to assess for malingering and to develop techniques by which to do so.

Although self-report scales existed at the time to broadly assess the validity of self-reported symptoms (Dahlstrom, Welsh, & Dahlstrom, 1972; Karson & O'Dell, 1976; Megargee, 1972), not much was available to objectively assess malingered cognitive symptoms (e.g., memory, attention) via performance measures. The earliest such techniques measured reaction time to stimuli (Goldstein, 1923; Langfeld, 1921; Spencer, 1929). The Swiss psychologist, Andre Rey (1941), then developed a dot counting test to measure poor motivation by assessing if completion time was associated with increased task difficulty (as it should be). Later, Rey (1964) also created a 15-item test to assess feigned memory impairment. The task was designed to be very easy but appear difficult, a common design of many performance-based effort tests. In the 1970s, the two alternative forced-choice technique was used to assess noncredible responding (indicated by less than chance [50%] responding), initially with a hysterically blind patient (Theodor & Mandelcorn, 1973) and later for any sensory deficit (Pankratz, 1979). With the publication of Pankratz's article, the term "symptom validity testing" (SVT) was born, and the technique was applied to detect feigned memory impairment (Pankratz, 1983). For a detailed review of early and modern SVT procedures, see Bianchini, Mathias, and Greve (2001).

Book publishing in the area of malingering in the modern area began with Rogers' (1988) classic text, *Clinical Assessment of Malingering and Deception*. Shortly thereafter, in the early 1990s, largely populated states such as Florida and California passed legislation to create workers' compensation fraud detection programs (CDI, 2010; Harger, 2010). Since that time, there has been a renewed interest in malingering detection in all situations in which secondary gain is possible and, as detailed in the following section, there has been a profound increase in the number and types of tests and other objective indicators designed to measure effort and the veracity of self-reporting.

The Evolution of Malingering in the *DSM*

In the original *Diagnostic and Statistical Manual of Mental Disorders* (*DSM;* American Psychiatric Association [APA], 1952), malingering was only listed as a supplementary term in an appendix, with no specific criteria provided. In *DSM-II* (APA, 1968), the only mention of malingering was that it is a conscious behavior and must be distinguished from a hysterical neurosis, conversion type. *DSM-II* also mentioned *Ganser syndrome* as an adjustment disorder of adult life but did not provide any other meaningful detail or criteria about it. Ganser syndrome was named after the German psychiatrist, Sigbert Josef Maria Ganser (1898), who described the condition in three male prisoners. The syndrome included sudden psychosis with hallucinations, providing concrete or approximate answers (e.g., 2 + 2 = 5), conversion-type sensory changes, altered mental status with amnesia for the episode, and complete return to normal mental status. Although Ganser conceptualized this syndrome as hysterical, others viewed it as a form of malingering (Resnick, 1984).

It was not until the publication of *DSM-III* in 1980 that malingering first appeared as one of the "V codes," which are conditions not attributed to a mental disorder that are a focus of attention and treatment (APA, 1980). The criteria that were provided for malingering in *DSM-III* have remained essentially unchanged in the most current version, *DSM-IV-TR* (APA, 2000).

The original *DSM-III* criteria stated that the essential feature of malingering was false or grossly exaggerated physical or psychological symptoms that were voluntarily produced. The goal of symptom production was presumed to be pursuit of an obviously recognizable goal "with an understanding of the individual's circumstances rather than of his or her individual psychology" (p. 379). Examples of obviously understandable goals include avoidance of military conscription or duty, avoidance of work, attempts to obtain financial compensation or drugs, and evading criminal prosecution. It was noted that malingering could be an adaptive behavior in some circumstances such as feigning an illness to escape a captor. According to *DSM-III*, high suspicion of malingering is warranted if the person presents in a medicolegal context, if there is a significant discrepancy between the person's claimed distress or disability and objective findings, if the person does not cooperate with the diagnostic evaluation and prescribed treatment, or if the person has antisocial personality disorder.

In *DSM-III*, malingering is listed as a differential diagnosis for conversion disorder, psychogenic pain disorder, psychogenic amnesia, psychogenic fugue, multiple personality disorder, psychotic disorder not otherwise specified (NOS), kleptomania, alcohol idiosyncratic intoxication, and factitious disorder. Thus, by the time of *DSM-III*, there was a clear recognition in psychiatry that malingering was a significant confound that needed to be considered in case conceptualization. Factitious disorder was added in *DSM-III* as a condition in which symptoms are voluntarily produced to assume the sick role as opposed to an effort to obtain a clear external gain. The language in *DSM-III* pertaining to symptoms being produced with an understanding of the individual's circumstances rather than his or her individual psychology was dropped in *DSM-III-R* (APA, 1987), and securing better living conditions were added as a possible external incentive. It was also noted elsewhere in the text of *DSM-III-R* that malingering can present a difficult diagnostic dilemma, which often can only be resolved by obtaining additional data from ancillary sources such as hospital and police records, family members, employers, and friends.

In *DSM-IV* (APA, 1994), it was stated that malingering should be ruled out when financial remuneration, benefit eligibility, and forensic determinations play a role. However, the securement of better living conditions was dropped as an external incentive example. The following descriptive language from *DSM-III* as it pertains to malingering was also dropped in *DSM-IV*: "The malingering individual is much less likely to present his or her symptoms in the context of emotional conflict, and the symptoms presented are less likely to be 'symbolic' of an underlying emotional conflict" (p. 332). Also dropped was a statement that symptom relief provided by malingering is not often obtained by suggestion, hypnosis, or intravenous barbiturates (cf. conversion disorder). In criteria one, "physician" was changed to "clinician," likely in recognition of the important role of psychologists in malingering detection. The criteria for malingering in *DSM-IV-TR* (2000) are unchanged compared to *DSM-IV*.

It is unclear how the criteria for malingering will change when *DSM-V* is published in 2013. However, Berry and Nelson (2010) criticized the *DSM-IV-TR* malingering criteria for (a) being categorical as opposed to dimensional; (b) having a pejorative and moralistic conceptualization as opposed to an adaptational function; (c) the (unwritten) assumption that malingerers will fake bad on most (if not all) procedures they undergo; (d) difficulty in proving intentionality; (e) difficulty distinguishing between internal and external motivations; and (f) low classification accuracy. They suggested that malingering should be replaced with a more empirically grounded alternative known as "feigned psychiatric, psychological, and neuropsychological symptoms." As such, they recommended that the focus should be placed on identifying feigned symptoms rather than the intentionality or goals of the patient. They also suggested that the possibility of feigning cognitive symptoms be specifically mentioned in the *DSM-V* criteria. The more empirically grounded approach includes the use of multiple objective detection methods (e.g., SVT) and criteria for probabilistic language modeled off of the "Slick criteria" for malingered neurocognitive dysfunction that listed ways to distinguish between definite, probable, and possible subtypes (Slick, Sherman, & Iverson, 1999). They also suggested the use of cut-scores to minimize false positives and grading false symptom reports into mild, moderate, and severe ranges.

RECENT TRENDS IN MTBI AND MALINGERING

Scientific Research

Although the decade from 2000 to 2009 has not yet received a formal appellation by the U.S. Congress, in the neuropsychological community, it can perhaps best be summarized as "The Decade of Mild Traumatic Brain Injury." This description can be best appreciated by examining Tables 1.1 through 1.3. Beginning with reviews of the scientific literature on PubMed (http://www.ncbi.nlm.nih.gov/pubmed/), it can be seen that there was nearly a sixfold increase in articles with the search term "mild traumatic brain injury" in 2000–2009 (730 articles) compared to the prior decade (115 articles). Likewise, there was also a sevenfold increase in use of the term "concussion syndrome" or "concussive syndrome" from 35 to 259 articles over the past two decades. It is also during this time frame that the term mild traumatic brain injury became much more popular than the term "mild head injury," an important distinction that will be returned to later in this chapter.

Although malingering has long been discussed in the scientific literature, the number of articles on this topic was relatively stable between 1960 and 1989, with a noticeable increase between 1900 and 1999. However, the largest increase took place over the last two decades with an increase from 534 articles to 963. Although this increase is nearly twofold, there was more than a threefold increase across the past two decades for articles on malingering and any word beginning with "neu-

TABLE 1.1 PubMed: Search Terms and Number of Hits by Decade

	"Mild Head Injury"	"Mild traumatic brain injury"	Concussion	"Concussion syndrome" OR "Concussive syndrome"	Malingering	Malingering AND neuropsych*	Malingering AND "mild traumatic brain injury" OR malingering AND "mild head injury"
1960–1969	0	0	426	22	260	0	0
1970–1979	8	0	757	13	356	2	0
1980–1989	44	0	1070	16	317	18	1
1990–1999	210	115	1065	35	534	113	14
2000–2009	281	730	1664	259	963	369	32

Note: Search terms are written in the exact manner they were entered. Some search terms were placed in quotes to ensure that search results were returned containing the exact search phrase. The search phrase neuropsych* uses an asterisk to include all search words beginning with the letters neuropsych (e.g., neuropsychology, neuropsychological.) Source: http://www.ncbi.nlm.nih.gov/sites/entrez

ropsych." Articles addressing malingering and MTBI or mild head injuries more than doubled across the last two decades. Articles pertaining to both "malingering and neuropsychology" or "malingering and mild traumatic brain injury/mild head injury" first began to significantly increase between 1990 and 1999, which parallels the development of many freestanding and embedded measures of cognitive effort, as described later in this chapter. The trend in these areas has increased, with most articles written about these topics being published over the past 10 years.

U.S. Case Law and Federal Law

Because many patients who report persisting symptoms after MTBI are involved in disability claims or lawsuits, neuropsychologists may find that their reports are

TABLE 1.2 Google Scholar: Search Terms and Number of Hits by Decade for Case Law in All 50 States

	"Mild Head Injury"	"Mild traumatic brain injury"	Concussion	"Concussion syndrome" OR "Concussive syndrome"	Malingering	Malingering AND neuropsych*	Malingering AND "mild traumatic brain injury" OR malingering AND "mild head injury"
1960–1969	0	0	864	46	236	0	27
1970–1979	2	0	643	44	268	2	18
1980–1989	3	1	745	67	452	4	29
1990–1999	11	8	658	123	622	17	86
2000–2009	19	60	1380	292	1320	55	259

Note: Search terms are written in the exact manner they were entered. Some search terms were placed in quotes to ensure that search results were returned containing the exact search phrase. The search phrase neuropsych* uses an asterisk to include all search words beginning with the letters neuropsych (e.g., neuropsychology, neuropsychological.) Source: http://scholar.google.com

TABLE 1.3 Google Scholar: Search Terms and Number of Hits by Decade in All Federal Courts

	"Mild Head Injury"	"Mild traumatic brain injury"	Concussion	"Concussion syndrome" OR "Concussive syndrome"	Malingering	Malingering AND neuropsych*	Malingering AND "mild traumatic brain injury" OR malingering AND "mild head injury"
1960–1969	0	1	132	19	119	4	0
1970–1979	1	1	115	10	157	0	0
1980–1989	1	0	180	21	212	4	0
1990–1999	3	2	185	30	380	14	1
2000–2009	15	29	535	153	1850	64	1

Note: Search terms are written in the exact manner they were entered. Some search terms were placed in quotes to ensure that search results were returned containing the exact search phrase. The search phrase neuropsych* uses an asterisk to include all search words beginning with the letters neuropsych (e.g., neuropsychology, neuropsychological.) Source: http://scholar.google.com

subpoenaed and that they are asked to provide a deposition or court testimony under oath regarding the results of the neuropsychological examination. This issue is not limited to forensic neuropsychologists but is now a regular occurrence in clinical settings as well. For example, in a study based on a database of clinically referred adult patients with persisting symptoms after known or suspected MTBI ($n = 67$), 58% of the patients acknowledged retaining legal counsel, and 52% were applying for or receiving disability benefits (Carone, 2008).

Table 1.2 highlights the increased focus on MTBI and malingering in U.S. case law. Specifically, although the topic of MTBI in U.S. case law was not evident in a significant way until the Decade of the Brain (1990–1999), there was 7.5 times the number of citations on this topic over the past decade (from 8 to 60 citations). There was also a twofold increase over the past two decades in the case law using the term concussion, and nearly 2.5 times the number of citations using the term concussion syndrome or concussive syndrome—both of which reflect the largest decade-to-decade increase.

Table 1.2 shows that citations on malingering have steadily increased from 1960 to 2009, with the largest increase (i.e., twofold) over the past two decades. The table also reveals that neuropsychology has had a significantly increased role in helping the legal system regarding issues of malingering over the past two decades and that issues pertaining to malingering and MTBI/mild head injury have increased threefold from the 1980s to 1990s and from the 1990s to the 2000s. Similarly dramatic trends are also found in the federal court system (see Table 1.3). Overall, the information displayed in Tables 1.1 to 1.3 clearly demonstrates a powerful and largely parallel trend in both the scientific literature and the legal system with respect to MTBI, symptom persistence, and malingering assessment.

Textbook Publications

As shown in the chapter appendix, our book searches only revealed four text publications on concussion between 1927 and 1988, with no texts published using the terms mild head injury or mild traumatic brain injury. However, paralleling the renewed interest in malingering in the late 1980s and early 1990s, texts on concussion/MTBI/ mild head injury increased dramatically, beginning with the publication of *Mild Head Injury* (Levin, Eisenberg, & Benton, 1989) and *Mild to Moderate Head Injury* (Hoff, Anderson, & Cole, 1989). As shown in the appendix at the end of this chapter, between 1990 and 1999, there were 10 books published in this area, followed by 17 books between 2000 and 2009. The upward trend appears to be continuing because there have already been 10 books published in this area between 2010 and the present, with 3 more books in press. As shown in the chapter appendix, there were 7 books published in the 1990s that focused on malingering, followed by 15 such books from 2000 to 2009. Thus, there appears to be an increasing trend in this area as well. However, prior to the current volume, there was no book devoted to the topic of MTBI, symptom validity assessment, and malingering.

Reasons for Historical Trends

As noted previously, there has clearly been a dramatically increased interest in MTBI, malingering, and symptom validity assessment over the past two decades in the research literature, the U.S. legal system, and textbook publications. There has also been a simultaneous increase in participation by clinical neuropsychologists in all of these areas; neuropsychologists have authored many/most of the articles, books, and tests devoted to these topics and have played primary roles in the evaluation of these issues in clinical and forensic settings. The recent historical trends over the past two decades appear to be primarily because of several factors including (a) the U.S. Congressional designation of the Decade of the Brain (1990–1999), (b) the development of numerous freestanding and embedded symptom validity measures, (c) the publication of the American Congress of Rehabilitation Medicine (ACRM) criteria for MTBI, (d) endorsement of symptom validity assessment by national neuropsychological organizations, (e) increased media and congressional attention to sports concussion, (f) the wars in Iraq and Afghanistan from 2003 to the present, and (g) the establishment of state workers' compensation fraud detection departments. Because the last of these factors was previously described, only the remaining factors are addressed in more detail in subsequent sections of this chapter.

The Decade of the Brain

The years 1990–1999 were formally designated as the Decade of the Brain by the U.S. Congress in an effort to enhance public awareness of the benefits of brain research (Jones & Mendell, 1999). As a result, the National Institutes of Health (NIH) promoted neuroscience research; research findings about the brain were increasingly publicized through various media outlets (which paralleled the increased use of the Internet), brain injury advocacy groups became increasingly visible, Brain Awareness Week was initiated in 1996, and there was a significant increase in the number of scientists identifying themselves as neuroscientists (Jones & Mendell, 1999). These events all laid a foundation for an increased focus on TBI including MTBI.

With the diagnosis of Alzheimer's disease of former President Reagan being made public in 1994, actor Michael J. Fox revealing that he had Parkinson's disease in 1995, and former *Superman* actor Christopher Reeves suffering a debilitating cervical spinal cord injury in 1998, much of the public and scientific focus in the 1990s was on these three neurological conditions, even though the latter is not a brain injury. This increased focus was accentuated by public activism appearances that poignantly showed the dramatic manner by which these conditions had affected Mr. Fox (e.g., frequent involuntary movements during congressional testimony) and Mr. Reeves (e.g., the former "Man of Steel" shown to be wheelchair-bound with a breathing support tube). In these ways, public events, public images, and public figures intersect with politics and the media to impact scientific focus. These events laid a foundation for similar public appearances and congressional testimony regarding TBI and MTBI over the last decade, as noted in the following section in the area of sports concussion.

The Development of Modern Symptom Validity Tests

Although symptom validity measures existed prior to the Decade of the Brain (Bush, 1990), the 1990s saw a veritable explosion of measures to evaluate symptom validity and malingering. Some of the more popular freestanding effort measures developed during this time period include the Portland Digit Recognition Test (PDRT; Binder & Willis, 1991); Computerized Assessment of Response Bias (CARB; Conder, Allen, & Cox, 1992); Word Memory Test (WMT; Green & Astner, 1995); and the Test of Memory Malingering (TOMM; Tombaugh, 1996). In addition, numerous effort measures were developed which were extracted from or "embedded" in tests not originally developed for this purpose. Examples include Reliable Digit Span (RDS; Greiffenstein, Baker, & Gola, 1994); recognition hits on the California Verbal Learning Test (CVLT; Trueblood & Schmidt, 1993); indices on the Wechsler Adult Intelligence Scale-Revised (WAIS-R) and the Wechsler Memory Scale-Revised (WMS-R; Mittenberg, Azrin, Millsaps, & Heilbronner, 1993; Rawling & Brooks, 1990; Trueblood, 1994); and indices on the Halstead Reitan Battery (HRB; Mittenberg, Rotholc, Russell, & Heilbronner, 1996). Many, but not all, of the effort measures developed in the 1990s remain in popular use today.

Publication of the ACRM Criteria for MTBI

In the early 1990s, a very popular definition of MTBI emerged from the Mild Traumatic Brain Injury Committee of the ACRM Head Injury Interdisciplinary Special Interest Group (1993). Specifically, the ACRM criteria state that clinical manifestations of MTBI are demonstrated by (a) loss of consciousness (LOC); (b) loss of memory for events immediately before or after the accident; (c) altered mental state at the time of the accident (e.g., feeling dazed, disoriented, or confused); or (d) focal neurological deficit(s) that may or may not be transient. The criteria further specify that there cannot be more than 30 minutes of unconsciousness or 24 hours of posttraumatic amnesia (PTA). Furthermore, after 30 minutes, the Glasgow Coma Scale (GCS) score cannot be less than 13.

Prior to the ACRM criteria, researchers often relied on narrower criteria to define MTBI, primarily a GCS score between 13 and 15, and supported by LOC less than 20 minutes, hospitalization of less than 2 to 3 days, negative neurological examination upon admission and discharge, and/or no medical complications (Gentilini et al., 1985; Rimel, Giordani, Barth, Boll, & Jane, 1981; Ruff, Levin, & Marshall, 1986); some criteria included an absence of neuroimaging abnormalities (Gronwall & Wrightson, 1980, 1981; Levin et al., 1987; McLean, Temkin, Dikmen, & Wyler, 1983). Although the ACRM criteria were important for clarifying that a patient does not necessarily need to lose consciousness to have suffered an MTBI, they led to a much looser diagnostic standard that can easily result in misdiagnosis if applied in a literal manner. For example, a patient of the primary author was once misdiagnosed with MTBI after telling a provider that he was "dazed" after a piece of ice fell on his head. He had no other symptoms at the time and neuroimaging was negative. Detailed clinical interview revealed that his use of the term dazed only referred to him feeling surprised that something struck him from overhead but he did not actually experience disorientation, slowed thinking, memory loss, or any other formal alteration of mental status. Thus, it is important for health care providers to ask patients to explain what they mean by terms such as dazed, "confused," or "foggy" if they are to be relied on for an MTBI diagnosis.

Concerns about MTBI misdiagnosis based on the ACRM criteria began to increase among neuropsychologists and resulted in a study by Lees-Haley et al. (2001). The study included 24 claimants with MTBI reporting persisting symptoms and 66 claimants with other forms of traumatic injury (psychological and physical) that did not involve the brain. When asking these patients to report their symptoms immediately after their injury/trauma, the groups did not significantly differ in terms of reporting transient mental status changes (e.g., dazed, disoriented, confused). In fact, they found that 51% of their sample of litigating individuals with non-brain injuries reported feeling dazed immediately after the trauma, and 65% reported feeling confused. The authors concluded that such complaints are so nonspecific that they have little diagnostic specificity. In another investigation of symptom base rates, Lees-Haley and Brown (1993) found that 62% of outpatient family practice patients reported having headaches and 20% reported having memory problems. Thus, the physical (fatigue, dizzy spells), emotional (anger, impatience) and cognitive (memory, concentration) symptoms that comprise "postconcussion syndrome" occur frequently in the normal population (Putnam & Millis, 1994), and the symptoms increase in relation to stress, even for individuals without brain trauma (Gouvier, Cubic, Jones, Brantley, & Cutlip, 1992).

Findings such as those preceding indicate that clinicians need to avoid applying MTBI criteria in a rigid, cookbook-like manner without considering alternate possibilities for self-reported symptoms. For example, in cases where a patient reports simultaneous onset of significant anxiety symptoms (e.g., hyperventilation, trembling) with reported transient mental status change (e.g., mental confusion) after an event that included mild trauma to the head or rapid acceleration–deceleration (i.e., whiplash), clinicians should consider referring to such cases as *possible* MTBI because it is impossible to determine whether the mental status changes were caused by an injury to the brain, psychological factors, or both. In cases where it is clear that the patient did not actually have a transient mental status change after a mild trauma to the head, the injury is best referred to as a mild head injury in the literal sense (i.e., no brain injury). We have been involved in many cases where a patient has been diagnosed with MTBI based on the patient's inaccurate use of terminology or based on other providers only using a trauma to the head or rapid acceleration–deceleration and subsequent nonspecific physical symptom reporting (e.g., headache) as a basis for the diagnosis. Although a focal neurological symptom (e.g., focal weakness) can override the need for a transient mental status change after injury, these are rarely encountered after MTBI (Coello, Canals, Gonzalez, & Martin, 2010).

Endorsement of Symptom Validity Testing by National Neuropsychological Organizations

One of the most influential developments in symptom validity assessment was the formal position published by the Policy and Planning Committee of the National Academy of Neuropsychology (NAN; Bush et al., 2005). The official conclusion in the NAN position paper was that "Assessment of response validity, as a component of a medically necessary evaluation, is medically necessary. When determined by the neuropsychologist to be necessary for the assessment of response validity, administration of specific symptom validity tests are also medically necessary" (p. 419).

The position paper and statement was significant because it marked the first time that a national organization of health care professionals expressly endorsed the regular use of symptom validity assessment, not only in forensic contexts but in clinical contexts as well. Two years later, the American Academy of Clinical Neuropsychology (AACN) Board of Directors (2007) published practice guidelines and included a section on the assessment of motivation and effort, stating that "the assessment of effort and motivation is important in any clinical setting, as a patient's effort may be compromised even in the absence of any potential or active litigation, compensation, or financial incentives" (p. 221).

This position was reiterated and expanded on when AACN published a consensus conference statement on the neuropsychological assessment of effort, response bias, and malingering, concluding that "The assessment of effort and genuine reporting of symptoms is important in all evaluations" (p. 1121; Heilbronner, Sweet, Morgan, Larrabee, & Millis, 2009). These position statements echoed a view stated many years prior by Rogers (1988) that "the honesty, accuracy, and completeness of each patient's self-report should be considered an integral element of clinical assessment" (p. 3).

Increased Media Attention to Sports Concussion

Although articles about sports concussion have been published for decades (Buckley, 1988; Cantu, 1992; Sercl & Jaros, 1962; Yarnell & Lynch, 1970), the topic significantly gained more traction in the past decade because of highly publicized research involving concussions in the National Football League (NFL). This focus by the NFL resulted in a series of 16 NFL concussion studies published in the journal *Neurosurgery*, beginning with a biomechanics study in 2003 (Pellman, Viano, Tucker, Casson, & Waeckerle, 2003) and ending with an animal study in 2009 (Hamberger, Viano, Säljö, & Bolouri, 2009), which concluded that concussions resulted in minimal to no brain injury based on immunohistochemical results. Another one of these studies (Pellman, Lovell, Viano, Casson, & Tucker, 2004) concluded that there was no evidence of cognitive impairment in NFL players with three or more concussions out for more than 7 days and that neuropsychological functioning rapidly returned to normal within days postinjury.

Results such as these led to allegations of NFL bias and/or cover-up, given its sponsorship of the studies. The allegations were discussed widely in the national media and gained additional traction when former professional wrestler, Chris Nowinski (2006), published a popular book about the dangers of sport concussion entitled *Head Games: Football's Concussion Crisis from NFL to Youth Leagues*. The book, as well as a popular media campaign blitz that included autopsy reports of chronic traumatic encephalopathy (CTE) in former NFL players and alleged deaths from concussions in children, the founding of a national center to study the effects of sports concussion, and coordination with nationally prominent neuroscientists (e.g., Drs. Robert Cantu and Bennett Omaulu) resulted in a very effective counter argument and led to negative publicity for the NFL. The publication of studies casting doubt on the NFL's findings, most notably a study associating increased risk of cognitive impairment in retired NFL players after multiple concussions (Guskiewicz et al., 2005), led the NFL to adopt a concussion-safety awareness campaign and numerous rule changes designed to prevent concussions. The topic also resulted in televised congressional hearings on sports concussions in October 2009 and January 2010 in which the dangers of sports concussions were discussed by lawmakers, scientists, brain injury advocates, and former sports players (Committee on the Judiciary House of Representatives, 2010).

Although all of this publicity has helped to raise public awareness of sports concussions and has fueled additional research interest in the topic, it has also resulted in many in the public and in the professional health care community misapplying findings from NFL studies (where there is a career's worth of concussions and head trauma) to patients who suffered a single uncomplicated concussion. As a result, it is common for some patients suffering a single concussive injury to worry excessively about the long-term effects of the injury (e.g., "Will I develop Alzheimer's disease now?"), and patients run the risk of iatrogenic effects when these fears are reinforced by health care providers. For more information on ethical considerations in sport neuropsychology, see Bush and Iverson (2010). Thus, clinicians need to properly educate patients about the differences between NFL concussion studies and the limited generalizability to their particular situation.

U.S. Military Actions in the Middle East From 2003 to the Present

MTBI has been termed as "a signature injury" of U.S. combat operations in Iraq and Afghanistan (Operations Iraqi Freedom [OIF] and Enduring Freedom [OEF], respectively; Independent Review Group, 2007). The high prevalence of MTBI diagnoses seems to have resulted from (a) the extensive use of improvised explosive devices as a weapon of choice among opposition forces; (b) increasingly efficient medical response and procedures; and (c) the conceptualization of nonspecific symptoms as resulting from injury to the brain. Given the complexity of cognitive, physical, and emotional symptoms emerging during or following deployment and combat operations, efforts to understand the origin and course of such symptoms are essential so that appropriate services and benefits can be provided. Neuropsychologists play an important role in clarifying the nature and extent of post-deployment cognitive, physical, and emotional symptoms.

One of the first steps in assessing post-deployment neuropsychological functioning is to establish the credibility of the veteran's presentation and performance on cognitive and psychological tests. However, despite the importance of this step of the evaluation process, few studies have yet been published on suboptimal effort rates with veterans of OEF and OIF. In a study of 23 combat veterans, of which nine remained enrolled in active duty service, Whitney, Shepard, Williams, Davis, and Adams (2009) found a 17% failure rate on the Medical Symptom Validity Test (MSVT; Green, 2004), with all who performed poorly on the measure of being active duty personnel.

In the only study to examine SVT failure rates for OEF/OIF veterans who were referred for neuropsychological evaluation after positive scores on VHA (Veterans Health Administration) TBI screens, Armistead-Jehle (2010) obtained a 58% failure rate on the MSVT. The score profiles of those who failed the MSVT were more similar to groups of individuals simulating impairment than to patients with established memory impairment. The 58% failure rate surpasses established base rates for SVT failures in civil forensic contexts (Larrabee, 2003). Differences between study participants who obtained passing and failing scores were difficult to discern; failure could not be attributable to demographic differences, clinical diagnosis of PTSD, or substance abuse. The groups did differ in terms of depression, with those failing the MSVT having diagnoses of depression; however, the participants were all independently functioning, community-dwelling individuals who did not require inpatient treatment for depression and were, thus, not functionally impaired. Although the evaluations used for this study were not conducted as part of the VHA's compensation and pension process, the potential for pursuing service connection or increased service-connected benefits is always present in the VHA and is an external incentive that is difficult to eliminate. Although the failure rates in the Armistead-Jehle study were higher than in the Whitney et al. (2009) study, they were consistent with the 53% clear symptom exaggeration rate found in a sample of Vietnam veterans (Freeman, Powell, & Kimbrell, 2008).

In the first study to examine the relationships among multiple symptom validity tests in OEF/OIF forensic, clinical, and research samples, veterans with a history of concussion had much higher rates of insufficient effort when evaluated in a forensic, compared to research context, similar to the rates found in nonveteran forensic samples (Nelson et al., 2010). Suboptimal effort accounted for a significant proportion of variance in overall cognitive test performance (20.3%–33.6%) in the forensic sample. After the authors controlled for effort, the performance of OEF/OIF veterans with a history of concussion did not differ significantly from those with no history of concussion on neuropsychological tests. The authors determined that, after controlling for effort, "remote history of concussion does not typically contribute to meaningful neuropsychological impairment in the late stage of recovery" (p. 720). They concluded that "Clinicians should strongly consider employing the VSVT [Victoria Symptom Validity Test] or other forced-choice effort measures during neuropsychological assessment of OEF/OIF concussion groups, particularly in forensic settings" (p. 721).

Overall, to make appropriate determinations regarding the reliability and validity of neuropsychological data obtained from OIF/OEF veterans, neuropsychologists must employ multiple, psychometrically based symptom validity tests and indicators and consider all relevant diagnostic possibilities when improbable symptom reporting or performance are observed. Failure to do so interferes with the provision of appropriate services to veterans and wastes valuable resources.

SUMMARY AND CONCLUSIONS

Traumatic brain injuries of all severities have been documented throughout most of recorded history. Similarly, exaggeration and fabrication of medical and psychiatric problems have a long history. Despite prior historical publications and scholarly efforts directed toward understanding MTBI and malingering, research on these topics has increased significantly over the past 10 to 20 years, with a concurrent increase in attention by the media.

Neuropsychology has played a prominent role in the increased understanding of MTBI, malingering, and their assessment. Neuropsychologists provide clinical and forensic evaluation of persons who have sustained TBIs, with MTBIs being by far the most common. The assessment of symptom validity (i.e., honesty and effort) is typically an essential part of such evaluations or may be the primary goal of the evaluation. There is perhaps no clinical condition for which symptom validity concerns are more relevant for neuropsychology than MTBI.

REFERENCES

Ackerman, M. J. (2010). *Essentials of forensic psychological assessment* (2nd ed.). New York: John Wiley & Sons.

American Academy of Clinical Neuropsychology. (2007). American Academy of Clinical Neuropsychology (AACN) practice guidelines for neuropsychological assessment and consultation. *The Clinical Neuropsychologist*, 21(2), 209–231.

American Psychiatric Association. (1952). *Diagnostic and statistical manual of mental disorders*. Washington, DC: Author.

American Psychiatric Association. (1968). *Diagnostic and statistical manual of mental disorders* (2nd ed.). Washington, DC: Author.

American Psychiatric Association. (1980). *Diagnostic and statistical manual of mental disorders* (3rd ed.). Washington, DC: Author.

American Psychiatric Association. (1987). *Diagnostic and statistical manual of mental disorders* (3rd ed., rev. ed.). Washington, DC: Author.

American Psychiatric Association. (1994). *Diagnostic and statistical manual of mental disorders* (4th ed.). Washington, DC: Author.

American Psychiatric Association. (2000). *Diagnostic and statistical manual of mental disorders* (4th ed., text rev.). Washington, DC: Author.

Armistead-Jehle, P. (2010). Symptom validity test performance in U.S. veterans referred for evaluation of mild TBI. *Applied Neuropsychology*, 17(1), 52–59.

Atkinson, R. M., Henderson, R. G., Sparr, L. F., & Deale, S. (1982). Assessment of Viet Nam veterans for posttraumatic stress disorder in Veterans Administration disability claims. *The American Journal of Psychiatry*, 139(9), 1118–1121.

Bartholow, R. (1864). *A manual of instructions for enlisting and discharging soldiers: With special reference to the medical examination of recruits, and the detection of disqualifying and feigned diseases*. Philadelphia, PA: Lippincott.

Bazarian, J. J., Blyth, B., & Cimpello, L. (2006). Bench to bedside: Evidence for brain injury after concussion—looking beyond the computed tomography scan. *Academic Emergency Medicine*, 13(2), 199–214.

Belanger, H. G., & Vanderploeg, R. D. (2005). The neuropsychological impact of sports-related concussion: A meta-analysis. *Journal of the International Neuropsychological Society*, 11(4), 345–357.

Belanger, H. G., Vanderploeg, R. D., Curtiss, G., & Warden, D. L. (2007). Recent neuroimaging techniques in mild traumatic brain injury. *The Journal of Neuropsychiatry and Clinical Neurosciences*, 19(1), 5–20.

Bergan, M. (1959). *Functional examination for malingering and psychogenicity in impaired hearing*. New York, NY: National Hospital for Speech Disorders.

Berry, D. T., & Nelson, N. W. (2010). DSM-V and malingering: A modest proposal. *Psychological Injury and Law*, 3, 295–303.

Bianchini, K. J., Mathias, C. W., & Greve, K. W. (2001). Symptom validity testing: A critical review. *The Clinical Neuropsychologist*, 15(1), 19–45.

Bigler, E. D. (2008). Neuropsychology and clinical neuroscience of persistent post-concussive syndrome. *Journal of the International Neuropsychological Society*, 14(1), 1–22.

Binder, L. M. (1997). A review of mild head trauma. Part II: Clinical implications. *Journal of Clinical and Experimental Neuropsychology*, 19(3), 432–457.

Binder, L. M., Rohling, M. L., & Larrabee, G. J. (1997). A review of mild head trauma. Part I: Meta-analytic review of neuropsychological studies. *Journal of Clinical and Experimental Neuropsychology*, 19(3), 421–431.

Binder, L. M., & Willis, S. C. (1991). Assessment of motivation after financially compensable minor head trauma. *Psychological Assessment*, 3, 175–181.

Bitzer, R. (1980). Caught in the middle: Mentally disabled veterans and the Veteran's Administration. In C. R. Figlery & F. Leventman (Eds.), *Strangers at home: Vietnam veterans since the war* (pp. 305–323). New York, NY: Praeger Publications.

Bonne, O., Gilboa, A., Louzoun, Y., Kempf-Sherf, O., Katz, M., Fishman, Y., . . . Lerer, B. (2003). Cerebral blood flow in chronic symptomatic mild traumatic brain injury. *Psychiatry Research*, 124(3), 141–152.

Buckley, W. E. (1988). Concussions in college football. A multivariate analysis. *The American Journal of Sports Medicine*, 16(1), 51–56.

Burkett, B. G., & Whitley, G. (1998). *Stolen valor: How the Vietnam generation was robbed of its heroes and its history*. Dallas, TX: Verity Press.

Bush, G. (1990). *Presidential proclamation 6158*. Retrieved from http://www.loc.gov/loc/brain/pro claim.html

Bush, S., & Iverson, G. L. (2010). Ethical issues and practical considerations in sport neuropsychology. In F. M. Webbe (Ed.), *Handbook of sport neuropsychology* (pp. 35–52). New York, NY: Springer Publishing.

Bush, S. S., Ruff, R. M., Tröster, A. I., Barth, J. T., Koffler, S. P., Pliskin, N. H., . . . Silver, C. H. (2005). Symptom validity assessment: Practice issues and medical necessity NAN policy & planning committee. *Archives of Clinical Neuropsychology*, 20(4), 419–426.

California Department of Insurance. (2010). *Workers' compensation fraud*. Retrieved from http://www.ins-urance.ca.gov/0300-fraud/0100-fraud-division-overview/0500-fraud-division-programs/workers-comp-fraud/index.cfm

Cantu, R. C. (1992). Cerebral concussion in sport. Management and prevention. *Sports Medicine*, 14(1), 64–74.

Carone, D. A. (2008). Children with moderate/severe brain damage/dysfunction outperform adults with mild-to-no brain damage on the medical symptom validity test. *Brain Injury*, 22(12), 960–971.

Carone, D. A., & Bush, S. (in press). Dementia pugilistica and chronic traumatic encephalopathy. In R. Dean & C. Noggle (Eds.), *Cortical dementias*. New York, NY: Springer Publishing.

Chen, J. K., Johnston, K. M., Frey, S., Petrides, M., Worsley, K., & Ptito, A. (2004). Functional abnormalities in symptomatic concussed athletes: An fMRI study. *Neuroimage*, 22(1), 68–82.

Coello, A. F., Canals, A. G., Gonzalez, J. M., & Martin, J. J. (2010). Cranial nerve injury after minor head trauma. *Journal of Neurosurgery*, 113(3), 547–555.

Collie, J. S. (1917). *Malingering and feigned sickness*. London, England: Edward Arnold.

Collie, J. S. (1932). *Fraud in medico-legal practice*. London, England: Edward Arnold.

Committee on the Judiciary House of Representatives. (2010). *Legal issues relating to football head injuries (Part I & II)*. Retrieved from http://judiciary.house.gov/hearings/printers/111th/111-82_53092.PDF

Conder, R., Allen, L., & Cox, D. (1992). *Manual for the Computerized Assessment of Response Bias*. Durham, NC: CogniSyst.

Cooter, R. (1998). Malingering in modernity: Psychological scripts and adversarial encounters during the First World War. In R. Cooter, M. Harrison & S. Sturdy (Eds.), *War, medicine, and modernity* (pp. 125–148). Stroud, United Kingdom: Sutton.

Dahlstrom, W. G., Welsh, G. S., & Dahlstrom, L. E. (1972). *An MMPI handbook: Vol. 1 clinical interpretation* (Rev. ed.). Minneapolis, MN: University of Minnesota Press.

Dawson, W. H. (1906). *German workman: A study in national efficiency*. London, England: Scribner.

Denny-Brown, D., & Ritchie, R. W. (1941). Experimental cerebral concussion. *Brain*, 64, 93–164.

Dikmen, S. S., Machamer, J. E., Winn, R., & Temkin, N. R. (1995). Neuropsychological outcome at 1-year post head injury. *Neuropsychology*, 9, 80–90.

Feinsod, M. (1997). Three head injuries: The Biblical account of the deaths of Sisera, Abimelech and Goliath. *Journal of the History of the Neurosciences*, 6(3), 320–324.

Field, M. (1953). Structured strain in the role of the Soviet physician. *The American Journal of Sociology*, 58, 493–502.

Foda, M. A., & Marmarou, A. (1994). A new model of diffuse brain injury in rats. Part II: Morphological characterization. *Journal of Neurosurgery*, 80(2), 301–313.

Frayne, R., Goodyear, B. G., Dickhoff, P., Lauzon, M. L., & Sevick, R. J. (2003). Magnetic resonance imaging at 3.0 Tesla: Challenges and advantages in clinical neurological imaging. *Investigative Radiology*, 38(7), 385–402.

Freeman, T., Powell, M., & Kimbrell, T. (2008). Measuring symptom exaggeration in veterans with chronic posttraumatic stress disorder. *Psychiatry Research*, 158(3), 374–380.

Frencham, K. A., Fox, A. M., & Maybery, M. T. (2005). Neuropsychological studies of mild traumatic brain injury: A meta-analytic review of research since 1995. *Journal of Clinical and Experimental Neuropsychology*, 27(3), 334–351.

Ganser, S. (1898). Über einen eigenartigen hysterischen Dämmerzustand. *Archiv für Psychiatrie und Nervenkrankheiten*, 30, 633–640.

Gavin, H. (1843). *On Feigned and Factitious Diseases, Chiefly of Soldiers and Seamen; on the Means Used to Simulate or Produce Them, and on the Best Modes of Discovering Imposters; Being the Prize Essay in the Class of Military Surgery, in the University of Edinburgh Session, 1835-6, with Additions*. London, Engalnd: John Churchill.

Gennarelli, T. A. (1986). Mechanisms and pathophysiology of cerebral concussion. *The Journal of Head Trauma Rehabilitation*, 1, 23–29.

Gentilini, M., Nichelli, P., Schoenhuber, R., Bortolotti, P., Tonelli, L., Falasca, A., & Merli, G. A. (1985). Neuropsychological evaluation of mild head injury. *Journal of Neurology, Neurosurgery, and Psychiatry*, 48(2), 137–140.

Giza, C. C., & Hovda, D. A. (2001). The neurometabolic cascade of concussion. *Journal of Athletic Training*, 36(3), 228–235.

Goldstein, E. R. (1923). Reaction times and the consciousness of deception. *The American Journal of Psychology*, 34, 562–581

Gouvier, W. D., Cubic, B., Jones, G., Brantley, P., & Cutlip, Q. (1992). Postconcussion symptoms and daily stress in normal and head-injured college populations. *Archives of Clinical Neuropsychology*, 7(3), 193–211.

Gowda, N. K., Agrawal, D., Bal, C., Chandrashekar, N., Tripati, M., Bandopadhyaya, G. P., . . . Mahapatra, A. K. (2006). Technetium Tc-99m ethyl cysteinate dimer brain single-photon emission CT in mild traumatic brain injury: A prospective study. *American Journal of Neuroradiology*, 27(2), 447–451.

Green, P. (2004). *Green's Medical Symptom Validity Test (MSVT) for Microsoft Windows (user manual)*. Edmonton, Canada: Green.

Green, P., & Astner, K. (1995). *Manual for the Oral Word Memory Test*. Durham, NC: CogniSyst.

Greiffenstein, M. F., Baker, W. J., & Gola, T. (1994). Validation of malingered amnesia measures with a large clinical sample. *Psychological Assessment*, 6, 218–224.

Gronwall, D., & Wrightson, P. (1980). Duration of post-traumatic amnesia after mild head injury. *Journal of Clinical Neuropsychology*, 2, 51–60.

Gronwall, D., & Wrightson, P. (1981). Memory and information processing capacity after closed head injury. *Journal of Neurology, Neurosurgery, and Psychiatry*, 44(10), 889–895.

Guskiewicz, K. M., Marshall, S. W., Bailes, J., McCrea, M., Cantu, R. C., Randolph, C., & Jordan, B. D. (2005). Association between recurrent concussion and late-life cognitive impairment in retired professional football players. *Neurosurgery*, 57, 719–726; discussion 719–726.

Guskiewicz, K. M., & Mihalik, J. P. (2011). Biomechanics of sport concussion: Quest for the elusive injury threshold. *Exercise and Sport Sciences Review*, 39(1), 4–11.

Hamberger, A., Viano, D. C., Säljö, A., & Bolouri, H. (2009). Concussion in professional football: Morphology of brain injuries in the NFL concussion model—part 16. *Neurosurgery*, 64(6), 1174–1182; discussion 1182.

Harger, L. (2010). *Workers' compensation, a brief history*. Retrieved from http://www.myfloridacfo.com/wc/history.html

Heilbronner, R. L., Sweet, J. J., Morgan, J. E., Larrabee, G. J., & Millis, S. R. (2009). American Academy of Clinical Neuropsychology Consensus Conference Statement on the neuropsychological assessment of effort, response bias, and malingering. *The Clinical Neuropsychologist*, 23(7), 1093–1129.

Hoff, J. T., Anderson, T. E., & Cole, T. M. (Eds.). (1989). *Mild to moderate head injury*. Boston, MA: Blackwell Scientific.

Hofling, C. K. (1965). Some psychological aspects of malingering. *GP*, 31, 115–121.

Hofman, P. A., Stapert, S. Z., van Kroonenburgh, M. J., Jolles, J., de Kruijk, J., & Wilmink, J. T. (2001). MR imaging, single-photon emission CT, and neurocognitive performance after mild traumatic brain injury. *American Journal of Neuroradiology*, 22(3), 441–449.

Hughes, D. G., Jackson, A., Mason, D. L., Berry, E., Hollis, S., & Yates, D. W. (2004). Abnormalities on magnetic resonance imaging seen acutely following mild traumatic brain injury: Correlation with neuropsychological tests and delayed recovery. *Neuroradiology*, 46(7), 550–558.

Independent Review Group. (2007). *Rebuilding the trust: Report on rehabilitative care and administrative processes at Walter Reed Army Medical Center and National Naval Medical Center*. Retrieved from http://www.ha.osd.mil/dhb/recommendations/2007/IRG-Report-Final.pdf

Iverson, G. L. (2005). Outcome from mild traumatic brain injury. *Current Opinion in Psychiatry*, 18(3), 301–317.

Iverson, G. L., Lovell, M. R., Smith, S., & Franzen, M. D. (2000). Prevalence of abnormal CT-scans following mild head injury. *Brain Injury*, 14(12), 1057–1061.

Jeret, J. S., Mandell, M., Anziska, B., Lipitz, M., Vilceus, A. P., Ware, J. A., & Zesiewicz, T. A. (1993). Clinical predictors of abnormality disclosed by computed tomography after mild head trauma. *Neurosurgery*, 32(1), 9–15; discussion 15–16.

Jones, A. B. (1917). *Malingering or the simulation of disease*. London, England: William Heinemann.

Jones, E. G., & Mendell, L. M. (1999). Assessing the decade of the brain. *Science*, 284(5415), 739.

Kant, R., Smith-Seemiller, L., Isaac, G., & Duffy, J. (1997). Tc-HMPAO SPECT in persistent post-concussion syndrome after mild head injury: Comparison with MRI/CT. *Brain Injury*, 11(2), 115–124.

Karson, S., & O'Dell, J. W. (1976). *A guide to the clinical use of the 16 PF*. Champaign, IL: Institute for Personality and Ability Testing.

Keen, W. M., Mitchell, S. W., & Morehouse, G. R. (1864). On malingering, especially in regard to simulation of disease of the nervous system. *American Journal of Medical Science*, 48, 367–374.

King, W. P. (1906). *Perjury for pay: An expos of the methods and criminal cunning of the modern malingerer*. Kansas City, MO: The Burton.

Kshettry, V. R., Mindea, S. A., & Batjer, H. H. (2007). The management of cranial injuries in antiquity and beyond. *Neurosurgical Focus*, 23(1), E8.

Kurca, E., Sivák, S., & Kucera, P. (2006). Impaired cognitive functions in mild traumatic brain injury patients with normal and pathologic magnetic resonance imaging. *Neuroradiology*, 48(9), 661–669.

Langfeld, H. S. (1921). Psychophysiological symptoms of deception. *The Journal of Abnormal Psychology*, 15, 319–328.

Larrabee, G. J. (2003). Detection of malingering using atypical performance patterns on standard neuropsychological tests. *The Clinical Neuropsychologist*, 17(3), 410–425.

Lees-Haley, P. R., & Brown, R. S. (1993). Neuropsychological complaint base rates of 170 personal injury claimants. *Archives of Clinical Neuropsychology*, 8(3), 203–209.

Lees-Haley, P. R., Fox, D. D., & Courtney, J. C. (2001). A comparison of complaints by mild brain injury claimants and other claimants describing subjective experiences immediately following their injury. *Archives of Clinical Neuropsychology*, 16(7), 689–695.

Levin, H. S., Eisenberg, H. M., & Benton, A. L. (1989). *Mild head injury*. New York, NY: Oxford University Press.

Levin, H. S., Mattis, S., Ruff, R. M., Eisenberg, H. M., Marshall, L. F., Tabaddor, K., . . . Frankowski, R. F. (1987). Neurobehavioral outcome following minor head injury: A three-center study. *Journal of Neurosurgery*, 66(2), 234–243.

Lidvall, H. F., Linderoth, B., & Norlin, B. (1974). Causes of the post-concussional syndrome. *Acta Neurologica Scandinavia Supplementum*, 56, 3–144.

Livingston, D. H., Loder, P. A., Koziol, J., & Hunt, C. D. (1991). The use of CT scanning to triage patients requiring admission following minimal head injury. *The Journal of Trauma*, 31(4), 483–487; discussion 487–489.

Lund, F. B. (1941). Galen on malingering, centaurs, diabetes, and other subjects more or less related. *Proceedings of the Charaka Club, X*, 52–55..

Magonet, J. (1992). *Biblical Lives*. London, England: SCM Press.

Martland, H. S. (1928). Punch Drunk. *Journal of the American Medical Association*, 91, 1103–1107.

McCrea, M. (2008). *Mild traumatic brain injury and postconcussion syndrome: The new evidence base for diagnosis and treatment*. New York, NY: Oxford University Press.

McCrory, P. R., & Berkovic, S. F. (2001). Concussion: The history of clinical and pathophysiological concepts and misconceptions. *Neurology*, 57(12), 2283–2289.

McKendrick, A. (1912). *Malingering and its detection under the workmen's compensation and other acts*. Edinburgh, Scotland: E. & S. Livingstone.

McLean, A. Jr., Temkin, N. R., Dikmen, S., & Wyler, A. R. (1983). The behavioral sequelae of head injury. *Journal of Clinical Neuropsychology*, 5(4), 361–376.

Megargee, E. I. (1972). *The California Psychological Inventory handbook*. San Francisco, CA: Jossey-Bass.

Meltzer, M. L. (1959). *Countermanipulation through malingering*. Unknown: Bureau of Social Science Research.

Mild Traumatic Brain Injury Committee of the Head Injury Interdisciplinary Special Interest Group of the American Congress of Rehabilitation Medicine. (1993). Definition of mild traumatic brain injury. *Journal of Head Trauma Rehabilitation*, 8, 86–87.

Miller, H. (1961a). Accident neurosis. *British Medical Journal*, 1, 919–925.

Miller, H. (1961b). Accident neurosis: Lecture II. *British Medical Journal*, 1, 992–998.

Mittenberg, W., Azrin, R., Millsaps, C., & Heilbronner, R. L. (1993). Identification of malingered head injury on the Wechsler Memory Scale-Revised. *Psychological Assessment*, 5, 34–40.

Mittenberg, W., Patton, C., Canyock, E. M., & Condit, D. C. (2002). Base rates of malingering and symptom exaggeration. *Journal of Clinical and Experimental Neuropsychology*, 24(8), 1094–1102.

Mittenberg, W., Rotholc, A., Russell, E., & Heilbronner, R. (1996). Identification of malingered head injury on the Halstead-Reitan battery. *Archives of Clinical Neuropsychology*, 11(4), 271–281.

Myers, C. S. (1916). Contributions to the study of shell-shock. *Lancet*, 1, 65–69.

Nelson, N. W., Hoelzle, J. B., McGuire, K. A., Ferrier-Auerbach, A. G., Charlesworth, M. J., & Sponheim, S. R. (2010). Evaluation context impacts neuropsychological performance of OEF/OIF veterans with reported combat-related concussion. *Archives of Clinical Neuropsychology*, 25(8), 713–723.

Nowinski, C. J. (2006). *Head games: Football's concussion crisis from the NFL to youth leagues*. Plymouth, MA: Drummond.

Ommaya, A. K., & Gennarelli, T. A. (1974). Cerebral concussion and traumatic unconsciousness. Correlation of experimental and clinical observations of blunt head injuries. *Brain*, 97(4), 633–654.

Oppenheimer, D. R. (1968). Microscopic lesions in the brain following head injury. *Journal of Neurology, Neurosurgery, and Psychiatry*, 31(4), 299–306.

Pankratz, L. (1979). Symptom validity testing and symptom retraining: Procedures for the assessment and treatment of functional sensory deficits. *Journal of Consulting and Clinical Psychology*, 47(2), 409–410.

Pankratz, L. (1983). A new technique for the assessment and modification of feigned memory deficit. *Perceptual and Motor Skills*, 57(2), 367–372.

Parker, N. (1979). Malingering: A dangerous diagnosis. *The Medical Journal of Australia*, 1(12), 568–569.

Pellman, E. J., Lovell, M. R., Viano, D. C., Casson, I. R., & Tucker, A. M. (2004). Concussion in professional football: Neuropsychological testing—part 6. *Neurosurgery*, 55, 1290–1303; discussion 1303–1295.

Pellman, E. J., Viano, D. C., Tucker, A. M., Casson, I. R., & Waeckerle, J. F. (2003). Concussion in professional football: Reconstruction of game impacts and injuries. *Neurosurgery*, 53(4), 799–812; discussion 812–794.

Putnam, S. H., & Millis, S. R. (1994). Psychosocial factors in the developmental and maintenance of chronic somatic and functional symptoms following mild traumatic brain injury. *Advances in Medical Psychotherapy*, 7, 1–22.

Rawling, P., & Brooks, N. (1990). Simulation Index: A method for detecting factitious errors on the WAIS-R and WMR. *Neuropsychology*, 4, 223–238.

Resnick, P. J. (1984). The detection of malingered mental illness. *Behavioral Sciences and the Law*, 2(1), 21–38.

Rey, A. (1941). L'examen psychologique dans les cas d'encephalopathie traumatique. *Archives de Psychologie*, 28, 286–340.

Rey, A. (1964). *L'examen clinique en psychologie*. Paris, France: Presses Universitaires de France.

Rigler, C. (1879). *Uber die folgen der verletzungen auf eisenbhanen* (Concerning the consequences of injuries on railroads). Berlin, Germany: Reimer.

Rimel, R. W., Giordani, B., Barth, J. T., Boll, T. J., & Jane, J. A. (1981). Disability caused by minor head injury. *Neurosurgery*, 9(3), 221–228.

Rogers, R. (Ed.). (1988). *Clinical assessment of malingering and deception*. New York, NY: Guilford Press.

Rohling, M. L., Binder, L. M., Demakis, G. J., Larrabee, G. J., Ploetz, D. M., & Langhinrichsen-Rohling, J. (2011). A meta-analysis of neuropsychological outcome after mild traumatic brain injury: Reanalyses and reconsiderations of Binder et al. (1997), Frencham et al. (2005), and Pertab et al. (2009). *The Clinical Neuropsychologist*, 25(4), 608–623.

Romanis, W., & Mitchiner, P. (1934). *The science and practice of surgery: Vol. 2.* (5th ed.). Philadelphia, PA: Lea & Febiger.

Ruff, R. M., & Jamora, C. W. (2009). Myths and mild traumatic brain injury. *Psychological Injury and Law*, 2, 34–42.

Ruff, R. M., Levin, H. S., & Marshall, L. F. (1986). Neurobehavioral methods of assessment and the study of outcome in minor head injury. *Journal of Head Trauma Rehabilitation*, 1, 43–52.

Schretlen, D. J., & Shapiro, A. M. (2003). A quantitative review of the effects of traumatic brain injury on cognitive functioning. *International Review of Psychiatry*, 15(4), 341–349.

Sercl, M., & Jaros, O. (1962). The mechanisms of cerebral concussion in boxing and their consequences. *World Neurology*, 3, 351–358.

Shapiro, R., & Mintz, A. (1990). Head injuries in the Old Testament. *Radiology*, 174(1), 84.

Sherman, T. (1913). *Notes on malingering under workmen's compensation laws*. New York, NY: Unknown.

Slick, D. J., Sherman, E. M., & Iverson, G. L. (1999). Diagnostic criteria for malingered neurocognitive dysfunction: Proposed standards for clinical practice and research. *The Clinical Neuropsychologist*, 13(4), 545–561.

Spencer, C. E. (1929). Methods of detecting guilt: Word-association, reaction-time method. *Oregon Law Review*, 8, 158–166.

Spencer, R. J., Drag, L. L., Walker, S. J., & Bieliauskas, L. A. (2010). Self-reported cognitive symptoms following mild traumatic brain injury are poorly associated with neuropsychological performance in OIF/OEF veterans. *Journal of Rehabilitation and Research Development*, 47(6), 521–530.

Stedman, J. K. (2006). *Stedman's medical dictionary* (28th ed.). Baltimore, MD: Lippincott Williams & Wilkins.

Theodor, L. H., & Mandelcorn, M. S. (1973). Hysterical blindness: A case report and study using a modern psychophysical technique. *Journal of Abnormal Psychology*, 82, 552–553.

Tombaugh, T. (1996). *Test of memory malingering*. Los Angeles, CA: Western Psychological Services.

Trueblood, W. (1994). Qualitative and quantitative characteristics of malingered and other invalid WAIS-R and clinical memory data. *Journal of Clinical and Experimental Neuropsychology*, 16(4), 597–607.

Trueblood, W., & Schmidt, M. (1993). Malingering and other validity considerations in the neuropsychological evaluation of mild head injury. *Journal of Clinical and Experimental Neuropsychology*, 15(4), 578–590.

Umile, E. M., Plotkin, R. C., & Sandel, M. E. (1998). Functional assessment of mild traumatic brain injury using SPECT and neuropsychological testing. *Brain Injury*, 12(7), 577–594.

Varney, N. R., & Bushnell, D. (1998). NeuroSPECT findings in patients with posttraumatic anosmia: A quantitative analysis. *The Journal of Head Trauma Rehabilitation*, 13(3), 63–72.

Wessely, S. (2003). Malingering: Historical perspectives. In P. W. Halligan, C. M. Bass, & D. A. Oakley (Eds.), *Malingering and illness deception*. New York, NY: Oxford University Press.

Whitney, K. A., Shepard, P. H., Williams, A. L., Davis, J. J., & Adams, K. M. (2009). The Medical Symptom Validity Test in the evaluation of Operation Iraqi Freedom/Operation Enduring Freedom soldiers: A preliminary study. *Archives of Clinical Neuropsychology*, 24(2), 145–152.

Wrightson, P. (2000). The development of a concept of mild head injury. *Journal of Clinical Neuroscience*, 7(5), 384–388.

Yarnell, P. R., & Lynch, S. (1970). Progressive retrograde amnesia in concussed football players: Observation shortly postimpact. *Neurology*, 20(4), 416–417.

APPENDIX 1.1 Chronological History of Book Publications on Malingering (*Continued*)

Year	Author/Editor (Ed.)	Title	Publisher	City
		The Early Years		
1843	Gavin, H.	*On Feigned and Factitious Diseases, Chiefly of Soldiers and Seamen, on the Means Used to Simulate or Produce Them and on the Best Modes of Discovering Imposters*	John Churchill	London, England
1844	Acland, H. W.	*Feigned Insanity: How Most Usually Simulated, and How Best Detected*	R. Clay	London, England
1864	Bartholow, R.	*A Manual of Instructions for Enlisting and Discharging Soldiers: With Special Reference to the Medical Examination of Recruits, and the Detection of Disqualifying and Feigned Diseases*	Lippincott	Philadelphia, PA
1906	Dawson, W. H.	*The German Workman: A Study in National Efficiency*	Scribner	London, England
1906	King, W. P.	*Perjury for Pay: An Exposé of the Methods and Criminal Cunning of the Modern Malingerer*	The Burton Company	Kansas City, MO
1912	McKendrick, A.	*Malingering and Its Detection Under the Workmen's Compensation and Other Acts*	E. & S. Livingstone	Edinburgh, Scotland
1913	Sherman, T.	*Notes on Malingering Under Workmen's Compensation Laws*	Unknown	New York, NY
1917	Dumez, A. G.[a]	*The Simulation of Disease. Drugs, Chemicals, and Septic Materials Used Therefor*	U.S. Government Printing Office	Washington, DC
1917	Collie, J. S.	*Malingering and Feigned Sickness*	Edward Arnold	London, England
1917	Jones, A. B.	*Malingering or the Simulation of Disease*	W. Heinemann	London, England
1932	Collie, J.	*Fraud in Medico-legal Practice*	Edward Arnold & Company	London, England
1959	Bergan, M.	*Functional Examination for Malingering and Psychogenicity in Impaired Hearing*	National Hospital for Speech Disorders	New York, NY
1959	Meltzer, M. L.	*Countermanipulation Through Malingering*	Bureau of Social Science Research	Unknown
		The Modern Era		
1988	Rogers, R. (Ed.)	*Clinical Assessment of Malingering and Deception*	Guilford Press	New York, NY
1988	Rogers, R. & Resnick, P. (Eds.)	*Malingering and Deception: The Clinical Interview*	Guilford Press	New York, NY
1993	Gorman, W.	*Legal Neurology and Malingering: Cases and Techniques*	W. H. Green	St. Louis, MO
1996	Hall, H. V., & Pritchard, D. A.	*Detecting Malingering and Deception: Forensic Distortion Analysis*	St. Lucie Press	Unknown

(Continued)

APPENDIX 1.1 Chronological History of Book Publications on Malingering (*Continued*)

Year	Author/Editor (Ed.)	Title	Publisher	City
		The Modern Era (*Continued*)		
1997	Rogers, R. (Ed.)	*Clinical Assessment of Malingering and Deception (2nd ed.)*	Guilford Press	New York, NY
1997	Reitan, R. M., & Wolfson, D.	*Detection of Malingering and Invalid Test Scores*	Neuropsychology Press	Tucson, AZ
1998	Reynolds, C. R. (Ed.)	*Detection of Malingering During Head Injury Litigation*	Plenum Press	New York
1998	Pankratz, L.	*Patients Who Deceive: Assessment and Management of Risk in Providing Health Care and Financial Benefits*	Charles C. Thomas	Springfield, IL
1998	McCann, J. T.	*Malingering and Deception in Adolescents: Assessing Credibility in Clinical and Forensic Settings*	American Psychological Association	Washington, DC
2000	Hall, H. V. & Poirier, J. G.	*Detecting Malingering and Deception: Forensic Distortion Analysis (2nd ed.)*	CRC Press	Boca Raton, FL
2001	Hutchinson, G. L.	*Disorders of Simulation: Malingering, Factitious Disorders, and Compensation Neurosis*	Psychosocial Press	Madison, CT
2002	Hom, J., & Denney, R. (Eds.)	*Detection of Response Bias in Forensic Neuropsychology*	Haworth Medical Press	Binghamton, NY
2003	Halligan, P. W., Bass, C., & Oakley, D. A.	*Malingering and Illness Deception*	Oxford University Press	New York, NY
2004	Feldman, M.	*Playing sick?: Untangling the Web of Munchausen Syndrome, Munchausen by Proxy, Malingering and Factitious Disorder*	Brunner-Routledge	New York, NY
2004	Stephens, P.	*How to Fake a Back Exam!: A Medical Professional's Guide to Prescription Drug Diversion*	Corporate Publishing	Fairmont, NC
2005	Granhag, P. A., & Strömwall, L. A. (Eds.)	*The Detection of Deception in Forensic Contexts*	Cambridge University Press	New York, NY
2007	Boone, K. B. (Ed.)	*Assessment of Feigned Cognitive Impairment: A Neuropsychological Perspective*	Guilford Press	New York, NY
2007	Kitaeff, J. (Ed.)	*Malingering, Lies, and Junk Science in the Courtroom*	Cambria Press	Youngstown, NY
2007	Larrabee, G. J. (Ed.)	*Assessment of Malingered Neuropsychological Deficits*	Oxford University Press	New York, NY
2007	Friedman, R.	*Polarizing the Case: Exposing and Defeating the Malingering Myth*	Trial Guides	Portland, OR
2007	Miller, J. H.	*Faked Disability: A Shame of America: An Insult to the Medical Profession, a Disgrace to the Legal Profession*	AuthorHouse	Bloomington, IN
2008	Rogers, R. (Ed.)	*Clinical Assessment of Malingering and Deception (3rd edition)*	Guilford Press	New York, NY

(*Continued*)

APPENDIX 1.1 Chronological History of Book Publications on Malingering

Year	Author/Editor (Ed.)	Title	Publisher	City
		The Modern Era (*Continued*)		
2008	Morgan, J. E., & Sweet, J. J. (Eds.)	*Neuropsychology of Malingering Casebook*	Psychology Press	New York, NY
2009	Strauss, A,	*Malingery: Stealing the Truth*	Booksurge Publishing	Charleston, SC
2010	Morel, K. R.	*Differential Diagnosis of Malingering Versus Posttraumatic Stress Disorder: Scientific Rationale and Objective Scientific Methods (Psychiatry – Theory, Applications and Treatments)*	Nova Science	Hauppauge, NY

Note. Year refers to publication year. Books listed are restricted to those published in English and which are nonfiction. Books were identified by title and keyword searches at the Library of Congress online catalog (http://catalog.loc.gov/) and via Amazon.com. Dissertations or lengthy research papers published as books in the modern era are not included. Texts needed to be devoted to malingering to be included (i.e., a chapter on the topic in a more general text did not meet inclusionary criteria). Test manuals were not included.
[a]Indicates a public health report.

APPENDIX 1.2 Chronological History of Book Publications on MTBI/Concussion

Year	Author/Editor (Ed.)	Title	Publisher	City/State or Country
		The Early Years[a]		
1760	Pott, P.	Observations on the Nature and Consequences of Wounds and Contusions of the Head, Fractures of the Skull, Concussions of the Brain...	C. Hitch and L. Hawes	Unknown
1927	Miller, G. G.	Cerebral Concussion	McGill University Publications	Montreal, Canada
1953	Courville, C. B.	Commotio Cerebri: Cerebral Concussion and the Postconcussion Syndrome in Their Medical and Legal Aspects	San Lucas Press	Los Angeles, CA
1958	Seletz, E.	Brain injuries: Cerebral Concussion, Contusion, Laceration, and Hemorrage	Callaghan	Unknown
1974	Gronwall, D. M. A., & Sampson, H.	The Psychological Effects of Concussion	Auckland University Press	Auckland, New Zealand
		The Modern Era		
1989	Levin, H. S., Eisenberg, H. M., & Benton, A. L.	Mild Head Injury	Oxford University Press	New York, NY
1989	Hoff, J., Anderson, T., & Cole, T. (Eds.)	Mild to Moderate Head Injury	Blackwell Scientific Publications	Boston, MA
1993	Mandel, S., Sataloff, R. T., & Schapiro, S. R. (Eds.)	Minor Head Trauma: Assessment, Management, and Rehabilitation	Springer Publishing	New York, NY
1996	Rizzo, M., & Tranel, D.	Head Injury and Postconcussive Syndrome	Churchill Livingstone	New York, NY
1996	Denton, G. L.	Brainlash: Maximize Your Recovery From Mild Brain Injury	Attention Span Books	Niwot, CO
1997	Green, B. S., Stevens, K. M., & Wolfe, T. D. W.	Mild Traumatic Brain Injury: A Therapy and Resource Manual	Singular Publishing Group	San Diego, CA
1998	Stoler, D. R., & Hill, B. A.	Coping with Mild Traumatic Brain Injury	Avery Publishing Group	Garden City Park, NY
1999	Denton, G. L.	Brainlash: Maximize Your Recovery From Mild Brain Injury (2nd. ed)	Demos Medical Publishing	New York, NY
1999	Bailes, J. E., Lovell, M. R., & Maroon, J. C. (Eds.)	Sport-Related Concussion	Quality Medical Publishing	St. Louis, MO

(Continued)

APPENDIX 1.2 Chronological History of Book Publications on MTBI/Concussion (*Continued*)

Year	Author/Editor (Ed.)	Title	Publisher	City/State or Country
		The Modern Era (*Continued*)		
1999	Wrightson, P., & Gronwall, D.	*Mild Head Injury: A Guide to Management*	Oxford University Press	New York, NY
1999	Raymond, M. J., Bennett, T. L., Hartlage, L. C., & Cullum, C. M. (Eds.)	*Mild Traumatic Brain Injury: A Clinician's Guide*	PRO-ED	Austin, TX
1999	Varney, N. R., & Roberts, R. J. (Eds.)	*The Evaluation and Treatment of Mild Traumatic Brain Injury*	Lawrence Erlbaum Associates	Mahwah, NJ
2000	Reitan, R., & Wolfson, D.	*Mild Head Injury: Cognitive, Intellectual, and Emotional Consequences*	Neuropsychology Press	Tucson, AZ
2000	Raskin, S. A., & Mateer, C. A.	*Neuropsychological Management of Mild Traumatic Brain Injury*	Oxford University Press	New York, NY
2000	Jay, G. W. (Ed.)	*Minor Traumatic Brain Injury Handbook: Diagnosis and Treatment*	CRC Press	Boca Raton, FL
2001	Parker, R. S.	*Concussive Brain Trauma: Neurobehavioral Impairment and Maladaptation*	CRC Press	Boca Raton, FL
2003	McCrory, J.	*Sport Related Concussion*	Taylor & Francis	New York, NY
2004	Lovell, M. R., Echemendia, R. J., Barth, J. T., & Collins, M. W. (Eds.)	*Traumatic Brain Injury in Sports: An International Perspective*	Swets & Zeitlinger	Lisse, Netherlands
2004	Mason, D. J.	*The Mild Traumatic Brain Injury Workbook: Your Program for Regaining Cognitive Function & Overcoming Emotional Pain*	New Harbinger Publications	Oakland, CA
2006	Hossler, P., & Savage, R.	*Getting A-head of Concussion: Educating the Student Athlete's Neighborhood*	Lash & Associates Publishing	Wake Forest, NC
2006	Slobounov, S., & Sebastianelli, W. (Eds.)	*Foundations of Sport-Related Brain Injuries*	Springer Science and Business Media	New York, NY
2006	Echemendia, R.	*Sports Neuropsychology: Assessment and Management of Traumatic Brain Injury*	Guilford Press	New York, NY
2006	Solomon, G. S., Johnston, K. M, & Lovell, M. R.	*The Heads-Up on Sports Concussion*	Human Kinetics	Champaign, IL
2007	Nowinski, C.	*Head Games: Football's Concussion Crisis From the NFL to Youth Leagues*	Drummond Publishing Group	East Bridgewater, MA

(*Continued*)

APPENDIX 1.2 Chronological History of Book Publications on MTBI/Concussion

Year	Author/Editor (Ed.)	Title	Publisher	City/State or Country
		The Modern Era (*Continued*)		
2008	McCrea, M.	*Mild Traumatic Brain Injury and Postconcussion Syndrome: The New Evidence Base For Diagnosis and Treatment*	Oxford University Press	New York, NY
2008	Denton, G. L.	*Brainlash: Maximize Your Recovery From Mild Brain Injury (3rd. ed)*	Demos Medical Publishing	New York, NY
2008	Omalu, B.	*Play Hard, Die Young: Football Dementia, Depression, and Death*	Neo-Forenxis Books	Unknown
2009	Department of Defense	*2009 Management of Concussion/Mild Traumatic Brain Injury Clinical Practice Guideline by the VA—Coverage of Veterans Issues, Concussion, Research*	Progressive Management	Unknown
2009	Keatley, M. A., & Whittemore, L. L. (Eds.)	*Recovering from Mild Traumatic Brain Injury (MTBI): A Handbook of Hope for Our Military Warriors and Their Families*	Brain Injury Hope Foundation	Boulder, CO
2010	Hoge, C. W.	*Once a Warrior Always a Warrior: Navigating the Transition from Combat to Home—Including Combat Stress, PTSD, and mTBI*	GPP Life	Guilford, CT
2010	Keatley, M. A., & Whittemore, L. L. (Eds.)	*Understanding Mild Traumatic Brain Injury (MTBI): An Insightful Guide to Symptoms, Treatments and Redefining Recovery*	Brain Injury Hope Foundation	Boulder, CO
2010	Bickerstaff, L.	*Frequently Asked Questions About Concussions*	The Rosen Publishing Group	New York, NY
2010	Webbe, F. M. (Ed.)	*The Handbook of Sport Neuropsychology*	Springer Publishing	New York, NY
2010	Hossler, P., & Collins, M. W.	*Concussion Policy: A Construction Guide for Schools*	Lash & Associates Publishing	Wake Forest, NC
2010	Acimovic, M. L.	*Mild Traumatic Brain Injury: The Guidebook*	Lulu.com	None
2010	Roberts, R. J., & Roberts, M. A.	*Mild Traumatic Brain Injury: Episodic Symptoms and Treatment*	Plural Publishing Inc.	San Diego, CA
2011	Kamberg, M.	*Sports Concussions*	The Rosen Publishing Group	New York, NY
2011	Meehan, W. P.	*Kids, Sports, and Concussion: A Guide for Coaches and Parents*	Praeger Publishers, Inc.	San Diego, CA

(*Continued*)

APPENDIX 1.2 Chronological History of Book Publications on MTBI/Concussion

Year	Author/Editor (Ed.)	Title	Publisher	City/State or Country
		The Modern Era (*Continued*)		
2011	Parker, R. S.	*Concussive Brain Trauma: Neurobehavioral Impairment and Maladaptation (2nd ed.)*	CRC Press	Boca Raton, FL
2011	United States Government Accountability Office	*VA Health Care: Mild Traumatic Brain Injury Screening and Evaluation Implemented for OEF/OIF Veterans, but Challenges Remain*	BiblioGov	Washington, DC
2011	Carroll, L., & Rosner, D.	*The Concussion Crisis: Anatomy of a Silent Epidemic*	Simon & Schuster	New York, NY
2011 (in press)	Sedory, D.	*Cram Session in Evaluation of Sports Concussion: A Handbook for Students and Clinicians*	Slack Incorporated	Thorofare, NJ
In press	Apps, J. A. N. (Ed.)	*Handbook of the Neuropsychology of Pediatric Concussion*	Springer Publishing	New York, NY

Note. Year refers to publication year. Books listed are restricted to those published in English and which are nonfiction. Books were identified by title and keyword searches at the Library of Congress online catalog (http://catalog.loc.gov/) and via Amazon.com. Dissertations or lengthy research papers published as books in the modern era are not included. Texts needed to be devoted to MTBI/concussion to be included (i.e., a chapter on the topic in a more general text did not meet inclusionary criteria).

[a]Publications in the early years section sometimes used the word "concussion" to refer to TBIs that are more severe than MTBI as conceptualized by modern standards.

The Role of Clinical Judgment in Symptom Validity Assessment

2

Thomas J. Guilmette

The 1990s began the proliferation of forensic neuropsychology and the concomitant rise in substantial research efforts to assist clinicians in ascertaining the validity of neuropsychological test results, particularly in medicolegal evaluations where the subject might have an incentive to "fake bad." Prior to that time, there were very few evaluation methods designed specifically to identify suboptimal performance and malingering in neuropsychological assessments. For example, in the 1988 first edition of Richard Rogers's *Clinical Assessment of Malingering and Deception*, Pankratz described just four tests specifically for malingering detection in intellectual and neuropsychological assessments: (a) dot counting; (b) memorization of 15 items; (c) word recognition test; and (d) the two-alternative forced-choice technique that he had recently coined as "symptom validity testing" (SVT) for the assessment of the validity of sensory and memory complaints. However, at that time, the SVT technique was not standardized in administration or normed on nonclinical controls, persons with known brain injury without incentive to malinger, or experimental or clinical simulators and had to be "constructed precisely for the complaint of the individual" (Pankratz, 1988, p. 183). In addition, only scores that were significantly less than chance were considered to be clinically meaningful, which is now known to be a relatively rare event among persons who are judged to produce invalid test results (Gervais, Rohling, Green, & Ford, 2004; Greve, Binder, & Bianchini, 2009).

The SVT designation no longer applies solely to forced-choice techniques but rather is now applied to any specific technique designed to evaluate the validity of symptoms and test responses. However, at that time, given the paucity of available measures designed to assess negative response bias and the relative nascence of research in this domain, the greatest weight of evidence for detecting malingering was given to test interpretation (e.g., the interpretation of general neuropsychological test results without benefit of specific procedures designed to assess effort and motivation), which is the focus of this chapter. The sections that follow are meant to provide the reader with an overview of the strategies, accuracy, and limitations of clinical judgment in ascertaining the validity of neuropsychological test results in the absence of validated measures of effort and malingering.

CLINICAL JUDGMENT STRATEGIES FOR DETECTING MALINGERING

Although the terms *suboptimal effort*, *malingering*, and *negative response bias* have somewhat different meanings and connotations, there can be considerable overlap among them; and for the purposes of this chapter, they will be used interchangeably. In essence, they all refer to the production of neuropsychological test results that are not fully explained by brain dysfunction and that are not reasonably attributable to variables that may, in some instances, moderate or confound test performance (e.g., education, age, fatigue, psychological conditions; Heilbronner, Sweet, Morgan, Larrabee, & Millis, 2009). A critical issue for clinicians in assessing the neuropsychological sequelae of mild traumatic brain injury (MTBI) is in determining whether neuropsychological test results are caused by brain injury or non–brain injury factors, such as the exaggeration or faking of deficits, when secondary (financial) gain may be a prominent motivator for the examinee's performance. Assessment is further complicated because neurologic exams and procedures (e.g., brain imaging such as CT and MRI scans) are frequently negative, and symptoms can range in severity but are often subjective. More pointedly for this chapter is the issue of how accurately neuropsychologists are able to identify invalid or misrepresented neuropsychological abilities when relying on clinical judgment and without administering well-validated SVT procedures, either those that stand alone as individual measures (e.g., often but not always a forced-choice test developed specifically to assess effort) or those that are "embedded" within a standardized neuropsychological test; the latter referring to a number of commonly used clinical measures that have been validated to assess not only a specific aspect of cognitive functioning, such as memory or attention, but also have been shown to be sensitive in identifying examinees who produce non-credible results.

In conjunction with the development and use of specific malingering detection techniques and procedures, a multimodal approach to malingering assessment has been consistently advocated, and other sources of information should also be considered from background history, interview, observations, and neuropsychological test results (Heilbronner et al., 2009). Apart from SVT results, some malingering "signs" are obvious and identifiable (e.g., the patient who is observed under surveillance performing tasks that he or she denied he or she was able to perform during interview or testing), whereas other indicators require significantly greater interpretation and judgment (e.g., determining whether a patient's score exceeds the expected impairment level given his or her complaints and injury history).

Pankratz (1988) advocated a seven-criteria "threshold model of malingered neuropsychological impairment" (p. 190), which included the following: (1) near misses to simple questions; (2) gross discrepancies from expected norms; (3) inconsistency between present diagnosis and neuropsychological findings; (4) inconsistency between reported and observed symptoms; (5) resistance, avoidance, or bizarre responses on standard tests; (6) marked discrepancies on test findings that measure similar cognitive ability; and (7) failure on any specific measure of neuropsychological faking. Many of his criteria have been included in some form or another into subsequent malingering detection approaches, but apart from criterion 7, the other malingering indicators require clinical judgment to determine whether a response or finding is a "near miss," "gross discrepancy," "inconsistency," or "marked discrepancy." In 1997, Pankratz and Binder updated the aforementioned list by dropping numbers 1, 2, and 6 and replacing them with "lying to health care providers," "functional findings on orthopedic or neurological exams," and "late onset of cognitive complaints following an accident."

Nies and Sweet (1994) outlined several strategies for clinicians to consider in attempting to identify malingerers, some of which rely more on clinical interpretation than others. For example, in addition to encouraging the use of specific tests of malingering, they also advocated examining nonsensical test patterns that are not usually found in genuine psychiatric or neurologic patients, examining *excessive* (italics theirs) inconsistency of test scores within and across test sessions, seeking independent information that can confirm or refute the patient's self-report of his or her limited capabilities in managing everyday living or work activities, and determining whether the client has actually sustained a significant loss because of the injury (e.g., loss of house because of bankruptcy or divorce).

Many clinical approaches to identifying malingering employ a "pattern of performance method," which has been described as the most effective way to detect malingering with conventional neuropsychological measures (Slick, Sherman, & Iverson, 1999). This approach was outlined by Slick, Sherman, and Iverson (1999) who described at least four different procedures. The first is performance on very easy or "floor" items such as forgetting one's name. The second method is to determine if scores or score profiles within or across tests are consistent with known patterns of function or dysfunction. The third method is the application of statistical procedures, such as discriminant function analyses, to test scores obtained from known criterion groups such as experimental or clinical malingerers. The fourth method examines magnitude or level of errors.

In proposing definitions and criteria for malingered neurocognitive dysfunction (MND), Slick et al. (1999) suggested three levels: definite, probable, and possible. The criteria for definite MND require the most stringent evidence of negative response bias (e.g., a below chance performance on one or more forced-choice measures of cognitive functions) and relies much less on clinical judgment than the other less definitive levels. For example, criteria for possible or probable MND require multiple clinical judgments including evaluating the discrepancy between test data and known patterns of brain functioning, the discrepancy between test data and observed behavior, the discrepancy between test data and reliable collateral reports, and the discrepancy between test data and documented background history. However, the magnitude of these discrepancies necessary for significance is essentially left up to the discretion of the individual clinician. In addition, other behaviors can be considered indicators for both possible and probable MND, including significant inconsistencies or discrepancies between the patient's self-reported symptoms and documented history, known patterns of brain functioning, behavioral observations, or information obtained from collateral informants. Thus, within a model of identifying MND, although clinical judgment is required, clear and compelling evidence is derived from the results of forced-choice SVT procedures, reflecting less reliance on test pattern and discrepancy analyses.

In a survey of "expert" neuropsychologists (e.g., individuals who had published at least two articles on detecting malingering or suboptimal effort between 1996 and 2001), 79% of participants reported using at least one specialized technique for malingering detection in forensic evaluations (Slick, Tan, Strauss, & Hultsch, 2004). However, in a broader sample of practicing neuropsychologists from the National Academy of Neuropsychology (Sharland & Gfeller, 2007), only 56% reported that they often or always include a measure of effort in evaluations. Of note, among the 10 potential methods used by the participants to detect poor effort or malingering, the five most common relied exclusively on clinical judgment and did not involve the use of specific effort or malingering procedures. Those five methods, used often or always by 64% to 88% of the respondents, included the following (listed from most to least frequent): (a) severity of cognitive impairment inconsistent with the condition; (b) discrepancies among records, self-report, and observed behavior; (c) the pattern of cognitive impairment inconsistent with the condition; (d) implausible self-reported symptoms in interview; and (e) implausible changes in test scores across repeated examinations. Thus, in spite of multiple measures sensitive to poor effort and malingering that were available to clinicians, only about half of the survey respondents used those measures routinely in their evaluations, suggesting that practitioners tended to rely heavily on applying clinical judgment to evaluating discrepancies and inconsistencies among test findings, observations, history, condition, and symptoms.

Applying clinical judgment to identify suspect patterns of performance can be effective only if the patterns themselves reveal significant discrepancies. To test this issue, van Gorp and colleagues (1999) examined the extent to which the pattern or level of performance on traditional neuropsychological tests, without benefit of specific SVT measures, could meaningfully assist in identifying the protocols of probable malingerers. Based on a retrospective analysis of 81 patients with mild-to-moderate TBI who had been referred for a clinical neuropsychological evaluation, 20 subjects were classified as suspected malingerers and 61 subjects were classified as non-malingerers. Identification of the probable malingerers and non-malingerers was made by their performance on specialized SVT procedures and on the nature of their injuries and complaints without examining their performance on traditional clinical neuropsychological tests. A jackknifing procedure used as a means of cross-validating a discriminant function analysis revealed that the pattern of neuropsychological test performance alone was no more effective than chance in identifying malingerers from non-malingerers. Level of performance was somewhat more useful, with the malingering group obtaining significantly lower scores on 6 of 11 neuropsychological variables (e.g., Stroop color and interference, Trails B minus Trails A, Rey-Osterrieth Complex Figure, dominant minus nondominant hand on Grooved Pegboard, Visual Reproduction II on the Wechsler Memory Scale-Revised). There were no differences with full scale, performance, or verbal IQ scores between the two groups. The authors suggested that

> the clinician use abnormally low performance as merely one indicator to suggest possible malingering, but he or she should rely more heavily on neuropsychological measures which have either been designed to detect malingering or are clinical measures which have been validated for the detection of malingering. (p. 249)

EFFICACY OF CLINICAL JUDGMENT IN DETECTING INVALID TEST RESULTS

The empirical research examining clinicians' ability to detect falsified neuropsychological profiles is not extensive. Three studies have generally supported neuropsychologists' ability to detect malingering, although methodological problems are noteworthy. Bruhn and Reed (1975) reported a 90% accuracy rate in identifying malingerers using just one measure—the Bender-Gestalt, a test now considered obsolete—although the judges were given the base rates of malingering, which is an advantage not as readily available in clinical practice. Goebel (1983) reported that a clinical judge, Goebel himself, correctly identified 80% of a patient group, 100% of controls, and 98% of simulators (152 undergraduates faking specific brain disorders) using the Halstead-Reitan Neuropsychological Battery (HRNB). However, the patient group had relatively extreme deficits, and many of the simulators performed within or near normal limits. Moreover, the clinician-judge (Goebel) had prior exposure to all the actual patient cases.

Trueblood and Binder (1997) is the third study that described generally positive results with neuropsychologists' capacity to detect malingering based on neuropsychological data, although a careful review of their methodology is warranted. In this study, four clinical malingerers and two patients with severe TBI were included. The four clinical malingerers had histories of MTBI, as evidenced by brief loss or disturbance of consciousness, and were also involved in litigation and/or seeking workers' compensation. All obtained below chance performance on a forced-choice test (e.g., Portland Digit Recognition Test or the Hiscock forced-choice procedure) and demonstrated multiple other aspects of test data supporting malingering or poor effort. Two of the four had surveillance information also supporting malingering. Length of unconsciousness for the two patients with severe TBI, neither of whom was involved in litigation, was 11 days and 2 months. All of the individuals completed comprehensive neuropsychological test batteries that included either an expanded HRNB or a test battery not centered around the HRNB.

Four hundred and forty neuropsychologists were sent summary test data of either two of the four malingering cases or the two severe TBI cases along with their histories describing the injury, litigation status, the results of the forced-choice testing for half the malingerers, and a cover letter indicating that detecting malingering was the focus of the study (Trueblood & Binder, 1997). Eighty-six useable responses were returned. The authors reported that error rates for diagnosing "cerebral dysfunction due to head injury," which was one of the four diagnostic options given to the raters, across the four malingered cases ranged from 0% to 25%, with a mean error rate of 10%. However, this 10% error rate should not be interpreted as a mean accuracy rate of 90% for diagnosing malingering because the authors did not count diagnoses of "normal" or "nonvolitional functional factors" as diagnostic errors for the malingering cases, even for those respondents who were given the results of a below chance performance on the forced-choice testing. If those incorrect diagnoses are also included, then the mean error rate across the malingered cases is 28%, which reflects an accuracy rate of 72% for choosing correctly one of the four diagnostic options. Of note, all four malingered MTBI cases produced test profiles reflecting substantial impairments, which arguably made their simulation obvious. For example, each of the following highly abnormal test scores, which fall several standard deviations below the mean, was produced by at least one of the four malingerers: (a) California Verbal Learning Test (CVLT) recognition = 4; (b) CVLT Trial 5 recall = 3; (c) Rey Auditory Verbal Learning Test recognition = 5; and (d) Trails B = 356 seconds.

Other research has been less supportive of neuropsychologists' ability to detect malingering from test protocols alone. For example, Heaton, Smith, Lehman, and Vogt (1978) distributed 32 protocols of Wechsler Adult Intelligence Scale scores, HRNB test results, and Minnesota Multiphasic Personality Inventory (MMPI) profiles to 10 neuropsychologists. The protocols contained the results of 16 experimental malingerers and 16 actual patients with TBI. All the patients with TBI had sustained a minimum of 12 hours of unconsciousness, and none was in litigation. The judges were aware of the general design of the study but did not know how many of the 32 test protocols contained malingered versus genuine results. The accuracy of the judges' ability to sort the malingering from the TBI protocols ranged from chance level prediction to about 20% better than chance. There was no benefit of experience in diagnostic accuracy, but a discriminant function analysis based on neuropsychological test results and the MMPI, respectively, correctly classified 100% and 94% of the participants in both groups. Overall, the authors described the classification rates of the judges to be "rather modest" (p. 899).

In a study that examined the accuracy of neuropsychologists to detect adolescent malingerers (Faust, Hart, Guilmette, & Arkes, 1988), three 15- to 17-year-olds were asked to fake believable deficits on the Wechsler Intelligence Scale for Children-

Revised or the Wechsler Adult Intelligence Scale-Revised and the HRNB. In Part 1 of the study, practicing neuropsychologists were sent either one of the malingered protocols or test results of an actual adolescent with TBI along with a clinical history consistent with a MTBI from a motor vehicle accident. They were asked to judge first if the test protocol was normal or abnormal. If judged to be abnormal, the participant was asked to select one of three primary causes (e.g., cortical dysfunction, malingering, or functional factors). Of those clinicians who judged the malingering cases to be abnormal, 0% identified malingering as the cause. In Part 2, another group of neuropsychologists was sent either two malingerers' cases, two head injured cases, or a malingerer's case and a head injury case. The cover letter informed the participants that the base rate for malingering in the data was 50%. The accuracy in identifying the malingering cases did not surpass chance levels. Moreover, 49% to 70% of the clinician-judges expressed that they were highly to very highly confident in their decisions.

Faust, Hart, and Guilmette (1988) extended their adolescent malingering study described previously to include three children, ages 9 to 12 years, who were asked simply to perform less well on testing (e.g., IQ and the HRNB for older children) than usual but not to be so obvious that the person testing would know they were faking. Neuropsychologists received one of the three malingering test results along with a clinical history consistent with a MTBI caused by a motor vehicle accident. As in the adolescent malingering study, the clinicians were first asked to judge if the results were normal or abnormal and, if abnormal, then to indicate if caused by cortical dysfunction, malingering, or functional factors. Even though nearly three-fourths of the judges reported at least moderate confidence in their diagnoses, the detection rate for malingering was 0%. Thus, consistent with the adolescent malingering study, these results cast significant doubt on neuropsychologists' ability to detect simulated brain damage from neuropsychological test results alone.

Critics of the Faust et al.'s (1988) adolescent and pediatric malingering studies have asserted that the results do not generalize to actual clinical settings, and thus this research has not adequately assessed malingering detection by practitioners (Bigler, 1990; Schmidt, 1989). These criticisms have centered on the competency of the neuropsychologist judges, the use of the questionnaire format that may have biased the participants to overinterpret pathology, the lack of direct client interview or observation, and the lack of collateral information (e.g., other historical data, additional medical history, educational records, reports from employers or friends/family, or neurodiagnsotic studies). In reply, Arkes, Faust, and Guilmette (1990) and Faust and Guilmette (1990) asserted, in part, that the judgment literature generally does not support the claims that interview data enhance the detection of malingering, that diagnostic accuracy is aided by additional information, or that practitioners are capable of integrating effectively multiple sources of clinical data. However, irrespective of the debate regarding the validity of the Faust malingering studies, there can be little doubt that their publication prompted greater research in neuropsychology to develop more systematic and valid methods to detect malingering.

IMPEDIMENTS TO CLINICAL JUDGMENT IN ASSESSING MALINGERING

The debate over the accuracy and application of clinical judgment in psychology is not new (Meehl, 1954). Criticisms regarding the limits of clinical judgment have been raised in the areas of general clinical assessments (e.g., descriptions of personality and psychopathology, diagnosis, case formulation, behavioral prediction, and treatment decisions; Garb, 2005), forensic evaluations (Borum, Otto, & Golding, 1993), determining psychiatric disability (Harding, 2004), and within neuropsychology itself (Wedding & Faust, 1989). A meta-analytic review revealed that actuarial or mechanical judgments regarding human behavior are equal or superior to clinical prediction methods across a wide range of circumstances (Grove, Zald, Lebow, Snitz, & Nelson, 2000).

There are a number of specific influences on the decision making of clinicians that can interfere with their ability to detect suboptimal effort and malingering in MTBI cases. One of these influences is the use of heuristics as decisional simplification strategies (Tversky & Kahneman, 1974). Although heuristics can be helpful under some situations, they can also add error in decisions in other cases. For example, the representativeness heuristic is based on the similarity between events rather than more meaningful probability considerations (Harding, 2004). Diagnostic decisions can be affected when clinicians base their impressions on the degree to which an individual is believed to resemble those making up a diagnostic category (Garb, 1998). For example, if a clinician believes that significant cognitive morbidity is often present in persons with a history of MTBI, as represented by the erroneous clinical lore that 15% of patients with MTBI (e.g., the "miserable minority") are left with permanent disability (Greiffenstein, 2009), then he or she would tend to interpret any test failure as indicative of MTBI cognitive sequela.

Another limitation of the representativeness heuristic is the general exclusion of base rate information in making diagnostic judgments. If a clinician believes in a high base rate of cognitive deficits following MTBI and low base rates of malingering, even though residual deficits are relatively rare (Carroll et al., 2004; McCrea, 2008), and malingering within the personal injury litigating MTBI population is estimated to be as high as 40% (Larrabee, 2007b; Mittenberg, Patton, Canyock, & Condit, 2002), then relying on test results alone for identifying suboptimal effort will likely lead to false negative errors in malingering detection.

Related to the potential adverse effects of decisional heuristics, two other cognitive limitations to clinical judgment warrant a brief review. These limitations include confirmatory bias and the limitations of configural interpretation. With the former, humans tend to seek to confirm our hypotheses rather than try to refute them; but confirmatory bias within a clinical setting can pose special problems because of the overlap across disorders and symptoms (Wedding & Faust, 1989). For example, memory problems are very common neuropsychological complaints but can be caused by a myriad of causes. For the neuropsychologist who believes that the memory complaints of patient with TBI must be genuine and solely related to the patient's neurological trauma, he or she may seek to confirm this hypothesis and ignore other possible conflicting data (e.g., normal scores on some memory measures) or disregard other potential etiologies such as chronic pain (Melkumova, Podchufarova, & Yakhno, 2011; Oosterman, Derksen, van Wijck, Veldhuijzen, & Kessels, 2011) or mood disorders (Jaeger, Berns, Uzelac, & Davis-Conway, 2006; Landrø, Stiles, & Sletvold, 2001; Moore, Moseley, & Atkinson, 2010).

In general, evidence suggests a strong relationship between MTBI complaints and psychiatric disorders given the considerable frequency of postconcussive symptoms reported by patients with psychiatric illness (Fox, Lees-Haley, Earnest, & Dolezal-Wood, 1995). Iverson (2006) found that approximately nine out of 10 patients with depression met liberal self-report criteria for postconcussion syndrome, and more than five out of 10 met conservative criteria for the diagnosis. King and Kirwilliam (2011) reported that in an MTBI sample with a mean postinjury time of 6.9 years, anxiety accounted for the greatest amount of variance in the severity of postconcussive complaints.

Regarding processing configural data, studies have generally revealed that humans' capacity for complex cognitive operations, including analyzing multiple cues and their interactions, is rather modest (Wedding & Faust, 1989). Thus, humans generally have limited ability to consider and weigh large amounts of data simultaneously. However, relying on pattern analysis of neuropsychological test results, rather than on well-validated SVT procedures, requires this type of complex data integration.

Another general limiting factor to relying on clinical judgment alone rather than on malingering detection strategies with known error rates is the lack of corrective feedback. Unlike meteorologists who find out in short order whether their predictions were correct, the neuropsychologist who has been "fooled" into believing that simulated impairments were genuine will likely never know about the deception or be able to learn from them. Without benefit of that feedback, the neuropsychologist becomes more and more confident about his or her clinical decision making because there is no evidence to the contrary. Lack of feedback can obviously occur with assessments that employ either stand-alone or embedded SVT procedures also, but at least in most cases, clinicians have the benefit of knowing the sensitivities and specificities of those procedures and thus can estimate false negative and positive rates. These rates are unknown, however, with the application of clinical judgment to test results alone.

The pattern of performance model referred to earlier generally requires that the clinician detect "significant" or "marked" differences between aspects of an examinee's performance (e.g., generally between severity of injury and severity of deficits noted on testing). One problem with this methodology is that the judgment regarding the significance of the discrepancy is left to the discretion of the evaluator without empirical guidelines. How far do scores have to deviate from the norm, other test scores, or the expected impairment level based on the injury to be considered significant or marked and thus possibly reflecting malingering? Is a test score that falls 1.0, 1.5, 2.0, or 3.0 standard deviations below an "expected" result considered to be significant or marked enough?

The descriptors used in pattern analysis methods to depict differences among different types of data are qualitative and not quantitative, which adds confusion and contributes to the lack of standardization in this approach. The more that neuropsychologists rely on qualitative information or descriptors to depict patient performance rather than specific cutoff scores, then the greater variability there will be among clinicians and their interpretations. For example, Guilmette, Hagan, and Giuliano (2008) found a high degree of variability among board-certified neuropsychologists in assigning qualitative descriptors to standard scores, especially for those in the lower half of the distribution. Thus, it is unlikely that in some, or perhaps many, cases neuropsychologists will agree on whether to define impairment or a score discrepancy as mild, moderate, severe, marked, or significant.

The analysis of neuropsychological test patterns to identify invalid results is further hampered by the significant variability with which examinees may attempt to produce fabricated or exaggerated deficits. Research has not identified a typical malingering profile. As Sweet (1999) stated,

> Malingerers may choose many or just particular measures on which to display their deliberately poor effort based on their own idiosyncratic belief system regarding brain injury . . . consecutive malingerers seen in the same office may appear similar or quite different from one another on given tests. (p. 259)

Boone (2009) described four clinical cases that differed significantly in their presentations of negative response bias regarding which specific SVT procedures were failed and when the failures occurred during the course of the exam. Thus, when attempting to simulate brain damage from MTBI, examinees may produce neuropsychological test profiles that reflect a range of deficits or none at all but still perform less proficiently than they could have with full effort on most or few of the measures administered. This variability and unpredictability in anticipating a "typical" malingering test profile increases substantially the difficulty for the clinician in ascertaining its validity.

Another limitation to the pattern of performance method is the degree to which there is significant intertest variability even in a nonclinical population (Binder, Iverson, & Brooks, 2009). Although most of the limitations to clinical judgment described previously would tend to result in false negative errors in malingering detection, estimating the degree to which test discrepancies may reflect an invalid performance needs to account for normal intraindividual variation, particularly across a large test battery (Crawford, Garthwaite, & Gault, 2007). For example, Schretlen and colleagues (2003) derived 32 z-transformed scores from 15 tests administered to 197 healthy community dwelling adults and found that the difference between each person's highest and lowest scores ranged from 1.6 to 6.1 standard deviations. Eliminating each participant's highest and lowest test scores still resulted in 27% of their sample producing a discrepancy that exceeded three standard deviations. Within the Wechsler Adult Intelligence Scale–IV normative sample, a 9-point difference, or three standard deviations, between a person's highest and lowest subtest scores among the 10 core subtests was obtained by over 16% of participants (Wechsler, 2008). If all 15 subtests are administered, then a 9-point intersubtest scatter was noted in almost 30% of the sample. Thus, although van Gorp et al. (1999) suggested that level of performance may be a better indicator of potential malingering than pattern of performance per se, the degree of variability found in normal, nonclinical samples increases the complexity of trying to determine invalid results using test scores alone.

Last, although a primary role of neuropsychological testing with MTBI cases is to provide objective evidence of cognitive functioning, many of the symptoms in the postconcussive syndrome are subjective and include many noncognitive complaints. These symptoms include, but are not limited to, headache, fatigue, photophobia, sleep problems, and changes in mood and personality. In assessing the validity of a person's postconcussive complaints, neuropsychologists may need to rely not only on the objective evidence provided by standardized testing but also on the perceived veracity of the complainant, particularly when SVT methods are not incorporated into the assessment. Here, the literature is not reassuring that clinicians are able to detect the inaccurate or fabricated self-report of their patients. Beginning with the classic study by Rosenhan (1973) in which pseudopatients who feigned a single symptom (e.g., auditory hallucinations) were admitted to a psychiatric hospital and given major psychiatric diagnoses, research has consistently demonstrated that people judge the credibility of an informant based on the characteristics that have no relation to his or her actual truthfulness (Spellman & Tenny, 2010). For example, the attractiveness and confidence of informants, as well as providing compelling accounts of their stories, make them appear more honest. On the part of the listener, there is also a general "truth bias," the tendency to assume that people are telling the truth (Spellman & Tenny, 2010), which arguably is even more applicable to psychologists than the general public because psychologists have entered a helping profession with the goal of relieving the distress of others. In all, the overwhelming evidence supports that lie detection among untrained observers (e.g., individuals who have not received specialized instruction and practice in the detection of lies) is about as accurate as a coin toss (Bond & DePaulo, 2006; Edelstein, Luten, Ekman, & Goodman, 2006). As Bond and DePaulo (2008) summarized, "It has become virtually axiomatic that the mean lie detection performances among groups of people are barely above chance" (p. 485).

CONCLUSIONS

Over the last 20 years, advances in the detection of suboptimal effort and malingering in neuropsychological assessment in general and with MTBI cases in particular have been remarkable. Within the psychometric domain, essentially all of the progress has been confined to the standardization and validation of multiple stand-alone SVT procedures or to embedded indicators within ability tests (Heilbronner et al., 2009). With the latter, there are multiple indicators with proven validity that can be calculated from ability measures that are often administered in a neuropsychological battery throughout the testing process (Boone, 2007; Larrabee, 2007a). However, there have been no advances in facilitating the role of clinical judgment in detecting malingering from the use of standard neuropsychological tests alone and without the benefit of validated SVT procedures or methods.

Verifying the validity of neuropsychological results by relying exclusively on pattern analysis or discrepancy methods without incorporating embedded validity indicators has not been proven to be effective. There are likely many reasons for this, including the application of inappropriate decisional heuristics, confirmatory bias, cognitive limits of configural interpretation, lack of corrective feedback, lack of quantitative or empirical guidelines to establish discrepancy cutoffs (e.g., among test scores, between test scores and severity of injury, or between test scores and self-report or behavioral observations), the unpredictability and inconsistency of malingering profiles, intraindividual test variability even among normals, and the inability to detect deception by observation or interview.

Recognizing the substantial limitations of clinical judgment in detecting malingering from test results alone, the National Academy of Neuropsychology position paper on symptom validity assessment states that

> when the potential for secondary gain increases the incentive for symptom exaggeration or fabrication and/or when neuropsychologists become suspicious of insufficient or inaccurate or incomplete reporting, neuropsychologists can, and must, utilize symptom validity tests and procedures to assist in the determination of the validity of the information and test data obtained. (Bush, 2005, p. 426)

The American Academy of Clinical Neuropsychology Consensus Conference on the Neuropsychological Assessment of Effort, Response Bias, and Malingering (Heilbronner et al., 2009) recommended to practitioners that psychometric indicators are the most valid approach to identifying neuropsychological response validity and that "stand-alone effort measures and embedded validity indicators should both be employed" (p. 1106).

In the neuropsychological assessment of MTBI cases in which there is incentive for negative response bias, clinicians should not base their decisions on their clinical judgment alone in attempting to verify the validity of their test results. Rather, the evidence overwhelmingly supports the need to rely on well-validated SVT procedures in determining the veracity of the results. This need to employ standardized

SVTs does not preclude practitioners from using their clinical judgment to form opinions about assessment validity from test patterns or other inconsistencies in the patient's self-report, history, or other factors; but these opinions should also integrate the results of multiple measures or procedures designed specifically to identify inadequate effort or malingering.

REFERENCES

Arkes, H. R., Faust, D., & Guilmette, T. J. (1990). Response to Schmidt's (1988) comments on Faust, Hart, Guilmette, and Arkes (1988). *Professional Psychology: Research and Practice*, 21, 3–4.

Bigler, E. D. (1990). Neuropsychology and malingering: Comment on Faust, Hart, and Guilmette (1988). *Journal of Consulting and Clinical Psychology*, 58(2), 244–247.

Binder, L. M., Iverson, G. L., & Brooks, B. L. (2009). To err is human: "Abnormal" neuropsychological scores and variability are common in healthy adults. *Archives of Clinical Neuropsychology*, 24(1), 31–46.

Bond, C. F. Jr., & DePaulo, B. M. (2006). Accuracy of deception judgments. *Personality and Social Psychology Review*, 10(3), 214–234.

Bond, C. F. Jr., & DePaulo, B. M. (2008). Individual differences in judging deception: Accuracy and bias. *Psychological Bulletin*, 134(4), 477–492.

Boone, K. B. (Ed.). (2007). *Assessment of feigned cognitive impairment: A neuropsychological perspective*. New York, NY: Guilford Press.

Boone, K. B. (2009). The need for continuous and comprehensive sampling of effort/response bias during neuropsychological examinations. *The Clinical Neuropsychologist*, 23(4), 729–741.

Borum, R., Otto, R., & Golding, S. (1993). Improving clinical judgment and decision making in forensic evaluation. *Journal of Psychiatry & Law*, 21, 35–76.

Bruhn, A. R., & Reed, M. R. (1975). Simulation of brain damage on the Bender-Gestalt Test by college students. *Journal of Personality Assessment*, 39(3), 244–255.

Bush, S. S., Ruff, R. M., Tröster, A. I., Barth, J. T., Koffler, S. P., Pliskin, N. H., . . . Silver, C. H. (2005). Symptom validity assessment: Practice issues and medical necessity NAN policy and planning committee. *Archives of Clinical Neuropsychology*, 20(4), 419–426.

Carroll, L. J., Cassidy, J. D., Peloso, P. M., Borg, J., von Holst, H., Holm, L., . . . Pépin, M. (2004). Prognosis for mild traumatic brain injury: Results of the WHO Collaborating Centre Task Force on Mild Traumatic Brain Injury. *Journal of Rehabilitation Medicine*, (Suppl. 43), 84–105.

Crawford, J. R., Garthwaite, P. H., & Gault, C. B. (2007). Estimating the percentage of the population with abnormally low scores (or abnormally large score differences) on standardized neuropsychological test batteries: A generic method with applications. *Neuropsychology*, 21(4), 419–430.

Edelstein, R. S., Luten, T. L., Ekman, P., & Goodman, G. S. (2006). Detecting lies in children and adults. *Law and Human Behavior*, 30(1), 1–10.

Faust, D., & Guilmette, T. J. (1990). To say it's not so doesn't prove that it isn't: Research on the detection of malingering. Reply to Bigler. *Journal of Consulting and Clinical Psychology*, 58(2), 248–250.

Faust, D., Hart, K., & Guilmette, T. J. (1988). Pediatric malingering: The capacity of children to fake believable deficits on neuropsychological testing. *Journal of Consulting and Clinical Psychology*, 56(4), 578–582.

Faust, D., Hart, K., Guilmette, T. J., & Arkes, H. R. (1988). Neuropsychologists' capacity to detect adolescent malingerers. *Professional Psychology: Research and Practice*, 19, 508–515.

Fox, D. D., Lees-Haley, P. R., Earnest, K., & Dolezal-Wood, S. (1995). Post-concussive symptoms: Base rates and etiology in psychiatric patients. *The Clinical Neuropsychologist*, 9, 89–92.

Garb, H. N. (1998). *Studying the clinician: Judgment research and psychological assessment*. Washington, DC: American Psychological Association.

Garb, H. N. (2005). Clinical judgment and decision making. *Annual Review of Clinical Psychology*, 1, 67–89.

Gervais, R. O., Rohling, M. L., Green, P., & Ford, W. (2004). A comparison of WMT, CARB, and TOMM failure rates in non-head injury disability claimants. *Archives of Clinical Neuropsychology*, 19(1), 475–487.

Goebel, R. A. (1983). Detection of faking on the Halstead-Reitan Neuropsychological Test Battery. *Journal of Clinical Psychology*, 39(5), 731–742.

Greiffenstein, M. F. (2009). Clinical myths of forensic neuropsychology. *The Clinical Neuropsychologist*, 23(2), 286–296.

Greve, K. W., Binder, L. M., & Bianchini, K. J. (2009). Rates of below-chance performance in forced-choice symptom validity tests. *The Clinical Neuropsychologist*, 23(3), 534–544.

Grove, W. M., Zald, D. H., Lebow, B. S., Snitz, B. E., & Nelson, C. (2000). Clinical versus mechanical prediction: A meta-analysis. *Psychological Assessment*, 12(1), 19–30.

Guilmette, T. J., Hagan, L., & Giuliano, A. J. (2008). Assigning qualitative descriptions to test scores in neuropsychology: Forensic implications. *The Clinical Neuropsychologist*, 22(1), 122–139.

Harding, T. P. (2004). Psychiatric disability and clinical decision making: The impact of judgment error and bias. *Clinical Psychology Review*, 24(6), 707–729.

Heaton, R. K., Smith, H. H. Jr., Lehman, R. A., & Vogt, A. T. (1978). Prospects for faking believable deficits on neuropsychological testing. *Journal of Consulting and Clinical Psychology*, 46(5), 892–900.

Heilbronner, R. J., Sweet, J. J., Morgan, J. E., Larrabee, G. J., & Millis, S. (2009). American Academy of Clinical Neuropsychology consensus conference statement on the neuropsychological assessment of effort, response bias, and malingering. *The Clinical Neuropsychologist*, 23(7), 1093–1129.

Iverson, G. L. (2006). Misdiagnosis of the persistent postconcussion syndrome in patients with depression. *Archives of Clinical Neuropsychology*, 21(4), 303–310.

Jaeger, J., Berns, S., Uzelac, S., & Davis-Conway, S. (2006). Neurocognitive deficits and disability in major depressive disorder. *Psychiatry Research*, 145(1), 39–48.

King, N. S., & Kirwilliam, S. (2011). Permanent post-concussion symptoms after mild head injury. *Brain Injury*, 25(5), 462–470.

Landrø, N., Stiles, T. C., & Sletvold, H. (2001). Neurological function in nonpsychotic unipolar major depression. *Neuropsychiatry, Neuropsychology, and Behavioral Neurology*, 14(4), 233–240.

Larrabee, G. J. (Ed.). (2007a). *Assessment of malingered neuropsychological deficits*. New York, NY: Oxford University Press.

Larrabee, G. J. (Ed.). (2007b). Malingering, research designs, and base rates. In *Assessment of malingered neuropsychological deficits* (pp. 3–13). New York, NY: Oxford University Press.

McCrea, M. A. (2008). *Mild traumatic brain injury and postconcussion syndrome: The new evidence base for diagnosis and treatment*. New York, NY: Oxford University Press.

Meehl, P. E. (1954). *Clinical versus statistical prediction: A theoretical analysis and a review of the evidence*. Minneapolis, MN: University of Minnesota Press.

Melkumova, K. A., Podchufarova, E. V., & Yakhno, N. N. (2011). Characteristics of cognitive functions in patients with chronic spinal pain. *Neuroscience and Behavioral Physiology*, 41(1), 42–46.

Mittenberg, W., Patton, C., Canyock, E. M., & Condit, D. C. (2002). Base rates of malingering and symptom exaggeration. *Journal of Clinical and Experimental Neuropsychology*, 24(8), 1094–1102.

Moore, D. J., Moseley, S., & Atkinson, J. (2010). The influence of depression on cognition and daily functioning. In T. D. Marcotte & I. Grant (Eds.), *Neuropsychology of everyday functioning* (pp. 419–440). New York, NY: Guilford Press.

Nies, K. J., & Sweet, J. J. (1994). Neuropsychological assessment and malingering: A critical review of past and present strategies. *Archives of Clinical Neuropsychology*, 9(6), 501–552.

Oosterman, J. M., Derksen, L. C., van Wijck, A. J., Veldhuijzen, D. S., & Kessels, R. P. (2011). Memory functions in chronic pain: Examining contributions of attention and age to test performance. *The Clinical Journal of Pain*, 27(1), 70–75.

Pankratz, L. (1988). Malingering on intellectual and neuropsychological measures. In R. Rogers (Ed.), *Clinical assessment of malingering and deception* (pp. 169–192). New York, NY: Guilford Press.

Pankratz, L., & Binder, L. M. (1997). Malingering on intellectual and neuropsychological measures. In R. Rogers (Ed.), *Clinical assessment of malingering and deception* (2nd ed., pp. 223–236). New York, NY: Guilford Press.

Rosenhan, D. (1973). On being sane in insane places. *Science*, 179(4070), 250–258.

Schmidt, J. P. (1989). Why recent researchers have not assessed the capacity of neuropsychologists to detect adolescent malingering. *Professional Psychology: Research and Practice*, 20, 140–141.

Schretlen, D. J., Munro, C. A., Anthony, J. C., & Pearlson, G. D. (2003). Examining the range of normal intraindividual variability in neuropsychological test performance. *Journal of the International Neuropsychological Society*, 9(6), 864–870.

Sharland, M. J., & Gfeller, J. D. (2007). A survey of neuropsychologists' beliefs and practices with respect to the assessment of effort. *Archives of Clinical Neuropsychology*, 22(2), 213–223.

Slick, D. J., Sherman, E. M., & Iverson, G. L. (1999). Diagnostic criteria for malingered neurocognitive dysfunction: Proposed standards for clinical practice and research. *The Clinical Neuropsychologist*, 13(4), 545–561.

Slick, D. J., Tan, J. E., Strauss, E. H., & Hultsch, D. F. (2004). Detecting malingering: A survey of experts' practices. *Archives of Clinical Neuropsychology*, 19(4), 465–473.

Spellman, B. A & Tenny, E. R. (2010). Credible testimony in and out of court. *Psychonomic Bulletin & Review*, 17(2), 168–173.

Sweet, J. J. (Ed.). (1999). Malingering: Differential diagnosis. In *Forensic neuropsychology: Fundamentals and practice* (pp. 255–285). Lisse, The Netherlands: Swets & Zeitlinger.

Trueblood, W., & Binder, L. M. (1997). Psychologists' accuracy in identifying neuropsychological test protocols of clinical malingerers. *Archives of Clinical Neuropsychology*, 12(1), 13–27.

Tversky, A., & Kahneman, D. (1974). Judgment under uncertainty: Heuristics and biases. *Science*, 185(4157), 1124–1131.

van Gorp, W. G., Humphrey, L. A., Kalechstein, A., Brumm, V. L., McMullen, W. J., Stoddard, M., & Pachana, N. A. (1999). How well do standard clinical neuropsychological tests identify malingering? A preliminary analysis. *Journal of Clinical and Experimental Neuropsychology*, 21(2), 245–250.

Wechsler, D. (2008). Wechsler Adult Intelligence Scale—Fourth Edition: Administration and scoring manual. San Antonio, TX: Pearson.

Wedding, D., & Faust, D. (1989). Clinical judgment and decision making in neuropsychology. *Archives of Clinical Neuropsychology*, 4(3), 233–265.

Ethical Considerations in Mild Traumatic Brain Injury Cases and Symptom Validity Assessment

3

Shane S. Bush

Professional ethics represent the shared values of a profession. In health care, such values include (a) protecting the welfare of patients; (b) engaging in activities that are helpful to patients; (c) respecting the right of competent adult patients to make the decisions that govern their health care and other aspects of their life; and (d) promoting fairness and justice. The bioethical terms that represent these values are *nonmaleficence, beneficence, respect for autonomy,* and *justice,* respectively (Beauchamp & Childress, 2009). Additional general ethical principles have also been proposed, such as *general beneficence,* which covers an ethical responsibility to the public at large (Knapp & VandeCreek, 2006). These general bioethical principles serve as the foundation on which professions establish more specific ethical standards, and they help guide clinicians to make sound ethical and clinical decisions in situations in which the right course of action is unclear. Such lack of clarity regarding professional choices is most likely to be experienced when clinicians are confronted with disorders that are controversial and with procedures that have not been fully established within the profession.

Mild traumatic brain injury (MTBI) with persisting symptoms is one condition that has long been a subject of controversy, and, until relatively recently, symptom validity assessment (SVA) was an aspect of the neuropsychological evaluation that was not fully established within the profession. Even today, the manner in which symptom validity methods and procedures are employed and interpreted is met with disagreement among some neuropsychologists. Examining professional ethics can help neuropsychologists find clarity of purpose and action in the complex intersection of MTBI and SVA. The purpose of this chapter is to present the ethical principles and standards and the professional guidelines that govern this aspect of neuropsychological practice so that practitioners may have increased confidence in the appropriateness of their professional activities in this context. First, though, the chapter describes the importance of establishing and maintaining a commitment to ethical ideals and the value of using a structured approach to ethical problem solving.

ETHICAL IDEALS AND DECISION MAKING

Ethical practice requires effort; it cannot occur by chance or good intentions alone. Good intentions must not only exist, but they must also be matched by good effort to understand relevant ethical issues, identify ethical resources, and adopt a model for ethical decision making.

Ethical Ideals and Positive Ethics

Enforceable professional ethics codes are based on a remedial approach to ethical practice. The remedial approach requires clinicians to adhere to certain minimum standards of practice or risk being disciplined by the professional organization. However, there are typically higher standards of ethical practice to which clinicians can aspire. In the 2002 American Psychological Association (APA) Ethics Code, the general principles, which are not enforceable, represent higher ethical principles which can guide ethical and clinical decision making for clinicians wanting to do more than meet minimum ethical requirements. Knapp and VandeCreek (2006) described the voluntary pursuit of ethical ideals as *positive ethics*.

Positive ethics are personal and proactive. Clinicians invested in high standards of ethical practice consciously decide that their professional identity and the welfare of their patients require more than simply avoiding ethical misconduct; rather, they strive for exemplary professional behavior at all times. Although the pursuit of ethical ideals may be challenging even for the most well-meaning and determined clinicians, the process itself can benefit patients, clinicians, and the profession.

The 4 A's of Ethical Practice and Decision Making

High standards of ethical practice are developed and maintained by (a) attempting to *anticipate* and prepare for ethical issues and challenges commonly encountered in one's specific practice contexts; (b) striving to *avoid* ethical misconduct; (c) taking steps to *address* ethical challenges when they are anticipated or encountered; and (d) maintaining a commitment to *aspire* to the highest standards of ethical practice. Collectively, these 4 A's of ethical practice and decision making (Bush, 2009) provide a foundation for safeguarding and promoting patient welfare.

Ethical Decision-Making Resources and Process

Like clinical decision making, ethical decision making is facilitated by following a structured, logical, and evidence-based process (Bush, 2007). Ethical decision-making models (e.g., Bush, 2007) give clinicians an outline of important points to consider and structured method for reviewing salient information. As with clinical decision making, reviewing and consulting resources is an important step in the decision-making process. Resources that inform ethical decision making include the following: (a) jurisdictional laws; (b) professional ethics codes, particularly the APA Ethics Code (2002); (c) the *Code of Conduct* of the Association of State and Provincial Psychology Boards (ASPPB; 2005); (d) ethics committees, state licensing boards, and liability insurance carriers; (e) position papers of professional organizations; (f) scholarly publications; (g) institutional guidelines and resources; and (h) informed and experienced colleagues. Use of such resources reduces reliance on subjective impressions, which may not always be consistent with high ethical standards and the best interests of the parties involved. Where available, findings from empirical studies of ethical issues (e.g., the work of McCaffrey and colleagues [2005] on third-party observation of neuropsychological testing) can be an especially valuable resource when choosing a course of action. Clinicians benefit from maintaining familiarity with core ethical, legal, and professional resources throughout their careers, rather than attempting to obtain and review the resources when confronting an ethical dilemma.

ETHICAL ISSUES

The ethical issues that are most relevant for neuropsychological practice in general (Bush, 2007; Bush, Grote, Johnson-Greene, & Macartney-Filgate, 2008) are also important for neuropsychological practice with persons who have a history of MTBI. However, some ethical standards and principles are especially important or pose particular challenges for neuropsychologists who evaluate and treat persons who present with persisting symptoms following MTBIs. Those ethical issues are described in this section.

Informed Consent

The following sections of the 2002 APA Ethics Code describe, in part, the clinician's obligations regarding the informed consent process.

> **3.10 Informed Consent**
> (a) When psychologists conduct research or provide assessment, therapy, counseling, or consulting services in person or via electronic transmission or other forms of communication, they obtain the informed consent of the individual or individuals using language that is reasonably understandable to that person or persons except when conducting such activities without consent is mandated by law or governmental regulation or as otherwise provided in this Ethics Code.
> **9.03 Informed Consent in Assessments**
> Informed consent includes an explanation of the nature and purpose of the assessment, fees, involvement of third parties, and limits of confidentiality and sufficient opportunity for the client/patient to ask questions and receive answers.

The importance of having competent adults agree to undergo the neuropsychological evaluation or receive neuropsychological treatment after being informed of (a) the nature of the services; (b) the uses of the information obtained; and (c) the foreseeable risks and benefits is based on the fundamental bioethical principle of respect for patient autonomy. Clinicians have obligations to provide certain specific information during the informed consent process, but they also use their professional judgment when deciding what optional information to share and the exact wording to use. This issue is complicated by the lack of shared understanding (as well as bias) among clinicians about the nature and long-term effects of MTBI. For example, some neuropsychologists are of the opinion that patients *have* damaged brains months or years after sustaining an MTBI and that the brain damage continues to cause severe neuropsychological impairments and disability. These clinicians may feel compelled, when describing the risks and benefits of neuropsychological testing, to inform patients that the testing may reveal brain damage resulting from their single concussion. Other neuropsychologists, however, with a different knowledge base and/or different biases may take the position that giving a patient such information would, because of its inaccuracy, likely be harmful to the patient and would very possibly have iatrogenic effects.

Similarly, neuropsychologists differ regarding the detail with which they describe the assessment of symptom validity and the use of symptom validity measures. Patients have a right to understand the SVA process to an extent that is sufficient to allow them to make an informed decision about whether they want to undergo the evaluation. Although descriptions of specific symptom validity tests (SVTs) or methods are never indicated, informing patients that the evaluation will include measures of effort and honesty is appropriate and generally necessary. Providing such information is much different than coaching an examinee about how to achieve a desired result on a given test or tests. Other than reinforcing their understanding that they should provide their best effort and respond in a valid manner, examinees learn nothing that would facilitate manipulation of the test results by being informed that measures of effort will be used. A sample consent form published by the National Academy of Neuropsychology (NAN; Bush, Barth, Pliskin, et al., 2005) includes such language. Thus, although the informed consent process may seem straightforward on the surface, decisions about which information should be conveyed must be carefully considered because it can have significant effects on a patient's decision to participate or to benefit from the services.

Selection of Tests and Other Procedures

The use of SVTs in the neuropsychological evaluation of persons who have a history of MTBI is now a standard of practice. Failure to appropriately assess symptom validity with multiple quantitative measures reveals a failure to practice in a manner that has been deemed necessary by professional organizations (American Academy of Clinical Neuropsychology, 2007; Bush, Ruff, Troster, et al., 2005; Heilbronner et al., 2009). The following sections of the 2002 APA Ethics Code describe, in part, the clinician's obligations regarding the selection of tests and other procedures.

> **9.01 Bases for Assessments**
> (a) Psychologists base the opinions contained in their recommendations, reports and diagnostic or evaluative statements, including forensic testimony, on information and techniques sufficient to substantiate their findings.
> **9.02 Use of Assessments**
> (a) Psychologists administer, adapt, score, interpret or use assessment techniques, interviews, tests or instruments in a manner and for purposes that are appropriate in light of the research on or evidence of the usefulness and proper application of the techniques.

Case Example

A psychologist who is board certified in a specialty other than clinical neuropsychology performs a neuropsychological evaluation in a forensic context. He was retained and paid by the examinee at the recommendation of her attorney to render an opinion about her disability status 2 years following a motor vehicle accident in which she sustained (or at least met nonspecific diagnostic criteria for) an MTBI. The neuropsychological test battery addressed the main neuropsychological domains in the following manner:

Intelligence: No measure used. The examiner reported that the examinee's job change and decreased income following the collision was evidence of decreased intelligence as a result of the collision.
Language: No measures used. The examinee's self-report of word-finding problems was used as evidence of impaired language functions.
Attention/Working Memory: No measures used. The examinee's self-report of significant trouble focusing at work was used as evidence of severe problems with attention and concentration.

Processing Speed: Wechsler Adult Intelligence Scale-III Coding subtest.

Visuospatial Skills: House-Tree-Person Drawings, Clock Drawing Test, Bicycle Drawing Test, and Bender Visual-Motor Gestalt Test.

Memory: Memory Assessment Scales and recall of Bender Visual-Motor
Gestalt Test designs.

Executive Functions: Trail Making Test Parts A and B, Category Test (Booklet Category
Test actually used).

Symptom Validity: Rey 15-Item Memory Test, Franzen and Iverson Memory Test
(more commonly called the *21-Item Memory Test*)

Mood/Personality: Beck Anxiety Inventory, Beck Depression Inventory, Bender Visual-Motor Gestalt Test, and House-Tree-Person Drawings.

Based on the results of these tests and the clinician's creative interpretation,
the clinician offered opinions about the examinee's ability to work in her prior occupation and the causal relationship between the remote collision and the examinee's
current deficits. Most competent neuropsychologists would agree that this "battery"
was inadequate for the purposes of this evaluation (probably for any evaluation).
Some of the measures seem to have very limited, if any, research to support their
use for the purposes for which this examiner used them. Thus, the results of the
measures used in this evaluation could not substantiate the examiner's opinions,
and the examiner's professional behavior was inconsistent with ethical practice according to Ethical Standards 9.01 and 9.02.

In addition, this examiner chose measures that were outdated and/or obsolete
for the purposes of this evaluation. According to the APA Ethics Code:

> **9.08 Obsolete Tests and Outdated Test Results**
> (a) Psychologists do not base their assessment or intervention decisions or
> recommendations on data or test results that are outdated for the current
> purpose.
> (b) Psychologists do not base such decisions or recommendations on tests
> and measures that are obsolete and not useful for the current purpose.

Specifically, of the 20 most commonly used neuropsychological measures
(Rabin, Barr, & Burton, 2005), this examiner selected only the Trail Making Test. The
House-Tree-Person Drawings and the Bicycle Drawing Test are not among the 50
most commonly used neuropsychological tests. When considering only memory
measures, the Memory Assessment Scales, published in 1991, is 19th among memory
tests in terms of frequency of use of neuropsychologists. Similarly, the 21-Item Memory Test is not among the 29 most commonly used SVTs (Sharland & Gfeller, 2007).
In addition, the Rey 15-Item Memory Test, because of its extremely poor sensitivity
compared to newer SVTs, is no longer considered a useful measure of examinee
effort, despite its continued popularity among some clinicians.

Although frequency of use among clinicians does not, in and of itself, mean that
one test is better than another for a given patient, knowledgeable clinicians tend to
choose similar measures for use in their practices. Although there can be good reasons
for not immediately adopting the newest tests or versions of tests (Bush, 2010), most
clinicians tend to replace their outdated instruments with newer measures that have
improved psychometric properties for use with certain patient populations. Of course,
some measures that were developed many years ago remain valuable for use in
contemporary practice, although some of those measures benefit from updated or
otherwise improved normative data. In this case, the examiner should have selected
some additional and alternative measures that have better psychometric properties
for use with this examinee.

Data Interpretation and Reporting

The following section of the 2002 APA Ethics Code describes, in part, the clinician's obligations regarding the interpretation of assessment results.

9.06 Interpreting Assessment Results

When interpreting assessment results, including automated interpretations, psychologists take into account the purpose of the assessment as well as the various test factors, test-taking abilities, and other characteristics of the person being assessed, such as situational, personal, linguistic, and cultural differences, that might affect psychologists' judgments or reduce the accuracy of their interpretations. They indicate any significant limitations of their interpretations.

There is a lack of agreement among neuropsychologists regarding both the best statistical methods for making determinations of impairment and the meaning to assign to the findings (Lees-Haley & Fox, 2001). In fact, disagreements can be so frequent and so dramatic as to cause attorneys to "shake their heads and comment that neuropsychology is 'smoke and mirrors' by experts who 'almost seem to make it up as they go along'" (Lees-Haley & Fox, 2001, p. 267). For example, clinicians differ in their choice of score cutoffs for impairment. Some clinicians consider any score that is more than one standard deviation below the mean (of an appropriate normative group) impaired (e.g., Heaton et al., 2004 refer to a t score of 39 as mild impairment). Other clinicians use a more conservative cutoff score of two standard deviations below the mean to define impairment. And still other clinicians use scores between one and two standard deviations below the mean.

Unfortunately, in the context of data interpretation, disagreement only begins with the selection of a score to represent impairment. Some clinicians understand that in any given test battery, a certain number of scores are expected to fall into the "impaired" range because of normal measurement error even for persons with no history of neurological injury (Binder, Iverson, & Brooks, 2009). Given that fact, it is the number of scores in a valid data set that fall below a specified impairment cutoff that is important rather than the specific cutoff score that is selected (Iverson, Brooks, & Holdnack, 2008). In addition, once the clinician decides how many scores below a certain cutoff are needed to consider the examinee to have an impairment, there is disagreement about the meaning of such findings for a person who has a history of MTBI (Lees-Haley & Fox, 2001). The pattern of test scores must make neuropsychological sense, given what is known about the neuropathology of the condition (Larrabee, 2005; Schretlen, Munro, Anthony, & Pearlson, 2003). Having some significantly low scores scattered across cognitive domains does not necessarily reflect the effects of neurological injury. Schretlen and colleagues concluded that their "data reveal that marked intraindividual variability is very common in normal adults, and underscore the need to base diagnostic inferences on clinically recognizable patterns rather than psychometric variability alone" (p. 864).

Disagreements also exist among some clinicians about the meaning of SVT results. Such disagreements commonly, but not exclusively, correspond with the origin of the referral. That is, clinicians who provide services on referral from plaintiff attorneys commonly have very different opinions than clinicians whose work originates from defense attorneys. Clinicians from each side may genuinely believe that their understanding of the professional and scientific literature is the correct one and that those who disagree are either uniformed or biased. However, considerable variability exists among clinicians regarding the degree to which they are uninformed, biased, some combination of the two, or simply viewing information and events through different life lenses with the best of intentions. Consistent with Ethical Standard 9.06, Thompson (2002) stated, "It is essential that psychologists acknowledge limitations about the accuracy or precision of test interpretation" (p. 58).

In the case example previously described, the examiner did not specify his criteria for determining impairment, but he did describe some scores at the 32nd percentile (compared to demographically similar peers) as being impaired, which is an exceptionally liberal criterion for impairment. Using such a cutoff for a single test, nearly one third of the general (healthy) population would be considered impaired. In my opinion, the examiner did, as is required by Ethical Standard 9.06, "take into account the purpose of the assessment," and in doing decided that he would find the examinee to be impaired and disabled, which is the result that both the examinee (who paid the examiner) and her attorney (who referred the examinee to the examiner) were hoping to get. Such behavior is inconsistent with the spirit of Ethical Standard 9.06 and with General Principle C (Integrity).

Despite the disagreements that exist among some neuropsychologists about various aspects of practice, particularly with MTBI cases, neuropsychological methods and procedures do allow for reliable and valid diagnostic and clinical determinations to be made with a reasonable degree of certainty. Neuropsychological methods meet the Daubert standard for acceptability in court, and well-intentioned, competent neuropsychologists can use such methods to make sound decisions that help involved parties understand the nature and extent of cognitive, emotional, and behavioral problems experienced by persons who have sustained MTBIs and help to improve care for the patients themselves.

Feedback to Patients

The following section of the 2002 APA Ethics Code describes, in part, the clinician's obligations regarding the provision of feedback about evaluation results to patients.

9.10 Explaining Assessment Results
Regardless of whether the scoring and interpretation are done by psychologists, by employees or assistants or by automated or other outside services, psychologists take reasonable steps to ensure that explanations of results are given to the individual or designated representative unless the nature of the relationship precludes provision of an explanation of results (such as in some organizational consulting, preemployment or security screenings, and forensic evaluations), and this fact has been clearly explained to the person being assessed in advance.

In clinical (vs. forensic) contexts, patients have a right to know the results of their evaluations, and providing the information to patients is typically beneficial from a clinical perspective. However, challenges can arise when clinicians discuss with patients the probable etiology of persisting cognitive symptoms following an MTBI and/or findings of invalid responding. In the first instance, patients differ regarding their preferred cause for cognitive problems. Although many patients are relieved to learn that it is much more likely that emotional distress, physical pain, pain medications, or some other non-neurological factor or combination of factors, rather than brain trauma, is causing their persisting cognitive symptoms (Iverson, 2005), some patients have stated, "Please tell me that I have brain damage, that I'm not crazy." Clinicians must be sensitive to this variability in patient response to feedback and be prepared to address different reactions.

Regarding feedback about invalid symptom presentations, various reactions and responses may be expected. Whereas some patients readily acknowledge that they did not put forth their best effort or respond in a completely forthright manner (for whatever reason), other patients may be very defensive and agitated, threatening, or hostile. Experience suggests that the reactions of most patients fall somewhere in between these two extremes. A sensitive, educational, and clear presentation of the evaluation results with opportunity for dialogue often helps lead to a productive feedback session (Carone, Iverson, & Bush, 2010). These authors presented an approach to symptom validity feedback that takes into account the relevant information to be conveyed to patients and provides a way of presenting the information that most patients are likely to be receptive to, thus substantially reducing the potential for confrontation.

EXAMINER DECEPTION

Examinees who intentionally exaggerate or fabricate symptoms are attempting to deceive their examiners. It is the need to determine whether such deception is present in individual cases that leads examiners to use SVTs and other measures. For SVTs to be effective, examinees must believe that the tests measure the constructs that they appear to measure. For example, examinees must believe that forced choice recognition tasks following exposure to verbal or visual stimuli are actually assessing their memory, rather than their effort. Some SVTs even require examiners to state in the instructions that the tests are very difficult. In these ways, examiners are deceiving examinees. Some observers may note that there is more than a small degree of irony in situations in which one party chooses to deceive another to detect the other's deception. However, the nature and degree of examiner deception in SVA is justified.

Justification for examiner deception in SVA is found in two main points. First, examinees are informed during the informed consent process that measures to determine symptom validity (i.e., effort and honesty) will be used, and examinees who consent to the evaluation do so with such knowledge. Giving examinees more detailed information about specific symptom validity measures would invalidate their use for those patients, rendering good scores on these tests essentially meaningless. Clinicians who do not engage examinees and/or their proxy decision makers in an informed consent or assent (including "notification of purpose" in some forensic contexts) process are not practicing in a manner required by professional ethics (Ethical Standards 3.10, Informed Consent; 9.03, Informed Consent in Assessments). Second, deception may be ethically justifiable when the benefits of its use outweigh the potential risks. The 2002 APA Ethics Code addresses deception in the context of research but not clinical services.

8.07 Deception in Research
(a) Psychologists do not conduct a study involving deception unless they have determined that the use of deceptive techniques is justified by the study's significant prospective scientific, educational or applied value and that effective, nondeceptive alternative procedures are not feasible.
(b) Psychologists do not deceive prospective participants about research that is reasonably expected to cause physical pain or severe emotional distress.

Although psychologists generally strive to promote accuracy and truthfulness in their professional activities (General Principle C, Integrity), misrepresentation of fact may be acceptable in situations in which the information derived from the deception is of considerable value and cannot be obtained in a nondeceptive manner. With neuropsychological evaluations, objective, empirically based determinations of symptom validity are essential and cannot be made without misleading examinees about the true nature of SVTs. Symptom validity indicators embedded within neuropsychological ability tests reduce the degree of deception because the tests are both measuring cognitive constructs and providing information about examinee effort. However, the use of freestanding SVTs is necessary in nearly all forensic evaluation contexts and in many clinical evaluation contexts.

Ethical Standard 8.09 also addresses the potential for physical pain or severe emotional distress that may result from the use of deception. Although physical pain is not an expected outcome of examiner deception in the context of SVA, some patients or examinees may react with strong emotions, most commonly anger, when their symptom exaggeration or fabrication is detected. Findings of invalid performance can have significant implications for how family members, other professionals, and triers of fact think about examinees. Yet, for examinees who present in a valid manner, SVT results have no adverse consequences. Nevertheless, neuropsychologists must be mindful of the possible effects of deception on the sense of trust or the emotional state of examinees and, when strong negative effects are evident, provide emotional support, education, and/or referrals or recommendations for mental health services (Bush, 2005).

PATIENT POPULATIONS, EVALUATION CONTEXT, AND EXAMINER BIAS

Experience suggests that neuropsychologists who evaluate and/or treat persons who have sustained MTBIs are primarily doing so in one of the following contexts: sports concussion, military personnel and veteran settings, work-related injuries, motor vehicle collisions, and other forensic contexts such as those involving falls. The ethical issues and challenges that are relevant and confronted in those contexts overlap considerably but also have unique differences (Bush & Cuesta, 2010; Bush & Iverson, 2010; Bush & Iverson, 2012; Carone & Bush, 2012; Bush & Graver, this volume; Bush, Russo, & Cuesta, 2012).

Professional competence is the foundational ethical issue across practice contexts and patient populations. The APA Ethics Code states, in part:

> **2.01 Boundaries of Competence**
> (a) Psychologists provide services, teach and conduct research with populations and in areas only within the boundaries of their competence, based on their education, training, supervised experience, consultation, study, or professional experience.
> (e) In those emerging areas in which generally recognized standards for preparatory training do not yet exist, psychologists nevertheless take reasonable steps to ensure the competence of their work and to protect clients/patients, students, supervisees, research participants, organizational clients and others from harm.

Without adequate training with MTBI populations, clinicians are likely to arrive at conclusions or offer suggestions or treatments that are of no benefit to their patients and could well be harmful, which is inconsistent with General Principle A (Beneficence and Nonmaleficence). Nevertheless, there can be considerable personal or financial incentive for clinicians trained in other neuropsychological subspecialties to want to transition into clinical work with people who have a history of MTBI. The lay public generally is uninformed about whether a given clinician is appropriately qualified to provide the services that he or she is offering. This is particularly the case if the clinician is not board certified in a particular specialty area. As a result, the public is vulnerable to publishers of concussion tests and clinicians who offer concussion treatment programs who provide promotional materials or statements that lack scientific support. Clinicians have an ethical obligation to provide truthful, non-misleading information about their services to potential patients (General Principle C, Integrity; Ethical Standard 5.01, Avoidance of False or Deceptive Statements). Even otherwise well-meaning and highly credentialed clinicians can find themselves or their employers influenced by media reports that are strong on emotion but based on incomplete or factually incorrect information (e.g., see Carone & Bush, 2012). Professionals are wise to approach scientifically unsubstantiated reports, whether made by the media or other professionals, with a healthy degree of skepticism.

Clinician bias is also encountered in neuropsychological services provided to persons who have a history of MTBI. Some clinicians, even those who are appropriately trained and credentialed, provide improper advocacy for patients whom they have diagnosed with brain damage and functional impairment resulting from a single remote MTBI. Such clinicians often treat the *brain injuries* of such patients for extended periods and may refer for additional services within the same clinic (from which they receive financial reimbursement for the additional services) without incorporating and sharing with patients the evidence base to support such treatment or informing patients of the limits of the scientific evidence to support the services provided. Such treatment of brain trauma in a person with a history of a remote MTBI is not the same as treating such patients from a biopsychosocial approach that addresses the complexity of the persisting symptoms and includes a focus on psychological distress, the latter of which appears to be appropriate treatment for this population (McCrea, 2007).

Like treating clinicians, independent examiners can be subject to bias, pulled by an extreme position on otherwise controversial professional matters or by real or perceived financial incentive to satisfy the referring party. As Sweet (2005) stated in the context of forensic practice, ethical concerns can be raised on both sides. "Stated differently, being retained by one or the other side of a litigated case is, across experts, not systematically associated with being either less or more ethical" (Sweet, 2005, p. 59). Ethical Principle D (Justice) advises, in part, "Psychologists exercise reasonable judgment and take precautions to ensure that their potential biases, the boundaries of their competence and the limitations of their expertise do not lead to or condone unjust practices." The individual neuropsychologist has ethical and professional obligations to provide evidence-based services, arrive at evidence-based conclusions, and remain as objective as possible while respecting the dignity and worth of all those encountered in professional practice.

CONCLUSIONS

Ethical neuropsychological practice involving SVA of persons who have a history of MTBI requires a personal investment in maintaining high standards of professional conduct and a thoughtful, deliberate approach. Many ethical issues exist that clinicians need to consider and prepare to address. Clinicians benefit from thinking proactively about the types of ethical issues and challenges that may emerge and from taking steps to address the issues and challenges before they become dilemmas.

In this era of increased costs and decreased payments, where productivity and reimbursable activities are of paramount importance, it can be difficult to allocate time to professional tasks that do not directly generate income. However, some professional activities that are not reimbursable, such as discussing and reviewing professional ethics, can have substantial financial benefits through promotion of practice excellence and avoidance of ethical misconduct and disciplinary consequences. In short, although we do not get paid to spend time thinking about ethics, we will pay if we don't.

REFERENCES

American Academy of Clinical Neuropsychology. (2007). American Academy of Clinical Neuropsychology (AACN) practice guidelines for neuropsychological assessment and consultation. *The Clinical Neuropsychologist*, 21(2), 209–231.

American Psychological Association. (2002). Ethical principles of psychologists and code of conduct. *The American Psychologist*, 57(12), 1060–1073.

Association of State and Provincial Psychology Boards. (2005). *Code of conduct.* Retrieved from http://www.asppb.net/i4a/pages/index.cfm?paged=3353.

Beauchamp, T. L., & Childress, J. F. (2009). *Principles of biomedical ethics* (6th ed.). New York, NY: Oxford University Press.

Binder, L. M., Iverson, G. L., & Brooks, B. L. (2009). To err is human: "Abnormal" neuropsychological scores and variability are common in healthy adults. *Archives of Clinical Neuropsychology*, 24(1), 31–46.

Bush, S. S. (2005). Introduction to section 13: Ethical challenges in the determination of response validity in neuropsychology. In S. S. Bush (Ed.), *A casebook of ethical challenges in neuropsychology* (p. 228). New York, NY: Psychology Press.

Bush, S. S. (2007). *Ethical decision making in clinical neuropsychology.* New York, NY: Oxford University Press.

Bush, S. S. (2009). *Geriatric Mental Health Ethics: A Casebook.* New York: Springer Publishing Company.

Bush, S. S. (2010). Determining whether or when to adopt new versions of psychological and neuropsychological tests: Ethical and professional considerations. *The Clinical Neuropsychologist*, 24(1), 7–16.

Bush, S. S., Barth, J. T., Pliskin, N. H., Arffa, S., Axelrod, B. N., Blackburn, L. A., et al. . . . Silver, C. H. (2005). Independent and court-ordered forensic neuropsychological examinations: Official statement of the National Academy of Neuropsychology. *Archives of Clinical Neuropsychology*, 20(8), 997–1007.

Bush, S. S., & Cuesta, G. M. (2010). Ethical issues in military neuropsychology. In C. H. Kennedy & J. Moore (Eds.), *Military neuropsychology* (pp. 29–56). New York, NY: Springer Publishing.

Bush, S. S., & Graver, C. J. (in press). Symptom validity assessment of military and veteran populations following mild traumatic brain injury. In D. A. Carone & S. S. Bush (Eds.), *Mild traumatic brain injury: Symptom validity assessment and malingering.* New York, NY: Springer Publishing.

Bush, S. S., Grote, C., Johnson-Greene, D., & Macartney-Filgate, M. (2008). A panel interview on the ethical practice of neuropsychology. *The Clinical Neuropsychologist*, 22(2), 321–344.

Bush, S. S., & Iverson, G. L. (2010). Ethical issues and practical considerations in sport neuropsychology. In F. M. Webbe (Ed.), *Handbook of sport neuropsychology* (pp. 35–52). New York, NY: Springer Publishing.

Bush, S. S., & Iverson, G. L. (Eds.). (2012). Introduction. In *Neuropsychological assessment of work-related injuries* (pp. 1–6). New York, NY: Guilford Press.

Bush, S. S., Ruff, R. M., Tröster, A. I., Barth, J. T., Koffler, S. P., Pliskin, N. H., . . . Silver, C. H. (2005). Symptom validity assessment: Practice issues and medical necessity. Official position of the National Academy of Neuropsychology. *Archives of Clinical Neuropsychology*, 20(4), 419–426.

Bush, S. S., Russo, A. C., & Cuesta, G. M. (2012). Ethical considerations in the neuropsychological evaluation and treatment of veterans. In S. S. Bush (Ed.), *Neuropsychological practice with veterans* (pp. 331–354). New York, NY: Springer Publishing.

Carone, D. A., & Bush, S. S. (2012). Dementia pugilistica and chronic traumatic encephalopathy. In R. Dean & C. Noggle (Eds.), *Cortical Dementias.* New York, NY: Springer Publishing.

Carone, D. A., Iverson, G. L., & Bush, S. S. (2010). A model to approaching and providing feedback to patients regarding invalid test performance in clinical neuropsychological evaluations. *The Clinical Neuropsychologist*, 24(5), 759–778.

Heaton, R. K., Miller, S.W., Taylor, M. J., & Grant, I. (2004). *Revised comprehensive norms for an expanded Halstead-Reitan Battery: Demographically adjusted neuropsychological norms for African American and Caucasian adults. Professional manual.* Lutz, FL: Psychological Assessment Resources, Inc.

Heilbronner, R. L., Sweet, J. J., Morgan, J. E., Larrabee, G. J., Millis, S. and conference participants. American Academy of Clinical Neuropsychology consensus conference statement on the neuropsychological assesssment of effort, response bias, and malingering. *The Clinical Neuropsychologist,* 23, 1093–1129.

Iverson, G. L. (2005). Outcome from mild traumatic brain injury. *Current Opinion in Psychiatry,* 18(3), 301–317.

Iverson, G. L., Brooks, B. L., & Holdnack, J. A. (2008). Misdiagnosis of cognitive impairment in forensic neuropsychology. In R. L. Heilbronner (Ed.), *Neuropsychology in the courtroom: Expert analysis of reports and testimony* (pp. 243–266). New York, NY: Guilford Press.

Knapp, S., & VandeCreek, L. (2006). *Practical ethics for psychologists: A positive approach.* Washington, DC: American Psychological Association.

Larrabee, G. J. (Ed.). (2005). *A scientific approach to forensic neuropsychology. Forensic neuropsychology: A scientific approach* (pp. 3–28). New York, NY: Oxford University Press.

Lees-Haley, P. R., & Fox, D. D. (2001). Isn't everything in forensic neuropsychology controversial? *Neuro-Rehabilitation,* 16(4), 267–273.

McCaffrey, R. J., Lynch, J. K., & Yantz, C. L. (2005). *Third party observers: Why all the fuss? Journal of Forensic Neuropsychology,* 4, 1–16.

McCrea, M. A. (2007). *Mild traumatic brain injury and postconcussion syndrome: The new evidence base for diagnosis and treatment.* New York, NY: Oxford University Press.

Rabin, L. A., Barr, W. B., & Burton, L. A. (2005). Assessment practices of clinical neuropsychologists in the United States and Canada: A survey of INS, NAN, and APA Division 40 members. *Archives of Clinical Neuropsychology,* 20(1), 33–65.

Schretlen, D. J., Munro, C. A., Anthony, J. C., & Pearlson, G. D. (2003). Examining the range of normal intraindividual variability in neuropsychological test performance. *Journal of the International Neuropsychological Society,* 9(6), 864–870.

Sharland, M. J., & Gfeller, J. D. (2007). A survey of neuropsychologists' beliefs and practices with respect to the assessment of effort. *Archives of Clinical Neuropsychology,* 22(2), 213–223.

Sweet, J. J. (2005). Ethical challenges in forensic neuropsychology, part V. In S. S. Bush (Ed.), *A casebook of ethical challenges in neuropsychology* (pp. 15–22). New York, NY: Psychology Press.

Thompson, L. L. (2002). Ethical issues in interpreting and explaining neuropsychological assessment results. In S. S. Bush & M. L. Drexler (Eds.), *Ethical issues in clinical neuropsychology* (pp. 51–72). Lisse, NL: Swets & Zeitlinger.

Differential Diagnosis of Malingering 4

Daniel J. Slick & Elisabeth M. S. Sherman

This chapter covers the differential diagnosis of malingering and related clinical presentations in the context of independent neuropsychological assessment of compensation-seeking individuals (e.g., those with a history of mild traumatic brain injury [MTBI])—a far from trivial issue in light of survey data suggesting that 20%–40% of persons in this population are thought to present with exaggerated or fabricated neuropsychological problems and deficits (Mittenberg, Patton, Canyock, & Condit, 2002; Sharland & Gfeller, 2007; Slick, Tan, Strauss, & Hultsch, 2004). The focus is on conceptual issues rather than specific psychometric tests and assessment methods (which are covered in other chapters in this book); and in that regard, there are no special considerations unique to cases of alleged MTBI. Nevertheless, the information in this chapter is directly applicable to symptom validity assessment in alleged or actual MTBI cases, and some of the example case scenarios involve patients with MTBI.

DEFINITIONS OF MALINGERING

In 1999, Slick, Sherman, and Iverson provided a definition and a set of diagnostic criteria specific to malingering of cognitive dysfunction in the context of neuropsychological assessment. This set of criteria has since become the most commonly used diagnostic standard in neuropsychological research, although the extent of clinical use remains unknown. The authors defined *malingered neurocognitive dysfunction* (MND) as the volitional exaggeration or fabrication of cognitive dysfunction for the purpose of obtaining substantial material gain, or avoiding or escaping formal duty or responsibility. Per this criterion, substantial material gain includes goods, money, or services that are not of trivial value such as financial compensation for personal injury. *Formal duties* are defined as actions that people are legally obliged to perform (e.g., prison, military, public service, or child support payments or other financial obligations). Formal responsibilities are those involving accountability or liability in legal proceedings (e.g., competency to stand trial). It should also be noted that per *Diagnostic Statistical Manual of Mental Disorders–Fourth Edition Text Revision (DSM-IV-TR;* American Psychiatric Association [APA], 2000) the essential feature of malingering is false or grossly exaggerated physical or psychological symptoms that are voluntarily produced, motivated by external incentives such as avoidance of responsibility (e.g., military duty, work), obtaining financial compensation, evading criminal prosecution, or obtaining drugs.

UNDERLYING CONCEPTS AND CONSTRUCTS

Several important concepts underlie the definition and construction of diagnostic criteria for malingering and inform the process of differential diagnosis. Chief among these are *primary gain*, *secondary gain*, and *volition*. In addition, *effort*, although not a particularly important aspect of the definition and criteria for malingering, has become a common and often misunderstood construct, particularly with respect to psychometric tests and test results and so also merits further discussion.

Primary and Secondary Gain

Primary gain is the immediate relief from guilt, anxiety, tension, internal conflicts, or other unpleasant psychological states that are directly derived from engaging in a particular behavior. It is the core explanatory mechanism of conversion disorder, in which a severe emotional conflict is unconsciously converted into sensorimotor symptoms such as blindness or paralysis for purposes of relieving intense anxiety. In contrast, secondary gains are the external benefits or advantages that a person obtains from engaging in a particular behavior. In contrast to conversion, secondary gains are a core explanatory mechanism of malingering; exaggerated and/or fabricated symptoms of illness or injury are produced in an attempt to obtain material benefits or advantages.

The concept of primary gain is usually linked to unconscious psychological processes that produce nonvolitional behaviors (e.g., conversion disorder, somatoform disorder), whereas secondary gain is associated with conscious psychological processes and volitional behavior (e.g., malingering). However, these associations do not always apply. For example, although the goal of symptom fabrication is relief of anxiety (i.e., primary gain) in both conversion and factitious disorders, in the first case it is nonvolitional, whereas in the second case it is volitional.

Primary gain and secondary gain are not mutually exclusive. People may engage in symptom exaggeration or fabrication to obtain relief from anxiety arising from internal emotional conflicts and at the same time their behavior may be consciously and/or unconsciously motivated by and directed toward attainment of external rewards such as financial compensation. However, by definition, malingering cannot be unconscious because it is an intentional process.

Psychosocial Versus Material-Legal Secondary Gains

For purposes of differential diagnosis, secondary gains may be divided into two main types. First, *psychosocial secondary gains* are the interpersonal, social, and associated minor material benefits or reinforcements that a person seeks and/or obtains from feigning symptoms of illness or injury. This type of benefit includes both positive psychosocial reinforcement such as attention, affection, and gifts from others and negative reinforcement in the form of escape from or avoidance of unpleasant or aversive psychosocial situations or obligations such as interpersonal conflicts. For example, consider the following case: A man sustains an MTBI in a sports accident, after which his spouse becomes more attentive and emotionally involved with him. As the man recovers from his injury, he begins to feign continuing symptoms to maintain these psychosocial secondary benefits. Eventually, his illness feigning behavior becomes entrenched in an apparent case of persisting post-concussion syndrome. In this case, although the person's behaviors are volitional and directed toward attainment of secondary gains, it is not an instance of malingering according to our model because the secondary gains do not encompass substantial material benefits or avoidance of formal duties or responsibilities. The question then arises, what diagnosis is applicable? This issue shall be revisited later in the chapter.

In contrast to psychosocial secondary gains, *material-legal secondary gains* include substantial tangible material benefits such as a financial settlement or workers' compensation award. Material-legal secondary gains also include escape from or avoidance of onerous or aversive *formal* duties, responsibilities, and obligations, such as criminal responsibility and military service. The distinction between psychosocial and material-legal secondary gains is important to consider in the differential diagnosis in cases of feigned deficits according to our conceptual framework, as the latter type of goal and motivation more clearly defines malingering and separates it from other diagnoses. However, it must be kept in mind that *DSM-IV-TR* does not make this specific distinction regarding malingering. In addition, feigning may often be directed toward *both* psychosocial and material-legal secondary gains and in such cases dual or multiple diagnoses will need to be considered.

Secondary Losses

Secondary losses are the opposite of secondary gains; they are any external disadvantages, detriments, or other types of aversive or negative consequences that a person receives as a result of engaging in a particular behavior. As with secondary gains, secondary losses may be classified as either psychosocial or material-legal in nature. Secondary gains and secondary losses are not mutually exclusive; both can follow from the same behavior. For example, consider the case of a woman who sustains an MTBI in a motor vehicle accident for which she subsequently seeks substantial financial compensation. In the hope of increasing the amount of compensation, she begins to greatly exaggerate her symptoms. This behavior eventually leads to profound alienation of some family members and close friends. Nevertheless, the woman continues to feign symptoms in hopes of obtaining a large settlement. In this case, substantial psychosocial secondary losses are incurred in an attempt to obtain a material-legal secondary gain. In other cases, substantial material-legal secondary losses may be incurred in pursuit of potentially greater material-legal secondary gains. For example, individuals who feign injuries may trade off substantial reductions in income for extended periods of time in hopes of obtaining a financial settlement that exceeds the losses incurred. It is important to consider the possibility that in some cases of suspected symptom exaggeration or fabrication, secondary losses may appear to outweigh secondary gains. Although on the surface, excessive secondary losses would seem to rule out the possibility of malingering, the two are not mutually exclusive because there is considerable individual variability with respect to the reinforcement value of various psychosocial and material gains and losses, and in some cases even the positive/negative balance (i.e., gain vs. loss) of specific outcomes. In other words, individuals may sometimes deliberately feign injury or illness even when doing so does not seem to *make sense*. Such behaviors may in fact reflect diminished cognitive capacity, as is addressed later in this chapter.

Volition

Volition refers to the degree to which a behavior is both conscious and deliberate. Volition entails a subjective sense of free will, choice, and control over one's behavior. Therefore, the degree to which any behavior is volitional can only be directly established when a person reports having intentionally engaged in a behavior (e.g., symptom exaggeration). However, in most neuropsychological evaluation contexts, volition must be inferred from evidence such as statements, test results, and other behaviors. As with all other subjective experiences, such as happiness and pain, the assessment of volition is fraught with difficulties relating to quantification and interindividual comparisons. In addition, there may be some differences of opinion regarding how to define and apply the construct of volition in certain contexts, as for example, when consciously directed and purposeful behaviors occur in response to coercion, hallucinations, or delusions. There is also the issue of whether volition is an all-or-nothing attribute of behavior.

With respect to the diagnosis of malingering, the degree to which behaviors are volitional is ordinarily determined by ruling out plausible explanations for non-volitional behavior. In cases where there is evidence of symptom exaggeration or fabrication, it is not normally possible to obtain or rely on direct reports from examinees concerning volition, because examinees rarely admit to feigning symptoms, let alone report the degree to which such behaviors are conscious and deliberate. In more clear-cut cases such as below chance performance on forced-choice measures, the assumption is that an examinee cannot inhibit a correct response and substitute an incorrect one without conscious awareness of doing so, and that such behaviors must therefore be deliberate.

Effort

Effort is usually defined in terms of amount of exertion or expenditure of energy—the amount of mental and/or physical energy expended in performing a task defines the level of effort put forth. If a person is said to demonstrate low or poor effort on a task, a low degree of exertion is implied. Conversely, high or good effort implies a high degree of exertion. Task difficulty is often defined in terms of effort; easy tasks require less effort than more difficult tasks. It follows from this that if one wanted to measure the maximal level of effort that people are willing or capable of exerting in a given situation, then a very easy task would be a poor choice because the ceiling would be too low. At the individual level, task difficulty varies with ability level and thus the level of effort required for a given test score may vary considerably across examinees. For example, a very intelligent individual may expend little effort in obtaining a perfect score on a basic math test, whereas a developmentally disabled person may expend much more effort but nevertheless obtain a much lower score. In this case, the test results may accurately reflect ability levels but they do not accurately reflect effort expenditure. Furthermore, it is instructive to consider that the lower level of effort put forth by the intelligent examinee does not attenuate the validity of his test scores, nor does the difference in effort level between the two examinees attenuate the validity of a comparison of their scores. Of course, there are cases where effort level does attenuate the validity of test scores. Moreover, a third factor is also critical to test performance and the validity of test results, particularly regarding the differential diagnosis of malingering, namely an examinee's test-taking goal. With respect to diagnosis, *malingering* is defined by the goal to which effort is directed and not the level of effort expended. That is, any effort expended toward feigning deficits for purposes of obtaining material-legal secondary gain or avoiding material-legal secondary loss constitutes malingering.

Consider the following example of two examinees who deliberately feign cognitive deficits to obtain financial compensation. The first examinee spends a substantial amount of time and energy (i.e., effort) researching brain injury sequelae and assessment methods and then expends considerable additional effort on the application of a complex feigning strategy during a neuropsychological assessment. In contrast, the second examinee conducts no research ahead of time and then employs a very simple and undemanding feigning strategy during an assessment. The first examinee may stand a better chance of successfully feigning brain injury than the second one, but both are malingering.

Although there is a clear and important distinction between level of effort and the goals to which any degree of effort is directed, the term *effort* is often loosely applied in clinical and research discussions and writing. For example, it is common to see test results strongly suggestive of feigned cognitive deficits (e.g., very low scores on symptom validity tests) described instead as evidence of *poor* or *inadequate* effort, as if the issue at hand was simply one of not trying hard enough rather than a possible deliberate attempt to mislead. Along the same lines, *symptom validity tests* (SVTs) are frequently described or referred to as measures of effort when they are primarily designed and used for detecting feigned cognitive deficits rather than isolated instances of inadequate effort. Although the term effort is commonly used to mean effort to perform well on tests, clinicians and researchers use more specific language to help avoid misunderstandings.

Although *effort tests* are designed to measure the degree to which one exerts effort to perform well, clinicians should consider the possibility that low scores on effort tests may be the product of considerable effort to perform poorly. Consider the following scenario: Two healthy examinees undergo neuropsychological testing. One examinee seeks to obtain the best possible scores, whereas the other attempts to feign cognitive deficits. Both are administered SVTs. The nonfeigning examinee is confronted with a very easy forced-choice recognition task, which she passes with little effort. In contrast, the feigning examinee is confronted with several tasks in addition to those confronted by the nonfeigning examinee, including keeping a specific feigning strategy in mind, monitoring and assessing item difficulty, deciding when to make errors and inhibit correct responses, monitoring performance over time to maintain a target error rate, and controlling anxiety about getting caught. In addition, the feigning examinee feigns frustration and distress and monitors the examiner's reactions for clues about the believability of his feigning performance. Thus, goal differences fundamentally alter the nature and task demands of the SVT such that it is considerably more challenging for the feigning examinee. However, despite these efforts, the feigning examinee overestimates the difficulty of the SVT and obtains a score in a range consistent with feigning. In this case, the feigning examinee's test results are indicative of *low* or *poor* effort to do well and indicative of high effort to perform poorly. More generally, given the additional cognitive demands that may be self-imposed, it is possible if not likely that many examinee who feign deficits put more effort into deliberately performing poorly on some tests than would be required to obtain a best score.

Perhaps a better frame of reference for viewing and describing poor SVT results is that of noncompliance with test instructions. *Compliance*, in this context, is exerting effort toward completing tasks in accordance with the specific directions given for each test (e.g., attending well to stimuli during presentation and telling the examiner everything they can remember on a memory test). Conversely, examinees are noncompliant to the extent that they exert less than maximal effort and/or do not follow test directions (e.g., failing to attend to stimuli and not telling the examiner everything that they can remember). Examinees may be noncompliant by virtue of putting forth inadequate effort to do well or by putting forth maximal effort toward exaggeration or fabrication of symptoms. Tests that are designed to inform the differential diagnosis of malingering are usually sensitive to both forms of noncompliance and can therefore be categorized *noncompliance detection measures*.[1] Alternatively, such tests could be referred to as measures for detecting *noncredible performance* as per Boone and Lu (2003). This designation can be extended to validity scales on self-report measures because these are designed to detect noncompliance with directions to respond carefully and honestly.

DIAGNOSTIC CRITERIA FOR MALINGERING

The most frequently cited and applied criteria for diagnosing malingering in published neuropsychological research are those of Slick et al. (1999). They have also been adapted for use in other areas such as the assessment of malingered pain-related disability (Larrabee, Greiffenstein, Greve, & Bianchini, 2007). This is a valid point, and one that can only be addressed by large-scale actuarial studies of a kind that have yet to be carried out. Another significant issue noted by Larrabee et al. concerns the greater evidentiary weight given to objective test data relative to self-report data; this distinction is not as yet supported by any research. In light of these and other conceptual and pragmatic criticisms as well as developments in assessment methods, Slick and Sherman (2012) recently proposed several updates and modifications to the Slick et al. (1999) malingering criteria involving (a) criteria for definite malingering; (b) exclusionary criteria; and (c) the diagnostic utility of self-report data, particularly with respect to psychological or psychiatric symptoms. These new criteria are presented in detail in the following section and summarized in Table 4.1.

Broadening the Criteria for Definite Malingering

Compelling Inconsistencies

Bianchini et al. (2005) proposed that *compelling inconsistencies*—examinee-reported symptoms that are unambiguously incompatible with or directly contradicted by examinee test performance or behaviors—should be considered pathognomonic of malingering when other critical criteria are met (i.e., substantial external incentive and behavior not accounted for by legitimate neurological or psychiatric disorders). Examples include a litigating examinee reports severe pervasive memory deficits but clearly demonstrates good memory for recent events and new information during a discussion with a family member during a break in testing; or a litigating examinee who reports that since being struck by a car she is always too afraid to cross streets by herself, but is later observed crossing a street alone without any hesitation or apparent distress. In the context of potential material-legal secondary gain for feigned impairment, and in the absence of any other reasonable explanation, such patent contradictions between self-reported and observed abilities should be considered prima facie evidence of definite malingering. In addition to direct observation, other sources of information such as surveillance video, collateral reports, or performance records that are sufficiently unambiguous and reliable could also be used to establish that an examinee's self-reported symptoms are unequivocally incompatible with his or her demonstrated level of function.

---

[1] Note that complete compliance/credibility across the entire assessment cannot be inferred from normal SVT scores alone. Numerous studies have clearly demonstrated that examinees who attempt to feign deficits may obtain passing SVT scores while also suppressing their performance on other tests administered during the same assessment. Normal range SVT scores should properly be interpreted as *not indicative of problems with compliance/credibility* rather than indicative of good compliance/credibility.

TABLE 4.1 Proposed Diagnostic Criteria for Malingered Neuropsychological Dysfunction (MND): A Revision and Extension of the Slick et al. (1999) Criteria for Malingered Neurocognitive Dysfunction

Primary MND
Definite
1. Presence of a substantial external incentive for exaggeration/fabrication of symptoms (Criterion 1). 2. One or more very strong indicators of exaggeration/fabrication of neuropsychological problems or deficits (one or more of Criteria 2.0–2.3). 3. Behaviors meeting necessary criteria are not substantially accounted for by psychiatric, neurological, or developmental factors.
Probable
1. Presence of a substantial external incentive for exaggeration/fabrication of symptoms (medical-legal secondary gain). 2. Three or more indicators of possible exaggeration/fabrication of neuropsychological problems or deficits (three or more of Criteria 3.1–3.7).
Secondary MND (definite and probable)
Criteria for definite or probable MND are otherwise met, but there are compelling grounds to believe that at the time of assessment, the examinee did not have the cognitive capacity to understand the moral/ethical/legal implications of his or her behavior and/or was unable to control his or her behavior, secondary to immaturity (i.e., in childhood) or bona fide developmental, psychiatric, or neurological disorders or injuries of *at least* moderate severity. Secondary malingering cannot be diagnosed in persons with mild conditions such as MTBI.
MND by Proxy (definite and probable)
Criteria for definite or probable MND are otherwise met, but there are compelling grounds to believe that a vulnerable examinee acted primarily under the guidance, direction, influence, or control of another individual. Examinees may be vulnerable to the influence of others by virtue of immaturity, neurodevelopmental and cognitive disabilities, and psychiatric illness, or by perceived inability to escape or avoid substantial coercion such as threats of physical harm for failure to behave as directed.
Specific Criteria
1. Presence of a substantial external incentive for exaggeration/fabrication of symptoms (medical-legal secondary gain). 2. Very strong indicators of exaggeration/fabrication of neuropsychological problems or deficits. 2.1. Below chance performance ($\leq$ .05) on one or more forced-choice measures 2.2. High posterior probability ($\geq$ .95 that performance is substantially below actual ability level) on one or more well-validated psychometric indices 2.3. Self-reported symptoms are unambiguously incompatible with or directly contradicted by directly observed behavior and/or test performance 3. Possible indicators of exaggeration/fabrication of neuropsychological problems or deficits. 3.1. Data from one or more well-validated psychometric measures, although not sufficient to meet Criterion 2a or 2b, are on balance more consistent with noncompliance than compliance 3.2. Marked and implausible discrepancy between test performance and level of function expected based on developmental and medical history 3.3. Marked and implausible discrepancy between test performance and directly observed behavior and capabilities 3.4. Marked and implausible discrepancy between test performance and reliable collateral reports concerning behavior and capabilities 3.5. Marked and implausible discrepancy between self-reported and documented history, consistent with exaggeration of preinjury level of function and capabilities, minimization or preexisting injuries or neuropsychological problems, and/or exaggeration of the severity of new injuries 3.6. Marked and implausible discrepancy between self-reported symptoms and level of function expected based on developmental and medical history 3.7. Marked and implausible discrepancy between self-reported symptoms and information obtained from reliable collateral informants

High Posterior Probabilities

Recent psychometric advances, particularly with respect to methods for combining numeric data from multiple SVTs, have led to the derivation of increasingly accurate posterior probabilities (e.g., Larrabee, 2008), the probative value of which needs to be accounted for. More specifically, given a reasonable choice of prior probability (i.e., estimated base rate modified by relevant data such as evidence of feigning in previous assessments) and a well-validated process for deriving posterior probabilities (i.e., positive predictive power) that is applicable to a given examinee, very high positive predictive values of feigning (e.g., $\geq .95$) can be considered as diagnostically equivalent to below chance SVT performance (i.e., indicative of definite malingering). Furthermore, the data used for deriving posterior probabilities need not necessarily be limited to objective test scores but can also include any other reliable numerical data such as scores from self-report measures; demographic characteristics such as age, gender, and socioeconomic status (SES); and neurological data such as Glasgow Coma Scale scores, length of posttraumatic amnesia, and positive radiological findings.

Elimination of Exclusionary Criteria in Favor of a Diagnosis of Secondary Malingering

In the Slick et al. (1999) MND criteria, a diagnosis of malingering is excluded when feigning is fully accounted for by bona fide psychiatric, neurological, or neurodevelopmental syndromes or conditions. Thus, according to these criteria, an examinee who consciously and deliberately exaggerates or fabricates neuropsychological dysfunction in an attempt to obtain a substantial material gain (e.g., disability payments) as a result of bona fide impairment of reasoning, judgment, or other cognitive faculties (e.g., in response to command hallucinations or delusion that an insurance company stole money from him or her) is *not* given a diagnosis of malingering. Unfortunately, this exclusionary criterion raises some thorny issues with respect to what to label feigning behaviors in such cases. In addition, it may create unnecessary confusion by implying that persons with psychiatric illnesses, neurological injuries or disorders, and people with neurodevelopmental disorders are incapable of malingering. One solution to this problem is to eliminate the exclusion for cases in which feigning of illness or injury for purposes of obtaining material-legal secondary gains is thought to be symptomatic of or secondary to some type of bona fide neurological impairment. Instead, a person who otherwise meets criteria for probable or definite malingering but whose feigning behaviors are thought to wholly arise from *legitimate* cognitive/psychiatric dysfunction affecting self-control and/or the capacity to understand the moral/ethical nature or social/legal implications of feigning impairment would be given a diagnosis of secondary malingering (Slick & Sherman, 2012). For example, a person who exaggerates symptoms of a brain injury to receive a substantial financial reward but is judged to have done so as a result of impaired judgment, reasoning, and impulse control secondary to a severe frontal lobe injury would be given a diagnosis of malingering secondary to brain injury. It should be noted that secondary malingering can only result from a severe psychiatric (e.g., schizophrenia), neurological (e.g., severe TBI), or neurodevelopmental disorder (mental retardation) and cannot be caused by a mild neurological condition such as MTBI.

The Utility of Self-Report Data and Evidence of Feigned Psychological Dysfunction

As noted earlier, a revised set of malingering criteria must give greater weight to some types of self-report data—as exemplified by compelling inconsistencies and posterior probabilities derived from scores on self-report measures. A comprehensive set of diagnostic criteria applicable to neuropsychological assessment should also fully account for cases of malingering that primarily or exclusively involve exaggerated or fabricated psychological dysfunction rather than focusing primarily on malingering of neurocognitive dysfunction. This may necessitate development of additional criteria for the application of specifiers such as *cognitive* malingering, *psychological* malingering, and *mixed cognitive/psychological* malingering. Given these considerations, a more apt nomenclature for a revised set of diagnostic criteria would be MND. See Table 4.1 for a proposed framework for these diagnostic criteria.

DIFFERENTIAL DIAGNOSIS

When confronted with evidence of symptom exaggeration or fabrication, several diagnoses and/or explanatory constructs may need to be considered. These are listed in Table 4.2 and discussed in detail in the following section.

Malingering by Proxy

First coined by Cassar, Hales, Longhurst, and Weiss in 1996 and further elaborated upon by Lu and Boone in 2002, *malingering by proxy* (MBP) applies to cases in which minors meet criteria for malingering primarily as a result of the deliberate influence or control of an adult. In neuropsychological evaluations performed in personal injury litigation contexts, MBP applies to cases in which a minor plaintiff is induced to feign neuropsychological problems or deficits by one or more adults, who do so as part of an attempt to increase the settlement awarded to the minor. The adults in question do not have to be parents or guardians. An adult sibling or other adult relative may take on such a role. Clinicians evaluating children who have suffered an MTBI should be aware of MBP, particularly in litigating or other compensation-seeking contexts.

The concept of MBP may be extended to encompass compensation-seeking adults who volitionally exaggerate or fabricate deficits to obtain psychosocial second-

TABLE 4.2 Diagnoses and Constructs That May Need to Be Considered in Cases of Exaggerated or Fabricated Neuropsychological Dysfunction

Malingering
Malingering by proxy
Secondary malingering[a]
Conversion disorder
Dissociative amnesia
Factitious disorder
Adjustment problem/disorder with specious symptoms[a]
Cogniform condition/disorder
Neurocognitive hypochondriasis
Stereotype threat
Oppositional-defiant presentations

[a] Proposed new diagnoses.

ary gains such as affection or approval from other persons who encourage or direct their behavior to share in the material benefits derived from it. MBP in adults also includes cases in which deficits are volitionally feigned to avoid or escape from psychosocial or extralegal punishments (i.e., secondary losses), or what Slick, Tan, and Strauss (2010) called *coerced malingering*. This would include feigning deficits to escape from or avoid explicit or implied physical, sexual, or psychological harm or abuse. For example, a person in an abusive relationship may exaggerate or fabricate deficits in a neuropsychological assessment in response to explicit or implied directions from the abuser, with implied or explicit threats associated with failure to comply.

A diagnosis of definite MBP requires conclusive evidence that an examinee was acting under the influence of another person when he or she feigned impairment. Direct observations of a person in position of influence or control (e.g., parent or spouse) may provide data that suggests MBP or in some cases is strong enough to support a diagnosis of probable MBP. This can include activities such as prompting, directing, or encouraging an examinee to report or demonstrate "symptoms," and provision of collateral reports of examinee deficits that are clearly exaggerated. However, barring outright admission, one will rarely discover any strong or direct evidence bearing on the degree to which an examinee's behavior is deliberately being influenced or controlled by someone else. Regardless, whenever MBP is suspected, it is particularly important to systematically obtain and carefully evaluate collateral informant reports.

MBP should not be diagnosed when an examinee feigns cognitive dysfunction because he or she mistakenly believes it will please or help others or when a child erroneously believes that someone wants or expects him or her to do so, but who has not been told to do it. For example, a child or adult of limited capacity who is repeatedly exposed to comments from a parent concerning the need for a large settlement or the need for the plaintiff to be punished may decide to feign deficits to ensure such an outcome, even if the parent never wanted or intended for the examinee to do so.

Conversion Disorder and Dissociative Amnesia

The *DSM-IV* defines *conversion disorder* as the nonvolitional feigning of sensory or motor deficits, the primary purpose of which is the attainment of relief from anxiety arising from intrapsychic conflicts. Complaints of sensory-motor problems or impairment are not infrequent among compensation-seeking examinees seen for neuropsychological assessment, and so conversion disorder may need to be considered as a differential diagnosis when there is evidence of noncredible deficits in those domains. However, if one accepts the *DSM-IV* definition and criteria, it can be excluded whenever feigned deficits are limited to the cognitive domain (but see Boone & Lu, 1999 for a different perspective). There is ongoing debate regarding the validity of the construct of conversion disorder (cf. Miller, 1999; Turner, 1999), but it appears that it will be retained substantially intact in the *DSM-V*. No good epidemiological data on conversion disorder are available for North America, and published incidence and prevalence estimates vary considerably (from 11 to 500 per 100,000 in the general population, and from 1% to 14% of medical/surgical inpatients, according to the *DSM-IV*). There are no published data on the incidence and prevalence rates of conversion disorder among compensation-seeking persons.

Per the *DSM-IV*, *dissociative amnesia* is a condition in which someone has an inability to recall important information, typically of a traumatic or stressful nature, that is too extensive to be explained by ordinary forgetfulness. Individuals with dissociative amnesia may present with circumscribed amnesia for specific events, time periods, or types of information. In some cases, they may present with dense amnesia encompassing their entire past and continuing into the present. Other types of cognitive complaints or symptoms are not usually seen, or they are usually trivial when present. The highly circumscribed memory deficits that typically characterize dissociative amnesia contrast markedly with the broader spectrum of complaints and symptoms that are usually seen and reported in many bona fide neurological conditions and also many malingering cases. As with conversion disorder, the reported impairment in dissociative amnesia is not volitional, but rather arises from intrapsychic conflicts and processes for primary gain. Similarities in the *DSM-IV* definitions of conversion disorder and dissociative amnesia suggest that the latter should not be diagnosed whenever an individual obtains or stands to obtain secondary gains from feigning impairment, but this is not listed as an exclusionary criterion. Therefore, dissociative amnesia may sometimes need to be considered in the differential diagnosis of feigned *amnesia* in compensation-seeking cases.

Epidemiological data on dissociative amnesia are extremely limited. No good studies of prevalence or incidence in North America are available. It is considered a very rare disorder and is thus unlikely the actual reason for memory impairment in litigation cases. However, dissociative amnesia is sometimes claimed as a defense in criminal cases and so it must be considered more frequently by neuropsychologists who work in this area.

Factitious Disorder

The *DSM-IV* (APA, 2000) defines *factitious disorder* as the intentional production of physical or psychological signs or symptoms, the motivation for which is assumption of the sick role. External incentives for assuming a sick role (i.e., secondary gain) *must be absent* and therefore, although not stated explicitly, the *DSM-IV* definition implies that factitious behaviors provide some type of primary gain. That is, the feigning of illness—in and of itself—provides gratification or relief from anxiety and intrapsychic conflict, and this in turn is the primary motivation for factitious behaviors. Therefore, the feigning behaviors in persons with factitious disorder are not primarily directed toward obtaining psychosocial or material-legal secondary gains. A factitious presentation may include fabrication of subjective complaints, falsification of objective signs, self-inflicted conditions, exaggeration or exacerbation of preexisting general medical conditions, or any combination thereof. Unlike conversion disorder, there is no restriction in the types of symptoms that are feigned in factitious disorder and thus neuropsychological complaints may well be part of the presentation. Onset is usually in early adulthood, often after predisposed individuals have personally or vicariously experienced hospitalization or severe illnesses, and is typically precipitated by some type of loss, rejection, or abandonment. No good epidemiological data on the prevalence of factitious disorder in North America are available, but it is widely thought to be a relatively rare condition in the general population. More specifically, with respect to the differential diagnosis of malingering, no good data have been published concerning the prevalence of factitious disorder among compensation-seeking examinees seen for third-party neuropsychological assessment.

If one strictly adheres to the *DSM-IV* definition and criteria for factitious disorder, then it cannot be considered as a differential diagnosis for malingering because it is automatically ruled out whenever external incentives are present. However, it has been argued that persons with factitious disorders do, in fact, enter the civil litigation system in some numbers, and are often misdiagnosed as malingerers (Eisendrath, 1996). This is but one of several substantial criticisms that have been raised about the *DSM-IV* model of factitious disorder (cf. Bass & Halligan, 2007; Turner, 2006).

Adjustment Problem/Disorder With Specious Symptoms: A Proposed New Diagnostic Category

As previously described, examinees may deliberately exaggerate or fabricate deficits for purposes of obtaining psychosocial secondary gains. An example of this is feigning symptoms of persisting postconcussion syndrome to receive increased attention and affection from friends and family. Noting that this type of feigning is not adequately encompassed by any extant diagnostic entity, Slick and Sherman (2012) proposed new diagnostic categories of *adjustment problem/disorder with specious symptoms* (APSS/ADSS), for application to cases in which a person exaggerates or fabricates symptoms to obtain psychosocial secondary gains, rather than material-legal secondary gains. In APSS and ADSS, the feigning of symptoms is primarily directed toward (a) obtaining and maintaining psychological benefits such as increased attention, affection, and support from others; (b) managing problematic interpersonal relationships (e.g., controlling others); and/or (c) escaping from aversive interpersonal situations or avoiding informal obligations such as household chores or schoolwork. Classification as a *problem* versus *disorder* depends on the severity of the symptom presentation. Situational symptom feigning in response to a specific interpersonal need or dilemma would fall within the APSS side of the spectrum. In contrast, a severe, deeply entrenched and pervasive condition in which a person's life revolves around the sick role as a means of obtaining psychosocial reinforcement and managing interpersonal relationships, would fall within the ADSS end of the spectrum.

An APSS/ADSS diagnosis may be relatively clear-cut in cases where examinees do not stand to obtain any material-legal secondary gains for feigning symptoms. However, in medical-legal assessments, it is not at all unusual to encounter examinees whose feigning appears to be motivated by both psychosocial and material-legal secondary gains (e.g., increased attention and support from family members and a financial settlement). In such cases, both APSS/ADSS and malingering may be diagnosed as appropriate.

Cogniform Disorder and Cogniform Condition

Delis and Wetter (2007) proposed two new diagnoses, *cogniform disorder* and *cogniform condition* to "encompass cases of excessive cognitive complaints and inadequate test-taking effort in the absence of sufficient evidence to diagnose malingering" (p. 589). Cogniform disorder is the more severe and pervasive form of the two diagnoses and is characterized by excessive cognitive symptoms affecting many activities of daily life. More specifically, cogniform disorder is defined as follows: (a) a pattern of cognitive complaints or low scores on psychometric cognitive tests that cannot be fully explained by a neurological disorder, mental disorder, medical condition, effects of a psychoactive substance, or other factors known to affect cognitive functioning such as fatigue accompanied by (b) significant manifestations of cognitive dysfunction in widespread areas of everyday life. The essential features of cogniform condition are the same as those of cogniform disorder, except that individuals do not present with significant manifestations of cognitive dysfunction in widespread areas of everyday life. This disorder is similar to a somatoform disorder, as described in the *DSM-IV*, but the symptom focus is limited to cognition.

As proposed, signs of cogniform disorder/condition can include symptom validity test failure and other test-based and behavioral evidence of noncompliance. Delis and Wetter stated that cogniform disorder/condition may also be diagnosed in cases where material-legal secondary gains are present, if there is insufficient evidence of conscious intent to deceive. In such cases the specifier *with evidence of external incentive* is to be applied. However, no specific criteria are provided for determining that there is insufficient evidence of a conscious intent to deceive, which leads to problems in cases of symptom validity test (SVT) failure in the context of material-legal secondary gain. In contrast, the Slick et al. (1999) MND criteria define forced-choice SVT failure as prima facie evidence of probable or definite volitional effort to deceive,[2] and in the context of material-legal secondary gain, this entails a diagnosis of definite malingering unless a rule-out condition is met. The incompatibility of Delis and Wetter's (2007) criteria for cogniform disorder/condition and the Slick et al. criteria for MND, along with other problematic aspects of the proposed cogniform diagnoses, raises significant concerns about validity and applicability (Binder, 2007; Boone, 2007; Larrabee, 2007b). Given these issues, our view is that a cogniform diagnosis should not normally be considered in cases where an examinee meets criteria for probable or definite malingering.

Neurocognitive Hypochondriasis

Boone (2009) proposed a specific neurocognitive variant of hypochondriasis, in which a person has a fixed belief that he or she has neurologically-based cognitive impairment in the absence of any actual objective impairment. Neurocognitive hypochondriasis is characterized by hypervigilance to minor cognitive difficulties and failures, which are attributed to neurological injury or illness. This condition is described as typically developing in the context of other psychiatric or adjustment problems and problematic interpersonal relationships, and it is often precipitated by a real illness or injury. A diagnosis of neurocognitive hypochondriasis can only be made when there is no objective evidence of any impairment either real or feigned (i.e., test scores fall within the expected or normal range), and therefore it will rarely, if ever, need to be considered as a differential diagnosis for malingering. Nevertheless, it is usual to see hypochondriacal features such as hypervigilance and misattribution in compensation-seeking examinees, particularly among those with more mild injuries who have been led to believe that they have more serious and/or permanent brain injuries. Such tendencies should be noted if they are present and their contribution to any problems with adjustment in daily life taken into account.

Stereotype/Diagnosis Threat

Stereotype threat is defined as expectancy-based modulation of test performance (Kit, Tuokko, & Mateer, 2007; Steele, 1997; Suhr & Gunstad, 2002, 2005). Poor test performance differentiates stereotype threat from neuropsychological hypochondriasis in which beliefs do not negatively affect performance on objective measures. For example, Levy (1996) demonstrated that older adults' performance on cognitive tests can

---

[2] However, malingering is not diagnosed if such efforts are entirely symptomatic of neurological, psychiatric, or neurodevelopmental disorders. See also the discussion of secondary malingering in this chapter.

be affected by priming with positive and negative stereotypes about aging. Suhr and Gunstad (2002, 2005) demonstrated a similar effect, which they termed *diagnosis threat* in young adults who had suffered mild head injuries. They found that neuropsychological test performance was worse among individuals who were informed about the potential effects of head injury on cognition in comparison to those who were not reminded of their head injury history. However, the expectancy effects found in research to date have been relatively small, and there is no reason to believe that such effects could substantially account for findings consistent with probable or definite malingering in compensation-seeking cases. Therefore, stereotype/diagnosis threat will not usually need to be considered in the differential diagnosis of probable or definite malingering.

Oppositional Presentations

Examinees sometimes approach neuropsychological assessment with an idiosyncratic oppositional manner. The degree of oppositionality can range from subtle/mild to blatant/extreme. At the milder end of the oppositional spectrum are behaviors such as negative comments about the examiner and assessment, minimal responses, refusal to guess, and other signs of lack of engagement, motivation, and mental exertion. At the more extreme end of the oppositional spectrum are behaviors such as outright test refusal, nonsensical responses, and incompatible activities like looking away from or inappropriate use of test materials. Oppositional behaviors may arise from situational factors and/or be symptomatic of more pervasive or serious clinical conditions. Such behaviors will always have implications for the validity of assessment results, but the diagnostic significance may be more complex in compensation-seeking cases. In such circumstances, marked oppositional behaviors will often have the same implications as in regular clinical assessments, but they may occasionally constitute a naïve attempt to feign impairment, particularly in cases where there is no documented history of such problems. Alternatively, oppositional behaviors may be a way for an examinee who wishes to exaggerate or fabricate deficits to avoid the challenge of feigning impairment on tests.

MALINGERING VERSUS BONA FIDE IMPAIRMENT

There is a tendency, particularly among lay persons, to equate malingering and related diagnoses such as factitious disorder with complete fabrication of all symptoms. However, experienced clinicians understand and accept that in some cases examinee behavior and test results may reflect both bona fide neuropsychological problems or deficits and symptom exaggeration/fabrication. All of the diagnostic entities described in this chapter can co-occur with bona fide neurological illnesses and injuries and real neuropsychological problems or deficits. More specifically, legitimate neurological injuries and malingering are not mutually exclusive. Thus, whenever there is strong evidence of feigning, clinicians should nevertheless fully consider and, if possible with any accuracy, estimate the extent to which real deficits may also be present.

CONCLUSIONS

Examinee presentations in medical-legal and other third-party neuropsychological assessments are often complex. The presence of potential substantial medical-legal secondary gain necessitates consideration of malingering as a possible diagnosis, and neuropsychological assessments in such a context should always include well-validated noncompliance detection measures. Neuropsychologists who undertake such assessments should—among many other things—be well versed in the differential diagnosis of malingering. Whenever malingering is suspected, no matter how strongly, it is necessary to carefully consider any additional, alternate, or complimentary diagnoses that may be applicable. The possibility of coexisting bona fide dysfunction or impairment will usually need to be considered, especially in cases of unambiguous documented brain injuries. Even when a diagnosis of probable or definite malingering is warranted, all relevant aspects of an examinee's presentation and circumstances—such as the presence of psychosocial secondary gains that may be influencing examinee's behavior—should be noted as contributing or coexisting factors.

The differential diagnosis of malingering can be practically tricky and fraught with unique difficulties and clinical challenges. The ethical commitment to do no harm is sacrosanct to the profession of psychology and very strongly held by most clinicians. As a result, the negative implications for examinees, particularly in sympathetic cases, may lead to considerable hesitancy when it comes to diagnosing probable or definite malingering, even when the evidence is objectively unambiguous, and also there may be some reluctance to clearly communicate such a conclusion when it is reached. At other times, such as when retained by the defense and/or when an examinee arouses a negative emotional reaction, there may be temptation to stretch the data to fit a diagnosis of malingering. Positive and negative biases may easily creep in if there is lack of awareness or unwillingness to engage in self-examination. Good clinicians recognize and accept the presence of such influences, are vigilant about their reactions to them, step back as necessary, and strive to take a balanced and objective approach to the data.

REFERENCES

American Psychiatric Association (2000). *Diagnostic and statistical manual of mental disorders* (4th ed., text rev.). Washington, DC: Author.

Bass, C., & Halligan, P. W. (2007). Illness related deception: social or psychiatric problem? *Journal of the Royal Society of Medicine*, 100(2), 81–84.

Bianchini, K. J., Greve, K. W., & Glynn, G. (2005). On the diagnosis of malingered pain-related disability: Lessons from cognitive malingering research. *The Spine Journal*, 5(4), 404–417.

Binder, L. M. (2007). Comment on cogniform disorder and cogniform condition: Proposed diagnoses for excessive cognitive symptoms. *Archives of Clinical Neuropsychology*, 22(6), 681–682.

Boone, K. B. (2007). Commentary on "Cogniform disorder and cogniform condition: Proposed diagnoses for excessive cognitive symptoms" by Dean C. Delis and Spencer R. Wetter. *Archives of Clinical Neuropsychology*, 22(6), 675–679.

Boone, K. B. (2009). Fixed belief in cognitive dysfunction despite normal neuropsychological scores: Neurocognitive hypochondriasis? *The Clinical Neuropsychologist*, 23(6), 1016–1036.

Boone, K. B., & Lu, P. H. (1999). Impact of somatoform symptomatology on credibility of cognitive performance. *Clinical Neuropsychologist*, 13(4), 414–419.

Boone, K. B. & Lu, P. (2003). Noncredible cognitive performance in the context of severe brain injury. *The Clinical Neuropsychologist*, 17(2), 244–254.

Cassar, J. R., Hales, E. S., Longhurst, J. G., &Weiss, G. S. (1996). Can disability benefits make children sicker? *Journal of the American Academy of Child and Adolescent Psychiatry*, 35(6), 700–701.

Delis, D. C., & Wetter, S. R. (2007). Cogniform disorder and cogniform condition: Proposed diagnoses for excessive cognitive symptoms. *Archives of Clinical Neuropsychology*, 22(5), 589–604.

Eisendrath, S. J. (1996).When Munchausen becomes malingering: Factitious disorders that penetrate the legal system. *Bulletin of the American Academy of Psychiatry and Law*, 24(4), 471–481.

Kit, K. A., Tuokko, H. A., & Mateer, C. A. (2007). A review of the stereotype threat literature and its application in a neurological population. *Neuropsychology Review*, 18(2), 132–148.

Larrabee, G. J. (2007b). Commentary on Delis and Wetter, "Cogniform disorder and cogniform condition: Proposed diagnoses for excessive cognitive symptoms." *Archives of Clinical Neuropsychology*, 22(6), 683–687.

Larrabee, G. J. (2008). Aggregation across multiple indicators improves the detection of malingering: Relationship to likelihood ratios. *Clinical Neuropsychologist*, 22(4), 666–679.

Larrabee, G. J., Greiffenstein, M. F., Greve, K. W., & Bianchini, K. J. (2007). Refining diagnostic criteria for malingering. In G. J. Larrabee, (Ed.), *Assessment of malingered neuropsychological deficits* (pp. 334–371). New York, NY: Oxford University Press.

Levy, B. (1996). Improving memory in old age through implicit self-stereotyping. *Journal of Personality and Social Psychology*, 71(6), 1092–1107.

Lu, P. H., & Boone, K. B. (2002). Suspect cognitive symptoms in a 9-year-old child: Malingering by proxy? *Clinical Neuropsychologist*, 16(1), 90–96.

Miller, E. (1999). Conversion hysteria: Is it a viable concept? *Cognitive Neuropsychiatry*, 4(3), 181–191.

Mittenberg, W., Patton, C., Canyock, E. M., & Condit, D. (2002, February). *A national survey of symptom exaggeration and malingering base rates*. Poster presented at the Annual Meeting of the International Neuropsychological Society, Toronto, Canada.

Sharland, M. J., & Gfeller, J. D. (2007). A survey of neuropsychologists' beliefs and practices with respect to the assessment of effort. *Archives of Clinical Neuropsychology*, 22(2), 213–223.

Slick, D. J., & Sherman, E. M. S. (2012). Differential diagnosis of malingering and related clinical presentations. In E. M. S. Sherman & B. L. Brooks (Eds.), Pediatric forensic neuropsychology (pp. 113–135). New York, NY: Oxford University Press.

Slick, D. J., Sherman, E., & Iverson, G. L. (1999). Diagnostic criteria for malingered neurocognitive dysfunction: Proposed standards for clinical practice and research. *Clinical Neuropsychologist*, 13(4), 545–561.

Slick, D. J., Tan, J. E., Sherman, E. M. S., & Strauss, E. (2010). Malingering and related conditions in pediatric populations. In A. S. Davis, (Ed.), *Handbook of pediatric neuropsychology* (pp. 457–470). New York, NY: Springer.

Slick, D. J., Tan, J. E., Strauss, E. H., & Hultsch, D. (2004). Detecting malingering: A survey of experts' practices. *Archives of Clinical Neuropsychology*, 19(4), 465–473.

Steele, C. (1997). A threat in the air. How stereotypes shape intellectual identity and performance. *American Psychologist*, 52(6), 613–629.

Suhr, J. A., & Gunstad, J. (2002). "Diagnosis threat": The effect of negative expectations on cognitive performance in head injury. *Journal of Clinical and Experimental Neuropsychology*, 24(4), 448–457.

Suhr, J. A., & Gunstad, J. (2005). Further exploration of the effect of "diagnosis threat" on cognitive performance in individuals with mild head injury. *Journal of the International Neuropsychological Society*, 11(1), 23–29.

Turner, M. (1999). Malingering, hysteria, and the factitious disorders. *Cognitive Neuropsychiatry*, 4(3), 193–201.

Turner, M. A. (2006). Factitious disorders: Reformulating the DSM–IV criteria. *Psychosomatics*, 47(1), 23–32.

Noncredible Explanations of Noncredible Performance on Symptom Validity Tests

5

Paul Green & Thomas Merten

WHAT DO NEUROPSYCHOLOGICAL AND EFFORT TESTS MEASURE?

Neuropsychological Tests

Neuropsychologists measure brain function using standardized tests, or, at least that is the intention. For generations, it was assumed that differences in cognitive ability from one person to another were accurately mirrored by differences in cognitive test scores, although not perfectly because there was some random error. It was assumed that, in nearly all cases, people being administered cognitive tests were trying their best and that low scores reflected low abilities in nearly all cases. Scores in the impaired range were readily interpreted as signs of cognitive deficits and impaired brain function. Error was assumed to be just as likely to lead to an overestimate of brain function as to an underestimate.

Only relatively recently was it shown that the assumption that people are trying their best is often wrong, and that low scores frequently do not signify low ability at all because the data are simply invalid (e.g., Fox, 2011; Green, Rohling, Lees-Haley, & Allen, 2001; Meyers, Volbrecht, Axelrod, & Reinsch-Boothby, 2011; Stevens, Friedel, Mehren, & Merten, 2008). Invalid test results from poor effort or deliberate underachievement do not occur only in groups where there is an obvious external incentive to appear cognitively impaired, such as those seeking financial compensation for cognitive impairment. Even in groups previously assumed to be highly motivated to do well, effort may be poor, leading to invalid test results. For example, it was assumed that professional athletes being tested cognitively at baseline and then after concussions would try their best. Their motivation was to carry on playing and earning a living. The assumption of valid data and good effort was disproven when an American professional football player, Peyton Manning, admitted that he had deliberately performed poorly at baseline so that his scores after a concussion would look as if there was no impairment, and other players admitted that this was a commonly-used tactic to manipulate the test scores in their favor (Fox59 Sports Staff, 2011). Neuropsychologists now know that, in many different contexts, effort can be low to a degree that is sufficient to invalidate test results, especially if there is an incentive to appear impaired (e.g., Chafetz, 2008; Chafetz, Prentkowski, & Rao, 2011; Flaro, Green, & Robertson, 2007; Sullivan, May, & Galbally, 2007). For that reason, effort testing is increasingly recognized as an essential component of neuropsychological testing (Bush et al., 2005; Heilbronner, Sweet, Morgan, Larrabee, & Millis, 2009).

Effort Tests

Good effort tests are not sensitive to differences in ability between adults and children (e.g., Green & Flaro, 2003). They are unaffected by intelligence level except at the extreme low point (Demakis, Gervais, & Rohling, 2008). For example, several hundred children with developmental disabilities were tested clinically by Dr. Lloyd Flaro over a 15-year period, including children with seriously disabling conditions such as autism, childhood schizophrenia, fetal alcohol syndrome, and mental retardation (Green, Flaro, Brockhaus, & Montijo, 2012). In the whole sample, on average, only 3% of these children would be described as showing poor effort based on results from the Word Memory Test (WMT; Green, 2003/2005; Green & Astner, 1995), the Medical Symptom Validity Test (MSVT; Green, 2004), and the Nonverbal MSVT (NV-MSVT; Green, 2008). In a subgroup of the latter children with a full scale intelligent quotient (FSIQ) between 50 and 70, 6.5% of cases would be classified as having poor effort profiles, which stands in marked contrast to a greater than 40% failure rate of the WMT and MSVT in adults with mild traumatic brain injury (MTBI) in the same report. A quarter of the adults with an alleged history of MTBI failing the easy subtests had a poor effort profile on the WMT, which would be inconsistent with any form of genuine severe cognitive impairment.

Performance on effort tests that are based on very easy verbal recognition memory tasks is affected very little by brain trauma, even by hippocampal damage (Goodrich-Hunsaker & Hopkins, 2009). Such tests are rarely failed by people with most neurological diseases or with a history of severe TBI if the person makes an effort and produces reliable scores on neuropsychological tests (e.g., Carone, 2008). Hence, failure in a nondemented person is usually not a result of neurological injury or disease.

ALTERNATIVE ATTEMPTS TO EXPLAIN EFFORT TEST FAILURE

Whereas effort tests are designed, to the extent possible, not to be sensitive to differences in true ability, the habits of psychologists and psychiatrists do not change easily. As a result, traditional concepts that have been used to explain low scores on neuropsychological tests, which are sensitive to actual impairment of brain function, have sometimes been used in an attempt to explain effort test failure in terms of something other than poor effort. Often, such concepts are inappropriate and not based on empirical data. For example, it is sometimes argued in forensic cases that people with a history of MTBI fail tests like the NV-MSVT because they have impaired memory. This explanation might seem superficially reasonable, but it ignores the fact that such tests are extremely easy and that far more failures on such tests occur in those with very mild TBI than in those with severe TBI. On the NV-MSVT, the rate of failure of the easy subtests was zero in cases with severe TBI, but it was 26% in the MTBI group (Green, 2011). Impaired memory from brain injury cannot explain such a counterintuitive finding, but poor effort in the MTBI cases with compensation claims can do so.

Some clinicians have argued that an examinee was in pain, distracted, anxious, fatigued, or depressed and that it was one or more of these factors that led to the scores on traditional cognitive tests being suppressed. Clinical folklore has accommodated and promoted such interpretations, leading in years past to widespread acceptance in clinical practice of explanations for low test scores based on factors, which appear superficially reasonable but which have not been empirically shown to suppress test scores.

Depression

It is common to read in clinical reports by psychologists, psychiatrists, or other physicians that cognitive impairment is present because the person is depressed. In the *Diagnostic and Statistical Manual for Mental Disorders Fourth Edition, Text Revision* (*DSM-IV-TR*; American Psychiatric Association [APA], 2000), subjective cognitive impairment (e.g., concentration problems, indecisiveness) is listed as a possible symptom of depression. No requirement is made for actual cognitive impairment to be verified on objective cognitive tests, even though subjective symptoms and objective test scores are generally not correlated with each other. Past studies did suggest major cognitive impairment in depression, as reviewed in a meta-analysis by Veiel (1997), but none of those studies employed effort tests. As a consequence, the reliability and validity of the group data were questionable.

These studies probably led to the impression that the observed low test scores signified cognitive deficits, which were a result of depression; whereas the data were probably not valid because of poor effort in a substantial proportion of cases. It has now been established that effort test failure is present in about 30% of people with depression and disability claims and that poor effort has a much greater effect on all neuropsychological test scores than depression. In the Rohling, Green, Allen, and Iverson (2002) study, of those who were making a full effort, there was no difference in neuropsychological test scores between those with and without symptoms of depression.

Until researchers adequately control for poor effort, the profession will not know whether certain subtypes of depression involve impaired cognition or whether any impairment is lifelong or just a transient correlate of an episode of depression. Such studies need to be done in the future. In the meantime, attributing any objective cognitive deficits to depression has to be done with great caution. Explaining failure on extremely easy effort tests based on depression is not justified by the evidence. If people with depression fail effort tests that are failed only by people suffering from dementia or other very severe neurocognitive conditions, poor effort is the most likely cause. Of course, there may be individual exceptions at the extreme end of the spectrum, such as a patient in a severe vegetative depressive state with pronounced apathy; but even in such a case, failed symptom validity tests (SVTs) could accurately suggest that this person's test results are not reliable and not predictive of long-term potential.

In a very recent review of the cognitive effects of depression, McClintock, Husain, Greer, and Cullum (2010) stated, "Depression has been inconsistently associated with neurocognitive functioning and there is a limited understanding regarding the relationship between depression severity and neurocognitive sequelae" (p. 29). Their paper reviewed many studies but failed to note that, with only one exception, none of the studies ruled out symptom exaggeration by using SVTs or validity scales built into personality tests, nor did the authors recommend incorporating SVTs into future research on cognitive impairment in depression. Thus, there is still a need for increased awareness on how easily poor effort on testing can lead to spurious test results and why the use of SVTs is now considered necessary in clinical practice and in group research.

In the case of the WMT, MSVT, and NV-MSVT, there is a pattern of scores seen in extremely impaired people suffering from Alzheimer's disease, in which they fail easy subtests and score very much lower on harder subtests. Using simple rules based on profile analysis, no case with dementia was classified as showing poor effort on the WMT (Green, et al. 2012), and almost no case with dementia was classified as poor effort on the MSVT (Howe, Anderson, Kaufman, Sachs, & Loring, 2007) or the

NV-MSVT (Henry, Merten, Wolf, & Harth, 2010; Howe & Loring, 2009; Singhal, Green, Ashaye, Shankar, & Gill, 2009). In contrast, people asked to simulate impairment typically score lower than people with dementia on easy subtests and higher than dementia on the harder subtests, and they do not show the expected superiority on very easy versus hard subtests (Green, 2008; Singhal et al, 2009). In a database of 2,009 consecutive adults tested in the first author's office and in an even larger database of our colleague, Dr. Roger Gervais, about 30% of cases with a primary diagnosis of depression failed the easy subtests of the WMT, MSVT, or NV-MSVT. People with major depression and compensation or disability claims often scored as low as patients with dementia or lower on such very easy recognition memory subtests. However, the mean profiles of scores in such people with depression were similar to those of simulators. Their mean scores were not like those of people with dementia, and they were not explainable based on true impairment.

Pseudodementia After Mild Head Injury

There is a term, "pseudodementia," which refers to someone who appears to be suffering from dementia but is actually suffering from depression. Celinski and Tyndel (1988) selected patients who had been diagnosed with pseudodementia after suffering very mild head injuries. It was stated that one purpose of the study was to "document that a pseudo-dementive condition may develop as one of the sequelae to a minor or mild head injury with little indication of any brain injury" (p. 30). Although the study participants were previously working people with normal range intelligence, those who were diagnosed with pseudodementia produced IQ scores between 52 and 77. All 16 cases were said to have poor motivation for rehabilitation; 75% of cases failed to recognize the examiner on the second occasion and claimed no memory of having been assessed before by the same examiner; 56% of cases were thought to be making deliberate attempts to be perceived as seriously disabled; 37.5% of cases "displayed a Ganser syndrome or willful simulation of symptoms" (p. 37). Many psychological factors unrelated to head injury were noted to be present, such as feelings of entitlement or using the injury to achieve secondary goals. Nevertheless, it was stated that pseudodementia after very mild head injury "cannot be equated with malingering" (p. 35). It was assumed that their psychiatric condition actually suppressed their true ability, such that they could not have obtained higher scores, even if they had tried their best. It was as if depression from MTBI had frozen their cognitive aptitudes, producing a state resembling dementia or moderately severe mental retardation. Yet, in a meta-analysis of the effects of MTBI by Rohling et al. (2011), it was concluded that there is no measurable effect of MTBI on neuropsychological tests 3 months postinjury. In addition, in a meta-analysis by Iverson (2005), it was shown that the overall effect of malingering on neuropsychological test scores was considerably higher than that of a number of different conditions, including TBI, depression, and benzodiazepine withdrawal.

The primary author of the latter pseudodementia study now concedes that malingering was not considered a likely explanation for the low scores, partly because objective effort tests were not being widely used at that time, and the need for such tests was not yet appreciated (Celinski, M., personal communication, June 2011). Two years after the study, the Workers' Compensation Board called in Dr. Celinski to show him a video recording of two of his most impaired patients with pseudodementia working on top of houses as roof installers with no apparent impairment, although still collecting benefits and claiming to be unable to work. Had their brains unfrozen? Had their pseudodementia gone into remission as they recovered from MTBI? More likely is the suggestion that their extremely low IQ scores were invalid in the first place because they were malingering cognitive deficits to obtain money. It is not plausible that they actually underwent a drop in intelligence from average to as low as 52 merely as a result of a minor head injury "with little indication of any brain injury" (p. 30). It was proven after the study ended that two of these cases were malingering, and it is our opinion that the remainder of the group were probably also malingering cognitive deficits. The extremely low IQ scores in the latter "pseudodementia" cases represent just one isolated example of a very widespread phenomenon in which invalid and very low cognitive test scores are produced by the client as part of a deliberate strategy to obtain benefits for claimed impairment, and many professionals studying these people do not recognize malingering despite some very strong signs of its presence.

POOR EFFORT IN MILD TRAUMATIC BRAIN INJURY AND OTHER DIAGNOSES

This section describes the prevalence of poor effort in MTBI and other conditions and uses such information to explain why certain explanations of effort test failure are noncredible in MTBI cases.

Mild Traumatic Brain Injury

For people with an incentive to appear impaired and who fail effort tests, the observed test scores typically underestimate actual ability to a marked degree (Fox, 2011; Green, 2007; Meyers et al., 2011; Stevens et al., 2008). In groups of disability claimants or compensation claimants, including those who were already receiving financial disability benefits, it was found that about 30% of cases were not making enough effort to produce valid test results, and in the MTBI group, the figure was roughly 40% (Green et al., 2001). In the group as a whole, the effort made by the examinee was of far greater importance in determining test scores than was the severity of brain injury. Effort explained 50% of the variance in the whole neuropsychological test battery, whereas education explained only 12%, and brain injury severity explained a comparatively minor 4%.

This study outcome was at first a controversial finding because it was hard for clinicians to believe that the tests which they trusted as more or less direct indicators of brain function could be 10 times more powerfully affected by poor effort than by severe brain injury. However, this finding has subsequently been replicated in several studies in different countries, including those by Constantinou, Bauer, Ashendorf, Fisher, & McCaffrey (2005); Drane et al. (2006); Stevens et al. (2008); and, most recently, Fox (2011 and Meyers et al. (2011). These studies show that the magnitude of the suppressive effect of poor effort is so great that a person with a very mild head injury failing effort testing will typically score on a wide range of neuropsychological tests as low as or substantially lower than someone with a very severe brain injury who passes the same effort tests, as first reported by Green et al. (2001). Their scores may be so low that they seem to have pseudodementia but they do not; their data are invalid.

The phenomenon of major suppression of test scores by poor effort has been shown to be very widespread. It is estimated that about 40% of all mild head injury claimants fail effort or SVTs and produce invalid test results (Larrabee, Millis, & Meyers, 2009). In the current first author's (Paul Green's) database, the rate of failure on SVTs was greater for those with a history of MTBI than for those with severe TBI (e.g., Green, 2011; Green, Iverson, & Allen, 1999; Iverson, Green, & Gervais, 1999).

Analysis of the most recent data from 2,009 consecutive cases for this chapter showed that failure of the easy WMT subtests was greater for those from certain referral sources; the highest rate of 38% being found in those referred for assessment by the Workers' Compensation Board, compared with rates of 29% in cases referred by lawyers in personal injury litigation, both plaintiff and defense, and 30% in cases receiving medical disability payments. The failure rate was relatively low at 16% in cases who were employees of a large oil company in which the salaries of skilled and unskilled employees are about 4 times greater than the national average. The lowest failure rate of zero was found in healthy people applying to be police officers and in parents with multiple social and psychiatric problems whose children had been taken away and who were trying to regain custody of their children (Flaro et al., 2007).

The highest failure rate of all on the WMT was in 191 cases with a history of MTBI who were selected for having no computed tomography (CT) brain scan abnormality. Their mean Glasgow Coma Scale (GCS) was 14.7, and they were referred by the Workers' Compensation Board. Whereas the latter cases represented the group which sustained the mildest head injuries, 50% of these cases failed the extremely easy WMT subtests. In contrast, the failure rate was only 23% in 120 cases with moderate to severe brain injuries and a mean GCS of 5.6, all of whom had abnormalities on CT or magnetic resonance imaging (MRI) brain scans. In those TBI cases referred by lawyers, there was a WMT failure rate of only 9.5% in those with severe TBI and abnormal brain scans ($n = 21$), but the failure rate was 47% in those with a history of MTBI and with perfectly normal brain scans ($n = 64$). Thus, in those referred by lawyers, the failure rate on the very easy WMT subtests was 5 times higher in the MTBI cases than in those with severe TBI.

In both Workers' Compensation and lawyer-referred groups, failure on WMT effort subtests is far more frequent in those with a history of MTBI than in those with severe TBI. In itself, this finding rules out many alternative explanations of effort test failure, including impairment from actual brain lesions. M. D. Allen, Bigler, Larsen, Goodrich-Hunsaker, and Hopkins (2007) have argued that people taking the WMT showed certain changes in brain metabolism, and they concluded that the WMT really does correspond with brain function and requires effort. There is no disputing that the WMT is an effort test and that the brain must be active to perform even an easy task like the WMT recognition subtests, but M. D. Allen et al.'s (2007) findings do not explain many research findings with SVTs and brain injury. If brain lesions were the reason for failure on easy WMT subtests in people with TBI, there should be a positive dose-response relationship in which lower test scores are found in those with the most severe TBI and the most severe brain lesions. In fact, there is a dose-response relationship but it is negative, with a higher failure rate observed in those with the most minor injuries, as previously explained. Similar results revealing a negative dose-response relationship were reported by Bianchini, Curtis, and Greve (2006), and such results are contrary to what would be found if brain injury caused effort test failure. Instead, a general finding is that effort test failure is greatest in those with external incentives to appear impaired (Chafetz et al., 2011; Flaro et al., 2007), and this is why more failures are obtained by those with a history of the mildest TBIs; presumably their claims of severe impairment are more likely to be disputed than those with obvious very severe brain injuries.

The effects of effort frequently turn common sense expectations upside down, and alternative explanations of effort test failure must be dismissed unless they can account for such paradoxical results. Whereas it would be expected that severe brain injury would create more impairment than mild brain injury, poor effort can completely reverse this pattern on the WMT, MSVT, NV-MSVT, and other symptom validity measures. In the first author's database of 2,009 consecutive neuropsychological assessments, failure on the MSVT recognition subtests, which are even easier than those of the WMT, was present in 57% of 105 cases with a history of MTBI and normal brain scans, contrasted with only a 14% failure rate in those with severe TBI and abnormal brain scans ($n = 56$). In the same sample, reliable digit span (Greiffenstein, Baker, & Gola, 1994) showed the same pattern, with only a 15% failure rate in severe TBI but a 30% failure rate in a MTBI population. The Test of Memory Malingering (TOMM; Tombaugh, 1996) was failed by only 6% of the severe TBI cases but by 15% of those with a MTBI history. The relatively low TOMM failure rates are explainable by lower sensitivity of the TOMM than are other SVTs to poor effort (Gervais, Rohling, Green, & Ford, 2004; Green, 2011). When such paradoxical results are observed, it can be very confusing if clinicians try to explain the results as indicators of true brain dysfunction. However, if clinicians choose to address the latter data and not to ignore them, there is little alternative but to conclude that the greater frequency of effort test failure in those with a history of mild versus severe brain injury is contrary to what would happen if brain disease were the primary cause of SVT failure.

Poor Effort in Other Diagnoses

There is a growing awareness that in many other populations in whom we used to assume good effort on testing, erroneous test scores as a result of poor effort do occur and are sometimes pervasive. One example of such a group is university students pursuing accommodations for learning disabilities or hyperactivity for whom high failure rates on effort tests have been attributed to the presence of external gains for appearing to be learning disabled or being classified as having attention-deficit/hyperactivity disorder (ADHD; Harrison, 2006; Sullivan et al., 2007). Almost half of these adults at university failed the WMT, whereas on the same test there was only one failure out of 32 cases of institutionalized people with well-established mental handicaps in a study in Germany (Brockhaus & Merten, 2004). In the same manner, in children with developmental disabilities such as childhood schizophrenia, autism, and fetal alcohol syndrome, only a small subgroup failed effort tests including the WMT (e.g., Green et al., 2012). Poor effort in such children was very much less frequent than in adults seeking compensation for the allegedly disabling effects of MTBI.

Poor effort has been found to be widespread in people who are claiming to be disabled by many and varied conditions such as depression, anxiety, post-traumatic stress disorder (PTSD), chronic pain, or neurological disease (Chafetz, 2008; Green et al., 2001). When failure rates on SVTs are compared between adults (e.g., Green et al., 2001; Sullivan et al., 2007) and children (e.g., Carone, 2008; Green & Flaro, 2003; Green et al., 2012), the results reveal that SVT failure rates are much higher in adults than in children with similar diagnoses (e.g., schizophrenia, bipolar disorder, depression, ADHD, or TBI). This means that schizophrenia, bipolar disorder, depression, ADHD, and TBI are very unlikely to explain effort test failure in most cases, including adults, because such conditions are assumed to affect children more severely than adults, and children generally underperform adults when the data are valid.

There is resistance among some clinicians and researchers to accepting the findings summarized previously because these data suggest that invalid test results from poor effort are common. In fact, they are often present in more than 30% of the samples studied, severely contaminating group mean neuropsychological test scores, especially in adult groups. The available alternative explanations of effort test failure are limited by three factors: (a) the imagination and creativity of the psychologist or physician interpreting test results; (b) the sparse availability of properly controlled studies in which there is evidence of some factor other than effort, which can explain paradoxical effort test failure rates (i.e., mild vs. severe TBI; adults vs. children); and (c) the traditional practice in the medical profession of recognizing that malingering exists in theory but almost never diagnosing it in clinical practice.

Stone (2009) argued that malingering is indeed very rare. This statement is true if the estimate of the prevalence of malingering is based on the written diagnosis of "malingering" by physicians, because nearly all physicians studiously avoid using the term. Yet modern studies using effort tests suggest that malingering of cognitive deficits is very widespread indeed, with an estimated incidence of, for example, 40% in people with claims for disability based on mild head injury (Larrabee et al., 2009). Malingering is commonplace and widespread when there are secondary gains to be had for appearing impaired. It is just that, for reasons to be examined later in this chapter, physicians and other health care providers very rarely state that it is present.

Many attempts to explain low effort test scores apart from deliberately poor effort or gross symptom exaggeration have some appeal to some clinicians because they have been used for generations to explain deficits on conventional intellectual and neuropsychological tests. It is evident that they appear to "explain" why low neuropsychological test scores have occurred in particular cases. Examples already mentioned are those of pseudodementia, depression, and brain lesions. Others include anxiety, fatigue, headache, chronic pain, and other psychiatric disorders, including conversion or some other somatoform disorder. The problem is that most of these hypotheses never had much of an empirical basis to support them when they were applied to neuropsychological test scores in the first place. In retrospect, we can now see that past studies of cognitive deficits in groups of patients did not take account of poor effort. It is doubtful whether concepts such as anxiety, fatigue, headache, and so forth have any place at all in explaining failure on very easy effort tests (except perhaps in extreme cases). It is hard to imagine how such factors could account for the results summarized previously, including more effort test failures in mild than severe TBI cases and greater failure rates in adults than in children. In fact, the era of effort testing has prompted a fundamental reexamination of whether such concepts explain any cognitive deficits, and, in some cases, it has led to their rejection.

For example, consider the widely held notion that depression suppresses cognitive test scores and that the effect goes away when the depression lifts. Is this true? Apparently not. In a large sample of compensation claimants, it was shown that once poor effort cases were removed, depression had no effect on any neuropsychological test (Rohling et al., 2002). This is not to say that patients with depression do not have any cognitive deficits; in fact, it may be argued that cognitive deficits such as impaired immediate story recall and abnormal patterns of ear differences (on monaural vs. binaural story recall) in some people with depression are markers of an underlying brain dysfunction and vulnerability to depression (Green, 1987; Green & Kotenko, 1980). This effect is not the same as the idea that cognitive deficits come and go concurrent with transient changes in mood, which would trivialize the significance of cognitive deficits if it were true, nor does it imply that preexisting cognitive deficits can explain failure in the subgroup of patients with major depression who fail SVTs. It might be argued that those patients with depression who failed effort testing in the Rohling et al. (2002) study did so because they were genuinely unable to pass the easy WMT subtests. If so, we might ask how these patients with depression differed from most who easily passed the same effort subtests. It could be argued that those patients with depression who failed the WMT recognition subtests scored at the same level as patients with Alzheimer's disease because they were actually as impaired as such patients with dementia. This can be rejected because analysis of the WMT profiles showed that they were not the same as seen in patients with Alzheimer's disease. Their scores on harder subtests were not as low as found in patients with Alzheimer's (Green et al., 2012). See the following discussion on dementia for more specific information. In addition, it is not plausible that depression causes cognitive impairment as severe as observed in people with dementia. A more likely conclusion is that past literature on cognitive deficits in people with depression was misleading because invalid low test scores resulting from poor effort were never considered and were never ruled out.

It may be speculated that anxiety suppresses effort test scores, but the evidence is not supportive. People with PTSD have an anxiety-based condition, but when only those PTSD cases passing effort tests were considered, PTSD had no effect on any neuropsychological test score (Demakis et al., 2007). Fibromyalgia is a chronic pain condition associated with cognitive complaints, including impaired memory (sometimes colloquially called "fibro fog"), but those patients with fibromyalgia passing effort tests had no memory impairment on neuropsychological testing (Gervais et al., 2001). In the latter study, nearly all effort test failures were in the group claiming disability, and there were almost no failures in those without a financial disability claim. Failure on the effort tests could only be explained by an incentive to appear impaired and not by fibromyalgia. This finding is consistent with the fact that when there are positive incentives to pass effort tests, such as getting custody of children, even people with a full scale intelligence less than 70 or people with major psychiatric illness and drug abuse invariably pass effort tests (Chafetz et al., 2011; Flaro et al., 2007).

People with chronic pain syndromes failed effort tests at a rate of 42% in a study by Gervais, Green, Allen, and Iverson (2001). It could have been argued that they failed because of distraction by pain or because of associated conditions such as depression or fatigue. On the other hand, people in the next group of patients with chronic pain from the same Workers Compensation referral source were warned at the end of the day that the computerized assessment of response bias (CARB; L. M. Allen, Conder, Green, & Cox, 1997) was only measuring effort in their case. As a result of providing the latter information, the CARB failure rate dropped to 4%, which was 10 times lower than the failure rate observed when the pain patients were not told that it was an effort test. In contrast, the failure rate on the WMT, about which they were not warned, stayed at the same high level. In the third group of patients, no warning was given about the CARB being an effort test, as in the first phase, and the failure rate returned to baseline. Chronic pain, depression, fatigue, headache, or drug use cannot explain the major differences in effort test failure rates, which occurred merely as a function of telling or not telling the examinee that the test only measures effort. The fact that simply telling the patients with chronic pain that the CARB was an effort test almost eliminated failures suggests that failure was voluntary, externally motivated, and not because of chronic pain, depression, fatigue, or anxiety.

Effort Test Performance in Dementia

It has been established by a vast amount of research over more than the past 25 years that certain SVTs are extremely easy. In many cases, the tests were designed with the knowledge that recognition memory tests are extremely resistant to genuine memory impairment. For example, three people with bilateral hippocampal damage and amnesia passed the easy WMT subtests, which mainly measure effort, and yet they displayed severe memory deficits on the harder WMT subtests such as free recall of the word pairs (Goodrich-Hunsaker & Hopkins, 2009). As a consequence of such effort tests being extremely easy, these tests are rarely failed by those with severe impairment when the person sincerely wants to do well (Merten, Bossink, & Schmand, 2007).

One exception is that dementia of the Alzheimer's type can lead to failure even on extremely easy effort tests, such as the TOMM. In the TOMM test manual, 27% of patients with dementia listed on pages 43–45 failed the TOMM. In the same manner, the easy recognition subtests of the WMT, MSVT, and NV-MSVT are failed by some people with dementia. On the latter tests, however, the simplicity of recognition memory tasks is not the only principle used to determine whether the data are valid. Just as important is the fact that people with valid test results and good effort score higher on easier tasks than on harder tasks. This finding is the basis of profile analysis. Using this method, it has been shown that very few people with dementia are classified as having put forth poor effort, whereas most simulators are identified by anomalous profiles, which do not reflect the true relative difficulty of the various subtests for those making a genuine effort (Green et al., 2012; Henry et al., 2010; Singhal et al., 2009). This is especially true if more than one of the latter effort tests is used.

Also, using data from the series of children tested by Dr. Flaro, it was found that very few mentally retarded children failed the easy WMT subtests, and those who did mainly had a possible genuine memory impairment profile (GMIP) and not poor effort (Green, 2009). Out of 46 cases with a FSIQ between 50 and 70, only three cases would be classified as probable poor effort, and in two of these cases, the children's reading levels were lower than the minimum required level of Grade 3 for administering the computerized WMT. Even in the FSIQ range of 50–70, most developmentally disabled children are able to pass the easy WMT subtests. Those who fail the easy subtests are usually classified as having a GMIP. It is important to analyze the WMT profile and especially to calculate whether the easy–hard difference is at least 30 points.

If recognition memory tests are not failed by most mentally handicapped children and adults or by people with amnesia from bilateral hippocampal damage (Goodrich-Hunsaker & Hopkins, 2009), then clinicians might assume that failure on an SVT by someone with a history of a very mild head injury would automatically lead to the conclusion that effort is poor and that the person's test results cannot be assumed to reflect their actual capabilities. Logically, that is the correct conclusion because MTBI does not cause mental retardation or dementia and impairment equivalent to severe hippocampal damage (Iverson, 2005; Rohling et al., 2011), and, even if it did, it would still not explain SVT failure. However, some clinicians still explain low scores on SVTs the way they have explained low scores on far more difficult neuropsychological tests for many years. For example, a person who sustained a mild head injury might fail effort testing, and a psychologist hired by the person's attorney might claim that the person really was unable to pass the effort tests because he had a headache, was depressed or anxious, was under stress on the day of testing, had driven a long way to get to the appointment, was angry with the examiner, had back pain, was tired, or because he had actual memory impairment similar to that of people with Alzheimer's disease. There is no limit to the amount of possible alternative explanations that could be put forward to try to explain effort test failure.

Yet in each case, the question is, "What empirical evidence is there to support the alternative explanation of effort test failure, and can the evidence account for the already published research findings summarized above?"

Usually, the alternative explanations have no credible support. For example, Bowden, Shores, and Mathias (2006) claimed that the WMT effort subtests really measure ability in mild and severe TBI cases. This notion is contradicted by much of the data that have been presented previously, and it was very effectively rebutted by Rohling and Demakis (2010). They showed that Bowden et al.'s (2006) own data supported the general finding that the easy WMT subtests are unrelated to age and intelligence and that they measure effort. There was also no excess of failures in severe versus MTBI cases, which would have been expected if WMT effort subtests really measure ability. In addition, the sample size of the Bowden et al. (2006) study was small, and children were mixed with adults. In their paper, there was no information on how many of the sample were children and how many were adults. This distinction is important because children usually fail the WMT effort subtests far less often than adults, as noted earlier.

Drug Effects on Effort Testing

One alternative explanation for poor performance on SVTs is the idea that some drugs could affect SVT scores, which is an idea that is reflected in a study of the effects of Lorazepam on the WMT (Loring et al., 2011). In that study, some participants who passed the easy WMT subtests on placebo failed when they were on Lorazepam, although one case showed the opposite pattern. That is, one case passed the easy WMT subtests when on Lorazapem and failed when on placebo. Another case failed the WMT on placebo, suggesting poor effort, and then dropped out of the study. Thus two nondrug cases failed the easy WMT subtests, which is evidence that even volunteers with no apparent explanation for performing poorly sometimes do not make a full effort. The mean WMT Immediate Recognition (IR) score in the group taking Lorazepam was 92.1% correct, compared with a mean of 97.9% correct in the placebo group. For the delayed recognition (DR) subtest, the corresponding percent correct scores were 94.4% (Lorazepam) and 97.1% (placebo). Hence, the average effect of Lorazepam was quite small and not enough to push the mean score for the Lorazepam group below the cutoff for failure (82.5% correct).

In contrast, the mean WMT IR and DR scores in the original sample of 20 volunteer simulators described by Iverson et al. (1999) were more than 30 points lower, being 63% on IR and 62% on DR. In the same manner, 322 cases of MTBI in the first author's consecutive outpatient series scored lower than the latter Lorazepam group. The mean scores from all MTBI cases with no brain scan abnormality were 84% correct on IR and 82% correct on DR. In MTBI cases failing the WMT, the mean scores were 72% correct on IR and 68% correct on DR, much lower than the scores observed in the Lorazepam volunteers.

Loring et al. (2011) used all WMT subtests, which is the correct method of administration. This means that we may examine whether the seven cases on Lorazepam failing at least one easy WMT subtest had profiles, as a whole, resembling either those of people with dementia or those of simulators. In the 20 simulators described by Iverson et al. (1999), all cases failed the easy subtests, whereas most volunteers on Lorazepam passed. Reanalysis of the simulator data for this chapter showed that 11 simulators (55% of the group) had a profile that would be classified as poor effort irrespective of clinical diagnosis because their mean score on the easier subtests was not at least 30 points higher than the mean on the harder subtests. In the seven drugged volunteers who failed the easy subtests, three (43%) had such a profile that could not be explained by genuine impairment. Such profiles would automatically be taken to indicate poor effort and unreliable test results because the easy–hard difference was too small. In the remainder who failed with a possible genuine impairment profile, poor effort would only be concluded if dementia could be ruled out. There was a possible genuine memory impairment profile in 45% of the original 20 simulators and in 57% of the seven volunteers who failed the easy WMT subtests when on Lorazepam. The distribution of profiles of results in drugged WMT failures, therefore, differs little from what was found with known simulators. In the two cases on placebo who failed the easy WMT subtests, one had a poor effort profile and the other had a possible genuine memory impairment profile. In contrast, in people suffering from dementia, all of those cases who failed the WMT had a possible genuine memory impairment profile (Green, 2011).

How should we interpret the fact that seven out of 28 cases on Lorazepam were said to have failed by scoring 82.5% or lower on IR, DR, or consistency, and that the profile distribution of these failures resembles that seen in simulators, not in people with dementia? One interpretation is that Lorazepam might, in some cases, lead to a lowering of effort, giving rise to some degree of suppression of the WMT recognition memory test scores, although much less suppression than we see in simulators or in MTBI cases failing the WMT. If so, it could be argued that we should assume that the person's test results are probably not reliable and do not reflect their abilities when not drugged. The alternative argument put forward by the authors was that Lorazepam produces temporary brain dysfunction in healthy adults and that it thereby causes WMT failure. In fact, the data are not of the type seen in people with brain lesions. On the contrary, the aforementioned analysis of the WMT results suggests that Lorazepam minimally affects the mean WMT, IR, and DR scores in the whole group and that the overall pattern of results in the minority who failed the WMT on Lorazepam was most similar to that of the original simulator sample. Perhaps certain anxiety-reducing medications have the effect of reducing the effort applied to SVTs by a minority of volunteers. Perhaps Lorazepam leads to a state of amotivation in volunteers who have very little invested in doing well or poorly on the WMT. If so, this needs to be studied further with sample sizes larger than in the Loring et al. (2011) study and with various SVTs. On the other hand, the two subjects who failed the WMT when not on the drug and the subjects not on the drug who showed clear evidence of poor effort suggest that there is a problem with effort in some people who volunteer for such studies. They are either more impaired than the people with bilateral hippocampal damage who all passed the WMT (Goodrich-Hunsaker & Hopkins, 2009) and the mentally handicapped adults (Brockhaus & Merten, 2004), or they are simply not as motivated to do well. The latter seems more likely, and it better explains the WMT profiles observed. Ideally, two groups of drug-treated volunteers would be tested: one given a significant incentive to pass the WMT and one with no external incentive. How much money people would have to be paid to pass the easy WMT subtests when given an anxiety-reducing drug in a laboratory is an empirical question.

MALINGERING IN CLINICAL AND FORENSIC CONTEXTS

In clinical and forensic contexts, where there are major incentives to appear impaired, such as the availability of disability payments and time off work or large legal settlements, deliberately poor performance on cognitive tests is hypothetically called malingering. The word *hypothetically* is used here because in practice, malingering is concluded very rarely by physicians. This is not because malingering is rare but because it is the exceptional doctor who will take the risk of concluding in writing that a person is malingering, even if the evidence is overwhelming. Hence, readers of medical reports will gain the impression that malingering is very rare. The reality is that it is grossly underdiagnosed and not reported in most cases even when it is known to be present. We have heard some physicians claim that they do not see themselves as police officers, enforcing the law in cases of fraud against the disability insurance system. One occupational health physician stated that he did not want to go to work anticipating that 30% of the cases he was due to see that day might be malingering. It was too unpleasant. He told the first author in private, "I prefer not to know." The first author's own family doctor told him that physicians do not diagnose malingering because they would stand to lose a patient and open up the door to "all sorts of risks."

Whatever their rationale, in practice, physicians typically avoid using the word *malingering*, with the possible exception of some forensic psychiatrists. Such psychiatrists differ from treating physicians because they do not have a doctor–patient relationship with the claimant, and their main duty is to provide impartial evidence to the court. Such psychiatrists often work in highly secure conditions, with prison guards and police at the ready to defend them if needed. In noncriminal contexts, however, symptoms with no medical explanation, symptoms that are bizarre and nonanatomical, and grossly exaggerated claims of impairment are often explained away by physicians using medical-sounding or psychological concepts that have some superficial appeal but which have very little, if any, empirical support (e.g., nonphysiological findings, inconsistencies, Waddell signs). Going against this tide, the validity of the patient's presentation in clinical neuropsychology today is not taken for granted, and an attempt is made to measure the validity of cognitive deficits and other complaints objectively. Effort tests are required to determine whether test scores are valid or not, and validity checks are needed in self-report instruments to decide whether or not there is gross symptom exaggeration (Bush et al., 2005, Heilbronner et al., 2009).

Effort Test Failure and Compensation

A classic modern-day example of malingering would be an adult with a mild head injury, with no loss of consciousness, no posttraumatic amnesia, no neurological signs, and no brain scan abnormality, who pursues a large financial claim for brain injury and who, in the course of an independent assessment, fails extremely easy tests, such as reliable digit span (Greiffenstein et al., 1994), Meyers' built-in effort indicators (Meyers et al., 2011), the TOMM (Tombaugh, 1996), the Victoria Symptom Validity Test (Slick et al., 2003), or other SVTs (e.g., MSVT).

There are several studies showing that people with low abilities usually do not fail the easy MSVT subtests, except for some people with dementia or people with an external incentive to appear impaired. For example, healthy children in Grades 2–5 nearly all passed the MSVT (Blaskewitz, Merten, & Kathmann, 2008; Gill, Green, Flaro, & Puci, 2007). Children who do not speak French were tested in French and still scored almost 100% correct on the easy recognition subtests of the MSVT (Richman et al., 2006). MSVT failure, like most SVT failures, is far higher in cases of MTBI than in those with severe TBI, and adults fail the MSVT far more often than children (Carone, 2008). Out of more than 200 children with developmental disabilities, only 5% of cases failed the easy MSVT subtests, and, of those, only half would be classified as making a poor effort based on profile analysis (Green et al., 2012). Thus, poor effort would be concluded in, at the most, 2.5% of developmentally disabled children based on the latter study. In contrast, in the same study, the easy MSVT subtests were failed by 42% of the sample of adults with mild head injury who were claiming financial compensation. Poor effort would be the only reasonable explanation in all such cases.

The U.S. Social Security Administration dispenses hundreds of billions of dollars per year to people in various financial benefit programs. For example, the official report of the Social Security Administration (SSA; 2010) stated that 752 billion dollars were spent by the SSA in the year 2010. Hence, it is a financially important fact that 61% of adult claimants for Social Security disability payments were found to fail the easy recognition subtests of the MSVT, contrasted with 37% failure in children (Chafetz, 2008). Failure rates in children were greater in the children who had other family members receiving disability benefits, suggesting malingering by proxy. On the TOMM, the failure rates in the Social Security disability sample were 56% in adults and 28% in children. Chafetz et al. (2011) compared adult groups of low intelligence: one group with an incentive to look good to obtain custody of their children and one claiming disability. Failure on SVTs was nonexistent in the group trying to get custody of their children; but it was very high in the disability claimant group, showing that failure on SVTs, including the MSVT, was explained by motivation to appear impaired and not by low intelligence.

In people with financial compensation claims for soft tissue injuries or psychiatric presentations in the studies of Richman et al. (2006) in Canada and Gill et al. (2007) in Britain, there was approximately a 50% failure rate on the easy MSVT subtests, and yet mentally handicapped children easily passed the same subtests. There was a 58% MSVT failure rate in soldiers leaving the U.S. Army and being assessed within the veterans administration system (Armistead-Jehle, 2010). In each case, the authors concluded that failure on the MSVT was a function of poor effort, and by inference from the context, malingering was the underlying cause. The latter high rates of poor effort and malingering are consistent with data using other effort tests (Larrabee, 2003; Larrabee et al., 2009), and they suggest that disability and compensation systems are probably being placed under great strain by the multibillion dollar annual costs of supporting a large percentage of cases who are grossly exaggerating their symptoms in pursuit of financial compensation.

THE "UNCONSCIOUS" EXPLANATION FOR EFFORT TEST FAILURE

Malingering is inferred from evidence of symptom exaggeration in the context of external gain. However, in practice, when clinicians encounter such effort test failure in a forensic context, there will invariably be someone, often hired by the plaintiff lawyer, proposing alternative explanations for SVT failure apart from poor effort. Stone (2009), for example, speaking for many traditionalists, claims that malingering is rare and argues that in virtually all cases symptoms with no medical explanation are bona fide symptoms that can cause disability. This is a claim that appears to be counterintuitive, and the idea that such unexplained symptoms are unconsciously produced is based on no evidence or at least no data are presented to support this notion. Such medically unexplainable symptoms are grouped together under the term *somatoform disorders*, implying symptoms which appear physical but have no known anatomical or physiological explanation. Under that rubric would fall claims of severe, persistent, and disabling impairment of cognitive abilities by a person with only a MTBI.

People with somatoform disorders, including people with fibromyalgia (Gervais, Russell, et al., 2001) and pain disorder (Bianchini, Greve, & Glynn, 2005; Gervais, Green, et al., 2001), tend to have a high failure rate on SVTs. This should not be surprising because these conditions involve symptom reporting that has no known basis in any actual medical condition, and there are also no objective medical tests (e.g., biomarkers) to confirm the diagnosis. It is hard to disprove someone's claim of having subjective symptoms such as fatigue and pain, including headaches, back pain, neck pain, or limb pain. In many people with such symptoms, the symptoms are real, and gross exaggeration is not present. However, in people with "soft" conditions, which cannot be tested by objective medical methods, there are often external incentives for claiming to be impaired, such as avoidance of work, obtaining disability payments, or maintaining their status as disabled; and it is well established that such external incentives are often strongly linked with effort test failure. Malingering in a substantial portion of these cases would seem to be the most obvious explanation for effort test failure. This would be consistent with the fact that those who fail effort tests produce invalid and grossly exaggerated neuropsychological deficits, which also have no medical explanation (Constantinou et al., 2005; Fox, 2011; Green et al., 2001; Meyers et al., 2011; Stevens et al., 2008).

In medicine (especially psychiatry) and in psychology, rather than concluding that the person is voluntarily producing, grossly exaggerating, or faking these medically unexplainable cognitive deficits and sometimes impossible symptoms, there has been a tradition of inferring invisible unconscious processes that are presumed to be the causal factors. It is assumed that the person does not play any voluntary role in producing a large number of symptoms, such as cognitive deficits, pain, fatigue, or paralysis, even though clinicians only know of the symptoms because the person tells the clinicians about them or demonstrates them behaviorally. It is assumed but never proven that the patient is disabled by a medically unexplainable and scientifically untestable process, involving unconscious forces of a Freudian type. In such cases, a choice is made by the practitioner not to use the most obvious explanation of behavior, which is that the person chooses to display himself or herself as being disabled because there are external gains such as money, avoidance of responsibility, or some other desirable change in the environment.

Clinicians would not use unconscious mechanisms to explain away why a person defrauds social security by claiming to be separated from their spouse when they are not, so that the couple can collect more money per month. The courts would probably not accept unconscious forces as an explanation of why a person steals a car or shoes from a store. Recently, a Canadian court seems to have assumed that it was voluntary actions and the obvious financial motivation that best explained why a woman claiming to have cancer shaved her own head and collected large amounts of money from friends and well wishers, when it was proven that she never had cancer.

What is so different then, if a person claims to be disabled by pain, paralysis, or severe cognitive impairment when there is no known medical cause and when the person fails effort tests that are unaffected by pain? Even when the person uses symptoms to claim monetary benefits and when the claimed impairment is grossly inconsistent with history and known medical facts, most physicians prefer to avoid the most obvious explanation, which is malingering. Instead, they usually choose a term like *conversion disorder* or some other somatoform disorder in which it is assumed that the person is not voluntarily exaggerating symptoms and is not using them to secure financial or other external rewards. Here, we would not want to imply that all bizarre and nonsensical symptom complaints are best explained as malingering, just that physicians and psychologists tend to overuse the concept of involuntarily produced symptoms while overlooking or misrepresenting the many cases where voluntary manipulation and impression management are the main factors in operation.

The same problem of uncritically ascribing unconscious forces to claimed symptoms can be found with the concept of dissociative amnesia. Although dissociative amnesia may occur in people with particularly severe trauma exposure, this form of amnesia is often used as an explanation for why someone could not remember a violent crime that he or she committed (e.g., Cima, Nijman, Merckelbach, Kremer, & Hollnack, 2004; Pujol & Kopelman, 2003). Based on a literature review, Giger, Merten, and Merckelbach (2011) recently argued that, with claimed crime-related amnesia, possible malingering of memory loss has to be carefully investigated by the forensic expert, and malingering should be the preferential hypothesis to be tested. The diagnosis of dissociative amnesia cannot be made by mere exclusion of evidence for organic amnesia. Instead, malingering has to be ruled out on an explicit basis, and this priority, in turn, means that objective methods for identifying symptom exaggeration are required.

A Convenient Diagnosis

The chief physician from one medical disability assessment company, for whom the first author has assessed many people, pointed out that, whereas SVTs and associated observations served to identify malingering in approximately 20% of their cases using effort tests, less than one in a thousand of the same cases were classified as malingering by many specialist physicians employed by the same company. This physician believed that the difference was purely based on political–economic considerations. For example, if physicians began to identify 20%–50% of their cases as malingering, they might face massive opposition by unions representing government and city employees and strike action could ensue. Physicians doing independent medical examinations who labeled people as malingering would risk being blacklisted from seeing many clients, and this would represent the loss of a very lucrative source of income. Blacklisting by a union can mean that doctors contracted by insurance companies to perform independent medical examinations may be prevented from seeing union members.

A case can be made that in medical disability and personal injury claims, the tradition of using a diagnosis of somatoform disorder often describes the politically and economically motivated choices of physicians and other professionals more than it describes the actual condition of the patient. Physicians faced with symptoms that make no medical sense in a person claiming financial benefits on a medical basis either have to admit that they do not know what it is or they have to give it a name. If they call it malingering and attribute intentional symptom production to the patient, they will be obstructing the client's pursuit of what could be large financial benefits. They will, therefore, face a risk of complaints from patients who will strenuously object to being confronted with presenting in a dishonest way. In extreme cases, the physician will face physical threats or face legal action by the aggrieved patient. When faced with these possibilities, it is far more convenient for the physician to use what may appear to be a harmless and widely used label such as somatoform disorder, "cognitive disorder not otherwise specified (NOS)," or "postconcussion syndrome," than it is to conclude that the patient is malingering.

The scientific validity of a somatoform disorder diagnosis is compromised by the fact that physicians do not have any objective method to prove or disprove a central criterion of the diagnosis, which is that the symptoms are not voluntarily produced or exaggerated. However, rarely is this challenge raised. In contrast, the term malingering is used when there is objective evidence to support voluntary exaggeration or fabrication of symptoms for external gain.

The same motivation to avoid unpleasant outcomes and interactions affects any professionals evaluating the same patient, including neuropsychologists, psychologists, physical therapists, and occupational therapists. In some cases, when receiving money for treating the patient, money may be lost by the professional if the patient is labeled as malingering, so there is an added conflict. To understand how and why professionals adopt alternative explanations of malingered behavior, apart from the obvious one, it is necessary to study the real life context in which malingering occurs and the behavior of professionals who are called upon to make a diagnosis. The case of "the man with no hands" described next illustrates how a series of professionals failed to consider or acknowledge what would be very obvious to most laymen. The case shows how health care professionals ignored the most obvious explanation and made excuses for a patient who was eventually proven beyond any reasonable doubt to be malingering and, it could easily be argued, was committing insurance fraud.

The Man With No Use of His Hands

This is a real case, but certain details have been changed to conceal the identity of the person and agencies involved. The man with no use of his hands (MWNH) was a 39-year-old driver of a 2-ton delivery truck who was involved in a rear end collision in eastern Canada. When stopped at a traffic light, his vehicle was struck from the rear by a small car. Immediately, the driver of the car, who was uninjured, went to the front of MWNH's truck and asked him if he was alright. MWNH told him that he was not sure whether he was injured. MWNH worked as a driver for many months following the accident, but then he claimed that he had such severe pain that he could not use his hands. He made a workers' compensation claim for wrist pain, neck pain, and back pain from the accident. He also claimed severe and disabling cognitive impairment from a claimed mild head injury. He hired a lawyer to sue the other driver for financial losses from his impairment. He claimed to be unable to drive or do any manual work because he could not use his hands for even simple actions such as tying his shoelaces, lifting a fork, brushing his teeth, combing his hair, or opening a door. He claimed that his wife had to dress him, feed him, and assist in literally all toileting, and yet he appeared very physically fit. He claimed that he could not find any alternative to manual work because he had severe memory impairment, and yet there was no known cause for his cognitive deficits.

MWNH's hands appeared perfectly normal to look at, and one psychiatrist commented that he had calluses to suggest that he had been working. MWNH claimed that he could not push a doorbell with his finger, and he got the taxi driver to accompany him to ring the bell at the front door of the first author's office. Examinations by neurologists and other physicians revealed no explanation for his claimed inability to use his hands. By the time that he was flown from another city to be seen by the first author, he had already seen many different specialists—none of whom could find a medical explanation for his symptoms. However, one doctor diagnosed him with chronic regional pain syndrome (CRPS). A psychiatrist diagnosed him with a somatoform disorder and treated him for this condition for years using opiate medication and antidepressants with no apparent success.

When seen shortly after the collision by a psychologist, MWNH was complaining of impaired memory, and he was given memory testing, including the WMT.

He said that he was unable to use his hand to operate the computer mouse, so he was given an oral form of the test, which involves listening to the examiner reading word pairs and then being presented with various memory tasks, including two 50-50 forced-choice tasks. On the forced-choice tasks, he scored significantly worse than chance. If he had been trying to do well, there would have been no good reason why this patient should not have scored well above the chance range. Chance level scores can occur despite good effort, but this happens only in the most severely impaired people who are typically permanently institutionalized for some form of dementia. Such people are obviously very severely cognitively impaired, and even such severely impaired people very rarely score below chance (Green et al., 2012; Singhal et al., 2009).

The usual interpretation of worse than chance scores is that MWNH knew the correct answers and deliberately chose the incorrect responses. MNWH claimed memory impairment severe enough to prevent him from working. He claimed to be trying his best in the assessment, but this was contrary to the fact that he deliberately failed extremely easy subtests of the WMT. He was receiving financial support for being disabled from work, and he was pursuing a large monetary settlement in court in a personal injury lawsuit against the unfortunate driver of the car that struck his truck. The basis of his claim was that he was both severely cognitively impaired and unable to use his hands for any action whatsoever. MWNH's claimed impairment and his worse than chance test scores meet almost any definition of malingering. He met the Slick, Sherman, and Iverson (1999) criteria for definite malingered neurocognitive dysfunction.

The effort test results were reported, and each physician received a copy of that report. However, the psychologist who wrote the report did not conclude malingering. He mentioned the possibility of a "voluntary component to symptom production" but left open the possibility that it could be a somatoform disorder. This diagnostic ambiguity was allowed to exist on file despite the fact that evidence of voluntary exaggeration or faking of symptoms, such as worse than chance performance, rules out a diagnosis of a somatoform disorder. Avoidance of the word *malingering* by psychologists is not unusual because, just like physicians over the generations before SVTs were available, psychologists do not want to stand out as the only health care professional claiming that a client is malingering, when all others are using a label such as somatoform disorder. Doing so could risk a complaint to the licensing body, and responding to such complaints is time consuming, expensive, and aversive. It is easier not to conclude malingering.

A second psychiatrist saw MWNH and was unable to explain the complaint of nonfunctioning hands. As MWNH left his office, the psychiatrist reached out to shake hands and the client shook hands normally, apparently caught off guard. For this reason, the psychiatrist mentioned the possibility that "there was a voluntary component" to the syndrome. If so, then he could not be diagnosed as having a somatoform disorder based on *DSM-IV-TR* criteria, but the psychiatrist did not use the word *malingering*. This choice is understandable. Not long ago, within the workers' compensation system, the use of the term *malingering* by a physician would have been taboo and, in the event of a complaint, the college of physicians would frown on anyone using that term. In addition, one forensic psychiatrist who did conclude malingering when it was warranted faced a rally by an injured workers' group outside his office, accusing him of bias, and he has been blacklisted by at least one referral source under pressure from the union. Thus, there are not only external incentives for malingerers to exaggerate or fake their symptoms, but there are also powerful external incentives for physicians and psychologists not to use the term *malingering* in diagnostic reports.

A repeat assessment by the same psychologist led to passing scores on the effort tests, which he had taken the first time, proving, incidentally, that his test results were unreliable because one time he scored worse than chance and the next time he scored almost perfectly. Perhaps he had been coached by his lawyer on the conclusions of the previous psychological report in which worse than chance scores were described. This seems very likely, given that coaching by attorney's prior to neuropsychological assessment is known to happen (Wetter & Corrigan, 1995; Youngjohn, 1995).

In a neuropsychological assessment by the first author, which was requested by the defense lawyer in the accident claim, MWNH showed a pattern of failure on SVTs consistent with invalid data, but there were no worse than chance scores. He failed effort tests, which he had not been given before and which he could not have read about in prior reports. It was concluded that the claim of being unable to use his hands was not plausible based on past medical assessments and that he was malingering cognitive impairment, as shown by evidence of worse than chance scores on prior effort testing, memory complaints grossly out of proportion to the accident details, no evidence of any brain injury, a lack of any credible medical explanation for his physical or psychological symptoms, the lack of any understandable temporal association between the paralysis of his hands and the timing or mechanics of the minor motor vehicle accident, and a demonstrated ability to shake hands normally when off guard.

A panel of three psychiatrists was asked to review the case and decide whether the man was genuinely impaired and eligible for benefits within the workers' compensation system. His treating psychiatrist appeared before the panel and introduced himself as "an advocate for the patient," which is different from an impartial and objective witness. Although acknowledging that there was no medical explanation whatsoever for MWNH's inability to use his hands for simple actions or for his claimed severe cognitive impairment, the psychiatrist argued that, nevertheless, MWNH was genuinely severely disabled and that he was unable to use his hands for any actions because of a somatoform disorder. He ignored the evidence of significantly worse than chance test scores on effort testing and the fact that he demonstrated the ability to use his hands when caught off guard and stated that the man was not consciously producing any symptoms, which is simply not credible. After reviewing the file, including the report of worse than chance responding, the review panel of psychiatrists concluded that, although it was unusual, MWNH was indeed unable to use his hands and was totally disabled from work. They wrote, "We see no evidence of malingering."

The defense lawyer was more impressed than the review panel by the evidence of malingering and so he flew MWNH to see a medical specialist in a distant city. He was videotaped on the outward flight, acting disabled and being given special assistance for feeding and drinking. However, on his return, when he reentered the airport and presumably did not know that he was being watched, he demonstrated on videotape that he had full and free use of his hands when opening doors, carrying things, eating at a restaurant, and using the washroom without the assistance of his wife. The videotape proved beyond reasonable doubt that his claim of persistent and unremitting inability to use his hands for even simple actions, such as urinating, eating, or opening doors was utterly false.

Thus, the treating psychiatrist's hypothesis that his condition was involuntary was proven wrong. The idea that there was some unidentifiable, invisible, and unconscious force producing the symptoms was also rendered noncredible. The most obvious explanation was the best one, which was that he was faking symptoms to obtain money. The review panel members were proven to be wrong in their conclusion that he was actually unable to use his hands, and they were wrong in concluding that he was not malingering. At an informal event, it was suggested to one of the review panel members that even if the evidence of malingering were overwhelming and incontrovertible, as in this case, he would still avoid the conclusion of malingering in any case that he saw. His reply was "Right. It is not worth the risk."

The treating psychiatrist described his somatoform disorder as severely disabling, and the presumed underlying cause was an unconscious process outside of his control; but this was disproven by the videotape and by the worse than chance WMT scores. In this case, the explanation that MWNH's symptoms were driven by unconscious forces was impossible to accept once all the evidence was gathered. The story of MWNH illustrates how far many physicians and psychologists will go to avoid confronting the patient with the fact that their presentation is invalid and how personal considerations can take precedence over diagnostic accuracy when facing the prospect of stating that someone is malingering. Readers who are not very familiar with the adjudication of compensation and disability claims might be surprised to know that MWNH was not charged with fraud. Several lawyers were involved, each representing different parties. The lawyers agreed on an out-of-court settlement of hundreds of thousands of dollars, three quarters of which was claimed by one benefit agency in a subrogated claim. His own lawyer took roughly a third of the remaining money, and the client took the rest.

The defense lawyer reported that MWNH was still paid monthly compensation despite proven malingering. The defense lawyer was asked why no fraud charge was brought, and he explained the motivation of all parties involved. To the insurance company, the costs of settlements of this type are covered by their own insurance at an international level, but such insurance would *not* cover their own court costs if they charged the client with fraud. The defense lawyer explained that to prove that his claim was fraudulent, "a bevy of doctors who supported MWNH with the favorable diagnosis of somatoform disorder would have to be proven incompetent in court" and, as he said, "Judges do not like to do that." Lawyers themselves prefer out-of-court settlements, as long as their costs are covered and the agreement satisfies all the lawyers. The client's lawyer moved to a quick settlement, once he saw the video recording proving beyond any reasonable doubt that his client's claim was false and, probably from a legal perspective, also fraudulent. He knew that he could lose all financial returns if the case went to court, so he settled for a lesser but still substantial amount.

This case illustrates how a fictional and directly disproven concept of unconsciously produced symptoms can prevail in medicine, in the insurance system, and in the legal arena not because it is factually correct but because it satisfies the motivational needs of everyone involved. The physicians who suspected but did not state that MWNH was malingering did not have to face the anger of the client, and they were paid for their "expert opinions" even though they were all wrong. One psychiatrist carried on treating the presumed somatoform disorder with opiate medications and was well paid by the government for doing so. He presumably received no complaints from the patient. The psychologist was not the recipient of any complaint to the college about his assessments for which he was compensated. The lawyers on both sides were content, although the plaintiff lawyer would have been happier if the multimillion dollar claim of total disability had been accepted. One benefit-funding agency, which had paid MWNH for years, received a large sum and carried on making payments anyway. The defending insurance company had no out-of-pocket costs for a trial. The buck was passed or rather hundreds of thousands of bucks in liability were passed to an international insurance company thousands of miles away across the Atlantic. The doctors could carry on without having to revise their use of the concept of a somatoform disorder because they probably never saw the videotape or heard the evidence that it contained. This is because legal settlements and evidence from video recordings are usually kept private.

Wilkinson and Picket (2010) pointed out in their book on social equality, "While natural scientists do not have to convince atoms or cells to accept their theories, social theorists are up against a plethora of views and powerful vested interests" (page xi). Nowhere is this more apparent than where there are large amounts of money at stake. When studying malingering, there is a need to understand the motivation and external incentives of all persons involved in handling the claim, assessing the medical condition, performing neuropsychological assessment, conceptualizing and describing the person's impairment, making insurance decisions, and reaching a legal settlement. It is within this complex setting that most health care professionals avoid using the word malingering, and in which neuropsychologists encounter many forms of noncredible explanations for noncredible symptoms. The noncredible explanations sometimes serve to protect the physician or psychologist from potential retaliation and complaints by the client. However, neuropsychologists have an ethical obligation to report their findings accurately and honestly. As the American Psychological Association's Ethics Code (2002) states, "Psychologists seek to promote accuracy, honesty, and truthfulness in the science, teaching, and practice of psychology. In these activities psychologists do not steal, cheat, or engage in fraud, subterfuge, or intentional misrepresentation of fact" (Knapp & VandeCreek, 2003).

It is time to recognize that the responsibility for identifying malingering should not rest with any single physician or psychologist because, in practice, the potential personal risks will deter nearly all such examiners from reporting their suspicions of malingering. When all other professionals involved in a case are using euphemistic terms to describe the malingering patient's presentation, a single professional who identifies malingering in writing not only faces opposition from the client but also is isolated because of the choices of other professionals not to face and report the facts. Perhaps, responsibility needs to be taken by the insurance agencies, which should arrange for anonymous committees to adjudicate claims and offer protection to examiners who identify evidence of malingering. Otherwise, as is the case today, in practice, nearly all instances of malingering will not be identified, and misdiagnosis will be the norm as in the case of MWNH and most others like him.

Forms of Resistance Against Symptom Validity Assessment

The history of symptom validity assessment is partly a history of resistance against it at various levels from within the field of neuropsychology itself, from branches of medicine and other psychological fields, and within the legal arena. Many neuropsychologists who do forensic assessment and who have been working in the field of symptom validity assessment and symptom validity research have been subjected to attacks at various levels. In a presentation by the second author at the European Symposium on Symptom Validity Assessment in May 2011, a number of pitfalls in reinterpreting effort test failure were identified. They are summarized in Table 5.1.

Some of the pitfalls in the table have already been presented in this chapter, including "amelioration," "pathologism," and "mythologism," all of which are implicit in the case of MWNH, and Table 5.1 explains what they are. There is, of course, some overlap between different pitfalls. Thus, in a case of claimed retrograde amne-

TABLE 5.1 Potential Pitfalls for Opponents of Symptom Validity Assessment

Identified Pitfalls	Characteristics	Proposed Remedy
Amelioration (or Meliorativism)	Avoiding clear diagnostic statements about malingering and negative response bias; use of euphemistic or obscuring language.	Use clear and correct language; identify negative response bias when it is present according to diagnostic standards; do not try to obscure it.
Mythologism	Repeating traditional beliefs without questioning them in the light of accumulated empirical evidence.	Study carefully the rationality and the empirical basis of authority statements; do not repeat them in an uncritical way. Note that mythologism may, in fact, weaken the arguments used rather than strengthen them.
Pathologism	Detecting a disease or a mental disorder in all persons who claim symptoms or problems.	Accept the fact that there are healthy people and that healthy people may claim symptoms that cannot be confirmed; analyze the validity of claimed symptoms instead of accepting them at face value.
Authoritarianism	Considering the verdict of famous (mostly older) experts in the field as the highest degree of evidence, in neglect of accumulated empirical research and evidence-based assessment.	Remember what Douglas MacArthur said: "Old soldiers never die, they just fade away." In the end, evidence-based arguments will prevail.
Ignorism or global attack against psychology	Proclaiming generalized incompetence of psychologists in the field of forensic assessment.	The competence of a professional is not created by verdict. Have a close look at what psychologists and their arsenal of validated assessment methods may offer to improve the quality of differential diagnosis.
Trivialism	Assuming that psychological assessment can be done by anybody.	Remember that psychological assessment in general and symptom validity assessment in particular are complex professional tasks that require an adequate level of qualification.
Personal attack	Going beyond any rational argument and attacking your opponent personally.	Although this procedure may be very efficient in the short run, it will backfire. If there are no better arguments, refrain from scientific dispute.
False historicism	Evoking historical associations to underline ethical doubts about symptom validity assessment.	If history is called into the witness box, be careful to be historically correct. Consider that lessons from history may have been learned.
Pseudoethics	Applying ethical principles in a flawed, often populist way.	Analyze the ethical implications according to established bioethical principles (e.g., Bush, 2007; Bush, Connell, & Denney, 2006; Iverson, 2006).
Repetitivism	Assuming that a statement is true because it is made so often (e.g., that malingering is very rare).	Look for the empirical data that support or refute the claim.

sia without anterograde amnesia, with identified external incentives and below chance responding on a forced-choice SVT, a clinician may shy away from concluding that the results clearly indicate malingering and end up, instead, with the diagnosis of "dissociative amnesia." This failure can be characterized both in terms of ameliora-tion and pathologism. When the clinician then argues that, even if this may be a case of malingering, it was not his or her role to question the authenticity of the symptom claim, and he or she had to protect the patient's credibility by (wrongly) giving him a psychiatric diagnosis; the clinician may also be trapped in "pseudoethi-cal" considerations.

There is a legend holding that fraudulent, pure, and deliberate malingering is its most infrequent form and that it is truly rare. Instead, exaggeration of real symp-toms is the more common version of malingering. This hypothesis was formulated by Raecke (1919) and has been repeated many times (e.g., Braverman, 1978; Stone, 2009). Based on this traditional belief, it is sometimes argued that the whole database on negative response bias is flawed and does not reflect realities in European coun-tries or North America, but it epitomizes the errors of mythologism, "authoritarian-ism," and "repetitivism." The truth is that there is no sound methodological basis to determine what percentage of uncooperative patients' present *pure* forms of false symptom report or false symptom presentation. The basic problem is that in cases of uncooperativeness, it is often impossible to determine how much of the claimed symptomatology is authentic and how much is not. As a consequence, there is no reliable basis for estimating the base rate of *pure malingering* (Resnick, 1988). Today, the use of SVTs makes the task of identifying malingering a lot easier, although still it is not possible to prove based on sound methodology that all symptoms are malingered, even if it is proven that some are malingered. Forced-choice test scores that are significantly below chance provide the strongest evidence of intentional attempts to deceive the examiner.

CONCLUSIONS

It is fair to conclude that symptom validity assessment and the differential diagnosis of non-authentic symptom production remains an aspect of the field of neuropsychol-ogy, which, at times, is fiercely disputed both in the public and among clinical and forensic experts. Professionals may encounter different forms of resistance when they perform symptom validity assessment according to established standards of neuropsychology (e.g., Bush et al., 2005; Heilbronner et al., 2009). General recommen-dations for how to deal with resistance or personalized attacks are the following: (a) do not respond with the same strategy; (b) use sound and scientific arguments; and (c) favor evidence-based clinical and forensic assessment. In the end, logical argument and the empirical database will prevail.

There is a financial motivating factor that drives this symptom validity assess-ment process, and it will probably eventually lead to improved methods because of the scope and seriousness of the problem. Malingering is a multibillion-dollars-a-year problem for major institutions, agencies, and companies which provide financial support for those claiming impairment and disability. However, as methods for identifying invalid presentations and implausible disability claims become more ef-fective and more solidly research-based, the professionals who assess disability will face a looming ethical challenge. Should they face the facts now or continue to resist addressing the implications for their daily work of the voluminous research now available to support the use of symptom validity testing (Morgan and Sweet, 2009)? We strongly suggest the former.

REFERENCES

Allen, L. M., Conder, R., Green, P., & Cox, D. (1997) *Computerized assessment of response bias: A manual for computerized administration, reporting and interpretation*. Durham, NC: CogniSyst.

Allen, M. D., Bigler, E. D., Larsen, J., Goodrich-Hunsaker, N. J., & Hopkins, R. O. (2007). Functional neuroimaging evidence for high cognitive effort on the word memory test in the absence of external incentives. *Brain Injury*, 21(13–14), 1425–1428.

American Psychiatric Association. (2000). *Diagnostic and statistical manual of mental disorders* (4th ed., text rev.). Washington, DC: Author.

Armistead-Jehle, P. (2010). Symptom validity test performance in U.S. veterans referred for evaluation of mild TBI. *Applied Neuropsychology*, 17(1), 52–59.

Bianchini, K. J., Curtis, K. L., & Greve, K. W. (2006). Compensation and malingering in traumatic brain injury: A dose-response relationship? *The Clinical Neuropsychologist*, 20(4), 831–847.

Bianchini, K. J., Greve, K. W., & Glynn, G. (2005). On the diagnosis of malingered pain-related disability: Lessons from cognitive malingering research. *The Spine Journal*, 5(4), 404–417.

Blaskewitz, N., Merten, T., & Kathmann, N. (2008). Performance of children on symptom validity tests: TOMM, MSVT, and FIT. *Archives of Clinical Neuropsychology*, 23(4), 379–391.

Bowden, S. C., Shores, E. A., & Mathias, J. L. (2006). Does effort suppress cognition after traumatic brain injury? A re-examination of the evidence for the word memory test. *Clinical Neuropsychology*, 20(4), 858–872.

Braverman, M. (1978). Post-injury malingering is seldom a calculated ploy. *Occupational Health & Safety*, 47(2), 36–48.

Brockhaus, R. & Merten, T. (2004). Neuropsychologische Diagnostik suboptimalen Leistungsverhaltens mit dem word memory test [Diagnosing suboptimal effort with the word memory test]. *Der Nervenarzt*, 75(9), 882–887.

Bush, S. S. (2007). Ethische Aspekte der Diagnostik der Beschwerdenvalidität [Ethical considerations in symptom validity assessment]. *Praxis der Rechtspsychologie*, 17, 63–82.

Bush, S. S., Connell, M. A., & Denney, R. L. (2006). *Ethical practice in forensic psychology: A systematic model for decision making*. Washington, DC: American Psychological Association.

Bush, S. S., Ruff, R. M., Tröster, A. I., Barth, J. T., Koffler, S. P., Pliskin, N. H., . . . Silver, C. H. (2005). Symptom validity assessment: Practice issues and medical necessity NAN policy & planning committee. *Archives of Clinical Neuropsychology*, 20(4), 419–426.

Carone, D. A. (2008). Children with moderate/severe brain damage/dysfunction outperform adults with mild-to-no brain damage on the medical symptom validity test. *Brain Injury*, 22(12), 960–971.

Celinski, M., & Tyndel, M. (1988). Pseudo-dementia: A failure to recover from a mild head injury. *Rehabilitation Research/Recherche en Readaptation*, 29–39.

Chafetz, M. D. (2008). Malingering on the social security disability consultative exam: Predictors and base rates. *The Clinical Neuropsychologist*, 22(3), 529–546.

Chafetz, M. D., Prentkowski, E., & Rao, A. (2011). To work or not to work: Motivation (not low IQ) determines symptom validity test findings. *Archives of Clinical Neuropsychology*, 26(4), 306–313.

Cima, M., Nijman, H., Merckelbach, H., Kremer, K., & Hollnack, S. (2004). Claims of crime-related amnesia in forensic patients. *International Journal of Law and Psychiatry*, 27(3), 215–221.

Constantinou, M., Bauer, L., Ashendorf, L., Fisher, J. M., & McCaffrey, R. J. (2005). Is poor performance on recognition memory effort measures indicative of generalized poor performance on neuropsychological tests? *Archives of Clinical Neuropsychology*, 20(2), 191–198.

Demakis, G. J., Gervais, R. O., & Rohling, M. L. (2008). The effect of failure on cognitive and psychological symptom validity tests in litigants with symptoms of post-traumatic stress disorder. *The Clinical Neuropsychologist*, 22(5), 879–895.

Drane, D. L., Williamson, D. J., Stroup, E. S., Holmes, M. D., Jung, M., Koerner, E., . . . Miller, J. W. (2006). Cognitive impairment is not equal in patients with epileptic and psychogenic nonepileptic seizures. *Epilepsia*, 47(11), 1879–1886.

Flaro, L., Green, P., & Robertson, E. (2007). Word memory test failure 23 times higher in mild brain injury than in parents seeking custody: The power of external incentives. *Brain Injury*, 21(4), 373–383.

Fox, D. D. (2011). Symptom validity test failure indicates invalidity of neuropsychological tests. *The Clinical Neuropsychologist*, 25(3), 488–495.

Fox59 Sports Staff. (2011). *Manning admits scoring low on baseline concussion tests.* Retrieved from http://www.fox59.com/news/wxin-peyton-manning-manning-admits-scoring-low-on-baseline-concussion-tests-20110427,0,6104131.story

Gervais, R., Green, P., Allen, L. M., & Iverson, G. (2001). Effects of coaching on symptom validity testing in chronic pain patients presenting for disability assessments. *Journal of Forensic Neuropsychology,* 2(2), 1–19.

Gervais, R. O., Rohling, M. L., Green, P., & Ford, W. (2004). A comparison of WMT, CARB, and TOMM failure rates in non-head injury disability claimants. *Archives of Clinical Neuropsychology,* 19(4), 475–487.

Gervais, R. O., Russell, A. S., Green, P., Allen, L. M. III, Ferrari, R., & Pieschl, S. D. (2001). Effort testing in patients with fibromyalgia and disability incentives. *The Journal of Rheumatology,* 28(8), 1892–1899.

Giger, P., Merten, T., & Merckelbach, H. (2011). Tatbezogene Amnesien—authentisch oder vorgetäuscht? [Crime-related amnesia: Real or feigned?] *Fortschritte der Neurologie-Psychiatrie,* 80(7).

Gill, D., Green, P., Flaro, L., & Pucci, T. (2007). The role of effort testing in independent medical examinations. *The Medico-Legal Journal,* 75(Pt. 2), 64–71.

Goodrich-Hunsaker, N. J., & Hopkins, R. O. (2009). Word memory test performance in amnesic patients with hippocampal damage. *Neuropsychology,* 23(4), 529–534.

Green, P. (1987). Interference between the two ears and the effects of an earplug in psychiatric and cerebral-lesioned patients. In Takahashi et al. (Eds.), *Cerebral dynamics, laterality and psychopathology.* Holland, The Netherlands: Elsevier.

Green, P. (2003, revised 2005). *Manual for the word memory test.* Edmonton, Canada: Green's Publishing.

Green, P. (2004). *Manual for the medical symptom validity test.* Edmonton, Canada: Green's Publishing.

Green, P. (2007). The pervasive influence of effort on neuropsychological tests. *Physical Medicine and Rehabilitation Clinics of North America,* 18(1), 43–68.

Green, P. (2008). *Manual for the nonverbal medical symptom validity test.* Edmonton, Canada: Green's Publishing.

Green, P. (2009). *WMT profiles in children with a FSIQ of 50 to 70. Unpublished summary of data from Dr. Lloyd Flaro.* Retrieved from http://wordmemorytest.com/DISCUSSIONS/WMT_profiles_in_children_with_a_FSIQ_of_50_to_70.doc

Green, P. (2011). Comparison between the test of memory malingering (TOMM) and the nonverbal medical symptom validity test (NV-MSVT) in adults with disability claims. *Applied Neuropsychology,* 18(1), 18–26.

Green, P., & Astner, K. (1995). *Manual for the oral word memory test.* Durham, NC: Cognisyst.

Green, P., & Flaro, L. (2003). Word memory test performance in children. *Child Neuropsychology,* 9(3), 189–207.

Green, P., Flaro, L., Brockhaus, R., & Montijo, J. (2012). Performance on the WMT, MSVT, & NV-MSVT in children with developmental disabilities and in adults with mild traumatic brain injury. In C. R. Reynolds & A. Horton (Eds.) *Detection of Malingering During Head Injury Litigation* (2nd ed). New York, NY: Plenum Press.

Green, P., Iverson, G. L., & Allen, L. (1999). Detecting malingering in head injury litigation with the word memory test. *Brain Injury,* 13(10), 813–819.

Green, P., & Kotenko, V. (1980). Superior speech comprehension in schizophrenics under monaural versus binaural listening conditions. *Journal of Abnormal Psychology,* 89(3), 399–408.

Green, P., Rohling, M., Lees-Haley, P., & Allen, L. M. III, (2001). Effort has a greater effect on test scores than severe brain injury in compensation claimants. *Brain Injury,* 15(12), 1045–1060.

Greiffenstein, M., Baker, W., & Gola, T. (1994). Validation of malingered amnesia measures with a large clinical sample. *Psychological Assessment,* 6, 218–224.

Harrison, A. (2006). Adults faking ADHD: You must be kidding! *The ADHD report,* 14(4), 1–7.

Heilbronner, R. L., Sweet, J. J., Morgan, J. E., Larrabee, G. J., & Millis, S. R. (2009). American Academy of Clinical Neuropsychology consensus conference statement on the neuropsychological assessment of effort, response bias, and malingering. *The Clinical Neuropsychologist,* 23(7), 1093–1129.

Henry, M., Merten, T., Wolf, S. A., & Harth, S. (2010). Nonverbal medical symptom validity test performance of elderly healthy adults and clinical neurology patients. *Journal of Clinical and Experimental Neuropsychology,* 32(1), 19–27.

Howe, L., Anderson, A., Kaufman, D., Sachs, B., & Loring, D. (2007). Characterization of the medical symptom validity test in evaluation of clinically referred memory disorders clinic patients. *Archives of Clinical Neuropsychology,* 22(6), 753–761.

Howe, L., & Loring, D. (2009). Classification accuracy and predictive ability of the medical symptom validity test's dementia profile and general memory impairment profile. *The Clinical Neuropsychologist,* 23(2), 329–342.

Iverson, G. L. (2005). Outcome from mild traumatic brain injury. *Current Opinion in Psychiatry*, 18(3), 301–317.

Iverson, G. L. (2006). Ethical issues associated with the assessment of exaggeration, poor effort, and malingering. *Applied Neuropsychology*, 13(2), 77–90.

Iverson, G., Green, P., & Gervais, R. (1999). Using the word memory test to detect biased responding in head injury litigation. *The Journal of Cognitive Rehabilitation*, 17(2), 4–8.

Knapp, S., & VandeCreek, L. (2003). An overview of the major changes in the 2002 APA Ethics Code. *Professional Psychology, Research and Practice*, 34(3), 301–308.

Larrabee, G. J. (2003). Detection of malingering using atypical performance patterns on standard neuropsychological tests. *The Clinical Neuropsychologist*, 17(3), 410–425.

Larrabee, G. J., Millis, S. R., & Meyers, J. E. (2009). 40 plus or minus 10, a new magical number: Reply to Russell. *The Clinical Neuropsychologist*, 23(5), 841–849.

Loring, D. W., Marino, S. E., Drane, D. L., Parfitt, D., Finney, G. R., & Meador, K. J. (2011). Lorazepam effects on word memory test performance: A randomized, double-blind, placebo-controlled, crossover trial. *The Clinical Neuropsychologist*, 25(5), 789–811.

McClintock, S. M., Husain, M. M., Greer, T. L.& Cullum, C. M. (2010). Association between depression severity and neurocognitive function in major depressive disorder: A review and synthesis. *Neuropsychology*, 24(1), 9–34.

Merten, T., Bossink, L., & Schmand, B., (2007). On the limits of effort testing: Symptom validity tests and severity of neurocognitive symptoms in nonlitigant patients. *Journal of Clinical and Experimental Neuropsychology*, 29(3), 308–318.

Meyers, J. E., Volbrecht, M., Axelrod, B. N., & Reinsch-Boothby, L. (2011). Embedded symptom validity tests and overall neuropsychological test performance. *Archives of Clinical Neuropsychology*, 26(1), 8–15.

Morgan, J., & Sweet, J. J. (Eds.). (2009). *Neuropsychology of malingering casebook*. New York, NY: Psychology Press.

Pujol, M., & Kopelman, M. D. (2003). Psychogenic amnesia. *Practical Neurology*, 3(5), 292–299.

Raecke, J. (1919). Ueber aggravation und simulation geistiger störung [About exaggeration and malingering of mental disorder]. *European Archives of Psychiatry and Clinical Neuroscience*, 60, 521–603.

Resnick, P. (1988). Malingering of posttraumatic disorders. In R. Rogers (Ed.), *Clinical assessment of malingering and deception* (pp. 84–103). New York, NY: Guilford Press.

Richman, J., Green, P., Gervais, R., Flaro, L., Merten, T., Brockhaus, R., & Ranks, D. (2006). Objective tests of symptom exaggeration in independent medical examinations. *Journal of Occupational and Environmental Medicine*, 48(3), 303–311.

Rohling, M., Binder, L., Demakis, G., Larrabee, G., Ploetz, D., & Langhinrichsen-Rohling, J. (2011). A meta-analysis of neuropsychological outcome after mild traumatic brain injury: Re-analyses and reconsiderations of Binder etal. (1997), Frencham etal. (2005), and Pertab etal. (2009). *The Clinical Neuropsychologist*, 25(4), 608–623.

Rohling, M. L., & Demakis, G. J. (2010). Bowden, Shores, & Mathias (2006): Failure to replicate or just failure to notice. Does effort still account for more variance in neuropsychological test scores than TBI severity? *The Clinical Neuropsychology*, 24(1), 119–136.

Rohling, M. L., Green, P., Allen, L. M. III & Iverson, G. L. (2002). Depressive symptoms and neurocognitive test scores in patients passing symptom validity tests. *Archives of Clinical Neuropsychology*, 17(3), 205–222.

Singhal, A., Green, P., Ashaye, K., Shankar, K., & Gill, D. (2009). High specificity of the medical symptom validity test in patients with very severe memory impairment. *Archives of Clinical Neuropsychology*, 24(8), 721–728.

Slick, D. J., Sherman, E. M., & Iverson, G. L. (1999). Diagnostic criteria for malingered neurocognitive dysfunction: Proposed standards for clinical practice and research. *The Clinical Neuropsychologist*, 13(4), 545–561.

Slick, D. J., Tan, J. E., Strauss, E., Mateer, C. A., Harnadek, M., & Sherman, E. M. (2003). Victoria symptom validity test scores of patients with profound memory impairment: Nonlitigants case studies. *Clinical Neuropsychology*, 17(3), 390–394.

Social Security Administration. (2010). *Summary of performance and financial information*. Retrieved from http://www.ssa.gov/finance

Stevens, A., Friedel, E., Mehren, G., & Merten, T. (2008). Malingering and uncooperativeness in psychiatric and psychological assessment: Prevalence and effects in a German sample of claimants. *Psychiatry Research*, 157(1–3), 191–200.

Stone, J. (2009). The bare essentials: Functional symptoms in neurology. *Neurology in Practice*, 9, 179–189

Sullivan, B. K., May, K., & Galbally, L. (2007). Symptom exaggeration by college adults in attention-deficit hyperactivity disorder and learning disorder assessments. *Applied Neuropsychology*, 14(3), 189–207.

Sweet, J. J. (2009). Forensic bibliography: Effort/malingering and other common forensic topics encountered by clinical neuropsychologists. In J. E. Morgan & J. J. Sweet (Eds.), *Neuropsychology of malingering casebook*. New York, NY: Psychology Press.

Tombaugh, T. (1996). *Test of memory malingering*. Toronto, Canada: Multi Health Systems.

Veiel, H. O. (1997). A preliminary profile of neuropsychological deficits associated with major depression. *Journal of Clinical and Experimental Neuropsychology*, 19(4), 587–603.

Wetter, M. W., & Corrigan, S. K. (1995) Providing information to clients about psychological tests: A survey of attorney's and law students' attitudes. *Professional Psychology: Research and Practice*, 26(5), 474–477.

Wilkinson, R., & Pickett, K. (2010). *The spirit level: Why equality is better for everyone*. London, United Kingdom: Penguin Books.

Youngjohn, J. R. (1995). Confirmed attorney coaching prior to neuropsychological evaluation. *Assessment*, 2(3), 279–283.

Providing Feedback on Symptom Validity, Mental Health, and Treatment in Mild Traumatic Brain Injury

6

Dominic A. Carone, Shane S. Bush, & Grant L. Iverson

Evidence-based assessment of symptom validity is an important component of clinical and forensic neuropsychological evaluations (Bush et al., 2005; Heilbronner et al., 2009). Descriptions of symptom validity are most valuable when they are written in clear, unambiguous terms and use probabilistic language as appropriate (Iverson, 2003, 2010). Professional ethics require psychologists to provide feedback regarding assessment results to patients, unless the nature of the relationship prohibits such feedback and the examinee has been informed of that fact at the outset of the evaluation process (American Psychological Association [APA], 2002, Ethical Standard 9.10, "Explaining Assessment Results"). However, when assessment findings indicate that patients might have underperformed on testing and/or exaggerated symptoms and problems, neuropsychologists may find the discussion of such findings to be uncomfortable and challenging.

Carone, Iverson, and Bush (2010) presented a model on how to approach and provide feedback to patients about invalid test performance in clinical neuropsychological evaluations. The symptom validity feedback model consists of the following three phases: building rapport and obtaining informed consent, completing the evaluation and preliminary discussions, and the feedback session. The model was designed to be applicable to any diagnostic group but was largely developed from our work with patients reporting persisting symptoms after known or suspected mild traumatic brain injury (MTBI). This focus is reasonable because MTBI is the diagnostic group that is most likely to present with symptom validity failure, exaggeration, and/or malingering, according to a survey of board certified neuropsychologists (Mittenberg, Patton, Canyock, & Condit, 2002).

When working with patients who report longstanding problems following an MTBI, symptom validity test failure is one of many potential complex issues that might need to be addressed in a feedback session. These issues include (a) differential diagnosis; (b) possible misattribution of nonspecific symptoms to brain injury by the patient and/or other health care providers (Ferguson, Mittenberg, Barone, & Schneider, 1999; Gunstad & Suhr, 2001; Mittenberg, DiGiulio, Perrin, & Bass, 1992); (c) inaccurate information regarding the severity and course of MTBI (McCrea, 2008); (d) steadfast belief by the patient that he or she has suffered an "invisible injury" (i.e., one with no objective biomarkers or external signs of injury) that is disabling (Kennedy, Cullen, Amador, Huey, & Leal, 2010); (e) strong investment in one's identity as a "brain injury survivor" (Rozek Law Office, 2011); (f) self-validation of the seriousness of the injury and persistence of brain injury symptoms by citing media reports on military and sports concussion that are either misleading or inapplicable to the patient's case; (g) disenchantment and anger toward health care providers who have not validated the belief that brain injury is the primary or only cause of symptom persistence (Iverson, Zasler, & Lange, 2007); (h) frustration with, and anger toward, the insurance and legal systems; (i) the presence of comorbid psychiatric diagnoses (e.g., major depressive disorder: Iverson, 2006b); medical diagnoses (e.g., whiplash, chronic pain; Iverson & McCracken, 1997), and/or significant psychosocial stressors that contribute to symptom reporting; (Iverson, et al., 2007); (j) lack of mental health care despite extensive medical treatment; (k) overuse of medications and use of treatments that lack clinical validation (Department of Veterans Affairs & Department of Defense, 2009); (l) overuse of sensory reduction devices (e.g., sunglasses); (m) significant restrictions of independent activities imposed by the patient or well-meaning health care providers; and (n) excessive time off from work or other responsibilities in the context of compensation seeking (Reynolds, Paniak, Toller-Lobe, & Nagy, 2003).

These complex issues are often described in the reports of forensic neuropsychological evaluations, independent medical evaluations, or disability evaluations referred by nonclinical third parties (e.g., insurance companies, attorneys). However, they are not as easily written about or discussed with patients in the context of clinical neuropsychological evaluations referred by health care providers. Invalid symptom validity performance in clinical contexts is sometimes euphemistically and inaccurately described in reports and feedback sessions and is sometimes omitted entirely because of personal discomfort, fear of upsetting the patient or referral source, or fear of patient complaints to the provider and/or oversight authorities (Carone et al., 2010; Resnick, 1988; Ruff, Wylie, & Tennant, 1993). However, we believe that it is important to provide feedback about these issues to patients and to explain the issues in the neuropsychological report when they arise during clinical neuropsychological evaluations because they inform proper case conceptualization and diagnosis and have significant implications for management and treatment strategies.

In this chapter, we review our symptom validity feedback model and present updated information. We then describe our feedback approach with patients reporting persisting symptoms after MTBI. It is important to note that our feedback models are intended for use in clinical contexts and are not designed for evaluations performed for forensic purposes or for other nonclinical third parties.

INITIAL CONTACT WITH THE PATIENT

For effective feedback to take place, it is important to try to establish a good working relationship with the patient at the initial point of contact. After the evaluation has been scheduled, but before physically meeting the patient, we suggest sending the patient an informational brochure or pamphlet that describes the nature of the evaluation, including the anticipated length of the session(s), report turnaround time, whether to take medications as prescribed, and other frequently asked questions. This initial information can serve to relieve some anxiety about the evaluation before the patient arrives, because our experience is that most patients do not fully understand what a neuropsychological evaluation is or why they have been referred. This early step also helps show patients that you are interested in communicating with them before actually meeting with them. However, in some cases, patients do not read the information or they state they never received it, which means that the first contact is on the appointment date, when Phase 1 begins.

Phase 1: Building Rapport and Obtaining Informed Consent

The initial phase involves establishing rapport and obtaining informed consent. This phase is the most important because it is designed to establish a sense of openness, confidence, and trust in the provider while also helping to establish proper boundaries. This relationship is particularly important with patients who have chronic symptoms following an uncomplicated MTBI because, as previously noted, they sometimes feel resentment toward prior health care providers who have been (or were perceived to have been) quickly dismissive of the notion that their problems are neurologically based. As a result, some patients may feel the need to prove that they are neurologically compromised, and initially be wary, anxious, and/or mistrustful when meeting a new health care provider. If patients do not feel like they are being heard or understood, they will not trust the neuropsychologist, rapport will not develop (Vanderploeg & Belanger, 2009), and the patient will likely not trust the feedback when the evaluation is completed. In this sense, our model tries to improve patient responsiveness by conveying Rogerian warmth, genuineness, and understanding (Rogers, 1951). It is impractical to expect that one cannot successfully apply the feedback methods described later in our model if this initial phase is skipped or quickly glossed over.

When the patient arrives, we begin with a welcoming greeting, handshake, and some brief small talk to put the patient at ease. When beginning to segue to the informed consent process, it can be helpful to ask patients what their understanding is regarding why they have been referred for the evaluation. This question immediately shows patients that you are interested in their input, and the responses provided can help to quickly clarify misconceptions that may need to be addressed immediately. For example, one patient stated that the only reason he came for an evaluation was because he wanted a doctor's note stating he could not be evicted from his apartment because of a brain injury. Some patients report that their attorney encouraged the referral. Intervening at the outset regarding these types of issues helps triage patients to more appropriate providers (e.g., physician for injury documentation; forensic neuropsychologist for an independent evaluation). This triaging decreases the likelihood that the patient will be angry and upset after the evaluation is completed if they do not receive the desired outcome.

Once a determination has been made that referral for a clinical neuropsychological evaluation is appropriate, we then proceed to the informed consent process. We suggest summarizing the contents of the consent form or reading the consent form to patients in a conversational tone rather than handing it to them to quickly read and sign.[1] Although more time-consuming, this process provides the neuropsychologist with an opportunity to explain the nature of the evaluation in more detail (e.g., time commitment, types of abilities assessed and tests used, normative groups against which their results will be compared), convey that patient comfort is a priority (i.e., discussion of rest breaks, locations of bathrooms and vending machines), inform them of potential benefits (e.g., objective data, diagnostic clarification, possible treatment strategies), inform them of the importance of responding honestly and putting forth their best effort, and inform them of potential risks. Potential risks include the development of headaches, fatigue, and emotional distress; disagreement with existing diagnoses or assumptions that they hold about the cause of their problems; and a negative or neutral effect on compensation claims, disability applications, or lawsuits. Explaining these risks at the outset also helps triage patients to forensic

---

[1] For a sample informed consent form, contact the first author at caroned@upstate.edu

neuropsychologists if it becomes clear that they are primarily interested in the legal aspects, as opposed to the clinical aspects, of their case.

One aspect of the informed consent process for which consensus among clinicians is lacking involves whether to warn patients that techniques will be used to detect poor effort or exaggeration, because providing this warning might result in the patient taking a more sophisticated approach to trying to appear impaired when they are not (Youngjohn, Lees-Haley, & Binder, 1999). However, some take the position that a warning legitimately reduces the rate of malingering (Johnson & Lesniak-Karpiak, 1997), although this can depend on the degree of warning provided (i.e., subtle vs. overt) (Schenk & Sullivan, 2010). In addition, some researchers have found that certain effort-detecting methods (e.g., pattern of performance) are resistant (or relatively resistant) to the effects of coaching (Greub & Suhr, 2006; Suhr & Gunstad, 2000; Suhr, Gunstad, Greub, & Barrash, 2004).

Given these concerns and the mixed findings in the literature, our model encourages neuropsychologists to inform patients that they are expected to try their best and answer questions honestly, that there are "ways"[2] this will be evaluated, and that this topic will be commented upon in the final report. However, we do not mention any specifics about the ways symptom validity will be measured and make no mention of specific tests of effort or symptom validity (Boone, 2007; Iverson, 2006a). For all the patient knows, the way effort may be evaluated is by behavioral observation only, and some patients may believe the neuropsychologist is bluffing. An example of text that could be included in a consent form is as follows:

> It is important that you put forth your best effort and answer questions honestly. If your test performance suggests you are not putting forth your best effort or you are exaggerating symptoms, that situation can invalidate the test results and lead to inconclusive findings. This topic will be assessed and commented upon in the final report. If you do not think you can put forth your best effort during testing, please inform us immediately.

Once the consent process has been completed and testing has begun, rapport continues to be fostered; yet patients will also be aware that they are engaged in an evaluative process with inherent risks. Of course, patients are free to rescind their consent to be evaluated at any point during the examination. For patients who lack the cognitive capacity to provide consent, their assent (i.e., willingness to participate) is obtained and documented, consistent with APA (2002) Ethical Standard 3.10 (Informed Consent).

Phase 2: Completing the Evaluation and Preliminary Discussions (On the Day of Testing)

If sufficient evidence exists to indicate invalid performance, we suggest that the neuropsychologist initially explore how willing the patient is to acknowledge poor or variable effort when the testing is completed (i.e., prior to the patient leaving). However, this is a challenging undertaking because patients will rarely state that they put forth "poor effort" or "did not try my best" because these phrases have a negative personal connotation. For the same reason, we avoid specific inquiries about "faking," "lying," or "putting on a show" because these terms and phrases are

---

[2] Some neuropsychologists might use the expression "certain methods and procedures" for evaluating the accuracy of the test results.

accusatory, emotionally laden, and indicate that something socially unacceptable or immoral has occurred. Although these terms may accurately apply to a particular patient, it is important to help the patient feel comfortable enough to discuss this sensitive topic.

To facilitate a more open discussion, we utilize a variation of a cognitive restructuring technique (Mahoney & Arnkoff, 1978) that leads patients to think differently about a particular topic (i.e., poor effort) so as to alter the resultant emotional reaction. Specifically, we have found that patients are comfortable acknowledging that they "disengaged," were "not fully invested," or did not "stay motivated" on all of the tests. There are various ways to approach this topic, depending on the patient. Recounting behavioral observations and/or patient statements during the evaluation can be helpful in facilitating this discussion. For example, in cases where the patient displayed clear signs of frustration during testing (e.g., sighing, head shaking, negative self-statements), the following dialogue may ensue:

EXAMINER: There were several times during testing when you seemed to get very frustrated (anxious or upset). Do you remember that?

PATIENT: Yes. I did not think I was doing well, and some of those tests made me feel stupid.

EXAMINER: You seemed to be overwhelmed at times.

PATIENT: Yes, I was.

EXAMINER: So, can it be that when you feel overwhelmed, frustrated, or "stupid," you disengage somewhat from the task you are working on?

PATIENT: Yes, I think so.

In other cases, where there is no strong behavioral evidence of frustration or other ways to easily lead into the discussion, a way to broach this topic is to employ subjective task difficulty ratings once the examination is complete (Carone, 2008). This technique requires asking patients to rate the difficulty of memory tests and effort tests on a 10-point scale, with 10 being the most difficult. The effort tests are not described as such to the patient but the task is merely described (e.g., the test when you did such and such). Carone (2008) reported that adults with known or suspected MTBI who fail effort testing rated effort tests as much more difficult than those who pass (mean rating = 5.6 compared to 2.0; $SD = 1.3$ for both groups). This process gives the examiner the opportunity to ask what made the patient perceive the task as so difficult, which then leads to discussions of frustration and task disengagement. In some cases, however, an open-ended inquiry about task disengagement may need to ensue if there is no easy segue into the topic.

Obtaining acknowledgment about task disengagement is helpful because task disengagement might underlie effort test failure for many people, regardless of the etiology (e.g., malingering, oppositional attitude, severe apathy). The examiner can always choose to agree or disagree with the patient's stated reason for task disengagement (e.g., malingering vs. frustration), but the key is that the patient acknowledged that poor effort occurred. Such an acknowledgment can later be noted in the neuropsychological report and allows the examiner to discuss poor effort more freely in the feedback session because it has already been acknowledged. If the patient is unwilling to make this acknowledgment, our approach is to make a note of this and try to broach the topic again during a later feedback session.

When possible, we suggest holding the full feedback session on a date separate from the test administration so that the neuropsychologist has time to integrate all of the available information and consider how to best approach the particular issues of the case with the patient. However, there may be instances (e.g., patient lives very far away, urgency to a clinical situation) in which this scheduling option may not be possible. In such instances, the techniques described in Phase 3 can be applied immediately after testing has been completed.

Phase 3: The Feedback Session

This section describes general recommendations for the feedback session that can be tailored to individual cases. The authors acknowledge that every case is different and that there is no feedback model that can account for all of the wide-ranging situations that clinicians may encounter.

When patients arrive for feedback sessions, they may do so with considerable anxiety. For this reason, we suggest beginning the feedback session with social niceties to put the patient at ease. In some instances, examiners may then want to ask, "So, what were you expecting me to say today about your test performance?" or "How do you think you did on the testing?" This questioning again shows patients that they are being listened to, and it can help to quickly reduce anxiety. In our experience, some patients' initial concerns are that hyperbolic terms such as "crazy," "nuts," or "brain-dead," will be applied to them, or that a recommendation will be made to "lock me up." These concerns are quickly eliminated by emphasizing to patients that no such terms are used and that, with the exceptions involving harm to oneself or others, no such recommendations will be made. In most cases, however, patients state that they do not know what to expect and that they are open to hearing what the examiner has to say. Hearing this openness from the patient can be reassuring to the examiner (who may also be anxious about the feedback session), which in turn can make the feedback session easier and more pleasant for both parties.

If prior to the examiner's feedback the patient happens to raise a concern about a legitimate issue that is written about in the report, such as the presence of low cognitive test scores, we suggest acknowledging the concerns and saying something along the lines of, "All right, we are going to discuss your test scores in detail soon and go over what they mean." However, we also suggest adding, if true, something positive to this message such as "But don't worry, the scores are not as low as you may think" or "There may not be as many low scores as you think." If there are numerous low scores because of poor effort, it is often helpful to say something such as "There were some low scores, which is the bad news, but the good news is I think the scores could have been much better." The key at this initial point of the feedback session is to not only acknowledge the patient's stated concern(s) but to also provide reassurance.

For examiners who do not provide patients a copy of their report, the next step can be skipped. However, if the examiner is comfortable sharing their reports with patients, we suggest orienting the patient to the neuropsychological report. This process involves displaying a hard copy of the report and flipping through the pages sequentially, pointing to the various sections but not leaving enough time for them to read much of the content. The point of this exercise is to show the patient that a thorough and comprehensive document has been produced that combines an integration of interview data, medical records review, behavioral observations, and test data that all served as the basis for the conclusions and recommendations. This process is another aspect of the feedback session that can make the patient more receptive to the information provided.

The patient is informed that there is no need to review the history section of the report in detail at this point but that any relevant aspects from the history that helped form the conclusions will be discussed later in the session. Depending on the case, the examiner may not wish to visibly display the impression section or table of test results because the patient may quickly become upset at seeing a psychiatric diagnosis, a strong statement regarding poor effort or exaggeration, or test score interpretation. In cases where this is a particular concern, we suggest simply informing the patient that these sections are included but will be discussed later and then quickly displaying the section that narratively describes the test results and recommendations. The total time it takes to flip through the report with the patient should be relatively quick (i.e., less than a minute). The patient is then informed that the feedback is going to focus on the test results, interpretation, and recommendations. Although we describe a process of quickly orienting patients to their report, some clinicians may choose, after providing verbal feedback, to allow patients to read the report while in the office. This opportunity eliminates surprises when they get home, gives patients a chance to identify any factual errors in the history, and affords clinicians the opportunity to provide further clarification, particularly involving any professional jargon that was used.

When discussing effort test failure with patients, we utilize variants of the "bad news, good news approach" described earlier. That is, the "bad news" is that there were low test scores, but the "good news" is that there is evidence that the patient is capable of much better performance.

Although some neuropsychologists are opposed to providing any information to patients regarding symptom validity and how such determinations are made, our view is that patients seen in a clinical context have a right to know the results and conclusions of the evaluation and, *in general*, how such conclusions were made. However, when speaking with patients we agree that the examiner should make every attempt to avoid identifying the *specific* effort tests or methods that were used to assess symptom validity. When discussing the symptom validity issues, the patient is reassured that decisions about the validity of test scores are based largely on objective data as opposed to a subjective opinion (although subjective impressions can certainly play a role).

One method of discussing effort test failure in general terms, particularly with patients with chronic symptoms following an MTBI, is to ask them if they would agree that they should be more intellectually capable than a severely impaired clinical group (e.g., children with severe TBIs or older adults with advanced Alzheimer's disease). We have never had an instance where a patient who presents following an MTBI disagrees with this statement. This subjective comparison by the patient sets the stage for the next step, which is to inform the patient that his or her performance on some tests was so low that it was worse than patients in these severely impaired clinical groups. Displaying a visual aid comparing the patient's performance to these clinical groups can be a good way to convey this information (see Carone et al., 2010, Figure 1, for a sample visual aid).

Although the feedback model for invalid test performance is being presented separately from the MTBI feedback model described later, in reality, aspects of both models should be integrated. Thus, the next step involves explaining that because the history does not suggest the presence of a neurological condition that could explain such low performance, there must be other explanations. This is where incorporating information about expected MTBI recovery patterns can be helpful. The key at this point is to emphasize that examination results should be in accordance with the degree of neuropathology present, not in far excess of it (Larrabee, 1990, 1997; Stewart-Patterson, in press).

Lastly, the patient is informed that the other good news is that their test scores and perceived cognitive functioning will likely improve if they take some specific steps to address the factors that adversely affected his or her test performance. The patient can be informed that there are other patients (e.g., chronic severe TBI, multiple sclerosis) who do not have modifiable factors and have numerous areas of cognitive impairment that are permanent. It is conveyed as good news that they are not like these patients, while also emphasizing that you are not minimizing their reported distress. For patients who fail effort testing, a referral for psychotherapy may be made to improve coping, stress management, emotional stability, and motivation. This referral is particularly important for patients reporting persistent symptoms after MTBI who have typically not received evidence-supported psychotherapy (for anxiety, stress, depression, insomnia, or chronic pain) despite numerous medical visits for months to years. Referral for social worker services and case management may also be needed depending on the patient's available resources and the severity of psychosocial stressors. Despite these suggestions, it is unknown whether patients who fail effort testing are less likely to benefit from psychotherapy or other services (e.g., social work) than those who pass. Thus, psychotherapy for patients with the most dramatic form of effort test failure (e.g., worse than chance performance on effort testing) might be of little benefit to the patient and may not be an appropriate use of valuable resources.

In cases where there are known neurological factors that can lead to genuine cognitive impairment, yet effort tests are failed for reasons that are believed to be non-neurological, that patient is informed that cognitive impairment may be present but that the degree of such impairment cannot be precisely determined. It is noted that the obtained test scores are considered a reflection of the minimum level of the patient's true abilities, and an emphasis is again placed on addressing non-neurological factors.

Although clinicians have differing opinions on whether and when to use the term "malingering" in a neuropsychological report, use of the term malingering during a feedback session is especially challenging. We usually do not use the term malingering in clinical reports.[3] When used, it is often in a list of factors or differential diagnoses that might underlie the patient's exaggerated symptoms and suboptimal effort.[4] We will write that the results of the evaluation were confounded by poor effort and exaggeration. Using the term malingering for exaggerated symptoms and/or poor effort implies that we feel confident that the behavior is volitional and goal-directed. Therefore, our approach is to reserve use of the term for cases in which the convergence of evidence provides a high degree of diagnostic confidence (Tombaugh, 1996), couch the term in probabilistic language (Slick, Sherman, & Iverson, 1999), and emphasize that malingering does not always equate to feigning a nonexis-

---

[3] There are ways to write, clearly and unequivocally, that the results of the evaluation are not valid without using the term malingering. When there is strong evidence of suboptimal effort and symptom exaggeration, a clinician might use phrasing such as "I was unable to conduct a reliable and accurate evaluation of Mr. Smith's cognitive functioning. During this evaluation, there was strong evidence that he was providing poor effort. He appeared to be deliberately choosing wrong answers. As such, the test results are not valid. The results seriously underestimate his true cognitive abilities. In addition, there was evidence that he might have been over endorsing and exaggerating symptoms during psychological testing. As such, the results of the psychological testing have limited reliability and validity. Obviously, poor effort and possible exaggeration make it very difficult to accurately evaluate him."

[4] A clinician might write: "During this evaluation, there was considerable evidence of exaggerated symptoms and problems. There was also evidence of poor effort during testing. In any case involving significant exaggeration, there are several potential underlying explanations, causes, or motives, including frank psychosis, severe depression, a conversion disorder, a deep-rooted psychological need to be seen as sick and disabled (i.e., a factitious disorder), an extremely negative self-perception, a personality disorder, or malingering. Regardless of the underlying motivation, the presence of major exaggeration and poor effort makes it impossible to determine the true nature and extent of his psychiatric, psychological, or neurocognitive problems, and resultant disability (if any), through this evaluation."

tent condition for secondary gain (e.g., pure malingering) (Iverson, 2006a; Resnick, 1988). Most cases of malingering involve the intentional exaggeration, for an external incentive, of symptoms of a condition that actually exists or existed in the past (e.g., partial malingering). We suggest that the term malingering be used after the examiner has had a chance to explain the objective basis for the conclusions (e.g., failure on multiple effort tests, behavioral abnormalities, and inconsistencies). A sample explanation after explaining all of this information may go like this:

> The presence of all of these factors strongly indicates that there are times that you were aware of the correct answer and provided the wrong one. This behavior sometimes occurs when people are particularly concerned about their lawsuit or a disability evaluation. There is a technical term we use for this known as "malingering" (which can be combined with the modifier "possible or probable" if desired). It does not mean that you never suffered a concussion, never had symptoms, or do not still have some symptoms that legitimately bother you. Using the term means that it seems likely that some of your low scores on testing are not accurate because of suboptimal effort, not brain damage.

We agree with Tombaugh (1996) that use of the term malingering is typically of limited value to patients and referral sources without an attempt to determine the patient's possible motivations and suggest relevant interventions. Although there are no empirically validated treatments for malingering, it is possible that *some* malingering patients may reflect on their behaviors after being detected and work with a psychologist to develop a more prosocial way of achieving their goals (e.g., earning money by going back to work) and better coping mechanisms (e.g., improving self-confidence to enhance academic performance rather than relying on academic accommodations). Although such successful treatment may only occur in a minority of cases, there is not much else the neuropsychologist can suggest in such cases.

If the term exaggeration is used, our approach is to clarify from the outset to the patient that there are many factors that can cause an "exaggerated" presentation and that the term does not necessarily equate to willful deceit (although this of course remains a possibility). We suggest cautious use of a "cry for help" as a euphemistic explanation for exaggeration. This explanation has been exalted in mainstream clinical practice, not as a result of research evidence to support its accuracy, but simply because it is proffered in textbooks and computer scoring programs as a benign clinical explanation for this behavior. There are many potential singular or interwoven reasons why a person might exaggerate symptoms (e.g., personality characteristics, fear of not being taken seriously, wanting help that has not been forthcoming, depressive amplification, factitious behavior, or malingering).

Once the feedback has been provided, patients are debriefed and asked how they feel about the information they have received. This question provides an opportunity to correct any misperceptions. We recommend documenting the feedback process, including the patient's reactions and responses and how any concerns expressed by the patient were addressed. Some clinicians may also wish to have patients sign a brief form indicating their understanding of the information, their opportunity to ask questions, and their courteous and professional treatment by the clinician (see Appendix A at the end of this chapter for a sample form). Such documentation can be valuable later if the patient, independently or upon the recommendation of an advocate, challenges the findings in a formal venue (e.g., ethics committee, licensing board).

ANCILLARY ISSUES

There are numerous ancillary issues that emerge in the context of symptom validity assessment and feedback sessions, such as (a) whether to release the report; (b) whether to complete the evaluation if initial symptom validity tests are unequivocally failed; (c) whether to identify specific effort tests in the report; (d) how to handle the use of the terms "exaggeration" and "malingering"; (e) how to manage complaints; and (f) defensive, resistant, or aggressive reactions. We refer the reader to our original article (Carone et al., 2010) for further discussion of these issues as well as alternative views to our approach.

OTHER POTENTIALLY CHALLENGING FEEDBACK TOPICS

What follows is a description of some common issues that are also important to discuss during feedback sessions with patients reporting long-term symptoms following an MTBI, regardless of whether symptom validity tests were passed or failed. Many of these issues, in addition to being discussed in the feedback session, might also be the focus of treatment.

Diagnostic Clarification

An issue that sometimes emerges during feedback sessions with patients who have been previously diagnosed with MTBI is the need to clarify whether there is actually sufficient evidence for the diagnosis. In some cases, there is extremely weak evidence regarding whether even a very mild injury occurred (e.g., no evidence of loss of consciousness [LOC], minimal posttraumatic amnesia [PTA], and only brief "confusion"). The probability of having significant damage to the brain underlying symptom reporting in some of these cases is extremely low. Discussing this diagnostic issue with patients is much easier if they openly express uncertainty about the diagnosis. It is much more challenging if they have woven the diagnostic label into their self-concept (e.g., referring often to "my concussion" or "my brain injury"). These entrenched beliefs begin with an incorrect initial diagnosis and then get reinforced by subsequent health care providers who may be strong patient advocates. The longer the belief system is present and the greater the number of health care providers who have reinforced it, the more difficult it is to address and modify this belief system during feedback. In some cases, a feedback session is only the first step in this process. Gradually reconceptualizing problems as being related to other causes such as anxiety, life stress, sleep disturbance, somatic and cognitive preoccupation, and bodily pain becomes one component of treatment.

The diagnosis of MTBI is often made hastily, based on scant evidence, and without reviewing initial medical records. Moreover, it is underappreciated that some initial signs of MTBI, such as confusion or brief patchy amnesia, can be mimicked by acute traumatic stress and pain. Therefore, it is best to take a new careful history and review as many medical records as possible. Sometimes when obtaining a careful history and reviewing records, it becomes clear that the person had a relatively minor blow to the head, did not have appreciable amnesia, and the only evidence for an injury to the brain was feeling momentarily "off" or "confused." Although this could reflect a very mild concussion-related mental status change, it could easily be attributable to being surprised by an unexpected blow to the head and feeling sudden pain and psychological distress. It is very unlikely that a person would have long-term symptoms because of a "brain injury" in this scenario—yet that diagnosis is applied and mental health problems might be minimized or ignored. By combining a detailed clinical interview with a comprehensive medical records review, the primary author has found a substantial minority (about 30%) of patients with a primary diagnosis of MTBI actually appeared to be misdiagnosed (i.e., they had an injury to their head without clear evidence of an initial injury to their brain).

In discussing these issues with patients during feedback, it can be helpful to briefly explain how a concussion is diagnosed and why the patient, having not sustained mental status changes, does not actually meet operationally defined diagnostic criteria (American Academy of Neurology, 1997; Centers for Disease Control and Prevention, 2003; Defense and Veterans Brain Injury Center, 2006; Holm, Cassidy, Carroll, & Borg, 2005; Mild Traumatic Brain Injury Committee of the Head Injury Interdisciplinary Special Interest Group of the American Congress of Rehabilitation Medicine, 1993). In such cases, it is important to emphasize that it is good news that the person's current symptoms are unlikely to be caused by a serious brain injury. It is fortunate that the cause(s) and modifiers of the symptoms appear to be treatable (e.g., depression, anxiety, anger, somatization, cognitive distortions, poor sleep hygiene). This is described as "good news." It is also important to emphasize in such cases that because a concussion did not occur, one logically cannot have "post-concussion syndrome."

In other cases, it should be explained to the patient that it is unclear if they were truly concussed because there is a lack of objective medical documentation, lack of witnesses, transient symptoms at the time of injury that are difficult to clarify with further precision, or the strong possibility that other problems at the time of the injury (e.g., traumatic stress and pain) may account for the reported mental status change. We will often say we are not sure whether or not the patient sustained a very mild form of this injury in the original accident. We might say that if he or she was initially concussed, then it is likely that some initial symptoms in the acute to subacute stage of recovery might have been caused by this injury, but that the direct neurological effects of the trauma is very likely resolved over time.

Although many patients are relieved to learn that they do not "have" a brain injury, some patients become very distressed by such information because, in their minds, it means that they have a severe psychological disturbance. More than a few patients have stated something along the lines of, "Doc, please tell me that I have brain damage so that I know that I'm not crazy." Our role in such situations is to help properly educate the patients about brain trauma, psychological problems, and their potential improvement if they address their (sometimes minimized) emotional distress. This can be done following a discussion regarding expected recovery patterns.

Discussion of Expected Recovery Patterns

If it is concluded that the patient did suffer MTBI, it is often helpful to provide *accurate* patient education, such as discussing expected MTBI symptom recovery patterns and cognitive performance outcomes. Regarding expected cognitive performance outcomes, it can be helpful to note that many studies have shown that the measurable cognitive effects of an MTBI usually resolve by 3 months post injury (Belanger & Vanderploeg, 2005; Binder, 1997; Binder, Rohling, & Larrabee, 1997; Dikmen, Machamer, Winn, & Temkin, 1995; Frencham, Fox, & Maybery, 2005; Iverson, 2005; Rohling et al., 2011). Regarding symptom recovery expectations, we inform patients that this can be difficult to predict and highly variable. A substantial majority of concussed university athletes appear to be symptom-free within 10 days (McCrea, 2008), whereas civilians injured in their daily lives can experience symptoms for weeks or a few months (Caroll et al., 2004, Dikmen, Machamer, Winn, & Temkin, 2010). Having a pre-prepared PowerPoint presentation on a desktop computer can be helpful for these education sessions to help visualize the points being made. When the normal neurological recovery pattern from MTBI is discussed, the clinician can compare and contrast this with the symptom pattern of the particular patient. The farther a patient deviates from the normally expected pattern, the less likely that MTBI is the primary cause of the reported symptoms. This information naturally leads into a discussion into what other factors are present that can contribute to symptom persistence.

Discussion of Other Factors That Can Underlie Symptom Persistence

It is well established that post-concussion-like symptoms are nonspecific (Dunn, Lees-Haley, Brown, Williams, & English, 1995; Gunstad & Suhr, 2002; Iverson, 2006b; Iverson & Lange, 2003; Lees-Haley, Fox, & Courtney, 2001; Radanov, Dvorák, & Valach, 1992; Sawchyn, Brulot, & Strauss, 2000; Trahan, Ross, & Trahan, 2001; Wang, Chan, & Deng, 2006). There are many factors that can cause or maintain subjective symptoms long after an injury event. We suggest focusing initially on the explanations that have the strongest evidence and relevance for the particular patient. For example, it is common for people to have combinations of problems such as life stress, sleep disturbance, health-related anxiety and worry, and pain. These factors, especially when interwoven, can be mutually reinforcing and can cause a diverse range of post-concussion-like symptoms (see Figure 6.1).

In other cases, the potential impact of medical comorbidities on the patient's functioning needs to be discussed. For example, the impact of poorly treated sleep apnea, uncontrolled diabetes, and/or chronic pain conditions should be discussed regarding their possible effects; or the effects of the medications used to treat them,

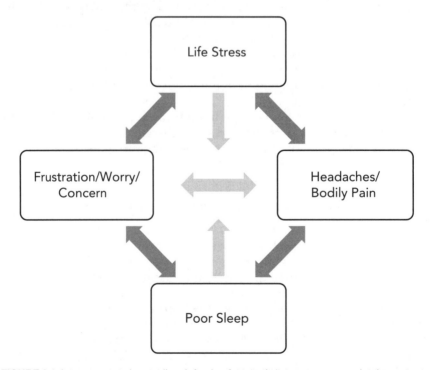

FIGURE 6.1 Interwoven and mutually reinforcing factors that can cause or maintain post-concussion-like symptoms.

upon cognitive functioning. Comorbid substance abuse is another relevant area that needs to be discussed if present. In older adults, an underlying mild cognitive impairment may be present, the symptoms of which were ignored until the MTBI served to focus the patient's attention on cognitive problems. Sometimes, the fact that it is normal for healthy individuals to have some low test scores also needs to be explained (Binder, Iverson, & Brooks, 2009; Brooks, Iverson, Holdnack, & Feldman, 2008; Iverson & Brooks, 2011; Schretlen, Testa, Winicki, Pearlson, & Gordon, 2008).

Depending on the patients' receptiveness to the above points, their intellectual capabilities, and the particulars of the case, the examiner may wish to enter into a brief discussion of some of the social-psychological research on patients' reports of persistent symptoms after MTBI. This includes research on the nocebo effect, "good old days" bias, and expectancy as etiology. In some cases, the first author has found it helpful to briefly summarize the classic findings on expectancy as etiology after MTBI (Mittenberg, et al., 1992), sometimes displaying the table of results.

Discussion of Treatment Options

One of the most important aspects to emphasize during the feedback session is that the patient has problems that are treatable; that there is hope. For patients with chronic symptoms after MTBI, it is important to focus on treatment that requires active participation that is motivated and directed toward change. This emphasis on active participation is necessary because many patients have engaged in prolonged inactivity and isolation from others. Occasionally, patients are advised to do things that are counterproductive. One unusual anecdotal example is a directive to stay in a dark room with little to no stimulation. Although time away from sports, school, and/or work (usually in the form of prescribed rest) may provide some limited benefit in the acute phase of neurological recovery after MTBI (de Kruijk, Leffers, Meerhoff, Rutten, & Twijnstra, 2002), this reduced activity is sometimes extended for months to years by well-meaning health care providers because the patient continues to report some symptoms. However, several authors have noted that prolonged enforced rest does not improve symptom recovery and may actually make the patient worse in numerous medical conditions, including MTBI (Allen, Glasziou, & Del Mar, 1999; Asher, 1947; de Kruijk et al., 2002). Sometimes, activity restrictions can also be continued when the patient reports being symptom-free because the health care provider wants to recheck them on a follow-up visit, just to be certain.

Although well-intentioned, extending activity restrictions or passive treatments past the normal MTBI recovery timeline risks creating a feeling of helplessness, over-identification with the disability role, and increased emotional distress. Thus, feedback sessions in the chronic phase should aim to empower patients by informing them that they are capable of doing something to change their situation, they should no longer view themselves as helpless victims of brain injury (e.g., "brain injury survivors"), and there is reason to believe that they can return to their premorbid level of functioning. The latter is a goal that patients are strongly encouraged to work toward.

Specific treatment recommendations depend on the most salient symptoms reported and what factors the clinician believes are causing the symptoms. For example, if a mood disorder and/or somatoform disorder appears central to the primary cause of the patient's problems, then a referral for psychotherapy is suggested. It is important to mention to patients that the treatment needs to be solution-focused and not merely supportive and cathartic. Thus, referral to doctoral level psychologists who specialize in cognitive behavioral therapy (CBT) is often preferred because of their extra education and training in specific intervention strategies. The principles behind CBT can be explained, and examples are provided as to how maladaptive thinking processes can contribute to psychological distress. It is emphasized that psychotherapy typically needs to occur weekly to biweekly and that the patient must be motivated to change for it to be effective.

If a psychiatric condition is significant enough to warrant consideration for psychotropic medication, this is conveyed to the patient as well. In this context, it is helpful to inform patients that a combination of psychotherapy and medication will likely be the most effective treatment compared to either psychotherapy or medication alone. For patients who prefer to only take psychotropic medication without psychotherapy, it is helpful to inform them that while medication may reduce the intensity of psychiatric symptoms, there is no medication that will teach them strategies to better cope with their problems. In some cases, we note that current treatment guidelines show that there are no empirically validated medication treatments for neurocognitive symptoms of MTBI (Department of Veterans Affairs & Department of Defense, 2009) despite the frequent prescription of such medications (e.g., neuro-stimulants) when cognitive problems are reported after MTBI. We emphasize to patients that their perceived cognitive difficulties will likely improve if they follow the treatments suggestions outlined above.

CONCLUSIONS

Professional ethics require psychologists to provide feedback regarding assessment results to patients, unless the nature of the relationship prohibits such feedback and the examinee has been informed of that fact at the outset of the evaluation process. However, when assessment findings indicate that patients responded or performed in an invalid manner, neuropsychologists may find the discussion of such findings to be challenging and uncomfortable. In this chapter we provided a model designed to assist clinicians when confronted with the need to provide feedback to patients regarding invalid performance during neuropsychological evaluations.

Clinicians are well served by considering such issues in advance and preparing their approach to such feedback session before meeting with patients. When provided in an educational and supportive manner, evidence-based education regarding MTBI and suboptimal performance can be constructive and advance patient well-being.

In addition, we discussed other issues that are important topics in feedback sessions, such as diagnostic clarification, typical and atypical recovery patterns, non-specificity of symptoms, comorbidities, and treatment options. In an open and respectful way, we might marvel at the complexity of the mind and body and eschew simplistic explanations for symptoms (e.g., "brain damage" vs. "crazy"). We might then discuss the large literature indicating that pain, anxiety, life stress, sleep disturbance, and mild depression, singly or especially in combination, can cause diverse post-concussion-like symptoms. We try to instill motivation and hope for improvement associated with lifestyle changes and treatment.

REFERENCES

Allen, C., Glasziou, P., & Del Mar, C. (1999). Bed rest: A potentially harmful treatment needing more careful evaluation. *Lancet*, 354, 1229–1233.

American Academy of Neurology. (1997). Practice parameter: The management of concussion in sports (summary statement). Report of the Quality Standards Subcommittee. *Neurology*, 48(3), 581–585.

American Psychological Association (2002). Ethical principles of psychologists and code of conduct. *American Psychologist*, 57(12), 1060–1073.

Asher, R. A. (1947). The dangers of going to bed. *British Medical Journal*, 2(4536), 967.

Belanger, H. G., & Vanderploeg, R. D. (2005). The neuropsychological impact of sports-related concussion: A meta-analysis. *Journal of the International Neuropsychological Society*, 11(4), 345–357.

Binder, L. M. (1997). A review of mild head trauma. Part II: Clinical implications. *Journal of Clinical and Experimental Neuropsychology*, 19(3), 432–457.

Binder, L. M., Iverson, G. L., & Brooks, B. L. (2009). To err is human: "Abnormal" neuropsychological scores and variability are common in healthy adults. *Archives of Clinical Neuropsychology*, 24(1), 31–46.

Binder, L. M., Rohling, M. L., & Larrabee, G. J. (1997). A review of mild head trauma. Part I: Meta-analytic review of neuropsychological studies. *Journal of Clinical and Experimental Neuropsychology*, 19, 421–431.

Boone, K. (2007). *Assessment of feigned cognitive impairment: A neuropsychological perspective*. New York, NY: Guilford Press.

Brooks, B. L., Iverson, G. L., Holdnack, J. A., & Feldman, H. H. (2008). Potential for misclassification of mild cognitive impairment: A study of memory scores on the Wechsler Memory Scale-III in healthy older adults. *Journal of the International Neuropsychological Society*, 14(3), 463–478.

Bush, S., Ruff, R., Troster, A., Barth, J., Koffler, S., Pliskin, N. et al. (2005). Symptom validity assessment: practice issues and medical necessity NAN policy & planning committee. *Archives of Clinical Neuropsychology*, 20, 419–426

Carone, D. A. (2008). Children with moderate/severe brain damage/dysfunction outperform adults with mild-to-no brain damage on the Medical Symptom Validity Test. *Brain Injury*, 22(12), 960–971.

Carone, D. A., Iverson, G. L., & Bush, S. S. (2010). A model to approaching and providing feedback to patients regarding invalid test performance in clinical neuropsychological evaluations. *The Clinical Neuropsychologist*, 24(5), 759–778.

Carroll, L. J., Cassidy, J. D., Peloso, P. M., Borg, J., von Holst, H., Holm, L., Paniak, C., et al. (2004). Prognosis for mild traumatic brain injury: Results of the WHO Collaborating Centre Task Force on Mild Traumatic Brain Injury. *Journal of Rehabilitation Medicine*, (Suppl. 43), 84–105.

de Kruijk, J. R., Leffers, P., Meerhoff, S., Rutten, J., & Twijnstra, A. (2002). Effectiveness of bed rest after mild traumatic brain injury: A randomised trial of no versus six days of bed rest. *Journal of Neurology, Neurosurgery and Psychiatry*, 73(2), 167–172.

Defense and Veterans Brain Injury Center. (2006). *Defense and Veterans Brain Injury Center Working Group on the acute management of mild traumatic brain injury in military operational settings: Clinical practice guidelines and recommendations*. Washington, DC: Author.

Department of Veterans Affairs, & Department of Defense. (2009). *Va/DoD Clinical practice guideline for management of concussion/mild traumatic brain injury*. Washington, DC: Author.

Dikmen, S. A., Machamer, J., Fann, J. R., & Temkin, N. R. (2010). Rates of symptom reporting following traumatic brain injury. *Journal of the International Neuropsychological Society*, 16(3), 401–411.

Dikmen, S., Machamer, J., Winn, R., & Temkin, N. R. (1995). Neuropsychological outcome at 1-year post head injury. *Neuropsychology*, 9, 80–90.

Dunn, J. T., Lees-Haley, P. R., Brown, R. S., Williams, C. W., & English, L. T. (1995). Neurotoxic complaint base rates of personal injury claimants: Implications for neuropsychological assessment. *Journal of Clinical Psychology*, 51(4), 577–584.

Ferguson, R. J., Mittenberg, W., Barone, D. F., & Schneider, B. (1999). Postconcussion syndrome following sports-related head injury: Expectation as etiology. *Neuropsychology*, 13(4), 582–589.

Frencham, K. A., Fox, A. M., & Maybery, M. T. (2005). Neuropsychological studies of mild traumatic brain injury: A meta-analytic review of research since 1995. *Journal of Clinical and Experimental Neuropsychology*, 27(3), 334–351.

Greub, B. L., & Suhr, J. A. (2006). The validity of the letter memory test as a measure of memory malingering: Robustness to coaching. *Archives of Clinical Neuropsychology*, 21(4), 249–254.

Gunstad, J., & Suhr, J. A. (2001). "Expectation as etiology" versus "the good old days": Postconcussion syndrome symptom reporting in athletes, headache sufferers, and depressed individuals. *Journal of the International Neuropsychological Society*, 7(3), 323–333.

Gunstad, J., & Suhr, J. A. (2002). Perception of illness: Nonspecificity of postconcussion syndrome symptom expectation. *Journal of the International Neuropsychological Society*, 8(1), 37–47.

Heilbronner, R. L., Sweet, J. J., Morgan, J. E., Larrabee, G. J., & Millis, S. R. (2009). American Academy of Clinical Neuropsychology Consensus Conference Statement on the neuropsychological assessment of effort, response bias, and malingering. *The Clinical Neuropsychologist*, 23, 1093–1129.

Holm, L., Cassidy, J. D., Carroll, L. J., & Borg, J. (2005). Summary of the WHO collaborating centre for neurotrauma task force on mild traumatic brain injury. *Journal of Rehabilitation Medicine*, 37(3), 137–141.

Iverson, G. L. (2003). Detecting malingering in civil forensic evaluations. In A. M. Horton,Jr. & L. C. Hartlage (Eds.), *Handbook of forensic neuropsychology* (pp. 137–177). New York, NY: Springer Publishing.

Iverson, G. L. (2005). Outcome from mild traumatic brain injury. *Current Opinions in Psychiatry*, 18, 301–317.

Iverson, G. L. (2006a). Ethical issues associated with the assessment of exaggeration, poor effort, and malingering. *Applied Neuropsychology*, 13(2), 77–90.

Iverson, G. L. (2006b). Misdiagnosis of the persistent postconcussion syndrome in patients with depression. *Archives of Clinical Neuropsychology*, 21(4), 303–310.

Iverson, G. L. (2010). Detecting exaggeration, poor effort, & malingering in neuropsychology. In A. M. Horton Jr. & L. C. Hartlage (Eds.), *Handbook of Forensic Neuropsychology* (2nd ed., pp. 91–135). New York, NY: Springer Publishing.

Iverson, G. L., & Brooks, B. L. (2011). Improving accuracy for identifying cognitive impairment. In M. R. Schoenberg & J. G. Scott (Eds.), *The Little Black Book of Neuropsychology: A Syndrome-Based Approach*. New York, NY: Springer Publishing.

Iverson, G. L., & Lange, R. T. (2003). Examination of "postconcussion-like" symptoms in a healthy sample. *Applied Neuropsychology*, 10(3), 137–144.

Iverson, G. L., & McCracken, L. M. (1997). 'Postconcussive' symptoms in persons with chronic pain. *Brain Injury*, 11(11), 783–790.

Iverson, G. L., Zasler, N., & Lange, R. T. (2007). Post-concussive disorder. In N. D. Zasler, D. I. Katz, & R. D. Zafonte (Eds.), *Brain Injury Medicine: Principles and Practice* (pp. 373–405). New York, NY: Demos Medical.

Johnson, J. L., & Lesniak-Karpiak, K. (1997). The effect of warning on malingering on memory and motor tasks in college samples. *Archives of Clinical Neuropsychology*, 12(3), 231–238.

Kennedy, J. E., Cullen, M. A., Amador, R. R., Huey, J. C., & Leal, F. O. (2010). Symptoms in military service members after blast MTBI with and without associated injuries. *NeuroRehabilitation*, 26(3), 191–197.

Larrabee, G. J. (1990). Cautions in the use of neuropsychological evaluation in legal settings. *Neuropsychology*, 4, 239–247.

Larrabee, G. J. (1997). Neuropsychological outcome, post concussion symptoms, and forensic considerations in mild closed head trauma. *Seminars in Clinical Neuropsychiatry*, 2(3), 196–206.

Lees-Haley, P. R., Fox, D. D., & Courtney, J. C. (2001). A comparison of complaints by mild brain injury claimants and other claimants describing subjective experiences immediately following their injury. *Archives of Clinical Neuropsychology*, 16(7), 689–695.

Mahoney, M. J., & Arnkoff, D. B. (1978). Cognitive and self-control therapies. In S. L. Garfield & A. E. Bergin (Eds.), *Handbook of psychotherapy and behavior change: An empirical analysis* (2nd ed., pp. 689–722). New York, NY: Wiley.

McCrea, M. (2008). *Mild traumatic brain injury and postconcussion syndrome: The new evidence base for diagnosis and treatment*. New York, NY: Oxford University Press.

Mild Traumatic Brain Injury Committee of the Head Injury Interdisciplinary Special Interest Group of the American Congress of Rehabilitation Medicine. (1993). Definition of mild traumatic brain injury. *Journal of Head Trauma Rehabilitation*, 8(3), 86–87.

Mittenberg, W., DiGiulio, D. V., Perrin, S., & Bass, A. E. (1992). Symptoms following mild head injury: Expectation as aetiology. *Journal of Neurology, Neurosurgery and Psychiatry*, 55(3), 200–204.

Mittenberg, W., Patton, C., Canyock, E. M., & Condit, D. C. (2002). Base rates of malingering and symptom exaggeration. *Journal of Clinical and Experimental Neuropsychology*, 24(8), 1094–1102.

National Center for Injury Prevention and Control. (2003). *Report to Congress on mild traumatic brain injury in the United States: Steps to prevent a serious public health problem*. Atlanta, GA: Centers for Disease Control and Prevention.

Radanov, B. P., Dvorák, J., & Valach, L. (1992). Cognitive deficits in patients after soft tissue injury of the cervical spine. *Spine (Phila Pa 1976)*, 17(2), 127–131.

Resnick, P. (1988). Malingering of posttraumatic disorders. In R. Rogers (Ed.), *Clinical assessment of malingering and deception* (pp. 84–103). New York, NY: Guilford Press.

Reynolds, S., Paniak, C., Toller-Lobe, G., & Nagy, J. (2003). A longitudinal study of compensation-seeking and return to work in a treated mild traumatic brain injury sample. *Journal of Head Trauma Rehabilitation*, 18(2), 139–147.

Rogers, C. R. (1951). *Client-centered therapy, its current practice, implications, and theory*. Boston, MA: Houghton Mifflin.

Rohling, M. L., Binder, L. M., Demakis, G. J., Larrabee, G. J., Ploetz, D. M., & Langhinrichsen-Rohling, J. (2011). A meta-analysis of neuropsychological outcome after mild traumatic brain injury: Reanalyses and reconsiderations of Binder et al. (1997), Frencham et al. (2005), and Pertab et al. (2009). *The Clinical Neuropsychologist*, 25(4), 608–623.

Rozek Law Office. (2011). *Mild TBI – The conspiracy between neuropsychology and the insurance industry – part II*. Retrieved from http://rozeklaw.com/blog/2011/traumatic-brain-injury/mild-tbi-conspiracy-between-neuropsychology-insurance-industry-part2/

Ruff, R. M., Wylie, T., & Tennant, W. (1993). Malingering and malingering-like aspects of mild closed head trauma. *Journal of Head Trauma Rehabilitation*, 8(3), 60–73.

Sawchyn, J. M., Brulot, M. M., & Strauss, E. (2000). Note on the use of the postconcussion syndrome checklist. *Archives of Clinical Neuropsychology*, 15(1), 1–8.

Schenk, K., & Sullivan, K. A. (2010). Do warnings deter rather than produce more sophisticated malingering? *Journal of Clinical and Experimental Neuropsychology*, 32(7), 752–762.

Schretlen, D. J., Testa, S. M., Winicki, J. M., Pearlson, G. D., & Gordon, B. (2008). Frequency and bases of abnormal performance by healthy adults on neuropsychological testing. *Journal of the International Neuropsychological Society*, 14(3), 436–445.

Slick, D. J., Sherman, E. M., & Iverson, G. L. (1999). Diagnostic criteria for malingered neurocognitive dysfunction: Proposed standards for clinical practice and research. *The Clinical Neuropsychologist*, 13(4), 545–561.

Stewart-Patterson, C. (in press). Detection of potential malingering indicators through document review. *International Association of Industrial Accident Boards and Commissions Journal*.

Suhr, J. A., & Gunstad, J. (2000). The effects of coaching on the sensitivity and specificity of malingering measures. *Archives of Clinical Neuropsychology*, 15(5), 415–424.

Suhr, J., Gunstad, J., Greub, B., & Barrash, J. (2004). Exaggeration index for an expanded version of the auditory verbal learning test: Robustness to coaching. *Journal of Clinical and Experimental Neuropsychology*, 26(3), 416–427.

Tombaugh, T. (1996). *Test of Memory Malingering* (TOMM). Los Angeles: Western Psychological Services.

Trahan, D. E., Ross, C. E., & Trahan, S. L. (2001). Relationships among postconcussional-type symptoms, depression, and anxiety in neurologically normal young adults and victims of mild brain injury. *Archives of Clinical Neuropsychology*, 16(5), 435–445.

Vanderploeg, R. D., & Belanger, H. G. (2009). Multifactorial contributions to questionable effort and test performance within a military context. In J. E. Morgan & J. J. Sweet (Eds.), *Neuropsychology of malingering casebook* (pp. 41–52). New York: Psychology Press.

Wang, Y., Chan, R. C., & Deng, Y. (2006). Examination of postconcussion-like symptoms in healthy university students: Relationships to subjective and objective neuropsychological function performance. *Archives of Clinical Neuropsychology*, 21(4), 339–347.

Youngjohn, J. R., Lees-Haley, P. R., & Binder, L. M. (1999). Comment: Warning malingerers produces more sophisticated malingering. *Archives of Clinical Neuropsychology*, 14(6), 511–515.

APPENDIX A

Neuropsychological Assessment Feedback Form

Name: _____ Today's Date: _____

Clinician Providing Feedback: _____

Your feedback regarding the neuropsychological evaluation process is important. Understanding your reaction to the evaluation provides an additional opportunity to meet your needs, and it can help identify areas where neuropsychological services might be improved. Please provide as much information as you are comfortable providing.

1. Were you given an opportunity to ask questions about the evaluation? [ ] yes [ ] no
2. Were you offered breaks during the evaluation? [ ] yes [ ] no
3. Were the results and recommendations explained to your satisfaction? [ ] yes [ ] no
4. Were you able to give your best effort and honest responses throughout this evaluation? [ ] yes [ ] no
5. Were you treated professionally, with courtesy and respect? [ ] yes [ ] no

If anything prevented you from giving your best and most honest effort, please describe.

_____
_____
_____

If you have any comments about your evaluation, please write them here.

_____
_____
_____

Patient's Signature:_____ Date: _____

Note. This form is adapted from one created by A. Chris Russo.

Research and Symptom Validity Assessment in Mild Traumatic Brain Injury Cases

7

Nathaniel W. Nelson & Bridget M. Doane

On review of clinical neuropsychology studies published within the last 20–30 years, it is difficult to identify any topic that has received quite as much attention as symptom validity assessment (SVA). Following the humbling revelation that clinical neuropsychologists are generally ineffective in discriminating feigned from genuine cognitive impairment on the basis of clinical intuition alone (cf., Faust, Hart, & Guilmette, 1988; Heaton, Smith, Lehman, & Vogt, 1978), the field has witnessed an exponential increase in research pertaining to SVA including the development of novel effort measures and self-report validity scales, as well as malingering and other forensic issues (Berry & Nelson, 2010; Sweet, King, Malina, Bergman, & Simmons, 2002). Special journal sections (e.g., *The Clinical Neuropsychologist*) and relevant texts (Boone, 2007; Larrabee, 2007; Morgan & Sweet, 2008) devoted to forensic neuropsychology are examples of how the field has accommodated the demand to report results of SVA research. Survey data reveal that most neuropsychologists typically include SVA instruments as a component of their evaluations (Sharland & Gfeller, 2007), and there is now a widespread consensus that SVA is fundamental to effective clinical neuropsychological practice (American Academy of Clinical Neuropsychology [AACN], 2007; Bush et al., 2005; Heilbronner, Sweet, Morgan, Larrabee, & Millis, 2009).

As documented, many, if not most, SVA studies in clinical neuropsychology have included mild traumatic brain injury (MTBI or concussion) samples. The inclusion of these samples may in part relate to the high frequency of MTBI encountered in clinical practice. According to the Centers for Disease Control and Prevention, about 1.5 million traumatic brain injuries (TBIs) of any severity are sustained in the United States each year (Langlois, Rutland-Brown, & Thomas, 2006), and MTBI is by far the most common severity of injury reported in emergent medical settings (Thurman & Guerrero, 1999). Relevant to military and veteran cohorts, MTBI is one of the most frequent injuries sustained in the recent conflicts in Iraq and Afghanistan (McCrea et al., 2008), with as many as 9%–23% of military personnel reporting a history of combat-related TBI (usually of mild severity) in recent surveys (Hoge et al., 2008; Polusny et al., 2011; Schneiderman, Braver, & Kang, 2008; Terrio et al., 2009). The incidence of blast-related concussion in the recent conflicts is believed to be unprecedented (Owens et al., 2008). TBI, presumably mild in most cases, is among the most frequently evaluated conditions in neuropsychological practice, only secondary to the dementias in older adults in two recent nationwide surveys of clinical neuropsychologists (Sweet, Meyer, Nelson, & Moberg, 2011; Sweet, Nelson, & Moberg, 2006).

Another tenable explanation for the frequent representation of MTBI in SVA research is that MTBI is among the most common conditions to be evaluated in personal injury litigation and other secondary gain contexts (Greiffenstein, 2009)—settings in which symptom exaggeration is common. SVA/MTBI studies do not typically include the majority group of patients with MTBI who demonstrate the usual pattern of rapid and favorable recovery soon after the injury (Belanger, Curtiss, Demery, Lebowitz, & Vanderploeg, 2005; Binder, Rohling, & Larrabee, 1997; Frencham, Fox, & Mayberry 2005; Iverson, 2005; McCrea, 2008; Rohling et al., 2011; Schretlen & Shapiro, 2003). It is true that some researchers conduct SVA in MTBI samples longitudinally, as in the case of athletes who are evaluated before and after sports-related injuries, to identify baseline suboptimal motivation followed by significant gains in scores following injury motivated by a strong desire to return to play (Bailey, Echemendia, & Arnett, 2006). But more often, SVA/MTBI studies include the minority of MTBI samples who endorse physical, psychological, and/or cognitive "postconcussive symptoms" (PCS) on a chronic basis and retrospectively attribute (or misattribute) these symptoms to a remote history of MTBI.

The current chapter addresses the role of research in SVA and MTBI and summarizes just a few of the most salient findings that have emerged in these areas in recent years. The reader is encouraged to consult additional references for further information pertaining to research on the topics of SVA (Boone, 2007; Larrabee, 2007; Morgan & Sweet, 2008; Rogers, 2008) and MTBI (e.g., McCrea, 2008). We begin by discussing a few essential themes for clinicians to consider from the general MTBI research in clinical neuropsychology, including the importance of accurate MTBI assessment and diagnosis, usual recovery patterns following MTBI, and factors that may complicate or extend the recovery process following MTBI including, but not limited to, secondary gain. We then turn to factors that are most relevant to SVA in MTBI samples and conclude with a discussion of areas for future SVA/MTBI research.

MILD TRAUMATIC BRAIN INJURY (CONCUSSION): GENERAL OVERVIEW

Before discussing the role of SVA research in MTBI samples, one should be familiar with more general research literature that describes assessment, diagnosis, and symptom recovery following uncomplicated MTBI. It is our belief that appreciation of this broader MTBI literature provides an important background for the practice of effective SVA with MTBI patients. In fact, it has been our experience that some individuals report a history of head injury that did not necessarily result in MTBI as supported by information documented through external record review. In this sense, verification of MTBI diagnosis might be regarded as the first and the most important step in conducting SVA in this group. Clinicians and researchers are encouraged to develop an intimate understanding of

- MTBI assessment and diagnosis,
- usual course of recovery,
- nonspecificity of chronic PCS, and
- factors that may complicate or extend recovery (including, but not limited to, secondary gain and symptom exaggeration).

Mild Traumatic Brain Injury Assessment and Diagnosis

Accurate MTBI assessment and diagnosis in SVA research or otherwise is essential to maintaining study quality and the meaningfulness of study findings. Of particular importance is the recognition that TBI severity is conventionally rated according to *acute* injury parameters or symptoms/response patterns that are observed immediately after brain injuries are sustained. As discussed subsequently, chronic physical, cognitive, and emotional symptoms are highly nonspecific and cannot be reliably linked with injury severity on the basis of self-report in the late stage of injury recovery (i.e., months or years postinjury).

Although various schemes have been developed to rate TBI severity, most schemes emphasize acute injury parameters such as loss of consciousness (LOC) and duration, posttraumatic amnesia (PTA) and duration, and Glasgow Coma Scale (GCS; Teasdale & Jennett, 1974) status. For example, according to the American Congress of Rehabilitation Medicine (ACRM; Kay et al., 1993), MTBI consists of a "traumatically induced physiologic disruption of brain function" that results in one or more of the following: (a) LOC (of approximately 30 min or less); (b) period of PTA (not more than 24 hr); (c) alteration in mental status; and/or (d) focal neurological deficit(s). MTBI, according to the latter scheme, may or may not be associated with varied physical (e.g., dizziness, headache, blurred vision), cognitive (e.g., diminished attention, memory, executive function), and/or behavioral or emotional changes (e.g., irritability, emotional lability), but should not have an initial GCS score less than 13. Researchers who are able to identify participants' acute injury indicators are able to provide a reasonable and informed opinion regarding the likelihood that an individual sustained a TBI of any severity. Access to records that describe GCS responses (eye opening, verbal, and motor responsiveness) and other acute injury characteristics can be of assistance in identifying whether MTBI was likely to have been sustained. These records are of most use when they are generated closer to the time of the injury scene (e.g., paramedic notes from the injury scene).

As important as these acute injury parameters are in arriving at an accurate diagnosis of MTBI, it is noteworthy that many MTBI researchers have limited access to primary records that pertain to the injury events themselves, and diagnoses and group assignments may be based on patient's self-report information alone. This situation has been especially true in the case of military and veteran MTBI samples. Related to the questionable reliability of retrospective reports, sole reliance on self-report information pertaining to historical injury events has been identified as perhaps the single most striking limitation of neuropsychology research in military and veteran samples (Nelson, Lamberty, Sim, Doane, & Vanderploeg, in press). Individuals with histories of MTBI may exhibit understandable difficulty estimating duration of LOC or PTA in the acute stage of injury. Self-report information may also vary from one point in time to the next (e.g., between clinical interviews). Individuals may also vary in presentation style when discussing previous concussive events, ranging from forthright to exaggerated to minimized depending on the circumstances associated with injuries (e.g., sports concussion, combat-related) and the context of the evaluation (Nelson, Hoelzle, Sweet, Arbisi, & Demakis, 2010). The true composition of MTBI groups included in MTBI/SVA studies is obscured when researchers are unable to corroborate self-report information with primary records obtained soon after injuries are sustained.

In short, the quality of MTBI (and MTBI/SVA) research is enhanced when researchers have a clear understanding of acute injury symptoms and signs that inform the plausibility that previous injury events did or did not likely contribute to MTBI. This is one of the reasons that the sports concussion context is ideal for studying the natural history of concussion (McCrea, 2008). Sports concussion researchers are aware when injuries are most likely to transpire (i.e., during participation in sporting events), are able to assess acute injury symptoms very soon after injury, and continue to follow cognitive and symptom recovery patterns longitudinally after injuries are sustained. When the true nature of reported injury events cannot be verified through collateral records or other external information, it may be more accurate to conceive of "MTBI" groups as "purported MTBI" or "suspected MTBI" groups in SVA research. Alternatively, Carone (2008) has classified such patients as "mild head injury" in the literal sense, with the word "head" being used to refer to a trauma or injury above the neck (most typically the scalp) but not the brain. This is different from some terminology on the literature in which the word head is used synonymously and with the word "brain," even though the two are not the same.

Usual Course of Recovery

An extensive literature documents the natural history of cognitive and symptom recovery that typically follows uncomplicated MTBI, and detailed review of this extensive literature transcends the scope of the current chapter. In general, this literature demonstrates that common acute injury cognitive deficits resolve within initial days of injury (McCrea et al., 2003), with the most individuals attaining baseline level of cognitive function within a matter of weeks to no more than a few months postinjury (Belanger et al., 2005; Binder et al., 1997; Frencham et al., 2005; Iverson, 2005; McCrea, 2008; Rohling et al., 2011; Schretlen & Shapiro, 2003). As a whole, the concussion literature suggests that lasting subjective symptoms and/or objective cognitive impairments are exceptional. Symptoms or impairments that persist beyond a few months postinjury are often reflective of factors other than the neurological effects of the MTBI itself (McCrea, 2008).

Nonspecificity of Chronic "Postconcussion" Symptoms

Physical, cognitive, and emotional symptoms akin to those described within the *Diagnostic and Statistical Manual of Mental Disorders Fourth Edition Text Revision (DSM-IV-TR)* "postconcussional disorder" criteria are common in non–head-injured clinical samples and healthy samples alike. As such, researchers cannot provide an accurate diagnosis of MTBI based on symptoms that are reported months or years after injuries have been sustained. As Iverson, Lange, Brooks, and Rennison (2010, p. 18) stated, "It would be a mistake to assume uncritically that these self-reported symptoms are causally related to a distant MTBI because most individuals with MTBI recover relatively quickly and fully, and because postconcussion symptoms are nonspecific."

The nonspecific nature of chronic PCS is illustrated by various studies, which have shown that these same symptoms are present among individuals *without* a history of MTBI. For example, Iverson and McCracken (1997) found that 39% of a chronic pain sample (without history of MTBI) met criteria for the *DSM-IV* postconcussion syndrome. Physical symptoms such as headache and fatigue are also common in psychiatric groups (Iverson, 2006), as well as in healthy samples (Iverson & Lange, 2003; Paniak et al., 2002), without a history of MTBI.

Incidentally, some researchers have asserted that as many as 15%–20% of individuals continue to show prolonged symptoms following concussion (Alexander, 1995; McLean, Temkin, Dikmen, & Wyler, 1983; Rutherford, Merrett, & McDonald, 1979). However, these studies did not control for key nonconcussive variables, such as involvement in litigation or symptom exaggeration, when reporting their findings (Greiffenstein, 2009). More methodologically sound studies suggest that the prevalence of chronic PCS is much lower, more likely in the range of 3%–5% in MTBI samples (McCrea, 2008). This minority of patients with MTBI is the cohort for whom SVA is often most relevant, given reports of chronic symptoms that are frequently in excess of injury severity and increased risk of symptom exaggeration that may be motivated by a desire to obtain an external incentive (e.g., monetary award) and/or avoid responsibility (e.g., return to work, family responsibilities).

Factors That May Complicate or Extend Recovery

If most individuals who sustain MTBI show a favorable course of recovery within weeks to no more than a few months postinjury, what unique factors might account for persisting symptoms or cognitive impairments for the minority of MTBI samples? A great deal of neuropsychology research has been developed with the intention of addressing this very question, some of which are summarized in the following text.

Premorbid/Comorbid Psychological Difficulties

Various researchers have discussed the role of premorbid and comorbid psychopathology and symptom outcomes following MTBI (Fann, Katon, Uomoto, & Esselman, 1995; Fenton, McClelland, Montgomery, MacFlynn, & Rutherford, 1993; Greiffenstein & Baker, 2001; King, 1996; Robertson, Rath, Fournet, Zelhart, & Estes, 1994; Wood, 2004). For some individuals, depression, anxiety, and other forms of emotional distress experienced before and/or after the injury event may complicate recovery following MTBI and contribute to, or largely account for, persisting PCS. Maladaptive personality traits and Axis II pathology may also contribute to poor outcomes for selected TBI samples (Hibbard et al., 2000), particularly among those with both Axis I and Axis II conditions (Evered, Ruff, Baldo, & Isomura, 2003).

Some researchers have offered a diathesis-stress model to account for chronic symptoms following MTBI (Metalsky, Halberstadt, & Abramson, 1987; Wood, 2004). According to this model, premorbid emotional difficulties contribute to vulnerability for poor outcome following MTBI, and chronic symptoms after MTBI may, for some, reflect an interaction between psychological and physiological factors. This possibility highlights the importance of locating the onset and the course of reported symptoms through a detailed and chronological psychosocial history. Such investigation may help to identify factors that may have predated the injury event and may have extended or exacerbated symptoms during the recovery stage.

Greiffenstein and Baker (2001) examined serial Minnesota Multiphasic Personality Inventory (MMPI) and MMPI-2 profiles among 23 claimants administered before and after participants had sustained MTBI. Each of the claimants was evaluated in relation to a history of MTBI and claimed having significant personality changes as a result of their injuries. The sample as a whole showed significant patterns of psychopathology before the MTBI had been sustained, and the sample showed particular elevations on scales associated with somatic symptoms (e.g., hypochondriasis and hysteria). Although postinjury profiles were also suggestive of diagnostically relevant psychological symptoms, the magnitude of symptoms was on average less severe relative to the preinjury profiles. Participants also showed a more defensive approach to testing in the postinjury assessment. The authors interpreted these findings as supporting the notion of a diathesis-stress model and the notion of poor outcome following MTBI. The individuals adopted a more defensive approach and reported relatively less psychopathology after MTBI was believed to have been reflective of an attempt to minimize problems that pre-dated MTBI and emphasized that current symptoms were directly related to MTBI.

Evidence further exists that psychological and emotional difficulties significantly mediate chronic PCS among military and veteran samples who reported a history of MTBI (Hoge et al., 2008; Polusny et al., 2011). Hoge et al. surveyed 2,525 U.S. Army infantry soldiers 3–4 mos after they had returned from deployment to Iraq. Of the full sample, 384 reported a history of combat-related injury that contributed to either LOC or altered mental status. Although PCS, such as cognitive difficulty, tinnitus, and irritability, were commonly reported among those who reported MTBI histories, with exception of headache, these symptoms were no longer associated with MTBI after adjusting for depression and PTSD symptoms.

Similar findings were reported by Polusny et al. (2011) who surveyed 953 U.S. National Guard soldiers 1 month before their return from Iraq and 1 year later. Rate of self-reported MTBI was 9.2% at Time 1 and 22.0% at Time 2. Although respondents with reported MTBI histories reported more PCS than those without MTBI histories, MTBI was no longer associated with PCS after controlling for PTSD symptoms. Taking these findings, together with those of Hoge et al. (2008), the authors concluded that PTSD and emotional distress play a significant role in the long-term report of PCS among military personnel with histories of MTBI. In sum, most available research suggests that psychiatric factors, rather than the neurological effects of MTBI alone, account for a significant proportion of PCS experienced by those studied.

Misattribution, False Expectations, and Self-Report Bias

Research suggests that persisting symptoms after MTBI may, for some individuals, reflect misattribution or false expectations regarding outcomes following such an event. This line of research suggests that some individuals develop erroneous cognitive beliefs regarding a connection between MTBI and chronic PCS, one of the themes being an overly pronounced expectation that remote MTBI has an untoward effect on subsequent function.

Mittenberg, DiGiulio, Perrin, and Bass (1992) proposed an "expectation as etiology" theory for symptom maintenance in MTBI samples with chronic PCS. The authors administered a PCS checklist to a group of 223 individuals without history or knowledge of MTBI and instructed the participants to provide responses based on "imagining" having sustained MTBI. Symptom responses were then compared with a group of 100 individuals with history of head injury, most with remote history of MTBI. With few exceptions, rates of self-reported PCS in the non–head-injured expectation group were strikingly consistent with those reported in the head-injured group, with approximately 67% shared variance in symptoms expected by the control group and the symptoms reported by the head-injured group. Furthermore, the head-injured group significantly underestimated frequencies of premorbid nonspecific symptoms relative to the non–head-injured group, suggesting that the head-injured group failed to appreciate the common and nonspecific nature of PCS and misattributed their symptoms to head injury. The authors suggested that expectation may play a causal role in symptom persistence.

In a related study, Gunstad and Suhr (2001) further explored the expectation as etiology hypothesis as well as retrospective report of PCS in a sample of 141 undergraduates assigned to one of six groups: prospective and retrospective healthy controls, a depression group, athletes with history of concussion, athletes without history of head injury, and individuals with chronic headaches. In support of the expectation as etiology theory, the authors found that the depressed group reported more current nonspecific symptoms than comparison groups. In addition, healthy controls, healthy athletes, and depressed participants all anticipated that they would experience more PCS following MTBI than they experienced in the present. Healthy athletes also anticipated having fewer post-MTBI PCS than healthy controls and depressed groups, which the authors offered may reflect the athletes' more realistic expectations related to previous experiences in sporting events or desire to recover based on the desires of their peers or coaches.

Consistent with the findings of Mittenberg et al. (1992), Gunstad and Suhr (2001) found that head-injured athletes reported significantly more current than preinjury PCS. However, participants with chronic headaches also reported more current than past nonspecific symptoms. As such, the authors offered that the

> experience of any negative event, be it accident or illness, head injury, or non–head-injury, may be required for one to focus on the past as 'better' than one's current state, for one to think about the 'good old days' prior to the negative event. (p. 330)

Subsequent researchers have reported similar findings supporting the "good old days bias" in independent samples, confirming that many individuals who sustain MTBI and report chronic PCS misperceive and minimize the frequency at which they experienced PCS prior to injury (Iverson et al., 2010; Lange, Iverson, & Rose, 2010). Beliefs regarding one's relative "health" prior to MTBI may serve as an important reinforcing source of ongoing PCS.

Negative expectations regarding recovery following MTBI may also contribute to diminished performances on formal neuropsychological measures. Suhr and Gunstad (2002) identified 36 undergraduates with history of MTBI, assigning 17 of the participants to a "diagnosis threat" group and 19 to a neutral condition group. In the diagnosis threat condition, specific reference was made to the history of MTBI, and participants were informed that neuropsychological research suggests that head injuries and concussions may result in cognitive deficits. The control group completed neuropsychological testing under neutral instructions. Although the diagnosis threat group demonstrated performances on measures of attention and cognitive efficiency that were comparable with the neutral condition group, the diagnosis threat performed significantly worse on measures of general intellect and memory function. Moreover, on completion of testing, the diagnosis threat group rated themselves as having put forth less effort, rated tasks as more difficult, and perceived that they had performed worse than the neutral condition group. Relevant to the current discussion of SVA in MTBI, self-perceived effort was, in turn, significantly correlated with overall performance on selected tasks in the diagnosis threat group, whereas perception of effort was not significantly correlated with performance in the neutral control group. The role of negative expectations and diagnosis threat on neuropsychological performances has been further examined in follow-up studies (Ozen & Fernandes, 2011; Suhr & Gunstad, 2005).

Secondary Gain and Symptom Exaggeration

In light of literature reviewed so far, it would be spurious to assume that all patients who report chronic symptoms after sustaining MTBI necessarily engage in motivated or intentional exaggeration of symptoms. It is essential to recognize that symptom *persistence* following MTBI does not necessarily connote purposeful symptom *exaggeration* following MTBI. Nevertheless, the reality is that a substantial proportion of MTBI cases who report chronic PCS frequently do exaggerate their symptoms (whether purposely or unpurposely) as described subsequently.

Rates of symptom exaggeration are known to increase dramatically within secondary gain contexts (e.g., personal injury litigation, workers' compensation, disability claim settings), and MTBI is among the most common conditions to be evaluated in secondary gain contexts (Greiffenstein, 2009). Litigation and secondary gain issues have been identified as significant moderators of long-term neuropsychological performances in MTBI samples (cf., Belanger et al., 2005; Binder & Rohling, 1996). One can expect that feigned cognitive performance may account for diminished neuropsychological performances for a proportion of litigating MTBI samples.

In fact, survey data illustrate the high rates of symptom exaggeration and malingering in litigating MTBI samples (Mittenberg, Patton, Canyock, & Condit, 2002). The authors surveyed 144 neuropsychologists who were board certified by the American Board of Clinical Neuropsychology (ABCN) regarding rates of probable symptom exaggeration or malingering in their practices. Illustrating the significant role of secondary gain context on symptom exaggeration, probable malingering was reported to transpire in approximately 19% of criminal cases, 29% of personal injury cases, and 30% of disability or workers' compensation cases, compared with a rate of only 8% in routine medical or psychiatric cases. Among the various conditions associated with litigation or compensation seeking, rates were highest for MTBI (38.5%), followed by fibromyalgia/chronic fatigue (34.7%), pain/somatoform disorders (31.4%), and neurotoxic disorders (26.5%). Of note, probable malingering and symptom exaggeration were reported to transpire in only 8.8% of litigating moderate-to-severe TBI cases.

The role of secondary gain and increased rates of symptom exaggeration is also illustrated by studies that observe neuropsychological performances among MTBI samples across various evaluation contexts (cf., Bianchini, Curtis, & Greve, 2006; Green, Rohling, Lees-Haley, & Allen, 2001). For example, Bianchini et al. (2006) examined symptom validity outcomes in a sample of 332 TBI (178 MTBI) cases according to levels of financial incentive to perform poorly. This study is unique in that it is among the few to adopt a dimensional approach to financial incentive status. Participants were identified as having no incentive, limited incentive (state-level workers' compensation law), or high incentive (federal law). The authors observed a "dose-response relationship" between potential financial compensation incentive and symptom validity indicators, with the high incentive group showing the broadest range of symptom invalidity. The authors concluded that clinicians should be especially attuned to possible exaggeration and malingering among individuals with high financial incentives, especially among individuals with histories of MTBI.

Rates of insufficient effort and symptom exaggeration have also been identified as varying by evaluation context in veteran MTBI samples (Nelson, Hoelzle, McGuire, et al., 2010; Nelson et al., 2011). Nelson, Hoelzle, McGuire, et al. (2010) examined neuropsychological performances of 44 veterans who were evaluated in the context of disability claim related to a remote history of MTBI. Performances of this secondary gain sample were compared with those of a veteran MTBI sample evaluated in a research context ($n = 38$) and a veteran research control group without history of MTBI ($n = 37$). Veterans evaluated in the disability context demonstrated a much higher rate of insufficient effort relative to veterans evaluated in the research group. For instance, 26 of the 44 (59.1%) veterans evaluated in the disability context demonstrated at least one indication of insufficient effort, seven (15.9%) showed two indications, and four (9.1%) showed three indications. This finding is notable when compared with eight of 75 (10.7%) research participants showing one indication of insufficient effort, and 0% showing any more than one indication of insufficient effort.

To summarize, although secondary gain and symptom exaggeration represent just one factor that may complicate or extend recovery following MTBI, the reality is that symptom exaggeration occurs with great frequency in MTBI samples, particularly among those who claim chronic PCS in the context of litigation or other secondary gain proceeding. As such, SVA is an essential component to neuropsychological evaluation in MTBI samples. It is in this context that we now discuss some of the more important findings that have emerged from the SVA/MTBI literature in recent years.

SYMPTOM VALIDITY ASSESSMENT RESEARCH IN MILD TRAUMATIC BRAIN INJURY CASES

Having reviewed some of the broader contextual issues that relate to recovery following MTBI and common factors that complicate or extend symptom recovery, we now turn to a discussion of the role of SVA itself in MTBI research. How do researchers typically conduct SVA/MTBI studies, and what important findings have been derived from SVA/MTBI research in recent years? We provide a relatively general overview of this research and refer the reader to Chapters 8, 9, and 10 of this volume for specific SVA measures and their respective strengths and weaknesses. This portion of the chapter specifically reviews

- common approaches to SVA/MTBI research,
- the impact of effort on cognitive performance in MTBI samples,
- the role of SVA in understanding MTBI outcomes,
- "paradoxical severity effect,"
- research on SVA of self-reported symptoms in MTBI,
- insufficient effort and psychological exaggeration in MTBI, and
- future directions.

Common Approaches to Symptom Validity Assessment/Mild Traumatic Brain Injury Research

Modern SVA/MTBI researchers have implemented several strategies to examine response validity issues in MTBI samples. The general form of these approaches has been described at length elsewhere (in particular, see Rogers, 2008 for an excellent review). The four most common designs implemented in SVA/MTBI research include simulation (analogue) research, "known groups" designs, "combined" groups, and differential prevalence designs.

Simulation Research

Some SVA/MTBI studies explore questions related to symptom exaggeration and malingering of MTBI-related deficits through simulation or analogue research. Simulation researchers typically instruct healthy community volunteers (e.g., college students) and/or clinical groups to exaggerate symptoms or feign cognitive deficits while completing cognitive testing and/or self-report measures. Results are then compared with those of a control group and/or clinical group that complete the same measures under conventional standardized ("honest") instructions. Participants who are instructed to simulate are often incentivized to successfully feign with a small monetary award, extra credit (for college students), or other reward.

A benefit of simulation research is that it allows researchers to better understand the quality of feigned MTBI-related cognitive deficits and symptoms as well as the magnitude of change in cognitive performance and self-reported symptoms that are associated with feigning. Simulation researchers are also able to apply statistical approaches (e.g., logistic regression, discriminant function analyses) that optimally differentiate the simulation groups from comparison groups according to appropriate cut scores (see Millis, 2008 for a fine review of statistical analyses in SVA research). Inspection of receiver–operator characteristics allow researchers to describe classification accuracies (e.g., specificity, sensitivity) that clinicians might consider in "real-world" forensic settings—settings in which feigned cognitive deficits and/or symptoms are most relevant. In addition, base rates of symptom validity are also known in simulation studies, which allows for clear understanding of classification accuracies that vary with base rates of a given condition such as positive and negative predictive power.

A classic example of an early SVA/TBI simulation study was conducted by Heaton et al. (1978), who were among the first to systematically investigate neuropsychologists' ability to discriminate feigned cognitive deficits from deficits associated with brain injury. The authors administered a neuropsychological test battery to a group of 16 participants with documented TBI histories (mostly severe TBI) under standardized conditions. Neuropsychological testing was also conducted on a group of 16 community volunteers who were instructed to feign cognitive deficits as if they had sustained an accident-related head injury to obtain a monetary award ($30). Overall level of impairment was comparable between the simulation and TBI groups, although some differences were observed on selected measures (e.g., motor function, MMPI presentation). Ten neuropsychologists were then requested to offer "blind" interpretations of the protocols and render an opinion as to whether protocols were more likely produced by simulators or TBI participants. Diagnostic accuracies of the neuropsychologists' judgments were modest, ranging from approximately 50% (chance level) to 68.8%. Results also suggested a weak relationship between one's confidence in detecting feigning and actual classification accuracy.

Results of simulation studies such as those reported by Heaton et al. (1978) and similar studies (e.g., Faust et al., 1988) played a pivotal role in raising clinicians' awareness regarding the importance of SVA in neuropsychological assessment and promoting research that improves detection of feigning and symptom exaggeration. In more recent years, SVA researchers have continued to implement simulation designs to explore various important issues such as (a) the effect of coaching on effort performance when simulating TBI (Brennan et al., 2009; Cato, Brewster, Ryan, & Giuliano, 2002); (b) malingering strategies among those instructed to feign impairment following TBI (Tan, Slick, Strauss, & Hultsch, 2002); and (c) the aforementioned role of misattribution in symptom presentation following MTBI (e.g., Mittenberg et al., 1992). One of the most tangible benefits of these simulation studies is the awareness of which participants are and are not exaggerating or feigning their MTBI-related impairments. Short of admission by test takers or arguably below-chance performance, clinicians are rarely able to state with complete confidence that patients and claimants with MTBI are feigning impairment. In other words, simulation research inherently includes high levels of internal validity (Arnett, Hammeke, & Schwartz, 1995).

However, what is gained in the way of *internal validity* through simulation research is lost in the way of *external validity* (Haines & Norris, 2001) or "generalizability to real-world settings" (Larrabee, 2007, p. 7). How can SVA/MTBI researchers be sure that the results of a study conducted under artificial conditions necessarily translate to real-world claimants? For example, the experiences of healthy college students is likely to vary substantially from claimants or litigants with a history of MTBI, comorbid psychological and emotional difficulties, and other factors that may contribute to one's approach to neuropsychological testing. In addition, claimants with histories of MTBI may be involved in a legal proceeding whose outcome may very well include substantial monetary awards that are significantly greater than the $50–$100 that may be offered to a college student who is instructed to feign difficulties.

In other words, the lack of generalizability of findings is a significant limitation of simulation research, and other approaches, such as the known-groups approach discussed subsequently, are typically preferable. Nevertheless, it is our belief that simulation research continues to play an important role in the study of SVA in MTBI under the assumption that studies explore novel questions under well-controlled experimental conditions. In addition, we are in agreement with Rogers (2008) that it is essential that simulation researchers compare simulation results not only with matched control groups but also with clinical samples with genuine histories of the condition under study to verify that between-group performance differences reflect feigning or symptom exaggeration and not the clinical condition (e.g., TBI) itself (e.g., Dearth et al., 2005).

Known Groups Studies

Another common approach to the study of SVA in MTBI is the known groups design, which entails *a priori* classification of feigning as defined by an independent gold standard or criterion (e.g., stand-alone effort measure) and observation of various outcomes between these independently classified groups. The known groups approach is typically conducted among real-world participants, often personal injury litigants or disability claimants who undergo neuropsychological evaluation related to a purported history of MTBI. As such, a benefit of this design is that participants are likely to be motivated by real-world incentives (Rogers, 2008). Inclusion of claimants and patients, as opposed to volunteer participants in simulation research, is likely to promote the relevance of study findings to routine clinical practice. A limitation of the known groups approach is that unlike simulation research in which groups are randomly assigned to feigning and nonfeigning conditions, random assignment is not a possibility in known groups research (Larrabee, 2007). Researchers cannot be completely sure of precise base rates of symptom exaggeration in forensic and clinical evaluation contexts, which limits their ability to provide precise estimates of positive and negative predictive validity. To get around this issue, researchers may cite differential prevalence research that establishes base rates estimates of symptom exaggeration (e.g., Mittenberg et al., 2002), and then generate positive and negative predictive values at various cut scores at theoretical base rates of symptom exaggeration.

In many ways, the known groups approach is well suited to SVA/MTBI research in light of neuropsychologists' increasing recognition of the importance of establishing specific criteria to inform one's diagnostic confidence in classifying symptom exaggeration and malingering. Criteria to establish classification of malingered neurocognitive dysfunction (MND), as proposed by Slick, Sherman, and Iverson (1999), have been particularly helpful to known groups in SVA/MTBI research in recent years. In summary, the Slick et al. (1999) criteria include multiple forms of information (e.g., patterns of performance on symptom validity testing [SVT], presentation on self-report measures of psychological function, discrepancies in performance and daily function) that allow clinicians and researchers to consider the likelihood that a given individual may be malingering or exaggerating his or her symptoms. Designations of possible, probable, and definite MND can be offered depending on the extent of feigning or symptom exaggeration that is demonstrated on formal evaluation and to the extent that feigning is believed to represent an attempt to secure an external incentive (e.g., monetary award).

As discussed in more detail in Chapters 8 and 9 of this volume, the known groups approach (using Slick et al., 1999 MND as an independent criterion) has been implemented to explore the use of a host of embedded effort indicators in TBI samples, such as the Wechsler Adult Intelligence Scale-III (WAIS-III; Curtis, Greve, & Bianchini, 2009); the Wechsler Memory Scale-III (WMS-III; Ord, Greve, & Bianchini, 2008); California Verbal Learning Test (CVLT; Curtis, Greve, Bianchini, & Brennan, 2006); verbal fluency (VF; Curtis, Thompson, Greve, & Bianchini, 2008); and Wisconsin Card Sorting Test (WCST; Greve, Heinly, Bianchini, & Love, 2009). Known groups design with Slick et al. (1999), MND as an independent criterion has also been employed to study the classification accuracies of SVTs themselves in MTBI samples, as in the case of the Test of Memory Malingering (TOMM; Greve, Bianchini, & Doane, 2006) and Portland Digit Recognition Test (PDRT; Greve & Bianchini, 2006). SVA/MTBI researchers have also applied the known groups design to examine MMPI-2 validity scale presentations associated with known insufficient effort (e.g., Greve, Bianchini, Love, Brennan, & Heinly, 2006).

Combined Group Studies

Rogers (2008) also recommended "combined research models," which integrate simulation and known groups designs in the study of response styles. This combined approach essentially allows researchers to benefit from the strengths of simulation research (internal validity) and known groups research (external validity) to allow for a powerful understanding of outcomes. However, with a few recent exceptions (Stevens & Merten, 2010), relatively few SVA/MTBI researchers have adopted the combined approach relative to those who have conducted either simulation or known groups approaches, and this highlights a need for future SVA/MTBI research.

Differential Prevalence Designs

Another approach to the study of SVA in MTBI samples is the differential prevalence design. In general, this design allows researchers to describe outcome frequencies in a given population, even if predictors of the outcome are not systematically examined. In SVA/MTBI research, a common differential design entails the documentation of symptom exaggeration frequencies in a given forensic evaluation context to identify the presumed role that secondary gain may have on one's presentation while undergoing neuropsychological evaluation (e.g., Lees-Haley, 1997). Meta-analytic approaches such as those conducted to understand the effect of financial incentives on cognition (Binder & Rohling, 1996) also adopt a differential prevalence design to address questions of interest. Other differential prevalence studies observe discrepancies in symptom exaggeration or insufficient effort according to evaluation context (e.g., forensic vs. clinical vs. research) to explore the quality and magnitude of symptom exaggeration in a given condition.

The differential prevalence design has been recognized as among the weakest approaches to SVA research (Rogers, 2008), largely owing to the fact that base rates of symptom exaggeration are *inferred* and not assessed directly. For example, some researchers may use evaluation context (e.g., forensic vs. clinical) as a proxy for symptom exaggeration rather than an independent gold standard (e.g., stand-alone effort test) to classify feigning and nonfeigning groups a priori. This approach follows the assumption that base rates of exaggeration are typically much higher in forensic versus clinical groups, even though this is not demonstrated in each study through a separate gold standard. Using this methodology, MTBI participants evaluated in the context of litigation or other secondary gain settings are anticipated to show higher rates of exaggeration than other comparison groups. Hence, researchers often compare outcomes of litigating MTBI samples with a clinical comparison group without identifying the extent to which either group exhibits feigning or symptom exaggeration with an independent criterion (as is the case in known groups research).

However, this approach is problematic because many, if not most, individuals who undergo neuropsychological evaluation in a forensic context do not engage in symptom exaggeration or malingering. In contrast, a meaningful proportion of individuals who undergo neuropsychological evaluation in a clinical context may have incentive to feign deficits for reasons that are not always clear to the examiner.

At the same time, however, the differential prevalence design can be "quite important for demonstrating the average effects associated with financial compensation" (Larrabee, 2007, p. 8). The approach of Tsushima, Geling, and Fabrigas (2011) is illustrative. The authors compared selected MMPI-2 validity scales of 281 litigating participants (with predominately MTBI diagnoses) with a group of 161 patients evaluated in a clinical context. Although the authors did not include an independent gold standard of symptom exaggeration, the MMPI-2 Symptom Validity Scale (formerly entitled the Fake Bad Scale [FBS]), Henry-Heilbronner Index (HHI), and Response Bias Scale (RBS) were found to be significantly higher in the litigating group relative to the control group, with particularly high effect size (ES) difference noted on RBS (.938). Findings such as these assist clinicians to understand that, on the group level, symptom invalidity is much higher in secondary gain contexts and is more likely to be observed on scales sensitive to exaggerated cognitive complaints.

Further, we would argue that the differential prevalence design can be potentially useful as a preliminary approach in understanding the symptom presentations of understudied MTBI samples. For example, in spite of the widespread occurrence of combat-related MTBI in the recent conflicts in Iraq and Afghanistan (McCrea et al., 2008), relatively few studies have examined long-term psychological and emotional presentations of veterans who reported a history of MTBI in these conflicts. Even fewer studies have examined how presentations of these returning veterans vary according to the setting in which they undergo neuropsychological evaluation. In this context, Nelson et al. (2011) examined the Minnesota Multiphasic Personality Inventory-2-Restructured Form (MMPI-2-RF) profiles of 128 veterans with remote histories of combat-related MTBI evaluated across forensic ($n = 42$), clinical ($n = 43$), and research ($n = 43$) settings. Across contexts, participants with active disability claims were approximately four times more likely to elevate on validity scales sensitive to exaggeration of somatic symptoms (FBS) and three times as likely to exaggerate on validity scales sensitive to cognitive difficulties (RBS). Again, although an independent indicator of symptom exaggeration (e.g., effort measure) was not administered to these participants, findings provide a benchmark of how presentation varies with secondary gain status in this novel population. The quality of symptom exaggeration (i.e., somatic, cognitive) in this cohort also assists clinicians in recognizing that interpretation of more traditional validity scales (e.g., F-scale) is unlikely to reveal symptom exaggeration among those with active disability claims.

The Impact of Effort on Cognitive Performance in Mild Traumatic Brain Injury Samples

One of the most compelling findings of the recent SVA/MTBI research is the dramatic effect that insufficient effort has on cognitive performance. In fact, some researchers have found that insufficient effort has more untoward effect on cognitive performance than severity of TBI itself. Illustrating this point, Green and colleagues (2001) examined neuropsychological performances of 904 consecutive patients, 470 of whom sustained a head injury of varying severity. Participants were evaluated in the context of workers' compensation claim, disability claim, or personal injury litigation. Participants completed a comprehensive neuropsychological battery inclusive of 43 test scores that were transformed to an overall test battery mean (OTBM) performance represented as a combined z score across performances. In the full sample, effort correlated very highly with overall test performance (0.73). Most notably, MTBI participants with evidence of insufficient effort showed significantly lower OTBM performances than moderate-to-severe TBI participants with sufficient effort. Thus, effort accounted for more than four times greater variance in OTBM performance than moderate-to-severe TBI itself.

Similar findings were reported in a follow-up study conducted by Rohling and Demakis (2010). The authors examined the role of TBI severity and effort on cognitive performance (again, inclusive of a composite OTBM performance) in the initial Green et al. (2001) sample as well as a second sample of participants studied by Bowden, Shores, and Mathias (2006). Averaging TBI severity rating parameters (GCS, PTA) in both research samples, TBI severity accounted for approximately 5% of OTBM performance. In contrast, effort accounted for approximately 25% of OTBM performance in the full sample. The result suggested that effort accounted for five times greater variance than TBI severity on cognitive test performance—a finding that was similar to the findings of Green et al. (2001). In further support, a study examining effort using embedded SVTs with clinical and forensic MTBI referrals, Meyers, Volbrecht, Axelrod, and Reinsch-Boothby (2011) found that almost 50% of the variance in neuropsychological test performance was explained by effort.

The overall effect of insufficient effort on cognitive performance is also informed by the results of meta-analytic research. Summarizing results of several previously published meta-analyses, Iverson (2005) compared cognitive outcomes of MTBI with those of various other conditions (e.g., moderate-to-severe TBI, depression, bipolar disorder) and exaggeration and malingering. Whereas the overall effect of MTBI on cognitive function was very small after approximately 3 months, moderate-to-severe TBI contributed to large (ESs) at both 0–6 months (ES > 0.90) and 24 months (ES > 0.8) postinjury (all results reviewed by Schretlen & Shapiro, 2003). Perhaps unsurprisingly, the effect of exaggeration/malingering in overall cognitive function was very high (ES > 1.0) according to a meta-analysis conducted by Vickery, Berry, Inman, Harris, and Orey (2001).

The Role of Symptom Validity Assessment in Understanding Mild Traumatic Brain Injury Outcomes

In light of the significant effect that effort contributed to cognitive performance in their sample, Green et al. (2001) expressed concern that failure to detect insufficient effort could lead researchers to reach false conclusions regarding the possible effect of MTBI on cognitive performance. In fact, the authors criticized previous concussion research that had not considered effort in their outcome reports (Dikmen, Machamer, Winn, & Temkin, 1995; Volbrecht, Meyers, & Kaster-Bundgaard, 2000).

When attempting to explore cognitive residua of concussion, it is now relatively commonplace for MTBI researchers to consider effort as a potential confound, and indications of insufficient effort are often considered as an important exclusion criteria. For example, as mentioned previously, rates of combat-related concussion in the recent conflicts in Iraq and Afghanistan are very high, and researchers are interested in the unique cognitive residua that may be associated with a history of combat-related MTBI (Belanger et al., 2009; Brenner et al., 2010; Gordon, Fitzpatrick, & Hilsabeck, 2011; Nelson, Hoelzle, McGuire, et al, 2010). Each of the latter authors excluded participants who demonstrated insufficient effort according to conventional cutoffs so that low scores were not falsely and directly attributed to the history of MTBI.

Illustrating this point, the aforementioned Nelson et al. (2010) study examined the effect of evaluation context and effort on neuropsychological performance in a veteran sample with reported histories of combat-related MTBI. Similar to Green et al. (2001) and Rohling and Demakis (2010), Nelson et al. developed an OTBM of overall neuropsychological performance derived from several neuropsychological measures. In particular, effort did not correlate significantly with OTBM when MTBI samples were evaluated in a research setting, largely because of the relatively infrequent occurrence of insufficient effort in this group. However, effort indicators were significantly correlated with OTBM (ranging from 0.45 to 0.58) when MTBI samples were evaluated in a forensic disability setting. OTBM among veteran MTBI disability claimants ($z = -0.75$) was significantly lower than a non-MTBI veteran research control group ($z = 0.02$) when not controlling for effort. If one were to interpret this at face value, one might conclude that MTBI contributes to cognitive impairment in the late stage of concussive injury. However, overall performance between MTBI veteran claimants with sufficient effort ($z = 0.00$) was nearly identical with the performance of the non-MTBI veteran research control group. These results highlight the importance of SVA in MTBI samples and support the notion that insufficient effort has a much greater effect on cognitive performance than MTBI itself in the late stage of concussive injury. For these reasons, it is now commonplace for reviewers of study manuscripts submitted to journals for publication to reject MTBI studies that do not include appropriate (e.g., sensitive and specific) SVA methods.

Paradoxical Severity Effect

As discussed earlier, TBI severity is conventionally rated according to several acute injury parameters. For instance, individuals who sustain LOC or PTA for extended durations are usually assigned a TBI rating that is of greater severity than those who do not sustain LOC of any duration and/or report seamless recall for events that transpired before and after the injury (no PTA). On this basis, one might anticipate a direct relationship between injury severity and cognitive impairment; the greater the severity, the greater the expected impairment. In fact, some researchers have documented a dose-response relationship between TBI severity and cognitive impairment in certain samples (Dikmen et al., 1995; Rohling, Meyers, & Millis, 2003).

However, a theme of the SVA/MTBI literature, at least among a subsample of individuals who report *chronic* symptoms or exhibit persisting impairments following MTBI, is the apparent incongruity that exists between what may appear to be a very mild brain injury on one hand and for many chronic MTBI patients a subjective experience of profound and disabling symptoms and impairments on the other. The general tendency for individuals with MTBI histories to show greater symptom embellishment or exaggeration on self-report measures of psychological and emotional function than more severely injured TBI samples has been labeled a paradoxical severity effect (Youngjohn, Davis, & Wolf, 1997). There is evidence that this same paradoxical severity effect is observed in some chronically symptomatic MTBI samples on effort testing (Greiffenstein & Baker, 2006; Thomas & Youngjohn, 2009).

Youngjohn et al. (1997) compared MMPI-2 profiles of 30 participants with histories of moderate-to-severe TBI with those of 30 litigating participants with histories of MTBI and chronic symptoms. Three sets of MMPI-2 profiles were compared: litigating MTBI, litigating severe TBI, and nonlitigating severe TBI. Although the litigating severe TBI group showed significantly greater elevations on selected clinical scales (Hs, Hy, Sc) relative to the nonlitigating severe TBI group, the litigating MTBI group showed marked elevations on multiple scales relative to both severe

TBI groups. Elevations in the MTBI group were particularly apparent on Hs, D, Hy, and Pt. The authors offered that these "paradoxical severity effects" might be viewed as being consistent with a somatoform disorder—a notion that had been offered by previous researchers (Putnam & Millis, 1994). The authors emphasize that their results are relevant only to those MTBI samples who report chronic symptoms and not the most of MTBI patients who typically show favorable recovery soon after injury.

In a follow-up study, Thomas and Youngjohn (2009) examined MMPI-2-RF profiles among a litigating sample of 55 participants with uncomplicated MTBI, 13 participants with complicated MTBI, and 15 participants with moderate-to-severe TBI. Participants also completed effort testing (PDRT, Word Memory Test [WMT], Dot Counting Test [DCT]) as a component of litigation. Although mild, a paradoxical severity effect was nevertheless observed on selected validity scales (FBS), clinical scales (Hs, D, Hy), and restructured clinical (RC) scales (RC1, RC2), with greater elevations observed in the uncomplicated MTBI group relative to the other groups. The authors also found an inverse relationship between symptom report and effort performances on SVT, although effort performance was more significantly associated with MMPI-2 presentation than TBI severity itself. The authors concluded that "litigation may lead to increased symptom reporting and elevated clinical and RC scales profiles irrespective of TBI severity" (p. 1079).

The notion of a paradoxical severity or "inverse dose-response" effect in MTBI samples was also explored by Greiffenstein and Baker (2006). The authors examined effort, motor, and psychiatric response validity indicators in an archival data set of 759 claimants who are head-injured. The sample was further classified according to symptomatic MTBI ("late postconcussion syndrome;" $n = 607$) and moderate-to-severe TBI groups ($n = 152$). Overall, results supported the notion of an inverse dose-response effect; individuals who had sustained less severe injuries demonstrated significantly worse performances on effort and motor measures. For example, individuals with histories of "whiplash" showed higher rates of symptom invalidity on the Rey Word Recognition test relative to those with histories of MTBI and moderate-to-severe TBI. Individuals with MTBI (admitting GCS of 15) showed significantly lower grip strength and TOMM performances relative to those with moderate and severe injuries. There was less evidence of paradoxical severity effect on the MMPI-2, although the authors restricted their analysis to the F-scale.

Paradoxical severity effects, which may reflect intentional and deliberate feigning (as in the case of malingering) or subconscious subversion of performance (as in the case of somatoform disorders), are also indirectly apparent in SVA/MTBI research showing that litigating MTBI samples underperform on effort measures relative to persons with dementia (e.g., Green, Montijo, & Brockhaus, 2011). Indeed, this counterintuitive finding essentially defines the floor effect strategy that underlies so many of the effort tests and embedded indices that are relied on neuropsychological practice (see Chapters 8 and 9 of this volume).

Research on Symptom Validity Assessment of Self-Reported Symptoms in Mild Traumatic Brain Injury

Individuals who exhibit noncredible presentations may not only feign cognitive deficits on effort measures but also exaggerate/embellish symptoms on self-report measures. A growing literature suggests that MTBI samples who exaggerate are most likely to overendorse or embellish somatic, cognitive, and overall health symptoms to a greater degree than other symptom types (e.g., psychotic). For many individuals, overendorsement of these varied physical (e.g., headaches, fatigue) and cognitive (e.g., inattention, memory complaints) difficulties may reflect an attempt to maintain a presentation that presumably reflects a history of MTBI.

The MMPI-2 continues to be among the most common measures administered in neuropsychological practice (Camara, Nathan, & Puente, 2000; Rabin, Barr, & Burton, 2005). One can assume that this reflects the strong use that the MMPI-2 has shown in identifying not only psychological and emotional difficulties through various clinical scales, but also the use that MMPI-2 validity scales have shown in identifying the validity of self-reported symptoms. Although other extended personality inventories include scales intended to assess the response validity of self-reported symptoms (e.g., Personality Assessment Inventory [PAI]; Morey, 1991), the effectiveness of these scales in detecting exaggerated somatic and cognitive symptoms has not been examined as extensively as the MMPI-2 in MTBI samples, and we shall, therefore, restrict our discussion to recent MMPI-2 studies pertaining to SVA in MTBI samples.

Several MMPI-2 validity scales, as well as more recently developed validity scales included in the MMPI-2-RF (Ben-Porath & Tellegen, 2008), have been shown to be especially useful in detecting exaggerated somatic and cognitive symptoms in MTBI samples. The MMPI-2-RF literature suggests that MTBI samples evaluated in forensic neuropsychology settings show a pattern of exaggeration that is quite distinct from other samples. Rather than to exaggerate psychotic symptoms and other difficulties that are typically detected by F-family scales (e.g., F, Fb, Fp), MTBI samples appear to exaggerate somatic and cognitive symptoms that are more akin to chronic postconcussive difficulties. Three recent MMPI-2-RF validity scales have shown particular merit in identifying exaggerated somatic and cognitive symptoms in MTBI samples: MMPI-2 Symptom Validity Scale (FBS; Lees-Haley, English, & Glenn,1991); RBS (Gervais, Ben-Porath, Wygant, & Green, 2007); and MMPI-2-RF Infrequent Somatic Symptoms Scale (Fs; Wygant et al., 2007).

The FBS, recently renamed as the Symptom Validity Scale, is among the more frequently studied "postrelease" MMPI-2 validity scales to be examined in MTBI samples. Use of the scale has increased dramatically since the time of development in 1991, and survey data suggest that it is among the top five symptom validity measures interpreted in clinical neuropsychology (Sharland & Gfeller, 2007). Initially developed for use with personal injury litigants with histories of motor vehicle-related and other forms of injury, FBS was developed to identify malingerers who "paradoxically present a combined mixture of fake good and fake bad self-reports" (Lees-Haley et al., 1991, p. 204) or provide selective self-reported psychological difficulties that can be linked exclusively to the injury itself (and minimize premorbid or alternate factors that might explain their symptoms).

FBS literature from the 1990s and 2000s supported the notion that the scale was sensitive to exaggeration of somatic symptoms (Larrabee, 1998; Greiffenstein, Baker, Axelrod, Peck, & Gervais, 2004), a pattern of exaggeration that was not likely to be apparent according to F, Fp, and other F-family scales. Many of these FBS studies included MTBI samples who were evaluated in forensic contexts and other settings in which high rates of overreported somatic symptoms might be anticipated (e.g., Ross, Millis, Krukowski, Putnam, & Adams, 2004). An initial meta-analytic review of this FBS literature suggested that FBS at times showed superior ES differences between overreporting and comparison groups (Nelson, Sweet, & Demakis, 2006). The composite ES between overreporting and comparison groups was large (0.96), and ES differences were especially large among studies that included samples with known insufficient effort (1.50) and among overreporting TBI samples (1.21).

A follow-up FBS meta-analysis (Nelson et al., 2010) documented continued proliferation of FBS literature, with approximately 52% increase in FBS literature identified since the time of the Nelson et al. (2006) study. As before, a large composite ES was observed in FBS between overreporting and comparison groups (0.95). Relevant to the current discussion of SVA and MTBI, the authors found that FBS ESs continued to be very large when studies included samples with known insufficient effort (1.16) and when studies included samples with purported histories of TBI (1.28). The latter results contrasted with results of the F-scale, which yielded only moderate ESs when effort was known to be insufficient (0.59) and in TBI samples (0.53). Summarizing results of both meta-analyses (Nelson et al., 2006, 2010), results suggested that FBS is likely to show greater effectiveness in identifying symptom exaggeration when individuals present with clear evidence of insufficient effort and when TBI (primarily MTBI) is the condition associated with one's reason for undergoing neuropsychological evaluation.

Another recently developed MMPI-2 validity scale relevant to our discussion of SVA/MTBI is the RBS. Unlike FBS, which was developed "rationally" on the basis of item content, the developers of RBS were interested in identifying MMPI-2-RF items that were sensitive to insufficient effort on formal effort testing. Specifically, Gervais et al. (2007) conducted multiple regression analyses to predict effort performances on three common effort measures (WMT, Computerized Assessment of Response Bias [CARB], TOMM), resulting in a 28-item scale that showed predictive use above and beyond F, Fp, and FBS. Although the initial validation study did not include MTBI samples, an early iteration of the scale showed strong ability to discriminate secondary gain claimants (primarily chronic MTBI) from a nonsecondary gain comparison group (Nelson, Sweet, & Heilbronner, 2007), and more recent studies have shown RBS to be of use in samples that were at least partly inclusive of MTBI (Whitney, Shepard, Williams, Davis, & Adams, 2009; Wygant et al., 2009). RBS has recently been added to the formal MMPI-2-RF computer scoring software available through University of Minnesota Press (http://www.upress.umn.edu/test-division/MMPI-2-RF/mmpi-2-rf-50-scales).

Another scale that may be useful in the detection of symptom exaggeration in chronic MTBI samples is the MMPI-2-RF Fs scale. The scale was developed to identify unusual somatic complaints that are not typically endorsed in diverse medical samples and chronic pain samples. An initial study revealed a large ES difference (0.90) between a sample with history of head injury and a sample of simulators instructed to feign symptoms. ESs for Fs were not meaningfully different across evaluation contexts (forensic, clinical, research) or disability claim status (active or nonactive) in a sample of veterans with histories of combat-related MTBI (Nelson et al., 2011). The authors suggested that methodological differences and sample differences (e.g., greater psychiatric comorbidities) in their study may account for the contrasting nature of their findings relative to those of Wygant et al. (2009). Further research is clearly needed to identify the potentially unique qualities of Fs in identifying symptom exaggeration in chronic MTBI samples.

Summarizing this literature, SVA of self-reported cognitive, physical, and emotional symptoms is needed in any circumstance when MTBI samples report symptoms on a chronic basis. The MMPI-2 is the most commonly administered measure of self-reported psychological and emotional functioning and continues to be an effective means of SVA in MTBI groups. Traditional validity scales, such as F and other F-family scales, are unlikely to detect exaggerated MTBI symptoms. FBS, RBS, and Fs are far more relevant to the quality of symptoms that are reported in chronic MTBI samples.

Insufficient Effort and Psychological Exaggeration: Distinct Constructs

Although SVA/MTBI research suggests that certain self-report validity scales (e.g., FBS, RBS) are more relevant to exaggerated self-reported symptoms than others (e.g., F-family), it is important to recognize that self-report SVA and performance (effort)-based SVA are separate methods of understanding response validity styles in chronic MTBI samples. Effort-based feigning and self-reported symptom exaggeration are distinct SVA strategies, and "malingering in one domain does not automatically imply malingering in the other" (Greiffenstein, Baker, Gola, Donders, & Miller 2002, p. 1599). Individuals may demonstrate response invalidity on effort testing, self-report measures, or both (Nelson & Sweet, 2009).

To better understand the constructs of cognitive and psychological symptom validity, Nelson, Sweet, Berry, Bryant, and Granacher (2007) conducted an exploratory factor analysis of three forced-choice effort measures (TOMM, Victoria Symptom Validity Test [VSVT], Letter Memory Test [LMT]) and several MMPI-2 validity scales, including the aforementioned FBS and RBS, in a sample of 122 compensation-seeking participants (approximately 60% were evaluated in relation to TBI). Results were consistent with a four-factor solution representing (a) insufficient effort; (b) symptom underreporting (L, K, S); (c) overreporting of psychotic or rarely endorsed symptoms (F, Fp); and (d) overreporting of neurotic (somatic, cognitive) symptoms (FBS, RBS). The effort factor a correlated minimally with factors b and c, and showed modest correlation (-0.39) with factor d. In other words, effort was most relevant to the quality of symptoms contained by scales that are sensitive to exaggeration of somatic (FBS) and cognitive (RBS) symptoms, but not to a degree that would suggest redundancy between the effort and self-report response validity constructs. The relationship between effort and self-reported somatic and cognitive symptoms was certainly not significant enough to suggest that either form of response validity measure could be used as a proxy for the other. The authors concluded that "incremental use" of both cognitive and psychological symptom validity measures was warranted in forensic neuropsychology settings.

Other research further supports the notion that self-report validity scales sensitive to somatic and/or cognitive symptom exaggeration are more predictive of effort performance than the others, although the overall relationship between effort and self-reported symptoms is modest. Smart et al. (2008) implemented optimal data analysis (ODA; Yarnold & Soltysik, 2005) to understand the potential value of MMPI-2 validity scales in predicting effort status. The authors included a sample of 198 participants evaluated in a secondary gain setting, most of whom reported a history of TBI and 109 participants without known secondary gain. Using MMPI-2 scales as predictors, ODA allowed the researchers to develop "linear decision trees" to classify effort status (sufficient vs. insufficient) according to optimal MMPI-2 cut scores. Of the MMPI-2 validity and clinical scales included in the ODA, an early version of RBS, combined with the Hysteria clinical scale, showed the strongest ability to identify insufficient effort in the sample. However, although specificity was generally strong in the overall model, sensitivity was relatively weak. The authors concluded that "both types of response validity measures (i.e., psychological and cognitive) do not directly correspond with one another, and both are necessary to obtain an accurate understanding of response validity for an individual patient or litigant" (p. 850).

Similar findings have been reported in more recent research conducted in military samples. Jones and Ingram (2011) implemented ODA in a group of 288 military personnel who completed the MMPI-2 and effort testing. The authors found that MMPI-2 and MMPI-2-RF scales sensitive to somatic and cognitive symptom exaggeration (e.g., RBS, FBS) showed stronger prediction of insufficient effort relative to the F-family scales.

In sum, the SVA/MTBI literature supports the joint use of self-report validity measures and effort measures in the evaluation of response validity in chronic MTBI samples. Implementation of both strategies is integral to a comprehensive SVA of individuals with chronic MTBI symptoms. Effort and self-report response validity measures can be interpreted incrementally and increase one's confidence in arriving at a classification of malingering as described by Slick et al. (1999).

CONCLUSIONS

SVA research in MTBI samples has dramatically improved clinicians' ability to identify feigned cognitive impairment and exaggerated symptoms relative to a time when neuropsychologists' ability to detect feigning was determined to be limited (Heaton et al., 1978). However, continued SVA/MTBI research is needed in several areas. For instance, as discussed in more detail in Chapter 19 of this volume, ongoing SVA/MTBI research is needed to better understand the strengths and limitations of contemporary SVA measures in specific MTBI populations such as pediatric/adolescent samples (Carone, 2008), geriatric samples, and culturally diverse groups (e.g., Vilar-López, Gómez-Río, Caracuel-Romero, Llamas-Elvira, & Pérez-García, 2008).

Continued development of sophisticated SVA strategies is also needed to protect against coaching that may be done on the part of attorneys and claimants as a means of maintaining the effectiveness of contemporary effort and self-report measures. The development of multiple effort indices within stand-alone effort measures (e.g., correct responses paired with response latencies on computerized effort measures; Slick, Hopp, Strauss, & Spellacy, 1996), sophisticated intrameasure regression effort indices (e.g., Wolfe et al., 2010), and the aggregation of multiple self-report measures, effort measures, and embedded indices (Boone, 2009; Larrabee, 2008; Meyers & Volbrecht, 2003; Victor, Boone, Serpa, Buehler, & Ziegler, 2009) will likely play an important role in maintaining the effectiveness of SVA in the future.

SVA/MTBI researchers are also encouraged to continue to explore underlying theoretical explanations for persisting PCS and factors that may contribute to feigning impairments and exaggerated symptoms in some MTBI samples. It is hoped that researchers will continue to discuss the somatization/malingering distinction in chronic MTBI samples, offer suggestions for revision to modern taxonomies (Berry & Nelson, 2010), and develop alternate ways of defining and conceptualizing excessive cognitive difficulties (Delis & Wetter, 2007) in their efforts to maintain the effectiveness of SVA in MTBI samples.

REFERENCES

Alexander, M. P. (1995). Mild traumatic brain injury: Pathophysiology, natural history, and clinical management. *Neurology, 45*(7), 1253–1260.

American Academy of Clinical Neuropsychology. (2007). American Academy of Clinical Neuropsychology (AACN) practice guidelines for neuropsychological assessment and consultation. *The Clinical Neuropsychologist, 21*(2), 209–231.

Arnett, P. A., Hammeke, T. A., & Schwartz, L. (1995). Quantitative and qualitative performance on Rey's 15-item test in neurological patients and dissimulators. *The Clinical Neuropsychologist, 9,* 17–26.

Bailey, C. M., Echemendia, R. J., & Arnett, P. A. (2006). The impact of motivation on neuropsychological performance in sports-related mild traumatic brain injury. *Journal of the International Neuropsychological Society, 12*(4), 475–484.

Belanger, H. G., Curtiss, G., Demery, J. A., Lebowitz, B. K., & Vanderploeg, R. D. (2005). Factors moderating neuropsychological outcomes following mild traumatic brain injury: A meta-analysis. *Journal of the International Neuropsychological Society, 11*(3), 215–227.

Belanger, H. G., Kretzmer, T., Yoash-Gantz, R., Pickett, T., & Tupler, L. A. (2009). Cognitive sequelae of blast-related versus other mechanisms of brain trauma. *Journal of the International Neuropsychological Society, 15*, 1–8

Ben-Porath, Y. S., & Tellegen, A. (2008). *MMPI-2-RF (Minnesota Multiphasic Personality Inventory-2 Restructured Form): Manual for administration, scoring, and interpretation.* Minneapolis, MN: University of Minnesota Press.

Berry, D. T. R., & Nelson, N. W. (2010). DSM-5 and malingering: A modest proposal. *Psychological Injury and Law, 3*(4), 295–303.

Bianchini, K. J., Curtis, K. L., & Greve, K. W. (2006). Compensation and malingering in traumatic brain injury: A dose-response relationship? *The Clinical Neuropsychologist, 20*(4), 831–847.

Binder, L. M., & Rohling, M. L. (1996). Money matters: A meta-analytic review of the effects of financial incentives on recovery after closed-head injury. *The American Journal of Psychiatry, 153*(1), 7–10.

Binder, L. M., Rohling, M. L., & Larrabee, G. J. (1997). A review of mild head trauma. Part I: Meta-analytic review of neuropsychological studies. *Journal of Clinical and Experimental Neuropsychology, 19*(3), 421–431.

Boone, K. B. (Ed.). (2007). *Assessment of feigned cognitive impairment: A neuropsychological perspective.* New York, NY: The Guilford Press.

Boone, K. B. (2009). The need for continuous and comprehensive sampling of effort/response bias during neuropsychological examinations. *The Clinical Neuropsychologist, 23*(4), 729–741.

Bowden, S. C., Shores, E. A., & Mathias, J. L. (2006). Does effort suppress cognition after brain injury? A re-examination of the evidence for the Word Memory Test. *The Clinical Neuropsychologist, 20*(4), 858–872.

Brennan, A. M., Meyer, S., David, E., Pella, R., Hill, B. D., & Gouvier, W. D. (2009). The vulnerability to coaching across measures of effort. *The Clinical Neuropsychologist, 23*(2), 314–328.

Brenner, L. A., Terrio, H., Homaifar, B. Y., Gutierrez, P. M., Staves, P. J., Harwood, J. E., . . . Warden, D. (2010). Neuropsychological test performance in soldiers with blast-related mild TBI. *Neuropsychology, 24*(2), 160–167.

Bush, S. S., Ruff, R. M., Tröster, A. I., Barth, J. T., Koffler, S. P., Pliskin, N. H., . . . Silver, C. H. (2005). NAN policy & planning committee position paper: Symptom validity assessment: Practice issues and medical necessity. *Archives of Clinical Neuropsychology, 20*, 419–426.

Camara, W. J., Nathan, J. S., & Puente, A. E. (2000). Psychological test usage: Implications in professional psychology. *Professional Psychology: Research and Practice, 31*(2), 141–154.

Carone, D. A. (2008). Children with moderate/severe brain damage/dysfunction outperform adults with mild-to-no brain damage on the medical symptom validity test. *Brain Injury, 22*(12), 960–971.

Cato, M. A., Brewster, J., Ryan, T., & Giuliano, A. J. (2002). Coaching and the ability to simulate mild traumatic brain injury symptoms. *The Clinical Neuropsychologist, 16*(4), 524–535.

Curtis, K. L., Greve, K. W., & Bianchini, K. J. (2009). The Wechsler Adult Intelligence Scale-III and malingering in traumatic brain injury: Classification accuracy in known groups. *Assessment, 16*(4), 401–414.

Curtis, K. L., Greve, K. W., Bianchini, K. J., & Brennan, A. (2006). California verbal learning test indicators of malingered neurocognitive dysfunction: Sensitivity and specificity in traumatic brain injury. *Assessment, 13*(1), 46–61.

Curtis, K. L., Thompson, L. K., Greve, K. W., & Bianchini, K. J. (2008). Verbal fluency indicators of malingering in traumatic brain injury: Classification accuracy in known groups. *The Clinical Neuropsychologist, 22*(5), 930–945.

Dearth, C. S., Berry, D. T., Vickery, C. D., Vagnini, V. L., Baser, R. E., Orey, S. A., & Cragar, D. E. (2005). Detection of feigned head injury symptoms on the MMPI-2 in head injured patients and community controls. *Archives of Clinical Neuropsychology, 20*(1), 95–110.

Delis, D. C., & Wetter, S. R. (2007). Cogniform disorder and cogniform condition: Proposed diagnoses for excessive cognitive symptoms. *Archives of Clinical Neuropsychology, 22*(5), 589–604.

Dikmen, S. S., Machamer, J. E., Winn, H. R., & Temkin, N. R. (1995). Neuropsychological outcome at 1-year post head injury. *Neuropsychology, 9*, 80–90.

Evered, L., Ruff, R., Baldo, J., & Isomura, A. (2003). Emotional risk factors and postconcussional disorder. *Assessment, 10*(4), 420–427.

Fann, J. R., Katon, W. J., Uomoto, J. M., & Esselman, P. C. (1995). Psychiatric disorders and functional disability in outpatients with traumatic brain injuries. *The American Journal of Psychiatry, 152*(10), 1493–1499.

Faust, D., Hart, K., & Guilmette, T. J. (1988). Pediatric malingering: The capacity of children to fake believable deficits on neuropsychological testing. *Journal of Consulting and Clinical Psychology, 56*(4), 578–582.

Fenton, G., McClelland, R., Montgomery, A., MacFlynn, G., & Rutherford, W. (1993). The postconcussional syndrome: Social antecedents and psychological sequelae. *The British Journal of Psychiatry*, 162, 493–497.

Frencham, K. A., Fox, A. M., & Maybery, M. T. (2005). Neuropsychological studies of mild traumatic brain injury: A meta-analytic review of research since 1995. *Journal of Clinical and Experimental Neuropsychology*, 27(3), 334–351.

Gervais, R. O., Ben-Porath, Y. S., Wygant, D. B., & Green, P. (2007). Development and validation of a response bias scale (RBS) for the MMPI-2. *Assessment*, 14(2), 196–208.

Gordon, S. N., Fitzpatrick, P. J., & Hilsabeck, R. C. (2011). No effect of PTSD and other psychiatric disorders on cognitive functioning in veterans with mild TBI. *The Clinical Neuropsychologist*, 25(3), 337–347.

Green, P., Montijo, J., & Brockhaus, R. (2011). High specificity of the word memory test and medical symptom validity test in groups with severe verbal memory impairment. *Applied Neuropsychology*, 18(2), 86–94.

Green, P., Rohling, M. L., Lees-Haley, P. R., & Allen, L. M. III. (2001). Effort has a greater effect on test scores than severe brain injury in compensation claimants. *Brain Injury*, 15(12), 1045–1060.

Greiffenstein, M. F. (2009). Clinical myths of forensic neuropsychology. *The Clinical Neuropsychologist*, 23(2), 286–296.

Greiffenstein, M. F., & Baker, W. J. (2001). Comparison of premorbid and postinjury MMPI-2 profiles in late postconcussion claimants. *The Clinical Neuropsychologist*, 15(2), 162–170.

Greiffenstein, M. F., & Baker, W. J. (2006). Miller was (mostly) right: Head injury severity inversely related to simulation. *Legal and Criminological Psychology*, 11, 131–145.

Greiffenstein, M. F., Baker, W. J., Axelrod, B., Peck, E. A., & Gervais, R. (2004). The fake bad scale and MMPI-2 F-family in detection of implausible trauma claims. *The Clinical Neuropsychologist*, 18(4), 573–590.

Greiffenstein, M. F., Baker, W. J., Gola, T., Donders, J., & Miller, L. J. (2002). The fake bad scale in atypical and severe closed head injury litigants. *Journal of Clinical Psychology*, 58(12), 1591–1600.

Greve, K. W., & Bianchini, K. J. (2006). Classification accuracy of the Portland Digit Recognition Test in traumatic brain injury: Results of a known-groups analysis. *The Clinical Neuropsychologist*, 20(4), 816–830.

Greve, K. W., Bianchini, K. J., & Doane, B. M. (2006). Classification accuracy of the test of memory malingering in traumatic brain injury: Results of a known-groups analysis. *Journal of Clinical and Experimental Neuropsychology*, 28(7), 1176–1190.

Greve, K. W., Bianchini, K. J., Love, J. M., Brennan, A., & Heinly, M. T. (2006). Sensitivity and specificity of MMPI-2 validity scales and indicators to malingered neurocognitive dysfunction in traumatic brain injury. *The Clinical Neuropsychologist*, 20(3), 491–512.

Greve, K. W., Heinly, M. T., Bianchini, K. J., & Love, J. M. (2009). Malingering detection with the Wisconsin card sorting test in mild traumatic brain injury. *The Clinical Neuropsychologist*, 23(2), 343–362.

Gunstad, J., & Suhr, J. A. (2001). "Expectation as etiology" versus "the good old days": Postconcussion syndrome symptom reporting in athletes, headache sufferers, and depressed individuals. *Journal of the International Neuropsychological Society*, 7(3), 323–333.

Haines, M. E., & Norris, M. P. (2001). Comparing student and patient simulated malingerers' performance on standard neuropsychological measures to detect feigned cognitive deficits. *The Clinical Neuropsychologist*, 15(2), 171–182.

Heaton, R. K., Smith, H. H. Jr., Lehman, R. A., & Vogt, A. T. (1978). Prospects for faking believable deficits on neuropsychological testing. *Journal of Consulting and Clinical Psychology*, 46(5), 892–900.

Heilbronner, R. L., Sweet, J. J., Morgan, J. E., Larrabee, G. J., Millis, S. R. (2009). American Academy of Clinical Neuropsychology Consensus Conference Statement on the neuropsychological assessment of effort, response bias, and malingering. *The Clinical Neuropsychologist*, 23(7), 1093–1129.

Hibbard, M. R., Bogdany, J., Uysal, S., Kepler, K., Silver, J. M., Gordon, W. A., & Haddad, L. (2000). Axis II psychopathology in individuals with traumatic brain injury. *Brain Injury*, 14(1), 45–61.

Hoge, C. W., McGurk, D., Thomas, J. L., Cox, A. L., Engel, C. C., & Castro, C. A. (2008). Mild traumatic brain injury in U.S. soldiers returning from Iraq. *The New England Journal of Medicine*, 358(5), 453–463.

Iverson, G. L. (2005). Outcome from mild traumatic brain injury. *Current Opinion in Psychiatry*, 18(3), 301–317.

Iverson, G. L. (2006). Misdiagnosis of the persistent postconcussion syndrome in patients with depression. *Archives of Clinical Neuropsychology*, 21(4), 303–310.

Iverson, G. L., & Lange, R. T. (2003). Examination of "postconcussion-like" symptoms in a healthy sample. *Applied Neuropsychology*, 10(3), 137–144.

Iverson, G. L., Lange, R. T., Brooks, B. L., & Rennison, V. L. (2010). "Good old days" bias following mild traumatic brain injury. *The Clinical Neuropsychologist*, 24(1), 17–37.

Iverson, G. L., & McCracken, L. M. (1997). 'Postconcussive' symptoms in persons with chronic pain. *Brain Injury*, 11(11), 783–790.

Jones, A., & Ingram, M. V. (2011). A comparison of selected MMPI-2 and MMPI-2-RF validity scales in assessing effort on cognitive tests in a military sample. *The Clinical Neuropsychologist*, 25(7), 1207–1227.

Kay, T., Harrington, D. E., Adams, R. E., Anderson, T. W., Berrol, S., Cicerone, K., . . . Malec, J. (1993). Definition of mild traumatic brain injury. *Journal of Head Trauma Rehabilitation*, 8(3), 86–87.

King, N. S. (1996). Emotional, neuropsychological, and organic factors: Their use in the prediction of persisting postconcussion symptoms after moderate and mild head injuries. *Journal of Neurology, Neurosurgery & Psychiatry*, 61(1), 75–81.

Lange, R. T., Iverson, G. L., & Rose, A. (2010). Post-concussion symptom reporting and the "good old days bias" following mild traumatic brain injury. *Archives of Clinical Neuropsychology*, 25(5), 442–450.

Langlois, J. A., Rutland-Brown, W., & Thomas, K. E. (2006). *Traumatic brain injury in the United States: Emergency department visits, hospitalizations, and deaths*. Atlanta, GA: Centers for Disease Control and Prevention, National Center for Injury Prevention and Control. Retrieved from http://www .cdc.gov/ncipc/pub-res/TBI_in_US_04/TBI_ED.htm

Larrabee, G. J. (1998). Somatic malingering on the MMPI and MMPI-2 in litigating subjects. *The Clinical Neuropsychologist*, 12, 179–188.

Larrabee, G. J. (Ed.). (2007). *Assessment of malingered neuropsychological deficits*. New York, NY: Oxford University Press.

Larrabee, G. J. (2008). Aggregation across multiple indicators improves the detection of malingering: Relationship to likelihood ratios. *The Clinical Neuropsychologist*, 22(4), 666–679.

Lees-Haley, P. R. (1997). MMPI-2 base rates for 492 personal injury plaintiffs: Implications and challenges for forensic assessment. *Journal of Clinical Psychology*, 53, 745–755.

Lees-Haley, P. R., English, L. T., & Glenn, W. J. (1991). A fake bad scale on the MMPI-2 for personal injury claimants. *Psychological Reports*, 68(1), 203–210.

McCrea, M. A. (2008). *Mild traumatic brain injury and postconcussion syndrome: The new evidence base for diagnosis and treatment*. New York, NY: Oxford University Press.

McCrea, M., Guskiewicz, K. M., Marshall, S. W., Barr, W., Randolph, C., Cantu, R. C., . . . Kelly, J. P. (2003). Acute effects and recovery time following concussion in collegiate football players: The NCAA concussion study. *Journal of the American Medical Association*, 290(19), 2556–2563.

McCrea, M., Pliskin, N., Barth, J., Cox, D., Fink, J., French, L., . . . Yoash-Gantz, R. (2008). Official position of the military TBI task force on the role of neuropsychology and rehabilitation psychology in the evaluation, management, and research of military veterans with traumatic brain injury. *The Clinical Neuropsychologist*, 22(1), 10–26.

McLean, A. Jr., Temkin, N. R., Dikmen, S., & Wyler, A. R. (1983). The behavioral sequelae of head injury. *Journal of Clinical Neuropsychology*, 5(4), 361–376.

Metalsky, G., Halberstadt, L., & Abramson, L. (1987). Vulnerability to depressive mood reactions: Toward a more powerful test of the diathesis-stress and causal mediation components of the reformulated theory of depression. *Journal of Personality and Social Psychology*, 52(2), 386–393.

Meyers, J. E., & Volbrecht, M. E. (2003). A validation of multiple malingering detection methods in a large clinical sample. *Archives of Clinical Neuropsychology*, 18(3), 261–276.

Meyers, J. E., Volbrecht, M. E., Axelrod, B. N., & Reinsch-Boothby, L. (2011). Embedded symptom validity tests and overall neuropsychological test performance. *Archives of Clinical Neuropsychology*, 26(1), 8–15.

Millis, S. R. (2008). Assessment of incomplete effort and malingering in the neuropsychological examination. In J. E. Morgan & J. H. Ricker (Eds.), *Textbook of clinical neuropsychology* (pp. 891–904). New York, NY: Taylor & Francis.

Mittenberg, W., Canyock, E. M., Condit, D., & Patton, C. (2001). Treatment of post-concussion syndrome following mild head injury. *Journal of Clinical and Experimental Neuropsychology*, 23(6), 829–836.

Mittenberg, W., Patton, C., Canyock, E. M., & Condit, D. C. (2002). Base rates of malingering and symptom exaggeration. *Journal of Clinical and Experimental Neuropsychology*, 24, 1094–1102

Mittenberg, W., DiGiulio, D. V., Perrin, S., & Bass, A. E. (1992). Symptoms following mild head injury: Expectation as aetiology. *Journal of Neurology, Neurosurgery & Psychiatry*, 55(3), 200–204.

Morey, L. C. (1991). *Personality assessment inventory*. Odessa, FL: Psychological Assessment Resources.

Morgan, J., & Sweet, J. (Eds.). (2008). *Neuropsychology of malingering casebook*. New York, NY: Taylor & Francis.

Nelson, N. W., Hoelzle, J. B., McGuire, K. A., Ferrier-Auerbach, A. G., Charlesworth, M. J., & Sponheim, S. R. (2010). Evaluation context impacts neuropsychological performance of OEF/OIF veterans with reported combat-related concussion. *Archives of Clinical Neuropsychology*, 25(8), 713–723.

Nelson, N. W., Hoelzle, J. B., McGuire, K. A., Sim, A. H., Goldman, D. J., Ferrier-Auerbach, A. G., . . . Sponheim, S. R. (2011). Self-report of psychological function among OEF/OIF personnel who also report combat-related concussion. *The Clinical Neuropsychologist, 25*(5), 716–740.

Nelson, N. W., Hoelzle, J. B., Sweet, J. J., Arbisi, P. A., & Demakis, G. J. (2010). Updated meta-analysis of the MMPI-2 symptom validity scale (FBS): Verified utility in forensic practice. *The Clinical Neuropsychologist, 24*(4), 701–724.

Nelson, N. W., Lamberty, G. J., Sim, A. H., Doane, B. M., & Vanderploeg, R. A. (in press). Traumatic brain injury in veterans. In S. S. Bush (Ed.), *Neuropsychological practice with veterans.* New York, NY: Springer Publishing.

Nelson, N. W., & Sweet, J. J. (2009). Malingering of psychiatric disorders in neuropsychological evaluations: Divergence of cognitive effort measures and psychological test validity indicators. In J. Morgan & J. Sweet (Eds.), *Neuropsychology of malingering casebook* (pp. 195–213). New York, NY: Taylor & Francis.

Nelson, N. W., Sweet, J. J., Berry, D. T. R., Bryant, F. B., & Granacher, R. P. (2007). Response validity in forensic neuropsychology: Exploratory factor analytic evidence of distinct cognitive and psychological constructs. *Journal of the International Neuropsychological Society, 13*(3), 440–449.

Nelson, N. W., Sweet, J. J., & Demakis, G. J. (2006). Meta-analysis of the MMPI-2 fake bad scale: Utility in forensic practice. *The Clinical Neuropsychologist, 20*(1), 39–58.

Nelson, N. W., Sweet, J. J., & Heilbronner, R. L. (2007). Examination of the new MMPI-2 response bias scale (Gervais): Relationship with MMPI-2 validity scales. *Journal of Clinical and Experimental Neuropsychology, 29*(1), 67–72.

Ord, J. S., Greve, K. W., & Bianchini, K. J. (2008). Using the Wechsler Memory Scale-III to detect malingering in mild traumatic brain injury. *The Clinical Neuropsychologist, 22*(4), 689–704.

Owens, B. D., Kragh, J. F. Jr., Wenke, J. C., Macaitis, J., Wade, C. E., & Holcomb, J. B. (2008). Combat wounds in Operation Iraqi Freedom and Operation Enduring Freedom. *The Journal of Trauma, 64*(2), 295–299.

Ozen, L. J., & Fernandes, M. A. (2011). Effects of "diagnosis threat" on cognitive and affective functioning long after mild head injury. *Journal of the International Neuropsychological Society, 17*(2), 219–229.

Paniak, C., Reynolds, S., Toller-Lobe, G., Melnyk, A., Nagy, J., & Schmidt, D. (2002). A longitudinal study of the relationship between financial compensation and symptoms after treated mild traumatic brain injury. *Journal of Clinical and Experimental Neuropsychology, 24*(2), 187–193.

Polusny, M. A., Kehle, S. M., Nelson, N. W., Erbes, C. R., Arbisi, P. A., & Thuras, P. (2011). Longitudinal effects of mild TBI and PTSD comorbidity on postdeployment outcomes in national guard soldiers deployed to Iraq. *Archives of General Psychiatry, 68*(1), 79–89.

Putnam, S. H., & Millis, S. R. (1994). Psychosocial factors in the development and maintenance of chronic somatic and functional symptoms following mild traumatic brain injury. *Advances in Medical Psychotherapy, 7*, 1–22.

Rabin, L., Barr, W., & Burton, L. (2005). Assessment practices of clinical neuropsychologists in the United States and Canada: A survey of INS, NAN, and APA Division 40 members. *Archives of Clinical Neuropsychology, 20*(1), 33–65.

Robertson, E. J., Rath, B., Fournet, G., Zelhart, P., & Estes, R. (1994). Assessment of mild brain trauma: A preliminary study of the influence of premorbid factors. *The Clinical Neuropsychologist, 8*, 69–74.

Rogers, R. (Ed.). (2008). Researching response styles. In *Clinical assessment of malingering and deception* (3rd ed., pp. 411–434). New York, NY: Guilford Press.

Rohling, M. L., Binder, L. M., Demakis, G. J., Larrabee, G.J., Ploetz, D.M., & Langhinrichsen-Rohling, J. (2011). A meta-analysis of neuropsychological outcome after mild traumatic brain injury: Reanalyses and reconsiderations of Binder et al. (1997), Frencham et al. (2005), and Pertab et al. (2009). *The Clinical Neuropsychologist, 25*(4), 608–623.

Rohling, M. L. & Demakis, G. J. (2010). Bowden, Shores, & Mathias (2006): Failure to replicate or just failure to notice. *Does effort still account for more variance in neuropsychological test scores than TBI severity? The Clinical Neuropsychologist, 24*(1), 119–136.

Rohling, M. L., Meyers, J. E., & Millis, S. R. (2003). Neuropsychological impairment following traumatic brain injury: A dose-response analysis. *The Clinical Neuropsychologist, 17*(3), 289–302.

Ross, S. R., Millis, S. R., Krukowski, R. A., Putnam, S. H., & Adams, K. M. (2004). Detecting probable malingering on the MMPI-2: An examination of the fake bad scale in mild head injury. *Journal of Clinical and Experimental Neuropsychology, 26*(1), 115–124.

Rutherford, W. H., Merrett, J. D., & McDonald, J. R. (1979). Symptoms at one year following concussion from minor head injuries. *Injury, 10*(3), 225–230.

Schneiderman, A. I., Braver, E. R., & Kang, H. K. (2008). Understanding sequelae of injury mechanisms and mild traumatic brain injury incurred during the conflicts in Iraq and Afghanistan: Persistent postconcussive symptoms and posttraumatic stress disorder. *American Journal of Epidemiology, 167*(12), 1446–1452.

Schretlen, D. J., & Shapiro, A. M. (2003). A quantitative review of the effects of traumatic brain injury on cognitive functioning. *International Review of Psychiatry*, 15(4), 341–349.

Sharland, M. J., & Gfeller, J. D. (2007). A survey of neuropsychologists' beliefs and practices with respect to the assessment of effort. *Archives of Clinical Neuropsychology*, 22(2), 213–223.

Slick, D. J., Hopp, G., Strauss, E., & Spellacy, F. J. (1996). Victoria symptom validity test: Efficiency for detecting feigned memory impairment and relationship to neuropsychological tests and MMPI-2 validity scales. *Journal of Clinical and Experimental Neuropsychology*, 18(6), 911–922.

Slick, D. J., Sherman, E. M., & Iverson, G. L. (1999). Diagnostic criteria for malingered neurocognitive dysfunction: Proposed standards for clinical practice and research. *The Clinical Neuropsychologist*, 13(4), 545–561.

Smart, C., Nelson, N. W., Sweet, J. J., Bryant, F. B., Berry, D. T., Granacher, R. P., & Heilbronner, R. L. (2008). Use of MMPI-2 to predict cognitive effort: A hierarchically optimal classification tree analysis. *Journal of the International Neuropsychological Society*, 14(5), 842–852.

Stevens, A., & Merten, T. (2010). Psychomotor retardation: Authentic or Malingered? A comparative study of subjects with and without traumatic brain injury and experimental simulators. *German Journal of Psychiatry*, 13, 1–8.

Suhr, J. A., & Gunstad, J. (2002). "Diagnosis threat": The effect of negative expectations on cognitive performance in head injury. *Journal of Clinical and Experimental Neuropsychology*, 24(4), 448–457.

Suhr, J. A., & Gunstad, J. (2005). Further exploration of the effect of "diagnosis threat" on cognitive performance in individuals with mild head injury. *Journal of the International Neuropsychological Society*, 11(1), 23–29.

Sweet, J. J., King, J. H., Malina, A. C., Bergman, M. A., & Simmons, A. (2002). Documenting the prominence of forensic neuropsychology at national meetings and in relevant professional journals from 1990 to 2000. *The Clinical Neuropsychologist*, 16(4), 481–494.

Sweet, J. J., Meyer, D., Nelson, N. W., & Moberg, P. J. (2011). The TCN/AACN 2010 "salary survey": Professional practices, beliefs, and incomes of U.S. neuropsychologists. *The Clinical Neuropsychologist*, 25(1), 12–61.

Sweet, J. J., Nelson, N. W., & Moberg, P. (2006). The TCN/AACN 2005 "salary survey": Professional practices, beliefs, and incomes of U.S. neuropsychologists. *The Clinical Neuropsychologist*, 20, 325–364.

Tan, J. E., Slick, D. J., Strauss, E., & Hultsch, D. F. (2002). How'd they do it? Malingering strategies on symptom validity tests. *The Clinical Neuropsychologist*, 16(4), 495–505.

Teasdale, G., & Jennett, B. (1974). Assessment of coma and impaired consciousness: A practical scale. *Lancet*, 2, 81–83.

Terrio, H., Brenner, L. A., Ivins, B. J., Cho, J. M., Helmick, K., Schwab, K., . . . Warden, D. (2009). Traumatic brain injury screening: Preliminary findings in a U.S. Army Brigade combat team. *The Journal of Head Trauma Rehabilitation*, 24(1), 14–23.

Thomas, M. L., & Youngjohn, J. R. (2009). Let's not get hysterical: Comparing the MMPI-2 validity, clinical, and RC scales in TBI litigants tested for effort. *The Clinical Neuropsychologist*, 23(6), 1067–1084.

Thurman, D., & Guerrero, J. (1999). Trends in hospitalization associated with traumatic brain injury. *The Journal of the American Medical Association*, 282(10), 954–957.

Tsushima, W. T., Geling, O., & Fabrigas, J. (2011). Comparison of MMPI-2 validity scale scores of personal injury litigants and disability claimants. *The Clinical Neuropsychologist*, 25(8), 1403–1414.

Vickery, C. D., Berry, D. T., Inman, T. H., Harris, M. J., & Orey, S. A. (2001). Detection of inadequate effort on neuropsychological testing: A meta-analytic review of selected procedures. *Archives of Clinical Neuropsychology*, 16(1), 45–73.

Victor, T. L., Boone, K. B., Serpa, J. G., Buehler, J., & Ziegler, E. A. (2009). Interpreting the meaning of multiple symptom validity test failure. *The Clinical Neuropsychologist*, 23(2), 297–313.

Vilar-López, R., Gómez-Río, M., Caracuel-Romero, A., Llamas-Elvira, J., & Pérez-García, M. (2008). Use of specific malingering measures in a Spanish sample. *Journal of Clinical and Experimental Neuropsychology*, 30(6), 710–722.

Volbrecht, M. E., Meyers, J. E., & Kaster-Bundgaard, J. (2000). Neuropsychological outcome of head injury using a short battery. *Archives of Clinical Neuropsychology*, 15(3), 251–265.

Whitney, K. A., Shepard, P. H., Williams, A. L., Davis, J. J., & Adams, K. M. (2009). The medical symptom validity test in the evaluation of Operation Iraqi Freedom/Operation Enduring Freedom soldiers: A preliminary study. *Archives of Clinical Neuropsychology*, 24(2), 145–152.

Wolfe, P. L., Millis, S. R., Hanks, R., Fichtenberg, N., Larrabee, G. J., & Sweet, J. J. (2010). Effort indicators within the California Verbal Learning Test-II (CVLT-II). *The Clinical Neuropsychologist*, 24(1), 153–168.

Wood, R. L. (2004). Understanding the "miserable minority": A diathesis-stress paradigm for post-concussional syndrome. *Brain Injury*, 18(11), 1135–1153.

Wygant, D. B., Ben-Porath, Y. S., Arbisi, P. A., Berry, D. T., Freeman, D. B., & Heilbronner, R. L. (2009). Examination of the MMPI-2 restructured form (MMPI-2-RF) validity scales in civil forensic settings: Findings from simulation and known groups samples. *Archives of Clinical Neuropsychology, 24*(7), 671–680.

Wygant, D. B., Sellbom, M., Ben-Porath, Y. S., Stafford, K. P., Freeman, D. B., & Heilbronner, R. I. (2007). The relation between symptom validity testing and MMPI-2 scores as a function of forensic evaluation context. *Archives of Clinical Neuropsychology, 22*(4), 488–499.

Yarnold, P. R., & Soltysik, R. C. (2005). *Optimal data analysis: A guidebook with software for Windows.* Washington, DC: American Psychological Association.

Youngjohn, J. R., Davis, D., & Wolf, I. (1997). Head injury and the MMPI-2: Paradoxical severity effects and the influence of litigation. *Psychological Assessment, 9,* 177–184.

Freestanding Cognitive Symptom Validity Tests: Use and Selection in Mild Traumatic Brain Injury

8

Leslie M. Guidotti Breting & Jerry J. Sweet

Symptom validity assessment (SVA) is an important part of the neuropsychological evaluation and subsequent clinical interpretation to assess the reliability and validity of test results. Studies have shown that clinical observation of effort alone cannot reliably differentiate examinees giving best effort from those who are not (Millis & Volinsky, 2001; see Chapter 2 for a detailed review of this topic). Objective measurement of effort in the evaluation of forensic patients has been the standard of practice for over a decade (Iverson & Binder, 2000; Sweet, 1999).

SVA is especially important in the context of secondary gain when external incentives may be associated with poor effort or exaggeration of cognitive deficits and symptoms, yielding worse performance on neuropsychological testing. In the context of cognitive performance, psychometrically-based SVA consists of using free-standing tests (separate tests specifically designed to assess effort) and examining empirically derived indicators embedded within cognitive ability tests. The primary purposes of this chapter are to explore the use of freestanding cognitive symptom validity tests (SVTs) with a mild traumatic brain injury (MTBI) population and to aid the clinician in deciding which SVTs to use. This particular group of patients is important because it has been estimated that about 40% of MTBI cases in litigation or seeking compensation fail effort tests, producing neuropsychological test findings that are invalid and suspicious for malingering (Flaro, Green, & Robertson, 2007; Larrabee, 2005; Mittenberg, Patton, Canyock, & Condit, 2002).

BRIEF HISTORY OF FREESTANDING COGNITIVE SYMPTOM VALIDITY TESTS

SVTs constitute a category of measures developed to evaluate response validity. At first, the category of SVT included primarily forced-choice tests, but over time, the appellation of SVT has broadened to include embedded validity indicators within tests of cognitive ability and validity scales within symptom-reporting inventories. Embedded effort measures assess the validity of performance within individual tests and have been examined within the traumatic brain injury (TBI) population. For example, validity indicators embedded within the California Verbal Learning Test-II (e.g., Bauer, Yantz, Ryan, Warden, & McCaffrey, 2005; Curtis, Greve, Bianchini, & Brennan, 2006) and the Wechsler Adult Intelligence Scale-III (e.g., Mathias, Greve, Bianchini, Houston, & Crouch, 2002) have been used with TBI samples. Validity indicators are also present within symptom-reporting inventories, such as the Minnesota Multiphasic Personality Inventory-II (Greve, Bianchini, Love, Brennan, & Heinly, 2006) and the Personality Assessment Inventory (Kurtz, Shealy, & Putnam, 2007) and have also been used with TBI samples. However, this chapter is focused exclusively on freestanding cognitive SVTs.

The term "symptom validity testing" was first introduced by Loren Pankratz in 1979 in the context of testing patients claiming gross memory and sensory impairment. Although the term was initially used narrowly to reference a dichotomous forced-choice format, it has subsequently been applied more broadly to include freestanding cognitive effort measures that employ any format. Within this chapter, we use the term SVT to refer to any one of various measures used to assess cognitive effort. Most freestanding cognitive SVTs were developed with TBI samples by examining performance of patients with varying severities of brain injury (i.e., mild, moderate, and severe).

Most freestanding cognitive SVTs use a forced-choice paradigm (see Iverson & Binder, 2000 for a review). Forced-choice SVTs were first introduced substantially to practitioners in the 1980s and have become widely used in forensic neuropsychological evaluations and increasingly with routine clinical referrals (Bianchini, Mathias, & Greve, 2001). By using this forced-choice paradigm, performance can be compared to that produced by chance alone. Most freestanding cognitive SVTs used with MTBI cases have been constructed to *appear* to be measuring memory *ability* because memory complaints are very common as a reason for referral. However, the tasks are so easy that they can be passed by most patients with severe cognitive impairment; they are actually measuring *effort* rather than memory.

Forced-choice tests are among the most extensively researched measures for the detection of response bias (Slick, Sherman, & Iverson, 1999). The development of forced-choice SVTs was based on the binomial theorem, which predicts that when there are only two responses possible, chance alone would produce a 50% correct response rate. Thus, if an examinee performs significantly below 50% correct, there is a strong suspicion that he or she is intentionally avoiding the correct answer (Frederick & Speed, 2007). Forced-choice tests can offer more than two responses, which affects the expected probability of a chance performance, although most offer only two. Most SVTs have empirically-derived cutoff scores that identify *insufficient effort* and identify significantly below-chance performance. Many forced-choice SVTs use a "90% correct rule" to determine poor effort (Sweet, 1999). Based on such cutoff scores, one can determine whether an examinee is exhibiting compromised effort as well as establishing the probability of malingering (i.e., definite, probable, possible; Slick et al., 1999).

SELECTION AND USE OF SYMPTOM VALIDITY TESTS

As elaborated on in a lengthy discussion of these topics, the American Academy of Clinical Neuropsychology (AACN) Consensus Conference Statement on the neuropsychological assessment of effort, response bias, and malingering (Heilbronner, Sweet, Morgan, Larrabee, & Millis, 2009) delineates various methods and strategies for identifying invalid responding and for discriminating insufficient effort from malingering. Specifically, the consensus statement defined *invalid responding* on ability measures as (a) not fully explained by brain dysfunction; (b) not reasonably attributable to variables that may moderate (e.g., education, age) or may confound (e.g., fatigue, psychological conditions) performances on ability tests; and (c) are significantly worse than, or at least differ in degree or pattern from, performance standards that reflect genuine neurological disorder (Heilbronner et al., 2009).

SVTs are not, of course, the only means of identifying invalid responding. Moreover, the use of SVTs can result in diagnostic conclusions that range from valid effort to insufficient effort to malingering. Whereas a determination of *insufficient effort* refers to a narrow conclusion that a test result does not represent a valid performance level for the particular examinee, a determination of *malingering* reflects a "big picture" conclusion that the individual's insufficient effort represents a deliberate attempt to exaggerate or fabricate cognitive dysfunction for the purpose of obtaining an external reward and/or avoiding responsibility.

A multidimensional, multimethod approach in assessing malingering is commonly accepted. Such an approach suggested by Nies and Sweet (1994) included (a) the use of specific tests of malingering or standard neuropsychological tests with forced-choice formats; (b) examination of intratest and intertest performance for highly inconsistent or nonsensical patterns of scores; (c) systematic collection of self-report data on symptoms and history for evaluation of discrepancies with test performance, and; (d) systematic collection of collateral data and evaluation of extra test behavior for evaluation of discrepancies with test performance. Slick et al. (1999) later expanded on these suggestions and proposed specific criteria for classifying the patient as malingering, using probabilistic language.

Confidence in the conclusion that insufficient effort and/or malingering is present within an evaluation is strengthened by reliance on multiple tests of effort (Greve, Binder, & Bianchini, 2009; Victor, Boone, Serpa, Buehler, & Ziegler, 2009), which ideally are distributed throughout the evaluation (Boone, 2009; Heilbronner et al., 2009). The benefit of using multiple freestanding cognitive SVTs to detect malingering was further demonstrated in a study examining the Portland Digit Recognition Test (PDRT), the Test of Memory Malingering (TOMM), and the Word Memory Test (WMT) in patients with TBI, which showed that classification accuracy of individual tests was inferior to that of joint classification accuracy combining the results of all three SVTs (Greve, Ord, Curtis, Bianchini, & Brennan, 2008). Nelson et al. (2003) compared eight SVTs (Rey Memory for 15-Item Test [RMFIT], Rey Dot Counting Test, Rey Word Recognition Test, Rey Auditory Verbal Learning Test recognition trial, Rey Complex Figure Test effort equation, digit span, Warrington Recognition Memory Test for words, and the "b" Test) and concluded that these various tests generally provide nonredundant data regarding patient credibility in neuropsychological evaluations. These findings support the contention that malingerers may use different strategies specific to a particular cognitive domain, again reinforcing the concept and psychometric foundation for using multiple SVTs in a single forensic evaluation.

In 2005, the National Academy of Neuropsychology (NAN) published a position paper regarding SVA. This paper stated that "adequate assessment of response validity is essential to maximize confidence in the results of neurocognitive and personality measures" (Bush et al., 2005, p. 419) and that "the clinician should be prepared to justify a decision *not* to assess symptom validity as part of a neuropsychological evaluation" (Bush et al., 2005, p. 421). The AACN held a consensus conference on effort, response bias, and malingering that resulted in an official AACN Consensus Conference Statement (Heilbronner et al., 2009). The AACN Consensus Conference Statement recommended that neuropsychological evaluations involving the potential for secondary gain include stand-alone and embedded validity indicators, and when evaluation time is constrained, embedded measures should be examined at a minimum. Some of the areas outlined for future investigation by the AACN Consensus Conference include (a) cost-benefit analysis of response bias assessment; (b) application of effort measures to pediatric samples; and (c) the need for examination of clinical populations at risk for failing effort and embedded validity indicators. For a recent summary on the current status and implications of SVT usage, see Sweet and Guidotti Breting (in press).

Sharland and Gfeller (2007) surveyed the use of SVTs among clinical neuropsychologists and found that 57% of respondents frequently included measures of effort when conducting a neuropsychological evaluation. Since that time, the frequency of SVT use has likely increased in part because of the NAN and AACN position statements. This study also found that the five most frequently used measures of effort or response bias included only two freestanding cognitive SVTs, which were the TOMM and the RMFIT. In the same manner, a study 3 years earlier also found the TOMM and RMFIT to be the most frequently used measures to detect insufficient performance (Slick, Tan, Strauss, & Hultsch, 2004). These findings also correlate with a third study that showed the TOMM and RMFIT to be ranked within the top 40 memory assessment instruments (Rabin, Barr, & Burton, 2005). SVT experts recognize that the TOMM has much more research suggesting effectiveness as a measure of effort than the RMFIT, which is widely viewed as insensitive and, therefore, ineffective. This lack of sensitivity explains why, when Sharland and Gfeller (2007) asked neuropsychologists to rate tests on accuracy of detecting insufficient effort, the RMFIT was not ranked highly. They found that the most frequently used tests were all freestanding cognitive SVTs, which included the (a) TOMM, (b) Validity Indicator Profile (VIP), (c) WMT, (d) Victoria Symptom Validity Test (VSVT), and (e) Computerized Assessment of Response Bias (CARB). Although this study was not specific to SVT use with MTBI populations, it is likely that the results would have been similar because a large portion of the evaluations conducted by neuropsychologists are related to MTBI.

MILD TRAUMATIC BRAIN INJURY, LITIGATION/COMPENSATION, AND FREESTANDING COGNITIVE SYMPTOM VALIDITY TESTS

By far, the most common reason for neuropsychologists to become involved in civil litigation is related to MTBI cases. Knowledge of MTBI outcome and recovery is important because it has been found that persisting symptoms may be attributable to factors not associated with the brain injury, including demographic, psychosocial, and situational (i.e., litigation, disability, compensation-seeking) factors. A review of the expected outcomes and recovery of MTBI is outside of the realm of this chapter, but extensive reviews can be found in McCrea (2008), McCrea et al. (2009), and the results of the World Health Organization Collaborating Centre Task Force on Mild Traumatic Brain Injury (Carroll et al., 2004). In summary, the empirical evidence from well-designed studies indicates that the initial cognitive effects of a single MTBI in a previously healthy individual are relatively mild, with recovery (i.e., returning to preinjury baseline) occurring within days to weeks (Dikmen, Machamer, Winn, & Temkin, 1995; Iverson, 2005). Meta-analytic studies have shown that patients with a history of MTBI are indistinguishable from normal controls by 3 months following the injury (Belanger, Curtiss, Demery, Lebowitz, & Vanderploeg, 2005; Frencham, Fox, & Mayberry, 2005; Iverson, 2005; Schretlen & Shapiro, 2003). Therefore, it is essential that a differential diagnosis be carried out, in that the initial occurrence of MTBI is much less likely a factor in creating persistent symptom complaints and behavioral dysfunction (i.e., beyond three months, assuming normal structural neuroimaging) than are non-brain injury factors (e.g., psychosocial, situational) (McCrea, 2008).

Since the early 1990s, clinical researchers have published an impressive number of peer-reviewed articles related to the increased risk of symptom exaggeration and malingering during forensic neuropsychological examinations. Textbooks fully devoted to this topic have appeared (e.g., Boone, 2007; Larrabee, 2007; Morgan & Sweet, 2009), as have the previously referenced professional organization position statements (Bush et al., 2005; Heilbronner et al., 2009), stating that in secondary gain contexts, neuropsychologists should evaluate motivation and effort using multiple SVTs.

It is important for clinical neuropsychologists who do not typically see patients within a forensic context to be familiar with this information because of the high incidence of MTBI and the likelihood of providing services to patients who have had an MTBI. Even within the clinical realm, it is important to examine effort to accurately interpret cognitive test results because there are many reasons, other than malingering, why patients may not put forth full effort on neuropsychological tests and because these patients are sometimes referred to neuropsychologists with ongoing compensation claims (e.g., litigation, workers' compensation, no-fault insurance). Moreover, examinees initially seen as *patients* can become *plaintiffs* and end up involving clinicians in forensic proceedings.

TYPES OF FREESTANDING COGNITIVE SYMPTOM VALIDITY TESTS

It is important to keep in mind that patients with TBI after a brief window of time measured in days to weeks are considered very likely, barring complication, to return to their preinjury neuropsychological and health status. Most TBIs resolve quickly and seemingly completely within days, but in a small number of cases with negative neuroimaging, recovery can take up to 3 months (McCrea, 2008). Recovery can sometimes take longer if there is a documented neuroimaging abnormality (e.g., contusion, hemorrhage) that is believed to be related to the trauma (Kashluba, Hanks, Casey, & Millis, 2008). With this understanding, there are numerous cognitive SVT studies illustrating the fact that patients with serious neurological conditions (i.e., severe TBI, mild dementia, learning disability) that have caused well-documented cognitive impairment, nevertheless easily pass freestanding cognitive SVTs. Therefore, when a patient with a history of TBI fails a freestanding cognitive SVT, the accepted perspective is that the likelihood of the TBI having been the neurological cause of failure is no greater than the risk of failure with a noninjured healthy normal individual. In other words, MTBI does not cause SVT failure. By extension, when research on freestanding SVTs has demonstrated acceptable sensitivity and specificity with other more cognitive impairment-inducing neurological conditions, it is a safe assumption that SVT research with MTBI would show the same sensitivity and specificity as with normal controls. For this reason, some established and frequently used cognitive SVTs have not focused much attention on MTBI samples specifically, such as the b test and the VSVT.

Aside from the normative data contained in each individual manual demonstrating that the specific cognitive SVT is passed at high rates even by those with severe TBIs, for each there is an additional scientific literature, which in some instances is quite extensive, examining these measures specifically with MTBI samples. The following sections describe the findings of these studies organized by type of stimuli that form the basis of freestanding cognitive SVT, namely (a) digit recognition, (b) letter or word recognition, and (c) visual or mixed verbal-visual tasks. Because the SVT literature is vast, we provide only limited citations as examples of relevant research to remain within space constraints. The reader can refer to the extensive bibliography by Sweet (2009) for numerous additional references.

Digit Recognition Cognitive Symptom Validity Tests

Freestanding digit recognition SVTs have been studied for more than two decades. Etcoff and Kampfer (1996) examined 23 studies for the use of specific SVTs in the forensic TBI context and found that at the time of their review, the stand-alone SVTs shown to have the most use were digit recognition procedures, specifically the PDRT and the 72-item and 36-item Hiscock Digit Memory Test (HDMT). Vickery, Berry, Inman, Harris, and Orey (2001) conducted a meta-analysis that examined 32 studies of the Digit Memory Test (DMT), PDRT, RMFIT, 21-Item Test, and the Rey Dot Counting Test and concluded that because of "less than perfect" (i.e., poor to moderate) sensitivity levels of each test, they should not be used in isolation as malingering screening devices. The more frequently used and studied digit recognition SVTs with the MTBI population are described in the following section. Readers should note that the Multi-Digit Memory Test (MDMT; Niccolls & Bolter, 1991) is a version of the Hiscock SVT that is no longer commercially available.

Computerized Assessment of Response Bias

The CARB (Allen, Conder, Green, & Cox, 1997) is a computerized forced-choice digit recognition task that presents a five-digit number to the examinee for a few seconds. The CARB is similar to the Hiscock and Hiscock's (1989) HDMT and the PDRT. It is an easier task than the PDRT because the correct five-digit number can more easily be remembered because only the first two digits are necessary to identify the correct choice. Green and Iverson (2001) examined performance on the CARB for 119 patients in litigation who were separated into three groups: alleged TBI ($n = 45$), presumed TBI ($n = 49$), and moderate-to-severe TBI ($n = 25$). They found that 29% of the alleged TBI group scored below the cutoff on the CARB, which is less than 90% correct. Twenty-four percent of the presumed TBI group scored below the cutoff, whereas only 4% of the moderate-to-severe TBI group scored below the cutoff. In addition, the moderate-to-severe TBI group demonstrated briefer response latencies than those with a history of MTBI.

Hiscock Digit Memory Test

The HDMT (Hiscock & Hiscock, 1989) was one of the first widely used SVTs. There are two versions of this test: a 72-item version and 36-item version. These tasks employ a design such that a five-digit number is presented, followed by increasing time intervals (5, 10, 15 secs) before responding using a forced-choice presentation of two five-digit numbers, one of which was seen before. This SVT has been studied extensively in various patient population groups, including patients who are brain injured or who have psychiatric illnesses, revealing that even a few errors on this test should raise concern regarding poor effort. Moreover, Prigitano and Amin (1993) found that even patients with severe TBI who had experienced a Glasgow Coma Scale between 3 and 8 were later able to perform at perfect or near-perfect levels. We were unable to find any HDMT studies specifically examining performance in an MTBI group.

Portland Digit Recognition Test

The PDRT (Binder, 1993) is a visual recognition task of auditorily presented five-digit number strings, which includes both "easy" and "hard" items. Binder and Kelly (1996) found a 0% false positive error rate in non–compensation-seeking patients with moderate-to-severe TBI and found that 30% of litigating patients with MTBI failed the PDRT. In a separate study of persons with a history of TBI, Greve and Bianchini (2006) separately examined MTBI and moderate-to-severe TBI groups that were further classified by malingering status based on the Slick (1999) et al.'s criteria to examine the specificity and sensitivity of the PDRT. They found that the original cutoff scores demonstrated excellent specificity and sensitivity in this known-group analysis but that they were quite conservative and that higher scores are able to detect more malingerers without increasing the false positive rate substantially.

Victoria Symptom Validity Test

The VSVT (Slick, Hopp, Strauss, & Thompson, 1997) is a computerized forced-choice digit recognition test that contains both "easy" and "hard" items. Few studies have specifically examined the use of the VSVT in identifying insufficient effort in the MTBI population other than the standardization study (Slick, Hopp, Strauss, & Spellacy, 1996). One such study compared VSVT performance of compensation-seeking patients with MTBI and non–compensation-seeking patients with intractable seizures (Grote et al., 2000). This study found that 100% of the non–compensation-seeking patients with intractable seizures scored in the "valid" range on the VSVT difficult memory items, compared to only 58.5% of the compensation-seeking patients with MTBI.

Letter- and Word-Based Cognitive Symptom Validity Tests

A number of freestanding cognitive SVTs exist that employ letter or word stimuli in their design. The most commonly used SVTs that are discussed individually in the following section include the Medical Symptom Validity Test (MSVT) and the WMT. Less frequently used SVTs that involve letter or word stimuli are the Letter Memory Test (LMT; Inman et al., 1998) and the 21-Item Test (Iverson, Franzen, & McCracken, 1991). Orey, Cragar, and Berry (2000) found the LMT to have good specificity and moderate sensitivity in a sample of college students with mild head injury. The LMT has proven to be very promising based on available research, but usage continues to be limited by the test not being commercially available. Another letter-based cognitive SVT is the b Test, which has been found to have an 85% specificity rate for nonlitigating patients with moderate-to-severe head injury (Boone et al., 2000).

Medical Symptom Validity Test

The MSVT (Green, 2004) is a computerized cognitive effort measure that displays 10 common word pairs and then assesses immediate forced-choice recognition, delayed forced-choice recognition, and consistency of responses. The MSVT also examines memory through the paired associates and free recall components of the test (see Carone, 2009 for a review). The MSVT is similar to the WMT, but is less complex and requires less time to administer. Armistead-Jehle (2010) found that 58% of veterans with a history of MTBI failed the MSVT (Green, 2004). This study found that of those who failed, their profile more closely resembled that of the simulators than those with genuine memory impairment, and they had uncharacteristic patterns of scores, such as better performances on more difficult subtests. The 58% failure rate was greater than the reported base rate of SVT failures of 30%–40% generally reported in civil forensic settings (Larrabee, 2005). Another study demonstrated the use of the MSVT in the evaluation of Operation Iraqi Freedom/Operation Enduring Freedom soldiers with MTBI histories who had been exposed to multiple blasts, except for one soldier who experienced a fall (Whitney, Shepard, Williams, Davis, &

Adams, 2009). They found that 17% of the sample scored below the cutoff scores on the MSVT, but none performed at below-chance levels. These studies highlight the importance of using SVTs when assessing brain injury within the military population (see Chapter 18 for more information on SVT use with patients with MTBI in a military setting).

The use of the MSVT was also examined in a heterogeneous group of 38 children with neurological injuries or disorders with more than half of the sample having sustained a moderate or severe TBI and in a sample of adults with MTBI/mild head injury (Carone, 2008). Carone (2008) found that most *children* with moderate-to-severe brain damage from various causes were able to pass the MSVT (95% passed), whereas only 79% of the *adult* MTBI/mild head injury group passed the MSVT. Moreover, the adult MTBI/mild head injury group rated the MSVT as being much more difficult than the children who are moderate-to-severely brain damaged did. These results demonstrated symptom exaggeration in a subset of adult patients with MTBI/mild head injury as detected by the MSVT. These results are consistent with another study that found failure on the MSVT was more frequent in adults with a history of MTBI than children with developmental disabilities (Green, Flaro, & Courtney, 2009).

In general, the research investigating insufficient effort in children with a history of MTBI is less well established than the adult MTBI literature. However, some research exists. Kirkwood and Kirk (2010) examined MSVT performance in children with a history of MTBI and found that 17% failed the test, demonstrating inadequate effort. Differences between this study of children and the adult studies include the most common cause of MTBI in children being recreation and sports, and most children with a history of MTBI not having a readily apparent external incentive that might decrease effort, such as litigation. Chapter 19 discusses SVT within the pediatric population.

Word Memory Test

The WMT (Green, 2005) is currently formatted as a computerized test designed to measure verbal memory of word pairs and biased responding. Green, Iverson, and Allen (1999) found that the WMT was failed more often by MTBI litigants than by nonlitigating patients with moderate-to-severe brain injury. In addition, those with an MTBI history who failed the WMT performed worse across a large neuropsychology test battery than those with severe brain injury who demonstrated good effort (Green, Rohling, Lees-Haley, & Allen, 2001).

Flaro, Green, and Robertson (2007) found that failure on the WMT was 23 times higher in MTBI claimants than parents seeking custody, which could not be explained by cognitive deficits but rather by differences in external incentives. That is, parents seeking custody are highly motivated to appear fully capable, whereas some litigants are motivated to appear less capable than they truly are. The false positive rate of the WMT has been questioned by some plaintiff experts who examine adults with a history of MTBI. However, a well-designed study found that false positives on the WMT in adults with MTBI histories are very rare (Green et al., 2009).

Visual or Mixed Verbal-Visual Cognitive Symptom Validity Tests

Several freestanding cognitive SVTs employing a visual or mixed verbal-visual format have been developed. Some of the more frequently used and studied SVTs with visual or mixed stimuli are described in the following section. A few of the less frequently used SVTs include the Amsterdam Short-Term Memory Test (ASMT;

Schagen, Schmand, de Sterke, & Lindebloom, 1997), Dot Counting Test (DCT; Boone, Lu, & Herzberg, 2002), and the VIP (Frederick, 1997).

Nonverbal Medical Symptom Validity Test

The Nonverbal Medical Symptom Validity Test (NV-MSVT; Green, 2008) is a visually-based, computerized test that is based on forced-choice recognition memory of 10 color image pairs. A study comparing the use of the NV-MSVT and the TOMM in patients seeking disability with a history of MTBI, and a group of patients with moderate-to-severe TBI, found that 100% of the moderate-to-severe TBI group passed both SVTs, whereas 26% of the MTBI group failed the NV-MSVT, and 10% of the MTBI group failed the TOMM (Green, 2011). This study concluded that the NV-MSVT was considerably more sensitive to poor effort than the TOMM in an MTBI group.

Rey Memory for 15 Items Test

The RMFIT (Rey, 1964) is a freestanding SVT that does not employ a forced-choice design. Rather, it involves showing the patient 15 different items for a brief period of time and then asking the patient to reproduce as many items as they can remember. Caution should be used when using the RMFIT because many objections to the test have been raised, which are largely related to the original cutoff scores having poor sensitivity (Greiffenstein, Baker, & Gola, 1994). Nevertheless, the test is still widely used, likely only because it was one of the earliest SVTs, is very quick to administer, and is in the public domain (i.e., free to administer). Reznek (2005) conducted a meta-analysis of 13 studies to demonstrate that the RMFIT has low sensitivity (36%) but good specificity (85%) when using a cutoff score of nine; however, when people with mental retardation are excluded and the cutoff is changed to be at seven correct items, the specificity becomes 95%, but the sensitivity decreases to 9%. A recognition memory procedure was later developed for the RMFIT, which has aided in increasing the measures of sensitivity (Boone, Salazar, Lu, Warner-Chacon, & Razani, 2002).

Test of Memory Malingering

The TOMM (Tombaugh, 1996) is a visually-based effort test that involves forced-choice recognition memory for 50 line drawings that typically are presented manually in paper booklets, although there is a computerized version available. Greve, Bianchini, and Doane (2006) examined the use of the TOMM in MTBI ($n = 103$), moderate-to-severe TBI ($n = 58$), and memory disorder ($n = 22$) samples. This study employed a "known-groups" design separating the patients into malingering and nonmalingering groups, finding that more than 90% of the nonmalingering patients with MTBI were correctly classified as passing the TOMM, whereas 60% of the malingering patients with MTBI were detected as failing the TOMM. When the MTBI and moderate-to-severe TBI groups were collapsed to examine only those with incentive to perform poorly, they found that 19.0% scored below the cutoff of 45 on Trial 2, and 21.1% scored below the cutoff on the retention trial. Another study that attempted to replicate the original validation study of the TOMM reported moderate sensitivity (64%) and good specificity (93%) for compensation-seeking patients with MTBI by examining Trial 2 of the TOMM with the traditional cutoffs, which allows the clinician to have high confidence that positive scores reflect inadequate effort (Haber & Fichtenberg, 2006). Haber and Fichtenberg concluded their article with a discussion as to whether a cutoff score of five errors is too lenient in a TBI population. Effort, as measured by the TOMM, explained 47% of the variance in the summary score from the Halstead-Reitan battery in MTBI litigants (Constantinou, Bauer, Ashendorf, Fisher, & McCaffrey, 2005).

CONCLUSION

Freestanding cognitive SVTs are an important part of a thorough forensic and clinical neuropsychological evaluation, particularly in patients with MTBI. A frequent finding in the SVT literature is that patients with MTBI histories (particularly those seeking compensation for their injuries) perform worse on cognitive SVTs than patients with moderate-to-severe TBIs. This inverse relationship is consistent with a well-known observation that the less severe the head/brain injury, the more numerous the patient's subjective complaints. This has been referred to as "compensation neurosis" (Miller & Cartlidge, 1972).

In conclusion, neuropsychologists use their own clinical judgment and knowledge of relevant peer-reviewed research in selecting SVTs but should rely on free-standing and embedded effort measures throughout evaluation of a patient with MTBI (Boone, 2009). The clear recommendation to rely on both SVTs and embedded measures also can be found in the AACN Consensus Conference on Effort, Response Bias, and Malingering (Heilbronner et al., 2009). When the concern is that of identifying malingering, an additional means of strengthening conclusions regarding intentionality can be to readminister failed SVTs with strong encouragement regarding an expected improvement in performance. If the second performance is worse than the first, the examinees intention has been clearly revealed. However, the clinician should be careful when using this approach not to identify the test as an effort measure or otherwise inform that effort is being measured. To reduce identification of effort tests using this approach, readministering a few other brief ability tests can be helpful. Some litigants and claimants will use this second opportunity to illustrate dysfunction by performing even more poorly than on the initial administration, thereby confirming the diagnosis of definite malingering (see case report by Sweet & Giuffre Meyer, 2011).

REFERENCES

Allen, L. M., Conder, R. L., Green, P., & Cox, D. R. (1997). *CARB '97 manual for the computerized assessment of response bias.* Durham, NC: CogniSyst.

Armistead-Jehle, P. (2010). Symptom validity test performance in U.S. veterans referred for evaluation in mild TBI. *Applied Neuropsychology*, 17(1), 52–59.

Bauer, L., Yantz, C. L., Ryan, L. M., Warden, D. L., & McCaffrey, R. J. (2005). An examination of the California verbal learning test II to detect incomplete effort in a traumatic brain-injury sample. *Applied Neuropsychology*, 12(4), 202–207.

Belanger, H. G., Curtiss, G., Demery, J. A., Lebowitz, B. K., & Vanderploeg, R. D. (2005). Factors moderating neuropsychological outcomes following mild traumatic brain injury: A meta-analysis. *Journal of the International Neuropsychological Society*, 11(3), 215–227.

Bianchini, K. J., Mathias, C. W., & Greve, K. W. (2001). Symptom validity testing: A critical review. *The Clinical Neuropsychologist*, 15(1), 19–45.

Binder, L. M. (1993). Assessment of malingering after mild head trauma with the Portland digit recognition test. *Journal of Clinical and Experimental Neuropsychology*, 15(2), 170–182.

Binder, L., & Kelly, M. P. (1996). Portland digit recognition test performace by brain dysfunction patients without financial incentives. *Assessment*, 3, 403–409.

Boone, K. (Ed). (2007). *Assessment of feigned cognitive impairment: A neuropschological perspective.* New York, NY: Guilford Press.

Boone, K. B. (2009). The need for continuous and comprehensive sampling of effort/response bias during neuropsychological examinations. *The Clinical Neuropsychologist*, 23(4), 729–741.

Boone, K. B., Lu, P., & Herzberg, D. S. (2002). *The dot counting test.* Los Angeles, CA: Western Psychological Services.

Boone, K. B., Lu, P., Sherman, D., Palmer, B., Back, C., Shamieh, E., . . . Berman, N. G. (2000). Validation of a new technique to detect malingering of cognitive symptoms: The b Test. *Archives of Clinical Neuropsychology*, 15(3), 227–241.

Boone, K. B., Salazar, X., Lu, P., Warner-Chacon, K., & Razani, J. (2002). The Rey 15-item recognition trial: A technique to enhance sensitivity of the Rey 15-item memorization test. *Journal of Clinical and Experimental Neuropsychology*, 24(5), 561–573.

Bush, S. S., Ruff, R. M., Tröster, A. I., Barth, J. T., Koffler, S. P., Pliskin, N. H., . . . Silver, C. H. (2005). Symptom validity assessment: Practice issues and medical necessity NAN policy and planning committee. *Archives of Clinical Neuropsychology*, 20(4), 419–426.

Carone, D. A. (2008). Children with moderate/severe brain damage/dysfunction outperform adults with mild-to-no brain damage on the medical symptom validity test. *Brain Injury*, 22(12), 960–971.

Carone, D. A. (2009). Test review of the medical symptom validity test. *Applied Neuropsychology*, 16(4), 309–311.

Carroll, L. J., Cassidy, J. D., Peloso, P. M., Borg, J., von Holst, H., & Holm, L., . . . Pépin, M. (2004). Prognosis for mild traumatic brain injury: Results of the WHO Collaborating Centre Task Force on Mild Traumatic Brain Injury. *Journal of Rehabilitation Medicine*, (Suppl. 43), 84–105.

Constantinou, M., Bauer, L., Ashendorf, L., Fisher, J. M., & McCaffrey, R. J. (2005). Is poor performance on recognition memory effort measures indicative of generalized poor performance on neuropsychological tests? *Archives of Clinical Neuropsychology*, 20(2), 191–198.

Curtis, K. L., Greve, K. W., Bianchini, K. J., & Brennan, A. (2006). California verbal learning test indicators of malingered neurocognitive dysfunction: Sensitivity and specificity in traumatic brain injury. *Assessment*, 13(1), 46–61.

Dikmen, S., Machamer, J. E., Winn, H. R., & Temkin, N. R. (1995). Neuropsychological outcome at 1-year post head injury. *Neuropsychology*, 9, 80–90.

Etcoff, L. M., & Kampfer, K. M. (1996). Practical guidelines in the use of symptom validity and other psychological tests to measure malingering and symptom exaggeration in traumatic brain injury cases. *Neuropsychology Review*, 6(4), 171–201.

Flaro, L., Green, P., & Robertson, E. (2007). Word memory test failure 23 times higher in mild brain injury than in parents seeking custody: The power of external incentives. *Brain Injury*, 21(4), 373–383.

Frederick, R. I. (1997). *Manual for the validity indicator profile*. Minnetonka, MN: NCS Assessments.

Frederick, R. I., & Speed, F. M. (2007). On the interpretation of below-chance responding in forced-choice tests. *Assessment*, 14(1), 3–11.

Frencham, K. A., Fox, A. M., & Maybery, M. T. (2005). Neuropsychological studies of mild traumatic brain injury: A meta-analytic review of research since 1995. *Journal of Clinical and Experimental Neuropsychology*, 27(3), 334–351.

Green, P. (2004). *Manual for the medical symptom validity test for Windows*. Edmonton, Canada: Green's Publishing.

Green, P. (2005). *Green's word memory test for Windows: Manual*. (Rev. ed.). Edmonton, Canada: Green's Publishing.

Green, P. (2008). *Green's nonverbal medical symptom validity test for Windows manual*. Edmonton, Canada: Green's Publishing.

Green, P. (2011). Comparison between the test of memory malingering (TOMM) and the nonverbal medical symptom validity test (NV-MSVT) in adults with disability claims. *Applied Neuropsychology*, 18(1), 18–26.

Green, P., & Iverson, G. L. (2001). Validation of the computerized assessment of response bias in litigating patients with head injuries. *The Clinical Neuropsychologist*, 15(4), 492–497.

Green, P., Iverson, G. L., & Allen, L. (1999). Detecting malingering in head injury litigation with the word memory test. *Brain Injury*, 13(10), 813–819.

Green, P., Flaro, L., & Courtney, J. (2009). Examining false positives on the word memory test in adults with mild traumatic brain injury. *Brain Injury*, 23(9), 741–750.

Green, P., Rohling, M. L., Lees-Haley, P. R., & Allen, L. M.III. (2001). Effort has a greater effect on test scores than severe brain injury in compensation claimants. *Brain Injury*, 15(12), 1045–1060.

Greiffenstein, M. F., Baker, W. J., & Gola, T. (1994). Validation of malingered amnesia measures with a large clinical sample. *Psychological Assessment*, 6(3), 218–224.

Greve, K. W., & Bianchini, K. J. (2006). Classification accuracy of the Portland digit recognition test in traumatic brain injury: Results of a known-groups analysis. *The Clinical Neuropsychologist*, 20(4), 816–830.

Greve, K. W., Bianchini, K. J., & Doane, B. M. (2006). Classification accuracy of the test of memory malingering in traumatic brain injury: Results of a known-groups analysis. *Journal of Clinical and Experimental Neuropsychology*, 28(7), 1176–1190.

Greve, K. W., Bianchini, K. J., Love, J. M., Brennan, A., & Heinly, M. T. (2006). Sensitivity and specificity of MMPI-2 validity scales and inficators to malingered neurocognitive dysfunction in traumatic brain injury. *The Clinical Neuropsychologist*, 20(3), 491–512.

Greve, K. W., Binder, L. M., & Bianchini, K. J. (2009). Rates of below-chance performance in forced-choice symptom validity tests. *The Clinical Neuropsychologist*, 23(3), 534–544.

Greve, K. W., Ord, J., Curtis, K. L., Bianchini, K. J., & Brennan, A. (2008). Detecting malingering in traumatic brain injury and chronic pain: A comparison of three forced-choice symptom validity tests. *The Clinical Neuropsychologist*, 22(5), 896–918.

Grote, C. L., Kooker, E. K., Garron, D. C., Nyenhuis, D. L., Smith, C. A., & Mattingly, M. L. (2000). Performance of compensation seeking and non-compensation seeking samples on the Victoria symptom validity test: Cross-validation and extension of a standardization study. *Journal of Clinical and Experimental Neuropsychology*, 22(6), 709–719.

Haber, A. H., & Fichtenberg, N. L. (2006). Replication of the test of memory malingering (TOMM) in a traumatic brain injury and head trauma sample. *The Clinical Neuropsychologist*, 20(3), 524–532.

Heilbronner, R. L., Sweet, J. J., Morgan, J. E., Larrabee, G. J., & Millis, S. R. (2009). American Academy of Clinical Neuropsychology consensus conference statement on the neuropsychological assessment of effort, response bias, and malingering. *The Clinical Neuropsychologist*, 23(7), 1093–1129.

Hiscock, M., & Hiscock, C. K. (1989). Refining the forced-choice method for the detection of malingering. *Journal of Clinical and Experimental Neuropsychology*, 11(6), 967–974.

Inman, T. H., Vickery, C. D., Berry, D. T. R., Lamb, D. G., Edwards, C. L., & Smith, G. T. (1998). Development and initial validation of a new procedure for evaluating adequacy of effort given during neuropsychological testing: The letter memory test. *Psychological Assessment*, 10(2), 128–139.

Iverson, G. L. (2005). Outcome from mild traumatic brain injury. *Current Opinion in Psychiatry*, 18(3), 301–317.

Iverson, G. L., & Binder, L. M. (2000). Detecting exaggeration and malingering in neuropsychological assessment. *The Journal of Head Trauma Rehabilitation*, 15(2), 829–858.

Iverson, G. L., Franzen, M. D., & McCracken, L. M. (1991). Evaluation of an objective assessment technique for the detection of malingered memory deficits. *Law and Human Behavior*, 15(6), 667–676.

Kashluba, S., Hanks, R. A., Casey, J. E., & Millis, S. R. (2008). Neuropsychologic and functional outcome after complicated mild traumatic brain injury. *Archives of Physical Medicine and Rehabilitation*, 89(5), 904–911.

Kirkwood, M. W., & Kirk, J. W. (2010). The base rate of suboptimal effort in a pediatric mild TBI sample: Performance on the medical symptom validity test. *The Clinical Neuropsychologist*, 24(5), 860–872.

Kurtz, J. E., Shealy, S. E., & Putnam, S. H. (2007). Another look at paradoxical severity effects in head injury with the personality assessment inventory. *Journal of Personality Assessment*, 88(1), 66–73.

Larrabee, G. (Ed.). (2005). Assessment of malingering. In *Forensic neuropsychology: A scientific approach* (pp. 115–158). New York, NY: Oxford University Press.

Larrabee, G. (Ed). (2007). *Assessment of malingered neuropsychological deficits*. New York, NY: Oxford University Press.

Mathias, C. W., Greve, K. W., Bianchini, K. J., Houston, R. J., & Crouch, J. A. (2002). Detecting malingered neurocognitive dysfunction using the reliable digit span in traumatic brain injury. *Assessment*, 9(3), 301–308.

McCrea, M. (2008). *Mild traumatic brain injury and postconcussion syndrome. The new evidence base for diagnosis and treatment*. New York, NY: Oxford University Press.

McCrea, M., Iverson, G. L., McAllister, T. W., Hammeke, T. A., Powell, M. R., Barr, W. B., & Kelly, J. P. (2009). An integrated review of recovery after mild traumatic brain injury (MTBI): Implications for clinical management. *The Clinical Neuropsychologist*, 23(8), 1368–1390.

Miller, H., & Cartlidge, N. (1972). Simulation and malingering after injuries to the brain and spinal cord. *Lancet*, 1(7750), 580–585.

Millis, S. R., & Volinsky, C. T. (2001). Assessment of response bias in mild head injury: Beyond malingering tests. *Journal of Clinical and Experimental Neuropsychology*, 23(6), 809–828.

Mittenberg, W., Patton, C., Canyock, E. M., & Condit, D. C. (2002). Base rates of malingering and symptom exaggeration. *Journal of Clinical and Experimental Neuropsychology*, 24(8), 1094–1102.

Morgan, J. E., & Sweet, J. J. (Eds.). (2009). *Neuropsychology of malingering casebook*. New York, NY: Psychology Press.

Nelson, N. W., Boone, K., Dueck, A., Wagener, L., Lu, P., & Grills, C. (2003). Relationships between eight measures of suspect effort. *The Clinical Neuropsychologist*, 17(2), 263–272.

Niccolls, R., & Bolter, J. F. (1991). *Multi-digit memory test*. San Luis Obispo, CA: Wang Neuropsychological Laboratories.

Nies, K. J., & Sweet, J. J. (1994). Neuropsychological assessment and malingering: A critical review of past and present strategies. *Archives of Clinical Neuropsychology*, 9(6), 501–552.

Orey, S. A., Cragar, D. E., & Berry, D. T. (2000). The effects of two motivational manipulations on the neuropsychological performance of mildly head-injured college students. *Archives of Clinical Neuropsychology*, 15(4), 335–348.

Pankratz, L. (1979). Symptom validity testing and symptom retraining: Procedures for the assessment and treatment of functional sensory deficits. *Journal of Consulting and Clinical Psychology*, 47(2), 409–410.

Prigitano, G. P., & Amin, K. (1993). Digit memory test: Unequivocal cerebral dysfunction and suspected malingering. *Journal of Clinical and Experimental Neuropsychology*, 15(4), 537–546.

Rabin, L. A., Barr, W. B., & Burton, L. A. (2005). Assessment practices of clinical neuropsychologists in the United States and Canada: A survey of INS, NAN, and APA Division 40 members. *Archives of Clinical Neuropsychology*, 20(1), 33–65.

Rey, A. (1964). *L'examen clinique en psychologie*. Paris, France: Presses Universitaires de France.

Reznek, L. (2005). The Rey 15-item memory test for malingering: A meta-analysis. *Brain Injury*, 19(7), 539–43.

Schagen, S., Schmand, B., de Sterke, S., & Lindeboom, J. (1997). Amsterdam short-term memory test: A new procedure for the detection of feigned memory deficits. *Journal of Clinical and Experimental Neuropsychology*, 19(1), 43–51.

Schretlen, D. J., & Shapiro, A. M. (2003). A quantitative review of the effects of traumatic brain injury on cognitive functioning. *International Review of Psychiatry*, 15(4), 341–349.

Sharland, M. J., & Gfeller, J. D. (2007). A survey of neuropsychologists' beliefs and practices with respect to the assessment of effort. *Archives of Clinical Neuropsychology*, 22(2), 213–223.

Slick, D. J., Hopp, G., Strauss, E., & Spellacy, F. J. (1996). Victoria symptom validity test: Efficiency for detecting feigned memory impairment and relationship to neuropsychological tests and MMPI-2 validity scales. *Journal of Clinical and Experimental Neuropsychology*, 18(6), 911–922.

Slick, D., Hopp, G., Strauss, E., & Thompson, G. (1997). *The victoria symptom validity test*. Odessa, FL: Psychological Assessment Resources.

Slick, D. J., Sherman, E. M., & Iverson, G. L. (1999). Diagnostic criteria for malingered neurocognitive dysfunction: Proposed standards for clinical practice and research. *The Clinical Neuropsychologist*, 13(4), 545–561.

Slick, D. J., Tan, J. E., Strauss, E. H., & Hultsch, D. F. (2004). Detecting malingering: A survey of experts' practices. *Archives of Clinical Neuropsychology*, 19(4), 465–473.

Sweet, J. J. (1999). Malingering: Differential diagnosis. In J. J. Sweet (Ed.), *Forensic neuropsychology: Fundamentals and practice* (pp.255–285). Lisse, The Netherlands: Swets & Zeitlinger.

Sweet, J. J. (2009). Forensic bibliography: Effort/malingering and other common forensic topics encountered by clinical neuropsychologists. In J. E. Morgan & J. J. Sweet (Eds.), *Neuropsychology of malingering casebook* (pp. 566–630). New York, NY: Psychology Press.

Sweet, J. J., & Giuffre Meyer, D. (2011). Well-documented, serious brain dysfunction followed by malingering. In J. E. Morgan, I. S. Baron, & J. Ricker (Eds.), *Casebook of clinical neuropsychology* (pp. 200–212). New York, NY: Oxford University Press.

Sweet, J. J., & Guidotti Breting, L. M. (in press). Symptom validity test research: Status and clinical implications. *Journal of Experimental Psychopathology*.

Tombaugh, T. N. (1996). *Test of memory malingering* (TOMM). New York, NY: Multi-Health Systems.

Vickery, C. D., Berry, D. T., Inman, T. H., Harris, M. J., & Orey, S. A. (2001). Detection of inadequate effort on neuropsychological testing: A meta-analytic review of selected procedures. *Archives of Clinical Neuropsychology*, 16(1), 45–73.

Victor, T. L., Boone, K. B., Serpa, J. G., Buehler, J., & Ziegler, E. A . (2009). Interpreting the meaning of multiple symptom validity test failure. *The Clinical Neuropsychologist*, 23(2), 297–313.

Whitney, K. A., Shepard, P. H., Williams, A. L., Davis, J. J., & Adams, K. M. (2009). The medical symptom validity test in the evaluation of Operation Iraqi Freedom/Operation Enduring Freedom soldiers: A preliminary study. *Archives of Clinical Neuropsychology*, 24(2), 145–152.

Use of Embedded Cognitive Symptom Validity Measures in Mild Traumatic Brain Injury Cases

9

Christian Schutte & Bradley N. Axelrod

The essential nature of symptom validity testing (SVT) during neuropsychological evaluations has become increasingly clear, prompting supportive position statements to this effect from the National Academy of Neuropsychology (NAN) (Bush et al., 2005) and the American Academy of Clinical Neuropsychology (AACN, 2007; Heilbronner, Sweet, Morgan, Larrabee, & Millis, 2009). According to the 2009 AACN position statement, the omission of symptom validity tests needs solid justification, especially within a forensic context. It has become a standard of practice to objectively assess effort on cognitive testing in forensic contexts, because the base rates for poor effort in patients involved in litigation or compensation-seeking have generally been reported to range from 30% to 40% (Howe, Anderson, Kaufman, Sachs, & Loring, 2007; Larrabee, 2003; Mittenberg, Patton, Canyock, & Condit, 2002). This incidence rate represents a substantial proportion of examinees, particularly in the case of mild traumatic brain injury (MTBI), which is commonly litigated and has been reported to be the group most commonly identified as malingering by board certified neuropsychologists (Mittenberg et al., 2002).

Although the use of SVTs has become a standard of practice in forensic contexts, Millis (2009) stated that "the assessment of effort should be a part of every neuropsychological examination, whether litigation or external incentive are present or not" because "the consequences of erroneously labeling someone as 'brain damaged' can be as egregious as labeling them as malingering" (p. 21). Thus, "effort testing has become a suggested standard in neuropsychological practice in both forensic and regular clinical practice" (Schutte, Millis, Axelrod, & Van Dyke, 2011, p. 455). Poor effort on cognitive testing may be evident for a variety of reasons outside of forensic referrals, such as poor engagement, lack of interest in the testing process, or an effort to maintain other external incentives (e.g., avoidance of responsibilities, care offered by other individuals in an examinee's life). Also, patients referred by health care providers may simultaneously be seeking compensation for brain injury even though they were not directly referred by an attorney, which can influence response styles during a clinical neuropsychological evaluation. For example, in a study in which nearly half of the MTBI patients were referred by physicians, Meyers, Volbrecht, Axelrod, and Reinsch-Boothby (2011) found that approximately 50% of the variance in cognitive performance was because of failure on SVTs. Additionally, Carone (2008) found that approximately 21% of clinically referred adults with a history of MTBI failed effort measures. Such data highlight the need to use effort measures in regular clinical evaluations in addition to forensic evaluations.

Measures of effort may broadly take two different forms: (a) stand-alone measures specifically designed to assess for effort that are typically based on a forced-choice paradigm (see Chapter 8); and (b) empirically derived embedded measures that are typically derived from commonly administered neuropsychological tests in clinical contexts. Measures such as the Test of Memory Malingering (TOMM) (Tombaugh, 1996), Word Memory Test (WMT) (Green, 2003), Medical Symptom Validity Test (MSVT) (Green, 2004), and Victoria Symptom Validity Test (VSVT) (Slick, Hopp, Straus, & Spellacy, 1996) are all well-validated stand-alone measures of effort. Although these measures are well validated with solid empirical foundations, there are various reasons that may prompt the examiner to seek additional methods for assessing effort; the reasons are as follows:

Efficiency: There are limitations to the amount of time and patient tolerance for testing (Howe, et al., 2007). Thus, embedded indices allow for efficient assessment of effort without placing further time constraints on the examination.

Identification and Coaching: Stand-alone forced-choice measures are based on the premise that the measure is actually not very cognitively challenging (although they are designed to appear challenging). As a result, even individuals who are significantly impaired tend to perform well on such measures. One of the difficulties with this format is that it can be easily identifiable, and with a little coaching the examinee could potentially know to perform well on measures that have binary answers. Suhr and Gunstad (2000) found that although coached simulators performed more poorly than a good effort group, they still performed better than the noncoached group. They concluded that performance on forced-choice measures can easily be altered by coaching, which is similar to findings from DiCarlo, Gfeller, and Oliveri (2000). Embedded indices have the potential benefit of avoiding this pitfall, particularly when more sophisticated methods of pattern analysis and statistical approaches are used.

Assessment in Multiple Domains: Stand-alone measures are typically designed to assess for poor effort on memory testing because poor effort is most common in that domain. However, use of embedded indices allows for assessment of effort in multiple domains, such as attention span, processing speed, motor speed, executive functioning, and memory. Further, the relative influence of performance in one domain on another can be assessed by using embedded indices (e.g., motor speed should be comparable across tasks such as Trail Making Test A and Digit Symbol).

Multiple Measures: Millis (2004) stated that performance that is statistically below chance is "persuasive evidence of response bias" (p. 1083). However, it is not common for individuals to actually perform at or below chance levels. As shown in a study by Greve, Binder, and Bianchini (2009), only about 12% of a litigating population in private practice performed below chance on any one measure, far below estimated base rates for poor effort in MTBI assessment in forensic settings. Although a below chance performance may be evidence of a "smoking gun" with regard to poor effort, the need for cut scores on multiple measures is necessary for adequate sensitivity. It has been consistently suggested that multiple measures of effort are needed for adequate assessment of response bias, which is easily accomplished with embedded measures.

Assessment at Multiple Time Points: Research has found that poor effort on one stand-alone measure is correlated with generally decreased performances on other measures (Constantinou, Bauer, Ashendorf, Fisher, & McCaffery, 2005; Green, 2007). However, Boone (2009) stated that assessing for effort at multiple time points across an evaluation is desirable because effort may be variable across testing for a variety of reasons. Heilbronner et al. (2009) stated that "effort level can be conceptualized as occurring on a continuum and can vary within and across tests" (p. 1097). Although stand-alone effort tests can be used at multiple time points across the evaluation, use of several embedded indices more easily allows for this to occur, which is suggested by Heilbronner and colleagues as a best practice.

FORMS OF EMBEDDED INDICES

It is important for clinicians to have a good foundational understanding about how embedded effort measures are developed and used in research and clinical settings so that they can make informed diagnostic decisions. Broadly, there are four methods of identifying poor effort through the use of embedded indices, although they can also be applied to stand-alone effort measures. These methods include forced choice tasks, consideration of floor effects, the "simulator" method, and criterion variable designs.

Forced Choice

Forced-choice tasks are well established and easily identified methods of assessing effort, as is clear by their use as stand-alone measures of effort. They are often readily available in multiple cognitive domains such as new learning and memory, including the California Verbal Learning Test-II (CVLT-II) (Delis, Kramer, Kaplan, & Ober, 2000), Rey Auditory Verbal Learning Test (RAVLT) (Schmidt, 1996), Warrington's Recognition Memory Test (RMT) (Warrington, 1984), and Seashore Rhythm Test (Heaton, Miller, Taylor, & Grant, 2004; Reitan & Wolfson, 1985). Although these measures are useful, they are often limited because of the low number of items, such as on the CVLT-II forced choice component (i.e., 16 items). Millis (2004) suggested that there should be at least 25 items, and preferably 50, on any forced-choice task because it is difficult to have a statistically significant below chance performance when there are fewer items.

Most forced-choice measures have empirically derived cut scores that have been found to be more sensitive to poor effort than using a worse than chance performance criterion while still maintaining solid specificity. In general, these cut scores are derived by statistically comparing measures to groups with known suspect effort or to groups with known pathology and deriving cut scores that are able to differentiate or predict group membership. These results are typically associated with higher cut scores than would be obtained from performance at a worse than chance level, which increases sensitivity. For example, a score on the RMT of 36% correct (18 out of 50) is significantly worse than chance when computed using the binomial method ($z = 1.98$, $p < .05$). However, a score of 68% correct has been demonstrated to be a valid cutoff in discriminating poor effort from intact performance (Iverson & Franzen, 1994).

Consideration of Floor Effects

It has been well established through prospective and meta-analytic research that there is a dose-response relationship between the severity of traumatic brain injury (TBI) and the outcome (Carroll et al., 2004; Dikmen, Machamer, Winn, & Temkin, 1995; Rohling, Meyers, & Millis, 2003; Schretlen & Shapiro, 2003). Assuming that the data is reliable and valid, individuals who have sustained a MTBI are unlikely to have neurologically-based cognitive deficits 1 year post-injury with the severity of cognitive deficits will generally be proportional to the degree of TBI sustained. In a meta-analysis, the World Health Organization reviewed 120 published articles concerning MTBI that were determined to be of adequate quality. They reached the conclusion that the "the most consistent predictors of delayed recovery after MTBI are compensation and litigation factors, independent of MTBI injury severity" (Carroll, et al., 2004, p. 97). Given that there is a clear dose-response relationship, we can therefore infer that an individual with a history of MTBI performing more poorly than an individual with a severe TBI would be indicative of poor effort unless there was a compelling medical or psychiatric comorbidity to indicate otherwise. For example, if an individual with a history of MTBI obtained a score of 6 on the commonly used embedded effort measure, Reliable Digit Span (RDS), 1 year post-injury, poor effort would be suggested because the vast majority of moderate-to-severe TBI patients providing good effort are able to perform superior to that (Axelrod, Fichtenberg, Millis, & Wertheimer, 2006).

The "Simulator" Method

"Simulator" designs include designs similar to floor effect models in which patients with documented injuries are evaluated. Clinical researchers can compare performance across the TBI severity continuum as well as other known groups with no history of TBI. Simulator designs use individuals who are asked to perform as if they were attempting to malinger. The advantage of using simulators is that there is a clearly defined standard with established criteria of who is attempting to malinger and who is not. One significant disadvantage of using simulators is limited generalizability for a variety of reasons. Simulator studies typically use samples of convenience such as university student populations who are educated about the sequelae of TBI, some of whom are then asked to feign poor performance and some of whom are asked to put forth their best performance. Such samples likely do not accurately represent the population at large who present to evaluations with their own set of unique personal stressors and problems that can lead to exaggerated performance. Simulator samples may also be significantly different from patient samples in terms of demographics, education, exposure to coaching, and malingering strategy. The motivation to feign cognitive impairment is also different because university students are typically feigning in such studies to earn extra credit in a class or a nominal amount of financial compensation, while those that are in litigation are likely suing for a much larger financial compensation. Such differences in incentive may impact test performance. For an example of such a design, see the study by Miller et al. (2010) in which they compared performance on memory testing among those with documented moderate-to-severe TBI to participants who were coached to simulate TBI.

Criterion Variable Designs

Criterion variable designs are useful in archival research or in mixed clinical samples that may be collected over time in a regular clinical setting. The researcher defines good versus poor effort using another well-validated measure or combination of measures, such as embedded measures that have previously been shown to differentiate good versus poor effort (Wolfe et al., 2010). For example, if a group of examinees perform below cutoff scores on the CVLT-II Forced-Choice subtest, then one could define that performance as poor. Other measures hypothesized to be sensitive to poor effort can be used to predict performance pass/failure on the CVLT-II with logistic regression. If the model is adequate, a receiver operating characteristics (ROC) curve analysis can be used to analyze the model's ability to differentiate good versus poor effort. Then, a cut score can be identified that optimizes sensitivity and specificity, or one that predetermines the level of specificity (typically around .90) a priori. One of the strengths of criterion variable designs is that the types of samples used are more readily available for researchers who collect data from regular clinical evaluations. Hence, this method is more efficient, and the sample may be more generalizable because the sample is an actual clinical sample. However, a significant problem with this type of research is that false negative and false positive errors may be more likely to occur depending on the strength of the criterion measure because the measure used as the criterion is not a perfect predictor of poor effort, which increases error. One way to reduce this problem is to combine multiple criterion variables together, such as using multiple embedded indicators.

INDIVIDUAL EMBEDDED EFFORT INDICATORS

There is a plethora of research on individual embedded indices ranging across multiple cognitive domains, including attention, processing speed, visuospatial processing, sensory abilities, motor functions, and executive functioning, as well as new learning and memory (see chapters 12 and 13 for additional description of research on numerous embedded symptom validity indicators in various cognitive domains). However, the application of that information should be deemed usable only if generated through research using forced choice, simulator, floor effect, or criterion variable designs. It is equally important to understand if there was a patient population included and how the samples were defined.

Tables 9.1–9.7 provide information summarized by cognitive domain for studies in which single embedded measures were used from a variety of tasks. A complete list of all known embedded measures is outside the scope of this chapter. Instead, we have selected variables taken from commonly used measures in neuropsychological assessment; and, consistent with the focus of this chapter, most measures were chosen that had specific research on MTBI. In keeping with the importance of knowing how generalizable a score may be, the research design used for each of the published studies is also noted.

For each score, readers will find not only the obtained cut scores but also the associated sensitivity (i.e., percentage of cases of poor effort from all cases falling below the cutoff score) and specificity (e.g., percentage of cases of good effort from all cases falling above the cutoff score) published by the authors. Using the sensitivity and specificity provided in the tables, the likelihood ratio (LR) for each measure can be computed in clinical practice relatively easily using common database programs such as Excel. This method allows for the rates of sensitivity and specificity to be combined into a single measure. Computation of the LR is equal to [sensitivity/(1 − specificity)]; that is, the number of people in the poor effort group identified by the test divided by those people with good effort falsely identified as having poor effort. A likelihood ratio greater than 1.0 suggests that the embedded measure is able to identify those who evidenced poor effort, and less than 1 indicates that the measure is associated with the absence of poor effort. As an example, the study by Ross, Putnam, Millis, Adams, & Krukowski (2006) presented in Table 9.1 identified a cutoff score of >9 errors on the Speech Sound Perception Test (SSPT), which results in .76 sensitivity and .74 specificity. The resulting LR is computed to be (.76)/(1 − .74) = .76/.26 = 2.92.

The benefit of a LR lies in the utility of deriving the probability that a performance is indicative of poor effort given a set base rate. First, convert the base rate to pretest odds; that is, the likelihood that an individual is offering poor effort in a

TABLE 9.1 Embedded Measures of Attention/Processing Speed

Source	Measure	Cut Score	Sensitivity	Specificity
Babikian, Boone, Lu & Arnold, 2006[b]	WAIS/digit span	ACSS < 7	.55	.82
Axelrod et al., 2006[c]			.50	.83
Babikian et al., 2006[b]		ACSS < 6	.42	.93
Axelrod et al., 2006[c]			.36	.97
Greffenstein, Baker, & Gola, 1994[f]	Reliable Digit Span	< 8	.86	.57
Larrabee, 2003[c]			.50	.94
Babikian et al., 2006[b]			.62	.77
Babikian et al., 2006[b]		< 7	.45	.93
Iverson, Lange, Green, & Franzen, 2002[c]	TMT-A	> 62 s	.17	1.00*
Ross et al., 2006[a]	SRT	> 7 errors	.76	.74
		> 8	.70	.86
		> 9	.59	.92
Curtis, Greeve, Bianchini, & Brasseux, 2010[d]		>9	.37	.96
Ross et al., 2006[a]	SSPT	> 9 errors	.72	.76
		> 12	.70	.90
Curtis et al., 2010[d]		>12	.59	.96
Ord, Boettcher, Greve, & Bianchini, 2010[e]	CPT-II/omissions	> 34 raw	.30	.97
		> 19 raw	.41	.90
	CPT-II/hit rate SE	> 15 raw	.41	.97
		> 13 raw	.52	.90

Note. WAIS = Wechsler Adult Intelligence Scale R and III; TMT-A = Trail Making Test Part A; SRT = Seashore Rhythm Test; SSPT = Speech Sounds Perception Test; CPT-II = Conners' Continuous Performance Test second edition.
[a]Mild TBI seeking financial compensation vs. moderate/severe TBI with no compensation.
[b]Mixed clinical group: suspect effort vs. good effort.
[c]TBI clinical sample and litigation: suspect effort vs. good effort.
[d]TBI litigation vs. clinical sample.
[e]TBI litigation vs. clinical sample.
[f]TBI: Suspect effort and moderate/severe TBI with good effort.
*Found to differentiate good vs. poor effort more strongly with MTBI than moderate/severe TBI.

given evaluation prior to any test being administered, by the formula "base rate/ (1 − base rate)." In a sample in which 31% of the population has poor effort, pretest odds would be (.31)/(.69) = .45. Posttest odds are computed by multiplying LR with pretest odds (e.g., 2.92 × .45 = 1.3). The resulting posttest odds indicate the likelihood that an individual will be correctly identified by the test. The probability that an individual score is associated with poor test performance is computed using the formula posttest odds/(1 + posttest odds). Using the same example, in a sample with a 31% estimated failure rate, the SSPT cutoff of more than 9 errors (.76 sensitivity and .74 specificity) results in a 57% probability of poor effort [probability of poor effort = 1.3 / (1+1.3) = 1.3/2.3 = 57%].

TABLE 9.2 Embedded Measures of Motor Functioning

Source	Measure	Cut Score	Sensitivity	Specificity
Arnold et al., 2005[a]	FTT*	< 34 men	.32	.94
		< 36 men	.41	.87
		< 33 women	.67	.00
		< 36 women	.67	.86
Larrabee, 2008[b]	FTT**	< 63	.40	.94
Binder, Kelly, Villanueva, & Winslow, 2003[b]	TFR	> 4 errors	.56	.82
Trueblood & Schmidt, 1993[a]	FNR	> 5 errors	.56	.84

Note. FTT = Finger Tapping; TFR = Tactual Form Recognition; FNR = Finger Number Writing.
[a]Mixed clinical group: suspect effort vs. good effort.
[b]TBI clinical sample and litigation: suspect effort vs. good effort.
*Finger tapping average of the dominant hand over three trials in a TBI sample.
**Finger tapping combined average left and right.

As a second example, assume that an individual is being seen for an independent medical examination (IME) related to litigation associated with an MTBI. Medical records show that the examinee had a Glasgow Coma Scale score of 15 in the ER, no amnesia for the event, and minimal posttraumatic confusion; and imaging of the brain was negative for intracranial pathology. The examinee is administered the Wechsler Adult Intelligence Scale, 3rd edition (WAIS-III) (Wechsler, 1997) Digit Span subtest and obtains an RDS of 7. Using Larrabee's (2008) work, we can determine the LR by .50/ (1 − .94) = 8.33. Given previous research in the area of MTBI, we know that the base rate of poor effort generally ranges from 30% to 40% in a similar population (Howe et al., 2007; Larrabee, 2003; Mittenberg et al., 2002). Being conservative, we choose a base rate of 30% so the pretest odds would be .30/(1 − .30) = .43. We then multiply the pretest odds of (.43) by the LR (8.33), which gives the posttest odds (3.58). In order to obtain the probability of poor effort in this case,

TABLE 9.3 Measures of Visuospatial Functioning

Source	Measure	Cut Score	Sensitivity	Specificity
Larrabee, 2003[a]	VFD	< 26	.48	.93
Whiteside et al., 2011[a]	JOLO	< 20 raw	.31	.87
		< 18 raw	.31	.90
	Benton FRT	< 41 raw	.40	.89
		< 40 raw	.40	.90
	Hooper VOT	< 22 raw	.45	.88
		< 21	.27	.92
	RCFT copy	< 25 raw	.30	.89
Lu et al., 2003[a]	RCFT copy	< 28 raw	.50	.91*
		< 26 raw	.45	.96*

Note. VFD = Visual Form Discrimination; JOLO = Judgment of Line Orientation; FRT = Facial Recognition Test; VOT = Visual Organization Test; RCFT = Rey Complex Figure Copy.
[a]Mixed clinical group: suspect effort vs. good effort.
*Suspect effort vs. mixed clinical group.

TABLE 9.4 Embedded Measures of Executive Functioning

Source	Measure	Cut Score	Sensitivity	Specificity
Greve & Bianchini, 2002[a]	WCST/unique	>0	.35	.94*
		>1	.22	1.00
Larrabee, 2008[b]	WCST/FMS	>1	.48	.87*
Greve, Bianchini, & Roberson, 2007***		> 2	.20	.96
		> 3	.12	1.00
Iverson et al., 2002[a]	TMT-B	>199	.071	.00*
Greve et al, 2007[c]	BCT/total errors[d]	> 82	.47	.84
		> 84	.47	.91
		> 103	.21	.95
	BCT/total errors[e]	> 86	.56	.85
		> 94	.44	.91
		> 1140	.0	.94
	BCT/I&II errors	>1	.16	.95*
Curtis, Thompson, Greve, & Bianchini, 2008[c]	FAS	T<34	.36	.90**
		T<36	.27	.95

Note. WCST = Wisconsin Card Sorting Test; BCT = Booklet Category Test; TMT-B = Trail Making Test part B; AUC = Area Under the Curve.
[a]TBI clinical sample: suspect effort vs. good effort.
[b]TBI litigation definite malingering vs. moderate/severe TBI no poor effort.
[c]TBI good effort, poor effort vs. clinical group.
[d]Mild TBI.
[e]Moderate/severe TBI.
*Found to differentiate good vs. poor effort more strongly with MTBI than moderate/severe TBI.
**AUC .72 with MTBI, AUC .53 with moderate/severe TBI.
***Cited Larrabee's 2003 data.

we calculate [posttest odds/(1 + posttest odds)] or 3.58/(1 + 3.58) = .78 or a 78% probability, which is an adequate indicator of poor performance given those test diagnostics.

One might incorrectly believe that we can simply add probabilities of multiple measures to combine the result from the different measures. Adding the probabilities together assumes that the tests are independent from each other, which is rarely the case. So, although finding a probability for one measure is helpful and easily done to assist in diagnostic certainty, there is no good way of directly adding these probabilities together. From a clinical point of view, calculating a probability is relatively easy because database programs (e.g., Excel or OpenOffice) now readily available allow for formulas to be entered so that the examiner can enter the raw data each time, and the program will easily calculate the probability at a set base rate.

COMBINING EMBEDDED EFFORT INDICES

Although there are advantages to embedded measures as noted above, to reduce the risk of inaccurate classification, no measure should be used in isolation to identify poor performance (Bush et al., 2005; Heilbronner et al., 2009). In fact, research on embedded indices has shown that failure on one measure is not uncommon (Dean,

TABLE 9.5 Embedded Measures of Visuospatial Memory (Rey Complex Figure Test)

Source	Measure	Cut Score	Sensitivity	Specificity
Lu et al., 2003[a*]	Immediate recall	< 11	.45	.86
		< 9	.36	.91
	True positive recog.	< 5	.52	.93
		< 4	.38	.96
		< 3	.24	.97
	False positive errors	> 3	.16	.94
		> 4	.071	.00
	Combination score	< 48	.76	.91
		< 45	.74	.94
Blaskewitz, Merten, & Brockhaus, 2009[b]		< 46	.52	.95
	Atypical recog. errors	> 1	.20	.93
Combination = copy score + [(true positive recognition − atypical recognition errors) × 3] atypical items: 1, 4, 6, 10, 11, 16, 18, 21				
Whiteside et al., 2011[a]	Recognition	< 16	.22	.91
		< 15	.19	.94

Note. Recog. = recognition.
[a]Mixed clinical group: suspect effort vs. good effort.
[b]TBI litigants vs. clinical patients.
*Suspect effort vs. mixed clinical group including memory impairment.

TABLE 9.6 Embedded Measures of Verbal Learning and Memory (Rey Auditory Verbal Learning Test)

Source	Measure	Cut score		Sensitivity	Specificity	
Meyers et al., 2001[a]	recognition	< 11		.50	1.00	
		< 12		.60	.86	
Boone et al., 2005[b]			**Clinic Patients**		**Controls**	
			Sens.	Spec.	Sens.	Spec.
	Trial 5	< 8	.48	.90	.48	.96
	Trial 1–5	< 30	.41	.91	.41	.96
	Trial 7	< 4	.30	.96	.30	1.00
	Trial 8	< 4	.44	.88	.44	.96
	Recognition	< 11	.77	.86	.77	.84
		< 10	.67	.93	.67	.92
	False +	> 2	.15	.86	.15	.88

Note. Sens. = sensitivity, Spec. = specificity
[a] mild TBI seeking financial compensation vs. moderate/severe TBI with no compensation.
[b] mixed clinical good vs. poor effort, control.

TABLE 9.7 Embedded Measures of Verbal Learning and Memory (California Verbal Learning Test-I & II)

Source	Measure	Cut Score	Sensitivity	Specificity
CVLT				
Sweet et al., 2000[a]	CVLT total 1–5	< 41	.72	.84
		< 35	.59	.89
Slick et al., 2000[b]		< 35	.39	.92
Millis, Putnam, Adams, & Ricker, 1995[c]		< 35	.74	.91
Sweet et al., 2000[a]	Recognition hits	< 13	.80	.87
		< 11	.63	.94
Slick et al., 2000[b]		< 11	.36	.93
Millis et al., 1995[c]		< 11	.87	.96
Sweet et al., 2000[a]	Long delay cued recall	< 8	.59	.81
		< 7	.52	.87
Slick et al., 2000[b]		< 7	.39	.92
Millis et al., 1995[c]		< 7	.83	.91
Sweet et al., 2000[a]	Discriminability	< 84	.65	.87
		< 81	.59	.90
Slick et al., 2000[b]		< 81	.36	.96
Millis et al., 1995[c]		< 81	.96	.91
Discriminability = [(1 − (False Positives + Misses)/33] × 100				
CVLT-II				
Root et al., 2005[d]	Forced choice recog.	< 15	.44	.93

Note. Recog. = recognition; CVLT = California Verbal Learning Test.
[a]TBI suspect effort, documented moderate/severe TBI, simulators and controls.
[b]TBI litigation: full range TBI good vs. poor effort.
[c]MTBI incomplete effort vs. mod/severe TBI.
[d]Mixed clinical and litigation sample: some TBI, not well defined.

Victor, Boone, & Arnold, 2008; Meyers, & Volbrecht, 2003). But what about combining results from several embedded effort measures? Some factors that compromise the combining of measures statistically include multicollinearity (the strength of the relationships between variables in the model), differing LRs across measures, and the different test batteries that are used among clinicians. These issues can change the meaning of the results. For example, strong relationships between variables (high multicollinearity) would likely lead to models that appear to be stronger than they actually are. Boone (2009) pointed out that empirical methods for combining measures are needed to avoid these statistical problems. It is fortunate that there are a few methods that have been developed to combine embedded indices. These methods are described below.

Additive Method

One method of combining multiple measures to assess overall effort on a test battery is to use failures on more than one test using individual cut scores, such as those presented in Tables 9.1–9.7. This method is intuitive and easy to use for the individual clinician. There is also a solid empirical foundation for examining effort in this way (Larrabee, 2008; Victor, Boone, Serpa, Buehler, & Ziegler, 2009). However, there are also limitations with this method. Similar to computing LR and the probability of group membership, this method essentially assumes that the embedded measures used are not strongly related to each other. Two studies demonstrate the intentional use of seemingly unrelated measures.

First, Larrabee (2003, 2008) used embedded indices derived from RDS, Failure to Maintain Set (FMS) on the Wisconsin Card Sorting Test (WCST) (Heaton, Chelune, Talley, Kay, & Curtiss, 1993); Visual Form Discrimination (VFD) (Benton, Sivan, Hamsher, Varney, & Spreen, 1994); finger tapping (FT) (Heaton et al., 2004); and the Fake Bad Scale (FBS) (Lees-Haley, English, & Glenn, 1991) from the Minnesota Multiphasic Personality Inventory, 2nd edition (MMPI-2) (Butcher, Dahlstrom, Graham, Tellegen, & Kaemmer, 1989). Second, Victor et al. (2009) included RDS and equations developed from the Rey Complex Figure Test (RCFT), RAVLT, and FT (formulas for RCFT and RAVLT can be seen in Tables 9.5 and 9.6). In both sets of studies, the selected measures were from different cognitive domains. Both Larrabee and Victor et al. found that two or more pairwise failures were indicative of poor effort. In one case, the self-report measure of the MMPI-2 was used, limiting the chance of strong relationships between these measures. Victor et al. showed that the measures used in their study were correlated between .23 to .63, with the strongest relationships between RAVLT, RCFT, and RDS. Thus, choosing measures from different domains on a rational basis may not be adequate to assure independence and may limit techniques to combine these measures together, such as chaining likelihood ratios, which assumes that the measures are independent.

Although the specific embedded measures that were published by Larrabee (2008) and Victor et al. (2009) perform well, that does not lead one to automatically conclude that the combination of any two or more embedded indices would hold up as well. In the presence of high multicollinearity among measures, one may be overly confident that there is evidence of poor overall test battery performance when simply using the number of failed embedded measures. Thus, efforts should be made to reduce the multicollinearity of embedded measures through research and/or clinical judgment if research does not exist regarding the embedded measures that have been chosen.

Choosing measures that are more or less independent of each other is not the only method of using an additive approach. Heilbronner et al. suggested that effort may vary within a single cognitive domain. In addition to assessing for overall poor performance on a test battery, it may be desirable to measure consistency over time by evaluating effort in one cognitive domain at multiple times throughout the assessment. One example might be if an individual showed significant impairment on RCFT delayed recall and then had a raw score of 14 on recognition (Whiteside, Wald, & Busse, 2011) (sensitivity = .19, specificity = .94), indicative of poor effort, early in the testing session. Later in the assessment, the same person has a forced choice of 16/16 on the CVLT-II with a solidly average Long Delay Free Recall (LDFR). This CVLT-II score would suggest adequate effort and intact free recall. Rather than suggesting that this individual is uniformly offering poor effort or that the individual has memory impairment, the alternative explanation may be that the examinee's verbal memory was intact but that his effort on visuospatial memory testing was poor. His variability in engagement on testing might have occurred for multiple reasons, such as lack of interest at different times of the day, worse effort on specific areas of cognition based on chief complaints, or medication effects. For example, Loring et al.'s (2011) work suggests that medications such as lorazepam can have a

TABLE 9.8 Additive Method

Source	Groups	Cut Score	Sensitivity	Specificity
Larabee (2008)	Definite MND[a]	> 1	.88	.89
		> 2	.54	1.00
	Probable MND[b]	> 1	.88	1.00
		> 2	.47	1.00
Victor et al., (2009)	Mixed clinical	> 1	.84	.94
		> 2	.51	.99

Note. MND = malingered neurocognitive dysfunction.
[a]Definite malingered neurocognitive dysfunction (as defined by Slick et al., 1999) vs. mod/severe TBI.
[b]Probable malingered neurocognitive dysfunction (as defined by Slick et al., 1999) vs. mixed neurologic and psychiatric samples.

negative impact on effort testing. Use of multiple embedded indices within the same domain assists in determining the validity of performance over the course of testing.

Larrabee (2003, 2008), Meyers and Volbrecht (2003), and Victor et al. (2009) all found that two or more failures on the embedded measures used in their studies were indicative of poor effort on the overall test battery. Larrabee used a cut score of < 26 on VFD, < 63 combined FT, > 1 FMS, < 8 RDS, and > 21 FBS. Victor et al. used RDS < 7, RCFT R-O effort equation < 48, RAVLT effort equation < 13, and FT dominant < 36 for men or < 29 for women. Sensitivity and specificity for these cut scores can be seen in Table 9.8.

Pattern of Performance

In addition to using individual indices that are thought to be sensitive to poor effort, the pattern of an examinee's performance can be useful in this regard. One informal method for assessing patterns of performance in MTBI cases is to compare performance on measures that are not likely to be affected by TBI to performance on those tasks known to be affected by cognitive impairment from TBI. For example, with the exception of patients with a history of certain neurological and/or neurodevelopmental comorbities (e.g., various learning disorders, expressive language disorder), verbal functioning, and academic abilities should not be relatively deficient in comparison to performance on tasks of processing speed, complex attention, executive functioning, or new learning and memory after MTBI. If one were to obtain a Wechsler Adult Intelligence Scale, 4th edition (WAIS-IV; Wechsler, 2008), Verbal Comprehension Index (VCI) of 70 (2nd percentile) and a Processing Speed Index (PSI) of 75 (5th percentile) in an MTBI patient reporting chronic symptoms, it would suggest that the individual may have had preexisting cognitive difficulties or was underperforming on testing. Although examining patterns of performance may raise concern about poor effort, there are few embedded approaches that directly examine simple contrast scores empirically.

One empirical method that does use contrast scores between embedded measures is to subtract Digit Span performance from Vocabulary on the Wechsler Adult Intelligence Scale-Revised (WAIS-R) or WAIS-III, which are both subtests that are unlikely to be strongly impacted by TBI, particularly in the chronic phase. Millis, Ross, and Ricker (1998) replicated Mittenberg, Azrin, Millsaps, and Heilbronner's (1993) Vocabulary minus Digit Span (V − DS) scaled score difference using the WAIS-R and found that using a cut score of V − DS of 2 or greater resulted in a sensitivity of .72 and a

TABLE 9.9 Embedded Measures of the RBANS (Effort Index)

Digit Span (Raw Score)	List Recognition (Raw Score)	Weighted Score
8–16	18–20	0
–	17	1
7	15–16	2
6	13–14	3
–	11–12	4
5	10	5
0–4	0–9	6

Cut Score	Sensitivity[a]	Sensitivity[b]	Sensitivity[c]	Specificity (MTBI)
>1	.67	.92	.75	.81
>2	.67	.79	.50	.91
>3	.53	.71	.46	1.00

Note. Adapted from "An Effort Index for the Repeatable Battery for the Assessment of Neuropsychological Status (RBANS)," by N. D. Silverberg, J. C. Wertheimer, and N. L. Fichtenberg, 2007, *The Clinical Neuropsychologist*, *21*(5), pp. 841–854.
[a]Clinical malingerers.
[b]Naïve simulators.
[c]Coached simulators.

specificity of .89 when comparing those with MTBI histories with the potential of financial compensation to those with documented moderate-to-severe TBI. A subsequent examination by Axelrod et al. (2006) found that V − DS was unable to differentiate poor effort among three groups of patients (TBI, probable malingerers, and non-litigating MTBI). The authors found that a cutoff score (7 or less) for the Digit Span age corrected scaled score (ACSS) was the best discriminator compared to other Digit Span measures (i.e., V − DS, RDS, raw score for Digit Span forwards and backwards) with classification rates of 69%, 75%, and 77%, respectively, in the above groups.

Another rationally derived method of pattern analysis was examined by Lu, Boone, Cozolino, and Mitchell (2003). They developed a formula derived from the RCFT to identify poor effort (see Table 9.5; the RCFT formula = copy score + [(true positive recognition − atypical recognition errors) × 3] atypical items, numbers 1, 4, 6, 10, 11, 16, 18, 21). Silverberg, Wertheimer, and Fichtenberg (2007) also developed a method of examining effort on the Repeatable Battery for the Assessment of Neuropsychological Status (RBANS) (Randolph, 1998) in a group of MTBI patients, healthy controls, clinical malingers, and simulators. They used a method of scoring performances on the RBANS Digit Span and verbal List Recognition subtests to derive a single Effort Index (EI) by weighing raw scores and adding the weighted scores together. It is notable that Armistead-Jehle and Hansen (2011) found that the RBANS-EI resulted in a high rate of false negatives, suggesting that it was not appropriate as a stand-alone effort measure and that stand-alone measures of effort outperformed this index. The method of weighing raw scores as well as sensitivity and specificity can be seen in Table 9.9.

Floor Effect

As described previously, it is known that there is a clear dose-response relationship between the severity of TBI and cognitive outcome. The floor effect method compares an individual examinee's performance to known groups, such as to a general clinical population or a TBI sample with documented moderate-to-severe TBI (Backhaus, Fichtenberg, & Hanks 2004; Killgore & DellaPietra, 2000; Langeluddecke & Lucas, 2003; Meyers & Volbrecht, 2003). Basing a cut score on an existing clinical sample (i.e., moderate-to-severe TBI patients correctly identified with good effort) provides an a priori specificity rate. Thus, performance on an entire neuropsychological battery can be examined to identify the worst performance in the group of moderate-to-severe TBI patients and to compare this with the performance of MTBI patients (who should not perform worse than more severely injured patients). This method assesses how atypical an individual score is based on comparison to the moderate-to-severe TBI group. Multiple areas of atypical performances become progressively rare in the MTBI group and provide increasing evidence of poor effort.

As an example of the floor effect method, assume that 90% of individuals with moderate/severe TBI have a Wechsler Memory Scale-Third Edition (WMS-III) General Memory Index (GMI) standard score above 70. One can then choose a GMI of 70 as a cut score, computing the number of individuals in the MTBI group who perform at 70 or below. The assumption is then made that a cut score has been preselected that will result in 90% specificity for moderate/severe TBI. A study by Ord, Greve, and Bianchini (2008) found when using this cutoff score on the WMS-III GMI that 52% of MTBI patients with malingered neurocognitive dysfunction performed below the cut score, whereas MTBI patients who were not malingering did not score below that cut score. In other words, 52% of the individuals with malingered MTBI (sensitivity) fell at a level worse than 90% of the people with moderate/severe TBI sample (specificity).

The benefit of using this method for examining poor effort is that a large number of measures can be empirically evaluated together, and an overall sensitivity and specificity can be derived. In addition, there does not need to be a single cut score for each measure. Hence, one does not need to sacrifice sensitivity for specificity because one can examine multiple measures simultaneously. For example, one can consider the number of test scores that are below the 75th percentile in a moderate-to-severe TBI group. Although it would not be prudent to choose a specificity of 75% for a single measure because of the risk of false positive identification of poor effort, one can examine the number of performances on a battery of tests that fall below this cutoff. Assume that no one in the moderate to severe group had more than 10 scores at this level on a large battery of tests. If an MTBI patient had more than 10 scores below the 75th percentile, this would suggest poor effort. Ord and colleagues (2008) presented WMS-III percentile scores in table format for samples of patients with moderate-to-severe TBI. Such data can be used to determine appropriate cutoff scores at or near 90% specificity as previously described for individual measures. When those cutoffs are applied to an individual with suspected poor effort, the utility of this method becomes apparent.

The Wechsler Advanced Clinical Solutions (ACS) package (Wechsler, 2008, 2009) provides an Effort Assessment Score Report in which the number of scores that fell below the 2nd, 5th, 10th, 15th, and 25th percentile are all computed. Although one could consider individual scores, as previously described, there is strength in the utility of the ACS because it examines the number of different scores that fall at an impaired level. Because this method differs somewhat from others in the literature, a detailed example is provided here.

Assume that four scores across the WAIS-IV and WMS-IV fall at the 8th, 12th, 19th, and 22nd percentile, respectively, on the Effort Assessment Score Report for an individual with a history of MTBI. That would mean that four tests fell below the 25%, two tests below the 15%, one test below 10%, and none below the 5%. The next step is to evaluate effort by looking at the Effort Assessment Score Report. The ACS printout provides tables, which include the number of scores falling below a particular percentage rank, comparing those numbers to other samples. A clinician might want to examine the number of tests that fell below the 10% cutoff because that seems to be a fairly restrictive rule.

Using the sample data above, one test fell below the 10% cutoff. In the available Effort Assessment Score Report table, 30% of the TBI group obtained one score which fell that low. By itself, the single score, which is arguably quite low, does not appear to clearly indicate overall poor effort because one score falling in that range happens relatively often (but see the next paragraph for possible limitations with this argument). Choosing to evaluate the number of tests which fell at or below the 25% cutoff will capture more scores together. Examining the 25% cut score alone might not seem like a particularly rigid cut score. However, when looking at the table with the ≤ 25% cutoff, we find that 3% of the overall clinical sample had four scores that fell below 25%. Further, none of the TBI patients had four scores that fell below the 25% cut scores. A clinician could then conclude that although any individual score below that level may be relatively normal, obtaining four scores—each of which fell below the associated 25% cut score—is exceedingly rare even in those with documented injuries and is likely indicative of poor effort, particularly in an individual with a MTBI history performing worse than those with documented moderate-to-severe TBI.

Much like other embedded indices, the value of this method is limited by how well the comparison groups are defined. For example, a neuropsychologist may compare an individual's performance on neuropsychological tests against a "TBI" group, but if it is unknown if the TBI group is composed of well-defined moderate/severe TBI or if the group includes persons with a history of MTBI or individuals providing poor effort, then it is not clear what the individual's scores mean in terms of effort. This is the case with the Wechsler ACS package, which does not define the nature of the comparison groups well in the technical manual. Groups that are not adequately defined significantly limit the application of this approach. Thus, in the absence of clearly defined comparison groups, approaches with these limitations should be used with caution, if at all.

Discriminant Function Analysis

The statistical technique of a discriminant function analysis (DFA) predicts group membership using one or a linear combination of continuous or binary independent variables. In the case of evaluating effort, group membership of good versus poor effort can be predicted using a combination of multiple measures on a battery of cognitive tests. Statistically, the DFA assumes variables are normally distributed and that groups have equal variances. This method allows one to identify group membership for an individual case using an entire model by multiplying the individual variables by the beta weights in the model. For example, if there are two variables in a model and one of them was found to be twice as important in the prediction of poor effort, then the weight for that variable would be twice as much. A significant limitation of this method is the assumptions of a normal distribution and equal variances, which is seldom the case in neuropsychological research. Table 9.10 includes a variety of DFA models, cut scores, and sensitivity and specificity values for the cut scores presented in the table.

TABLE 9.10 Discriminant Function Analysis Formulas Using Embedded Measures

Source	Measure	Cut Score	Sensitivity	Specificity
Millis, 1992[a]	RMT	−.253	.85	.82
DFA	*(.059 × faces) + (.103 × words) − 5.618*			
Mittenberg, Rotholc, Russell, & Heilbronner, 1996[b]	HRB	0	.84	.94
DFA	*(.01335924 × category test errors) + (−.04932242 × TPT time) + (−.1911619 × TPT memory) + (−.02631231 × seashore rhythm correct) + (.03914169 × speech perception errors) + (.01072021 × trail making A) + (−.01152765 × trail making B) + (.004032426 × finger tapping both hands) + (.02293813 × sensory suppressions) + (−.02050771 × finger tip number writing) + 1.80943*			
Sweet et al., 2000[c]	CVLT	0	.78	.91[d]
DFA	*(.010 × total) + (−.005 × long delay cued recall) + (.04 × discriminability[e]) + (.197 × recognition) − 6.135*			
Mittenberg et al., 2001[f]	WAIS-III	0	.57	1.00[g]
DFA (all subtests use scaled scores)	*(−.3288679 × digit span) + (.171452 × vocabulary) + (−.07195667 × arithmetic) + (−.08107555 × comprehension) + (.15800098 × similarities) + (−.07944288 × picture completion) + (.0780321 × digit symbol) + .9695551*			
Sherman, Boone, Lu, & Razani, 2002[f]	RAVLT/RCFT	0	.84	.85
DFA	*(.006 × AVLT trial 1) + (−.062 × RCFT delay) + (.354 × AVLT recognition) − 2*			

Note. RMT = Recognition Memory Test; HRB = Halstead Reitan Battery; CVLT = California Verbal Learning Test; WAIS = Wechsler Adult Intelligence Scale; RAVLT = Rey Auditory Verbal Learning Test; RCFT = Rey Complex Figure Test.
[a] mild TBI seeking financial compensation vs. moderate/severe TBI with no compensation.
[b] TBI vs. simulators.
[c] TBI with suspect effort, documented moderate/severe TBI, simulators, and controls.
[d] Replication of Millis et al., 1995.
[e] Discriminability is equal to [1 − (false positives + misses)/44 × 100].
[f] TBI with suspect evidence of poor effort and TBI with no evidence of poor effort vs. control group.
[g] Greve et al., 2003 sensitivity and specificity for MTBI using Mittenberg's cut score of 0.

Multiple Regression

Multiple regression, and more commonly, logistic regression, examines one or more linear variables in the prediction of a binary dependent variable. One of the benefits of this statistical technique is that it is more robust to heterogeneity of variance and non-normal distributions. Additionally, further diagnostics can examine multicollinearity problems and other model fit statistics. One of the strongest benefits of the logistic regression approach is that measures across testing can be included in a single model to identify patterns of performance at multiple time points on cognitive testing. Once a regression equation is verified, test data for an individual evaluation can be used with the equation by multiplying scores using corresponding beta weights and adding the constant, which is the y intercept of the regression line.

The resulting information can then be exponentiated to provide an estimation of the probability of effort test failure based on those test scores. Exponentiation involves raising the exponential function (also known as "e") to the power of the resulting multiple regression equation for an individual. In other words, the constant "e" is used to model a relationship in which it is assumed that change in the independent variable will result in the same proportional change in the dependent variable. Then, that number is divided by itself plus one. Although it may appear complicated conceptually, it is relatively easy to calculate these variables in clinical work with readily available spreadsheet programs. For example, in Excel one uses the formula command of "EXP" for the constant "e." It then becomes easy to have the regression first computed and totaled, then generate the exponentiated result with "EXP(formula)," and finally compute the probability of deficient performance with the quotient of EXP(formula) / [1+EXP(formula)].

Table 9.11 shows various regression models which have been published, demonstrating their utility in predicting group membership of good versus poor effort. For a detailed example, Wolfe and colleagues (2010) published a regression formula for the CVLT-II and found that the raw score for LDFR, d-prime, and the z score for Total Recall Discriminability worked together to create a viable prediction equation of poor effort. The corresponding beta weights for the scores and the constant appear below. The CVLT-II regression equation appears here:

$$p = \frac{e^{\,[(.32\,\times\,j)\,+\,(-.99\,\times\,k)\,+\,(-.693\,\times\,l)\,-\,1.092]}}{1 + e^{[(.32\,\times\,j)\,+\,(-.99\,\times\,k)\,+\,(-.693\,\times\,l)\,-\,1.092]}}$$

j = LDFR raw, k = d-prime raw score, l = total recall discriminability standard score

An individual's probability of poor effort can be calculated by entering performances on the CVLT-II. As a rule of thumb, a cut score of 0.5 or 50% probability is used. However, this cut score can be changed to address specific issues of base rates or empirically derived cut scores. Here is an example using a LDFR raw score of 4, d-prime of 2.3, and Total Recall Discriminability of -2.0:

$$p = \frac{e^{\,[(.32\,\times\,4)\,+\,(-.99\,\times\,2.3)\,+\,(-.693\,\times\,-2)\,-\,1.092]}}{1 + e^{[(.32\,\times\,4)\,+\,(-.99\,\times\,2.3)\,+\,(-.693\,\times\,-2)\,-\,1.092]}} = .33$$

Based on those data, there is a 33% probability that the individual's performance would be classified as poor effort. Hence, it appears that the individual was likely offering adequate effort on this measure.

Here is another data set, with LDFR of 1, d-prime of 0.7, and Total Recall Discriminability of -3.5:

$$p = \frac{e^{\,[(.32\,\times\,1)\,+\,(-.99\,\times\,.7)\,+\,(-.693\,\times\,-3.5)\,-\,1.092]}}{1 + e^{[(.32\,\times\,1)\,+\,(-.99\,\times\,.7)\,+\,(-.693\,\times\,-3.5)\,-\,1.092]}} = .72$$

Based on these data, there is a 72% chance that the individual's performance would be classified as poor effort. Thus, this type of performance would be more characteristic of malingering than the prior result (i.e., 33%). The regression method may be less intuitive than the additive method for detecting poor effort. However, performance patterns across tests are more difficult to coach and nearly impossible to predict by the examinee.

One significant weakness of regression, from a practical standpoint, is that it requires large samples (more than 200) in order to maximize stability. With smaller samples, there is risk of a model being overly optimistic and less predictive with future samples, meaning that the model may look stronger than it actually will be with other samples. That being said, some shrinkage—or reduction in the strength

TABLE 9.11 Regression Method Models Using Embedded Measures

Source	Measure	Cut Score[a]	Sensitivity	Specificity
Suhr & Boyer, 1999[b]	WCST	>1.90	.824	.933[c]
		>1.90	.47	.89[d]
		>3.68	.34	.94[de]
($-.75 \times$ number of categories) + ($1.01 \times$ failures to maintain set) + 3.16				
Meyers & Volbrecht, 2003[f]	RCFT/DSS/BD/FTT	-10		
FTT raw dominant $-$ [($.185 \times$ RCFT raw score) + ($.491 \times$ digit symbol scale score) + ($.361 \times$ block design scale score) + 31.34]				
Ross et al., 2006[g]	SRT/SSPT	.50[h]	.76	.80
		.60[h]	.70	.90
($.117 \times$ SSPT errors) + ($.245 \times$ SRT errors) -3.321				
Silverberg, Hanks, Buchanan, Fichtenberg, & Millis, 2008[i]	COWAT	.50[h]	.59	.89
		.47[h]	.47	.91
($-.679 \times$ declining output) + ($-.341 \times$ trial difficulty L $-$ J) + ($-.837 \times$ mean cluster size) + 4.63				
Ord et al., 2008[jl]	WMS-III	$-.5$[l]	.65	.93
(aud. Immediate $\times$ .012) + (verbal immediate $\times$ .0188) + (aud. Delayed $\times$ .0058) + (verbal delayed $\times$ $-.0241$) + (aud. Recog. $\times$ .0001) + (working memory $\times$ $-.1169$) + 10.89				
Miller et al., 2010[m]	WAIS-IV/ACS	.50[h]	.72	.89
($-.228 \times$ word choice) + ($-.007 \times$ logical memory recognition) + ($.238 \times$ verbal paired associates recognition) + ($-.951 \times$ visual reproduction recognition) + ($-.648 \times$ reliable digit span) + 10.615				
Wolfe et al., 2010[b]	CVLT-II	.50[h]	.66	.84
		.62[h]	.38	.87[kj]
($.32 \times$ LDFR raw) + ($-.99$ d-prime raw score) + ($-.693 \times$ total recall discriminability standard score) -1.092				
Schutte et al., 2011[f]	WMS-III/RCFT/ CVLT-II	.50[h]	.59	.95
($-.037 \times$ RCFT immediate memory standard score) + ($-.573 \times$ CVLT-II FC raw) + ($-.486 \times$ WMS-III verbal paired associates scale score) + ($1.082 \times$ CVLT-II trial 5 z score) + 15.25				

Note. WCST = Wisconsin Card Sorting Test; RCFT = Rey Complex Figure Test; FTT = Finger Tapping; SRT = Seashore Rhythm Test; SSPT = Speech Sound Perception Test; COWAT = Controlled Oral Word Association Test; WMS = Wechsler Memory Scale; WAIS = Wechsler Adult Intelligence Scale; ACS = Advanced Clinical Solutions; CVLT = California Verbal Learning Test; aud. = auditory; recog. = recognition.

[a] Cut scores are presented based on exponentiating the regression formula, which results in a probability of failure, and ROC analysis to determine sensitivity and specificity where available. A probability of .5 is a rule of thumb cut score in the absence of objectively derived cuts.

[b] TBI vs. simulators.

[c] Sensitivity and specificity for patients (*n* = 33) in this article are presented. This manuscript also examined simulators.

[d] Greve et al., 2002 replication.

[e] Greve et al., 2002 found inadequate specificity for this formula in a large mixed clinical sample

[f] Mixed clinical group: suspect effort vs. good effort.

[g] Mild TBI seeking financial compensation vs. moderate/severe TBI with no compensation.

[h] Exponentiated probability.

[i] TBI: suspect effort, documented moderate/severe TBI, simulators and controls.

[j] MTBI good vs. poor effort, mod/severe TBI and control.

[k] Donders et al., 2011 replication of the Wolfe et al. 2010 study.

[l] All scores in the Ord et al. (2008) study are index scores.

[m] All scores in the regression model are raw scores.

of the model—can be addressed using statistical techniques such as bootstrapping, which is a method of testing the model on a number of identically distributed samples. Additionally, Greve and Bianchini (2002) pointed out that regression assumes that people tend to offer poor effort or malinger in a uniform fashion, which may actually not be the case. As an example, Donders and Strong (2011) attempted to replicate the work of Wolfe et al. (2010). In their sample, the CVLT-II exponentiated formula previously presented showed that a cut score of 50% included too many false positives. As a result, they suggested a cut score of 62%. A 62% cut score reduced the sensitivity from .66 as reported by Wolfe et al. (2010) to .38, with a specificity of .87. Differences in the patient groups, research design, and other factors may have led to differing results on the two studies.

When using DFA and regression-based methods, the selection of individual variables is important because the selection method can significantly influence the outcome of the model. Three common methods of identifying variables in DFA are described here.

Rational: Rational identification of variables is one method that allows for prediction variables to be selected based on theory or hypothesis. The method is valuable in terms of face validity and construct validity. Schutte and colleagues (2011) and Meyers and Volbrecht (2003) used rational methods for model selection. The weakness of rational derivation is that it may not identify the strongest model. In addition, the identified model might not perform as expected with future samples.

Stepwise: There is more than one method of completing a stepwise regression model. A forward stepwise model starts with no variables in the model and selects the variable with the highest correlation with the criterion variable, which becomes the first variable in the model. A computerized statistical program (e.g., SPSS) then selects the variable with the next highest correlation and continues doing so until all variables with a statistically significant relationship to the criterion variable are chosen. A backward elimination stepwise model begins by entering all of the variables in the model and removing variables with the weakest relationship (i.e., not statistically significant) to the criterion variable. With forward and backward elimination procedures, a variety of variables of interest with the strongest relationships to the criterion can be kept; and those that are weak can be removed on an empirical basis, which rational selection is not able to do. However, the stepwise method has a significant weakness in its implementation in that it tends to overfit models because it capitalizes on chance findings, particularly in low sample sizes. Such models are subject to significant shrinkage, or in other words, the model is likely to be weaker on replication in other populations as a result of error or chance findings.

Bayesian Model Averaging: Bayesian Model Averaging (BMA) is a method of model identification that is able to account for uncertainty in models and treats uncertainties in terms of probabilities. This technique applies basic rules of probability to the selection of variables in the model. By averaging over many different competing models, BMA incorporates model uncertainty into conclusions about parameters and prediction. In most cases, "BMA selects the correct model and outperforms stepwise approaches at predicting an event of interest" (p. 158) (Wolfe et al., 2010; refer to Wolfe et al., 2010, for a discussion of the mathematical properties of BMA.).

CONCLUSIONS

The use of SVTs has become standard in forensic neuropsychological evaluations and is routinely used in clinical settings as well. Compared to free standing effort measures, embedded measures of effort are less face valid, should be more resistant to coaching, and are more efficient to use, which makes it easier to employ more of them across different time points in the evaluation. However, compared to stand-alone effort measures, weaknesses of embedded measures include the need for more statistical knowledge by the user and the fact that they were originally designed to measure ability as opposed to effort, which means that individuals with true cognitive deficits may legitimately perform poorly on these measures. For example, individuals with severe TBI may actually have significant deficits on executive functioning tasks, which underline the importance of medical records and good documentation. In addition, solid knowledge of the research used to derive these measures is important because sample and design characteristics are likely to have a significant impact on the meaning of failure on these measures. Weaknesses notwithstanding, the strength of embedded measures will likely lead to their continued use and importance in neuropsychological evaluations.

The use of embedded effort indices has shown significant evolution over time, from identification of individual cut scores to the sophisticated statistical approaches that allow for derivation of a probability of failure. There is no doubt that embedded indices will continue to take a more prominent role in the assessment of poor effort in neuropsychological examinations given their many advantages and will augment the use of stand-alone measures.

REFERENCES

American Academy of Clinical Neuropsychology. (2007). American Academy of Clinical Neuropsychology (AACN) practice guidelines for neuropsychological assessment and consultation. *The Clinical Neuropsychologist*, 21(2), 209–231.

Armistead-Jehle, P., & Hansen, C. L. (2011). Comparison of the Repeatable Battery for the Assessment of Neuropsychological Status effort index and stand-alone symptom validity tests in a military sample. *Archives of Clinical Neuropsychology*, 26(7), 592–601.

Arnold, G., Boone, K. B., Lu, P., Dean, A., Wen, J., Nitch, S., & McPherson, S. (2005). Sensitivity and specificity of finger tapping test scores for the detection of suspect effort. *The Clinical Neuropsychologist*, 19(1), 105–120.

Axelrod, B. N., Fichtenberg, N. L., Millis, S. R., & Wertheimer, J. C. (2006). Detecting incomplete effort with digit span from the Wechsler Adult Intelligence Scale-Third edition. *The Clinical Neuropsychologist*, 20(3), 513–523.

Babikian, T., Boone, K. B., Lu, P., & Arnold, G. (2006). Sensitivity and specificity of various digit span scores in the detection of suspect effort. *The Clinical Neuropsychologist*, 20(1), 145–159.

Backhaus, S. L., Fichtenberg, N. L., & Hanks, R. A. (2004). Detection of sub-optimal performance using a floor effect strategy in patients with traumatic brain injury. *The Clinical Neuropsychologist*, 18(4), 591–603.

Benton, A. L., Sivan, A. B., Hamsher, K. deS., Varney, N. R., & Spreen, O. (1994). *Contributions to neuropsychological assessment: A clinical manual* (2nd ed.). New York, NY: Oxford University Press.

Binder, L. M., Kelly, M. P., Villanueva, M. R., & Winslow, M. M. (2003). Motivation and neuropsychological test performance following mild head injury. *Journal of Clinical and Experimental Neuropsychology*, 25(3), 420–430.

Blasewitz, N., Merten, T., & Brockhaus, R. (2009). Detection of suboptimal effort with the Rey Complex Figure Test and Recognition Trial. *Applied Neuropsychology*, 16(1), 54–61.

Boone, K. B. (2009). The need for continuous and comprehensive sampling of effort/response bias during neuropsychological examinations. *The Clinical Neuropsychologist*, 23(4), 729–741.

Boone, K. B., Lu, P., & Wen, J. (2005). Comparison of various RAVLT scores in the detection of noncredible memory performance. *Archives of Clinical Neuropsychology*, 20(3), 301–319.

Bush, S. S., Ruff, R. M., Tröster, A. I., Barth, J. T., Koffler, S. P., Pliskin, N. H., . . . Silver, C. H. (2005). Symptom validity assessment: Practice issues and medical necessity NAN policy & planning committee. *Archives of Clinical Neuropsychology*, 20(4), 419–426.

Butcher, J. N., Dahlstrom, W. G., Graham, J. R., Tellegen, A. M., & Kaemmer, B. (1989). *Minnesota Multiphasic Personality Inventory–2 (MMPI-2): Manual for administration and scoring*. Minneapolis, MN: University of Minnesota Press.

Carone, D. A. (2008). Children with moderate/severe brain damage/dysfunction outperform adults with mild-to-no brain damage on the Medical Symptom Validity Test. *Brain Injury*, 22(12), 960–971.

Carroll, L. J., Cassidy, J. D., Peloso, P. M., Borg, J., von Holst, H., Holm, L., . . . Pépin, M. (2004). Prognosis for mild traumatic brain injury: Results of the WHO Collaborating Centre Task Force on Mild Traumatic Brain Injury. *Journal of Rehabilitation Medicine*, (Suppl. 43), 84–105.

Constantinou, M., Bauer, L., Ashendorf, L., Fisher, J. M., & McCaffery, R. J. (2005). Is poor performance on recognition memory effort measures indicative of generalized poor performance on neuropsychological tests? *Archives of Clinical Neuropsychology*, 20(2), 191–198.

Curtis, K. L., Greve, K. W., Brasseux, R., & Bianchini, K. J. (2010). Criterion groups validation of the Seashore Rhythm Test and Speech Sounds Perception Test for the detection of malingering in traumatic brain injury. *The Clinical Neuropsychologist*, 24(5), 882–897.

Curtis, K. L., Thompson, L. K., Greve, K. W., & Bianchini, K. J. (2008). Verbal fluency indicators of malingering in traumatic brain injury: Classification accuracy in known groups. *The Clinical Neuropsychologist*, 22(5), 930–945.

Dean, A. C., Victor, T. L., Boone, K. B., Philpott, L. M., & Hess, R. A. (2008). Dementia and effort test performance. *The Clinical Neuropsychologist*, 23(1), 133–152.

Delis, D. C., Kramer, J. H., Kaplan, E., & Ober, B. (2000). *California verbal learning test* (2nd ed.). San Antonio, TX: Psychological Corporation.

DiCarlo, M. A., Gfeller, J. D., & Oliveri, M. V. (2000). Effects of coaching on detecting feigned cognitive impairment with the Category Test. *Archives of Clinical Neuropsychology*, 15(5), 399–413.

Dikmen, S. S., Machamer, J. E., Winn, H. R., & Temkin, N. R. (1995). Neuropsychological outcome at 1-year post head injury. *Neuropsychology*, 9, 80–90.

Donders, J., & Strong, C. A. H. (2011). Embedded effort indicators on the California verbal learning test–second edition (CVLT-II): An attempted cross-validation. *The Clinical Neuropsychologist*, 25(1), 173–184.

Green, P. (2003). *Green's Word Memory Test for Microsoft Windows*. Edmonton, Alberta, Canada: Green's.

Green, P. (2004). *Green's Medical Symptom Validity Test (MSVT) for Microsoft Windows: User's manual*. Edmonton, Alberta, Canada: Green's Publishing Company.

Green, P. (2007). The pervasive influence of effort on neuropsychological tests. *Physical Medicine and Rehabilitation Clinics of North America*, 18(1), 43–68.

Greffenstein, M. F., Baker, J., & Gola, T. (1994). Validation of malingered amnesia measures with a large clinical sample. *Psychological Assessment*, 6, 218–224.

Greve, K. W., & Bianchini, K. J. (2002). Using the Wisconsin card sorting test to detect malingering: An analysis of the specificity of two methods in nonmalingering normal and patient samples. *Journal of Clinical and Experimental Neuropsychology*, 24(1), 48–54.

Greve, K. W., Bianchini, K. J., & Roberson, T. (2007). The Booklet Category Test and malingering in traumatic brain injury: Classification accuracy in known groups. *The Clinical Neuropsychologist*, 21(2), 318–337.

Greve, K. W., Binder, L. M., & Bianchini, K. J. (2009). Rates of below-chance performance in forced-choice symptom validity tests. *The Clinical Neuropsychologist*, 23(3), 534–544.

Heaton, R. K., Chelune, G. J., Talley, J. L., Kay, G. G., & Curtiss, G. (1993). *Wisconsin Card Sorting Test manual: Revised and expanded*. Odessa, FL: Psychological Assessment Resources.

Heaton, R. K., Miller, S. W., Taylor, M. J., & Grant, I. (2004). *Revised comprehensive norms for an expanded Halstead-Reitan Battery: Demographically adjusted neuropsychological norms for African American and Caucasian adults, professional manual*. Lutz, FL: Psychological Assessment Resources.

Heilbronner, R. L., Sweet, J. J., Morgan, J. E., Larrabee, G. J., & Millis, S. R. (2009). American Academy of Clinical Neuropsychology consensus conference statement on the neuropsychological assessment of effort, response bias, and malingering. *The Clinical Neuropsychologist*, 23(7), 1093–1129.

Howe, L. L. S., Anderson, A. M., Kaufman, D. A. S., Sachs, B. C., & Loring, D. W. (2007). Characterization of the medical symptom validity test in evaluation of clinically referred memory disorders clinic patients. *Archives of Clinical Neuropsychology*, 22(6), 753–761.

Iverson, G. L., & Franzen, M. D. (1994). The Recognition Memory Test, Digit Span, and Knox Cube Test as markers of malingered memory impairment. *Assessment*, 1, 323–334.

Iverson, G. L., Lange, R. T., Green, P., & Franzen, M. D. (2002). Detecting exaggeration and malingering with the trail making test. *The Clinical Neuropsychologist*, 16(3), 398–406.

Killgore, W. D. S., & DellaPietra, L. (2000). Using the WMS-III to detect malingering: Empirical validation of the rarely missed index (RMI). *Journal of Clinical and Experimental Neuropsychology*, 22(6), 761–771.

Langeluddecke, P. M., & Lucas, S. K. (2003). Quantitative measures of memory malingering on the Wechsler Memory Scale—third edition in mild head injury litigants. *Archives of Clinical Neuropsychology*, 18(2), 181–197.

Larrabee, G. J. (2003). Detection of malingering using atypical performance patterns on standard neuropsychological tests. *The Clinical Neuropsychologist*, 17(3), 410–425.

Larrabee, G. J. (2008). Aggregation across multiple indicators improves the detection of malingering: Relationship to likelihood ratios. *The Clinical Neuropsychologist*, 22(4), 666–679.

Lees-Haley, P. R., English, L. T., & Glenn, W. J. (1991). A fake bad scale for the MMPI-2 for personal injury claimants. *Psychological Reports*, 68(1), 203–210.

Loring, D. W., Marino, S. E., Drane, D. L., Parfitt, D., Finney, G. R., & Meador, K. J. (2011). Lorazepam effects on Word Memory Test performance: A randomized, double-blind, placebo-controlled, crossover trial. *The Clinical Neuropsychologist*, 25(5), 799–811.

Lu, P. H., Boone, K. B., Cozolino, L., & Mitchell, C. (2003). Effectiveness of the Rey-Osterrieth Complex Figure Test and the Meyers and Meyers Recognition Trial in the detection of suspect effort. *The Clinical Neuropsychologist*, 17(3), 426–440.

Meyers, J. E., Morrison, A. L., & Miller, J. C. (2001). How low is too low, revisited: Sentence repetition and AVLT-recognition in the detection of malingering. *Applied Neuropsychology*, 8(4), 234–241.

Meyers, J. E., & Volbrecht, M. E. (2003). A validation of multiple malingering detection methods in a large clinical sample. *Archives of Clinical Neuropsychology*, 18(3), 261–276.

Meyers, J. E., Volbrecht, M. E., Axelrod, B. N., & Reinsch-Boothby, L. (2011). Embedded symptom validity tests and overall neuropsychological test performance. *Archives of Clinical Neuropsychology*, 26(1), 8–15.

Miller, J. B., Millis, S. R., Rapport, L. J., Bashem, J. R., Hanks, R. A., & Axelrod, B. N. (2010). Detection of insufficient effort using the advanced clinical solutions for the Wechsler Memory Scale, fourth edition. *The Clinical Neuropsychologist*, 25(1), 160–172.

Millis, S. R. (1992). The Recognition Memory Test in the detection of malingered and exaggerated memory deficits. *The Clinical Neuropsychologist*, 6, 406–414.

Millis, S. R. (2004). Evaluation of malingered neurocognitive disorders. In M. Rizzo & P. Eslinger (Eds.), *Principles and practice of behavioral neurology and neuropsychology* (pp. 1077–1089). Philadelphia, PA: Saunders.

Millis, S. R. (2009). What clinicians really need to know about symptoms exaggeration, insufficient effort, and malingering: Statistical and measurement matters. In J. E. Morgan & J. J. Sweet (Eds.), *Neuropsychology of Malingering Casebook* (pp. 21–37). New York, NY: Psychology Press.

Millis, S. R., Putnam, S. H., Adams, K. M., & Ricker, J. H. (1995). The California verbal learning test in detection of incomplete effort in neuropsychological evaluation. *Psychological Assessment*, 7, 463–471.

Millis, S. R., Ross, S. R., & Ricker, J. H. (1998). Detection of incomplete effort on the Wechsler Adult Intelligence Scale-Revised: A cross validation. *Journal of Clinical and Experimental Neuropsychology*, 20(2), 167–173.

Mittenberg, W., Azrin, R., Millsaps, C., & Heilbronner, R. (1993). Identification of malingered head injury on the Wechsler Memory Scale-Revised. *Psychological Assessment*, 5, 34–40.

Mittenberg, W., Patton, C., Canyock, E. M., & Condit, D. C. (2002). Base rates of malingering and symptom exaggeration. *Journal of Clinical and Experimental Neuropsychology*, 24(8), 1094–1102.

Mittenberg, W., Rotholc, A., Russell, E., & Heilbronner, R. (1996). Identification of malingered head injury on the Halstead-Reitan battery. *Archives of Clinical Neuropsychology*, 11(4), 271–281.

Mittenberg, W., Theroux, S., Aguila-Puentes, G., Bianchini, K., Greve, K., & Rayls, K. (2001). Identification of malingered head injury on the Wechsler Adult Intelligence Scale – 3rd edition. *The Clinical Neuropsychologist*, 15(4), 440–445.

Ord, J. S., Boettcher, A., Greve, K. W., & Bianchini, K. J. (2010). Detection of malingering in mild traumatic brain injury with the Conners' Continuous Performance Test-II. *Journal of Clinical and Experimental Neuropsychology*, 32(4), 380–387.

Ord, J. S., Greve, K. W., & Bianchini, K. J. (2008). Using the Wechsler Memory Scale-III to detect malingering in mild traumatic brain injury. *The Clinical Neuropsychologist*, 22(4), 689–704.

Randolph, C. (1998). *The Repeatable Battery for the Assessment of Neuropsychological Status* (RBANS). San Antonio, TX: The Psychological Corporation.

Reitan, R. M., & Wolfson, D. (1985). *The Halstead-Reitan neuropsychological test battery: Theory and clinical interpretation*. Tucson, AZ: Neuropsychology Press.

Rohling, M. L., Meyers, J. E., & Millis, S. R. (2003). Neuropsychological impairment following traumatic brain injury: A dose-response analysis. *The Clinical Neuropsychologist*, 17(3), 289–302.

Ross, S. R., Putnam, S. H., Millis, S. R., Adams, K. M., & Krukowski, R. A. (2006). Detecting insufficient effort using the Seashore Rhythm and Speech-Sounds Perception Tests in head injury. *The Clinical Neuropsychologist*, 20(4), 798–815.

Root, J. C., Robbins, R. N., Chang, L. & VanGorp, W. G. (2006). Detection of inadequate effort on the California Verbal Learning Test—Second edition: forced choice recognition and critical item analysis. *Journal of the International Neuropsychological Society*, 12, 688–696.

Schmidt, M. (1996). *Rey Auditory and Verbal Learning Test: A handbook*. Los Angeles, CA: Western Psychological Services.

Schretlen, D. J., & Shapiro, A. M. (2003). A quantitative review of the effects of traumatic brain injury on cognitive functioning. *International Review of Psychiatry*, 15(4), 341–349.

Schutte, C., Millis, S. R., Axelrod, B. N., & Van Dyke, S. (2011). Derivation of a composite measure of embedded symptom validity indices. *The Clinical Neuropsychologist*, 25(3), 454–462.

Sherman, D. S., Boone, K. B., Lu, P., & Razani, J. (2002). Re-examination of a Rey auditory verbal learning test/Rey complex figure discriminant function to detect suspect effort. *The Clinical Neuropsychologist*, 16(3), 242–250.

Silverberg, N. D., Hanks, R. A., Buchanan, L., Fichtenberg, N., & Millis, S. R. (2008). Detecting response bias with performance patterns on an expanded version of the controlled oral word association test. *The Clinical Neuropsychologist*, 22(1), 140–157.

Silverberg, N. D., Wertheimer, J. C., & Fichtenberg, N. L. (2007). An effort index for the Repeatable Battery for the Assessment of Neuropsychological Status (RBANS). *The Clinical Neuropsychologist*, 21(5), 841–854.

Slick, D. J., Hopp, G., Strauss, E., & Spellacy, F. J. (1996). Victoria Symptom Validity Test: Efficiency for detecting feigned memory impairment and relationship to neuropsychological tests and MMPI-2 validity scales. *The Journal of Clinical and Experimental Neuropsychology*, 18(6), 911–922.

Slick, D. J., Sherman, E. M. S. & Iverson, G. L. (1999). Diagnostic criteria for malingered neurocognitive dysfunction: proposed standards for clinical practice and research. *The Clinical Neuropsychologist*, 13, 454–561.

Slick, D. J., Iverson, G. L. & Green, P. (2000). California Verbal Learning Test indicators of suboptimal performance in a sample of head-injury litigants. *Journal of Clinical and Experimental Neuropsychology*, 22, 569–579.

Suhr, J. A., & Boyer, D. (1999). Use of the Wisconsin card sorting test in the detection of malingering in student simulator and patient samples. *Journal of Clinical and Experimental Neuropsychology*, 21(5), 701–708.

Suhr, J. A., & Gunstad, J. (2000). The effects of coaching on the sensitivity and specificity of malingering measures. *Archives of Clinical Neuropsychology*, 15(5), 415–424.

Sweet, J. J. , Wolfe, P., Sattlberger, E., Numan, B., Rosenfeld, J. P. , Clingerman, S., Nies, K. J. (2000). Further investigation of traumatic brain injury versus insufficient effort with the California verbal learning test. *Archives of Clinical Neuropsychology*, 15(2), 105–113.

Tombaugh, T. N. (1996). *Test of Memory Malingering* (TOMM). Toronto, ON: Multi-Health Systems.

Trueblood, W., & Schmidt, M. (1993). Malingering and other validity considerations in the neuropsychological evaluation of mild head injury. *Journal of Clinical and Experimental Neuropsychology*, 15(4), 578–590.

Victor, T. L., Boone, K. B., Serpa, J. G., Buehler, J., & Ziegler, E. A. (2009). Interpreting the meaning of multiple symptom validity test failure. *The Clinical Neuropsychologist*, 23(2), 297–313.

Warrington, E. K. (1984). *Recognition Memory Test: Manual*. Berkshire, United Kingdom: NFER-Nelson.

Wechsler, D. (1997). *Manual for the Wechsler Adult Intelligence Scale* (3rd ed.). San Antonio, TX: Psychological Corporation.

Wechsler, D. (2008). *Wechsler Adult Intelligence Scale* (4th ed.). San Antonio, TX: Psychological Corporation.

Wechsler, D. (2009). *Wechsler Memory Scale – fourth edition (WAIS-IV): Technical and interpretive manual*. San Antonio, TX: Pearson.

Whiteside, D., Wald, D., & Busse, M. (2011). Classification accuracy of multiple visual spatial measures in the detection of suspect effort. *The Clinical Neuropsychologist*, 25(2), 287–301.

Wolfe, P. L., Millis, S. R., Hanks, R. A., Fichtenberg, N., Larrabee, G. J., & Sweet, J. J. (2010). Effort indicators within the California Verbal Learning Test-II (CVLT-II). *The Clinical Neuropsychologist*, 24(1), 153–8.

Psychological Assessment of Symptom Magnification in Mild Traumatic Brain Injury Cases

10

Robert L. Heilbronner & George K. Henry

Psychological and personality assessment predates the development of cognitive assessment by many decades. Indeed, the task of our early predecessors (e.g., Binet, Simon, Cattell) was to assess the psychological intelligence and personality constructs of human beings. It was not until later (e.g., 1940s) that Ward Halsted attempted to use cognitive instruments to assess "biological intelligence." With that step, neuropsychology as a formal field of study was born; however, with the realization that cognitive tests are sensitive and objective measures of brain–behavior relationships, the question arose, "Is there any value in including psychological assessment techniques (e.g., Rorschach, Thematic Apperception Technique [TAT]) as a component part of a neuropsychological evaluation?" To date, psychological inventories and questionnaires continue to be routinely used as part of a comprehensive neuropsychological evaluation, particularly in traumatic brain injury (TBI) and mild traumatic brain injury (MTBI) cases. Projective personality instruments such as the Rorschach and TAT are used much less frequently. Compared to the early projective techniques, current psychological assessment instruments are more standardized and objective, which explains their more common usage.

Research and clinical evidence suggest that the primary symptoms associated with MTBI from the acute to subacute phase include cognitive difficulties (e.g., reduced information processing speed, attention, concentration, and memory) and physical problems (e.g., headache, dizziness, fatigue). Although changes in psychological functioning (e.g., irritability, depression) and/or personality are sometimes described as postconcussive in nature, these symptoms can be easily exaggerated and are prone to response bias on psychological tests. In this chapter, we review measures of emotional states and personality traits that are among the most commonly used in neuropsychological evaluations, with a primary focus on the most recently developed validity scales for the Minnesota Multiphasic Personality Inventory (MMPI). The goal of this chapter is to identify which psychological tests and/or indices are most useful for identifying symptom magnification in patients with a history of MTBI. For discussion of other types of self-report scales (i.e., general symptom questionnaires) as measures of symptom validity, see Chapter 11.

PSYCHOLOGICAL INVENTORIES TO ASSESS SYMPTOM EXAGGERATION IN MILD TRAUMATIC BRAIN INJURY CASES

We have chosen to highlight those measures of mood and personality that are commonly used by neuropsychologists currently practicing in the United States. Brief screens were not included because they generally lack validity scales and have little or no research on their use for assessment of symptom validity with MTBI populations. The measures reviewed here include the following: 16 Personality Factors (16PF), Symptom Checklist-90-Revised (SCL-90-R), Millon Behavioral Health Inventory (MBHI), Million Clinical Multiaxial Inventory (MCMI), Personality Assessment Inventory (PAI), MMPI (various versions), and associated MMPI validity indices. Of these measures, only the MMPI/MMPI-2 is among the 25 tests (including cognitive tests) that are most commonly used by neuropsychologists (Rabin, Barr, & Burton, 2005). However, of the top 40 tests used for return-to-work assessments, the MMPI/MMPI2, PAI, MCMI/MCMI-II, and SCL-90/SCL-90-R were among the top 20.

16 Personality Factor

The *16PF*, now in its 5th edition (Cattell, Cattell, & Cattell, 1993; Russell & Karol, 2002), is a questionnaire designed to assess 16 personality factors. A PubMed search on the 16PF did not result in any research articles specifically devoted to patients with MTBI or symptom exaggeration.

Symptom Checklist-90-Revised

The SCL-90-R (Derogatis, 1994) is a 5-point rating scale checklist that evaluates a broad range of psychological problems and symptoms of psychopathology. The test has been evaluated specifically for sensitivity to malingered pain symptomatology with a group of patients with whiplash and chronic pain and to a group of persons who are noninjured asked to simulate chronic pain resulting from a whiplash injury (Wallis & Bogduk, 1996). Results showed that the simulating group produced greater elevations on the somatization, obsessive–compulsive, and depression scales than those produced by the genuine group as well as elevations across the range of clinical scales. McQuire and Shores (2001) compared the SCL-90 profiles of patients with chronic (primarily back) pain to a group of undergraduate psychology students who are noninjured asked to simulate pain disorder in the context of a compensation evaluation. They found that patients with pain produced their highest elevations on the same scales as the Wallis and Bogduk study (i.e., somatization, obsessive–compulsive, and depression), but the simulators scored higher on these scales than the genuine group. Both studies suggest that SCL-90 scores overestimate the degree of psychopathology experienced in people with chronic pain. No studies to date have been published examining the effectiveness of the SCL-90 in patients with MTBI.

Millon Behavioral Health Inventory

The MBHI (Millon, Green, & Meagher, 1982) was used in a study designed to assess personality traits in patients with MTBI and postconcussional sequelae at 1 week, 3 months, and 1 year following their accidents (Middleboe, Birket-Smith, Anderson, & Friis, 1992). This measure is a 150-item self-report inventory designed and standardized with a medical population, with the aim of providing the clinician with information on factors such as a patient's style of relating to health care personnel and treatment plans as well as major psychosocial stressors. Only 2 patients out of 51 had made a claim to an insurance company after the accident, and the interviewers had no suspicion of malingering in these two patients.

Findings from the study provided evidence for characteristic personality traits among patients reporting persisting symptoms after concussion during a 1 year follow-up. According to the authors, the results suggested that patients demonstrating high scores on the forceful personality style and sensitive personality style scales, because of their coping strategies, seemed at risk for developing persisting symptoms after concussion. Likewise, a risk group was constituted by patients with high scores on the scales of chronic tension and recurrent stress, both of which were possible predictors of poor outcome. The scales of introversive personality style and cooperative personality style were associated with fewer postconcussional symptoms. Results of the study were felt to be in accordance with previous studies (Kelly & Smith, 1981) examining the role of certain personality traits (e.g., psychogenesis) and iatrogenesis as predisposing factors for the development of postconcussional sequelae (Lishman, 1968; Lidvall, Linderoth, & Norlin, 1974). The authors reported that the MBHI could be used as an aid for the clinician in predicting outcome after MTBI. Because it relates to this chapter, compensation and litigation did not turn out to be of any major importance in this study, but this is a difficult conclusion to reach because only 2 of 51 patients were litigating. Thus, further investigation is needed on the MBHI and exaggeration after MTBI.

Millon Multiaxial Clinical Inventory-III

The MCMI, now in its third edition (Millon, Davis, & Millon, 1997), is a lengthy personality test that has been used by psychologists in assessing patients for personality disorders. It has also been used, to a lesser degree, in cases with a neuropsychological emphasis. One of the features that distinguishes the MCMI scales is the use of base rate scores that attempt to incorporate varying prevalences of psychiatric disorders, thereby offering a potential advantage over the fixed base rates that most standard scores implicitly assume. The MCMI-III also includes a validity index and three modifying scales: disclosure, desirability, and debasement, all intended to address response sets. Despite its widespread use in clinical psychology, very little research has been conducted with the MCMI in the context of malingering, and the operating characteristics of the MCMI-II validity index and modifying scales were determined to not be generalizable to the MCMI-III (McCann & Dyer, 1996; Rogers, Salekin, & Sewell, 1999).

According to Berry and Schipper (2007), the debasement index is the most directly applicable to the detection of overreporting of psychological problems. Using the MCMI-II, Lees-Haley (1992) demonstrated that disclosure and debasement differentiated patients with pseudo-posttraumatic stress disorder (PTSD) from patients with genuine PTSD. However, Schoenberg, Dorr, and Morgan (2003) found that the MCMI-III modifier indices were of little clinical use in distinguishing college student malingerers from bona fide psychiatric inpatients. These authors further stated that the MCMI-III appears to be less effective than the MMPI-II at discriminating nonpatient malingerers from inpatients with psychiatric illnesses.

With a mixed neuropsychology population, Ruocco et al. (2008) examined symptom validity test (SVT) failure rates on cognitive SVTs (Test of Memory Malingering [TOMM] and reliable digit span [RDS]) and MCMI-III validity indices. They found that 22.6% of the sample solely failed the neuropsychological SVT, 6.1% solely failed the psychiatric SVT, and only 3.5% of the sample failed SVTs in both domains. They concluded that the results supported a dissociation between exaggeration of cognitive and psychiatric symptoms.

In particular, in the context of patients with TBI, Aguerrevere, Greve, Bianchini, and Ord (2011) determined that scores from all MCMI-III modifier indices are useful for identifying intentional symptom exaggeration in TBI cases of mixed severity, with debasement being the most sensitive of the three indices. They found, "At scores associated with a 4% false positive (FP) error rate, sensitivity was 47% for disclosure, 51% for desirability, and 55% for debasement. Examination of joint classification analysis demonstrated 54% sensitivity at cutoffs associated with 0% FP error rate" (p. 497). In this study, the authors did not differentiate between mild and moderate-to-severe TBIs because based on analyses of variance (ANOVAs), there were no differences on the MCMI-III modifier indices as a function of injury severity.

Personality Assessment Inventory

The PAI (Morey, 1991) is another commonly used measure of personality traits and psychological functioning. Although, compared to the MMPI, relatively little research has been conducted with the PAI in TBI populations, some investigations have found the PAI to be of value in patients with TBI (Breshears, Brenner, Harwood, & Gutierrez, 2010; Demakis et al., 2007; Till, Christensen, & Green, 2009). Regarding the relationship between suboptimal cognitive effort and PAI clinical scales, Whiteside, Dunbar-Mayer, and Waters (2009) found that extreme elevations on the Somatic Complaint scale (SOM) are associated with TOMM failures. In particular, when using $T > 87$ as the cutoff score for the SOM to predict TOMM performance, the authors obtained adequate sensitivity (93%) and specificity (76%) with a positive predictive power (PPP) of 54% and a negative predictive power of 97%, resulting in a 91% correct classification rate.

In contrast to the findings of the Ruocco et al. (2008) study that supported a dissociation between exaggeration of cognitive and psychiatric symptoms, a study examining the relationship between the PAI validity scales and the TOMM found with a mixed clinical sample that elevations on the PAI's infrequency (INF) and Negative Impression Management (NIM) scales were often associated with decreased cognitive effort on the TOMM (Whiteside et al., 2009). Whiteside, Galbreath, Brown, and Turnbull (2012) examined PAI clinical response patterns using groups of compensation-seeking and non–compensation-seeking patients with MTBI. They found that the compensation-seeking patients with MTBI had significantly higher elevations on the scales related to somatic preoccupation (SOM), emotional distress (Anxiety scale [ANX]; Anxiety Related Disorders scale [ARD]; Depression scale [DEP]), and the NIM validity scale. In addition, the compensation-seeking group had elevations on all of the SOM subscales and the anxiety cognitive (ANX-C) and anxiety affective (ANX-A) subscales.

Minnesota Multiphasic Personality Inventory (MMPI, MMPI-2, and MMPI-2-RF)

Although principally developed for and used with psychiatric populations, there is little doubt that the MMPI (including the MMPI-2 and MMPI-2-RF) is the most widely used instrument to assess personality and psychological/emotional functioning in neuropsychology (Butler, Retzlaff, Vanderploeg, 1991; Lees-Haley, Smith, Williams, & Dunn, 1996; Rabin et al., 2005). The MMPI and its various versions have long played a role in the assessment of malingered symptom reporting (Berry, Baer, & Harris, 1991; Rogers, Sewell, & Ustad, 1995). In addition to traditional validity scales (L, F, K), other commonly used indices to assist in the detection of malingering/symptom exaggeration include F-K, Fb, Fp, obvious-subtle difference, and dissimulation-revised scores. The reader is referred to Larrabee (2005, pp. 133–142) for a review of these particular scales, particularly because they have been used in personal injury (PI) settings for litigants (not exclusively patients with MTBI) pursuing neuropsychological claims.

In the first study designed to assess the usefulness of the MMPI with mild closed head trauma populations (Diamond, Barth, & Zillmer, 1988), results demonstrated that MMPI findings for the mild head trauma sample showed elevations (> 60T) for all clinical scales, distinct from normative expectations for the general population, but markedly similar to the findings from a comparison sample of mixed adults who are neurologically impaired. The authors concluded that patients with a history of mild head injury showed significant emotional distress that is markedly similar to that seen in individuals with longstanding neurologic damage. They hypothesized that the emotional distress may reflect a posttraumatic stress reaction, antecedent personality factors, or a secondary response to the difficulty in resuming preinjury activities. Compensation-litigation issues were not formally addressed in this study, and only traditional validity indices (L, F, K) were investigated; the results of which were not significantly different between the two groups.

In a 1991 study, Leininger, Kreutzer, and Hill compared MMPI profiles of patients with minor and severe head injury. Results demonstrated that patients with minor head injury obtained mean elevations on clinical scales 1, 2, 3, 7, and 8, with the three highest elevations on scales 1, 2, and 8 indicative of depressive symptomatology, confusion, interpersonal alienation, and preoccupation with physical illness. In contrast, the patients with severe head injury obtained only one scale elevation (scale 2), with scale 8 approaching a *T* score of 70. The pattern of scale elevation was generally similar between the groups, with the mild head injury group obtaining higher scores on three of the scales (1, 2, and 7). In particular, there was a much larger proportion of females in the minor head injury sample. The authors concluded that the minor head injury group's relative preoccupation with somatic functioning should be anticipated considering the overlap between MMPI scale content (on scales 1 and 3) and commonly reported postconcussive sequelae. The paper did not include any information regarding litigation status, and only traditional validity indices (L, F, K) were investigated and found to not being significantly different between the two groups.

Since the publication of the MMPI-2 in 1989, there have been a number of empirically derived validity scales developed for detection of symptom overreporting. Before moving on to a discussion about specific MMPI, MMPI-2, and MMPI-2-RF indicators associated with symptom exaggeration in patients with MTBI, it is important to briefly address the Fake Bad Scale (FBS). The 43-item FBS was developed in 1991 (Lees-Haley, English, & Glenn, 1991) and subsequently revised as the 30-item FBS-r (Fake Bad Scale-revised; Symptom Validity Scale) and incorporated into the MMPI-2-RF in 2006. An excellent review of the FBS is available for interested readers (Greiffenstein, Fox & Lees-Haley, 2007). It is important to point out that FBS was first used in a sample of PI claimants claiming *emotional distress*. They were not patients with neuropsychological problems and did not include patients with histories of TBI or MTBI. However, early studies of FBS showed that it was sensitive in discriminating claimants with pseudo-PTSD from claimants with legitimate emotional distress. Later, Larrabee (1998, 2003) found FBS to be significantly more sensitive to detection of symptom exaggeration than F, Fb, or Fp in litigants compared to nonlitigating patients with TBI. For a review of other studies examining the FBS with other patient samples (e.g., multiple sclerosis, spinal cord injury, chronic pain, and depression), the reader is referred to Larrabee (2007) and Greiffenstein et al. (2007). It should be noted that FBS is not without its detractors (Bury & Bagby, 2002; Butcher, Arbisi, Atlis, & McNulty, 2003), and before anyone relies on results of the FBS score in his or her clinical and/or forensic opinions, he or she should be well aware of the criticisms of these authors. Some criticisms include the notion that the scale prejudicially labels patients as malingerers, that it is prone to FP labeling of patients as malingerers, and that common problems can lead to elevations on single items. However, the rejoinder has been that the scale is examined in totality as opposed to the individual items, that the test has been found not to overpathologize patients with legitimate medical condition, and that the scale has been renamed as the Symptom Validity Scale in the MMPI-2-RF.

The focus of this section is on a review of the research in the last 5 years that has witnessed the emergence and validation of a new generation of MMPI-2 special validity scales dedicated to evaluating psychological response validity, specifically the Henry-Heilbronner Index (HHI; Henry, Heilbronner, Mittenberg, & Enders, 2006), Response Bias Scale (RBS; Gervais, Ben-Porath, Wygant, & Green, 2007), Malingered Mood Disorder Scale (MMDS; Henry, Heilbronner, Mittenberg, Enders, & Roberts, 2008), and the Psychosocial Distress Scale (PDS; Henry et al., 2011). It should be noted that we developed all of these scales except for the RBS. Studies that included any subjects with a history of MTBI who had been administered the MMPI-2 were selected for review. An attempt was made to divide the literature review into separate sections dealing specifically with each new scale. However, since 2008, several studies have compared the ability of the HHI and RBS to discriminate between criterion groups. Thus, to avoid redundancy, a review of the literature involving either the HHI alone or both the HHI and RBS are addressed in the first section. In the subsequent section covering the RBS, research not including the HHI is reviewed.

Henry-Heilbronner Index

Initial research used a known-group design to empirically derive the 15-item HHI from the MMPI-2 (Henry et al., 2006). The scale was composed of items from the 43-item FBS and the 17-item Shaw and Matthews' Pseudoneurologic Scale (PNS; Shaw & Matthews, 1965). In the original study (Henry et al., 2006), two known groups were formed: A PI and disability claimants group ($n = 45$) composed of patients with MTBI (56%), other medical conditions (24%), and psychiatric disorders (20%), and a clinical control group composed of 74 nonlitigants composed of patients with MTBI (85%) and patients with moderate-to-severe TBI (15%). A series of logistic regression analyses showed that the HHI was superior to both the FBS and PNS in predicting group membership. A cut score of ≥ 8 on the HHI was associated with an 85.6% classification accuracy rate, good sensitivity (80%), and high specificity (89%). A score of ≥ 13 was associated with 100% PPP (i.e., no FP errors).

A comparative study of the HHI using a known-group design evaluated the predictive validity of the 27-item MMPI-2 Restructured Scale 1 (RC1), FBS, and HHI in identifying noncredible symptom response sets in 63 PI litigants and disability claimants compared to 77 nonlitigating head-injured controls (Henry, Heilbronner, Mittenberg, Enders, & Stanczak, 2008). Logistic regression analyses revealed that the HHI and FBS were better predictors of group membership than the RC1 indicating that the FBS, HHI, and RC1 may be measuring different constructs. Elevated scores on the HHI and FBS were conceptualized as reflecting exaggeration of disability or magnification of illness-related behavior.

Larrabee (2008a) presented unpublished data at the 36th Annual International Society Conference comparing the ability of several traditional MMPI-2 validity scales (F, FBS, Fp, and FBS-r) and newly developed validity scales (RBS, HHI, Fs and Fptsd) to discriminate between litigants and disability claimants ($n = 41$) and private clinical patients ($n = 54$). The litigants and disability claimants were composed of 24 subjects who met the Slick, Sherman, and Iverson (1999) criteria for definite malingered neurocognitive dysfunction, whereas 17 were diagnosed with probable malingered neurocognitive dysfunction. Embedded effort measures included RDS,

Wisconsin Card Sorting Test (WCST) failure to maintain set (FMS), total correct on Visual Form Discrimination (VFD), and mean dominant hand performance on the finger tapping test (FTT). The private clinical patient group was composed of subjects with TBI (50%), including 15 with severe TBI and 12 with moderate TBI. The remaining 50% of private clinical patients consisted of unspecified neurologic (24%) and psychiatric (26%) diagnoses. The number of MTBI cases, if any, was not specified.

Group differences were greatest for the FBS, RBS, FBS-r, and HHI with very large effect sizes (i.e., 1.99, 1.91, 1.85, and 1.77, respectively). Receiver operating characteristic (ROC) analyses of the FBS, RBS, FBS-r, and HHI showed an area under the curve (AUC) of 0.917, 0.901, 0.900, and 0.892, respectively. Larrabee reported that the RBS, FBS, and FBS-r added meaningfully to prediction of group membership between PI litigants and nonlitigant clinical patients. Although the HHI did not add additional predictive validity, it showed good discrimination between malingering versus clinical patients when used alone, and it shared significant variance with embedded SVTs (VFD, FTT, RDS, and FMS). An HHI cut score of ≥ 10 was associated with good sensitivity (70.7%) and fair specificity (83.3%). Raising the HHI cut score to ≥ 12 lowered the sensitivity to 64.3% but increased specificity to 96.3%, with only a 3.7% FP rate.

The Fptsd, F, Fs, and Fp scales did not add to the discrimination between the two groups. Of note, the 32-item Fptsd was developed by selecting MMPI-2 items infrequently endorsed ($< 20\%$) by both the normative sample and a sample of clinical patients diagnosed with PTSD (Elhai et al., 2002).

A study (Whitney, Davis, Shepard, & Herman, 2008) was undertaken in an attempt to confirm the validity of the RBS and to determine if the relationship between the TOMM and RBS could be replicated in an outpatient Veterans Administration (VA) clinical sample ($N = 46$). Two groups were formed on the basis of passing the TOMM ($n = 24$) and failing the TOMM ($n = 22$). The clinical sample consisted of mixed diagnoses including MTBI ($n = 12$); moderate-to-severe TBI ($n = 4$); psychiatric diagnoses ($n = 10$, including six with depression, three with PTSD, and one with schizoaffective disorder); and various neurologic diagnoses ($n = 20$) including coronary artery disease, meningitis, multiple sclerosis, transient ischemic attack/stroke, and encephalitis/seizure disorder. This study also looked at the relationship between the TOMM and two other empirically derived MMPI-2 validity indicators (i.e., the Fptsd scale and the HHI). Researchers predicted that the RBS would add significantly to the incremental validity of other MMPI-2 validity scales in predicting TOMM performance (pass vs. fail).

Independent t tests revealed that only the RBS, HHI, and Fb scale showed significant between-group differences. The RBS demonstrated the largest effect size ($d = 0.98$), followed by the HHI ($d = 0.90$), and the Fb ($d = 0.65$). An ROC analysis of the RBS revealed reasonably good predictive information (AUC = 0.75), although AUC values were not reported for the remaining validity scales. Regression analysis showed that the RBS added significantly to all of the MMPI-2 validity scales (except HHI) in predicting group membership, whereas none added significantly to the RBS in predicting TOMM performance when entered in the second block. Among the MTBI group, 67% failed the TOMM, and 17% scored above the RBS cutoff of > 19 This was compared to a 25% TOMM failure rate in the moderate-to-severe TBI group and none of these patients scoring above the aforementioned RBS cutoff. The authors opined that the RBS, and to some extent the HHI, were superior to all other MMPI-2 validity scales (including the FBS) in predicting SVT performance in an outpatient VA sample with mixed diagnoses referred for assessment of potential cognitive dysfunction.

A study by Dionysus, Denney, and Halfaker (2011) compared the ability of the FBS, RBS, and HHI to predict negative response bias in a sample of head-injured litigants ($N = 79$). Thirty-seven subjects who met the Slick et al. (1999) criteria for definite or probable malingered neurocognitive dysfunction formed the probable negative response bias (PNRB) group. Forty-two litigants who are head injured who passed SVTs and did not meet Slick et al. criteria formed the presumed valid (PV) group. Data on the severity of head injury was not available for all subjects, but 17 subjects in the PNRB group (46%) and 26 subjects in the PV group (62%) would have qualified for a diagnosis of MTBI based on acute neurologic indicators postinjury. Independent t tests revealed that the PNRB group scored significantly higher on the FBS, RBS, and HHI compared to the PV group. The FBS showed the largest effect size ($d = 1.34$), followed by RBS ($d = 1.31$), and HHI ($d = 1.11$). Correlations between the predictor variables (FBS, RBS, HHI) revealed the highest correlation between the HHI and FBS ($r = 0.71$), followed by HHI and RBS ($r = 0.65$) with a 0.51 correlation between scores on the RBS and FBS. An ROC curve was constructed for each scale, with excellent-to-acceptable area AUC for each scale. The FBS had the highest AUC (0.83), followed by the RBS (AUC = 0.82), and the HHI (AUC = 0.71). Logistic regression analyses were used to compare the RBS and HHI with the FBS in predicting group membership. The predictive validity of the FBS was increased with the addition of the RBS but not the HHI. Cut scores at 0.90 specificity for the three scales were FBS $\geq$ 25, RBS $\geq$ 14, and HHI $\geq$ 12.

A study by Young, Kearns, and Roper (2011) explored the ability of the MMPI-2 validity scales, RBS, and HHI to predict WMT failure and compensation status in a sample of 194 U.S. veterans composed mostly (81%) of males. Fifty-eight were assigned to a compensation context (CC) and 89 to a noncompensation context (NC). The veterans were referred for a neuropsychological evaluation that included the MMPI-2 and WMT. Most of the veterans had multiple Axis I psychiatric diagnoses without specification of primary diagnosis, whereas only four of the total sample (2.3%) were diagnosed with TBI.

Statistical analyses revealed that the RBS and F scale were significantly correlated with WMT failure ($r = 0.20$, respectively), followed by Fp ($r = 0.19$). The HHI trended toward significance ($r = 0.15$), whereas the HHI was significantly correlated with compensation status ($r = 0.24$), followed by FBS ($r = 0.18$), and Fb ($r = 0.16$), while the RBS was not significantly correlated ($r = 0.14$). A series of hierarchical logistic regressions showed that the RBS did not add significantly to the incremental validity over F, Fp, and FBS in predicting WMT failure. Stepwise regression was carried out to investigate the incremental validity of the HHI in predicting compensation status. The HHI in isolation was a significant predictor and added significantly to the predictive validity of Fb and FBS when entered in the second step.

Operational characteristics of the RBS were analyzed to assess classification accuracy in predicting WMT failure. At the original cutoff of 17, the RBS was associated with low specificity (0.81), and an increase to 19 was required to achieve acceptable specificity (0.91). Operational characteristics of the HHI to assess classification accuracy in predicting compensation status showed that the original cutoff of 8 was associated with low specificity (0.37), and an increase to 14 was required to achieve acceptable specificity (0.85). The authors cautioned that given the lower specificity values associated with the original RBS and HHI cutoff scores in their sample of U.S. veterans, these cutoffs may be too low for some settings because they were both developed within a context of external incentives (EIs) using PI litigants and disability claimants. Given that the HHI, but not WMT failure, was associated with CC group membership, the authors concluded, ''The HHI may have utility in the prediction of broader aspects of noncredible symptom report than those associated with performance-based SVTs" (Young et al., p. 201). However, the authors did not mention that more subjects in their noncompensation group (53.4%) failed the WMT compared to a 46.5% rate of WMT failure in their compensation group (C. Young, personal communication, September 16, 2011). This difference may have served to artificially inflate RBS and HHI cutoffs to maintain adequate specificity.

A recent study by Jones and Ingram (2011) used optimal data analysis (ODA) to compare the HHI, RBS, FBS, MMPI-2 F-family validity scales (F, Fb, Fp), and the FBS-r and Fs scales from the MMPI-2-RF in assessing overreporting of cognitive and/or somatic complaints in 288 active duty military members undergoing neuropsychological evaluations that included the VSVT, TOMM, and MMPI-2. The evaluations were performed on an outpatient basis secondary to head, blast, or heat injuries or other brain disease. Forty-three percent were diagnosed with closed head injury of which 40% were considered mild. The sample was divided into two known groups based on SVT performance: adequate effort group (AEG) by subjects who passed all SVTs ($n = 171$), and inadequate effort group (IEG) composed of subjects who failed > 1 SVT ($n = 117$).

Statistical analyses using principal component analysis (PCA) identified two components with HHI, RBS, and FBS composing of one component representing noncredible reporting of cognitive/somatic problems and a second component composed of F, FB, and Fp representing overreporting of psychological problems. Independent t tests showed that subjects in the IEG scored significantly higher on all validity scales compared to AEG subjects with the HHI demonstrating the greatest effect size ($d = 1.16$), followed by RBS ($d = 1.05$), FBS-r ($d = 0.89$), and FBS ($d = 0.98$). Medium effect sizes were shown for Fs ($d = 0.78$), F ($d = 0.76$), and Fb ($d = 0.61$), whereas Fp demonstrated a small effect size ($d = 0.25$).

The investigators employed ODA for determining the percentage accuracy classification (PAC) for each subject in the IEG and AEG samples. The HHI and RBS demonstrated the highest overall PAC (71.87%, respectively), followed by FBS (69.1%), Fs (67.71%), and FBS-r (67.01%). Fp had the lowest PAC of all the scales (57.64%). An ODA model efficiency analysis for each validity scale showed that the HHI and RBS performed better than the MMPI-2-RF family scales across all base rates in predicting noncredible cognitive/somatic symptom reporting. The HHI was the best-performing scale.

Hierarchical logistic regression was employed to examine whether the two best-performing F-family scales (F and Fb) added incremental predictive validity to the HHI and RBS. Neither F nor Fb added incrementally to HHI or RBS, whereas both HHI and RBS added incrementally to F in differentiating the IEG and AEG samples. The RBS did not add to the HHI, but the HHI added to the RBS. The authors concluded that the HHI performed the best, followed by RBS and FBS in discriminating veterans who failed SVTs from veterans who passed SVTs. The superiority of the HHI over the FBS in spite of the scales sharing 11 items was attributed to differences in scale development. In particular, the HHI was developed based on known groups of litigants and disability claimants who passed or failed SVTs, whereas the FBS was not.

The HHI was recently cross-validated (Henry et al., 2011a) on a new sample of 156 subjects. Subjects were assigned to one of two groups based on the presence or absence of external financial incentives. Seventy-eight subjects with external financial incentives who failed ≥ 2 freestanding performance-based measures of cognitive symptom validity were assigned to the litigant group (LG). Seventy-eight private clinical patients not in litigation, and with no known external financial incentives, were assigned to the nonlitigant group (NG). The LG was composed of 54 PI litigants and 24 disability claimants with an average age of 44.97 ± 11.66 years. The LG contained more males (57.4%) than females (42.6%), and the average educational level of the group was 14.47 ± 2.94 years. Diagnoses within the LG were mostly MTBI (49%), followed by depression (14%), toxic exposure (9%), anxiety (5%), electrical injury (4%), chronic pain, cancer, and moderate-to-severe TBI at 3%, respectively. The remaining 10% were composed of various medical diagnoses, including stroke, sleep apnea, multiple sclerosis, cardiac arrest, learning disability, burn injury, and cysticercosis. The NG was composed of 79 private clinical patients with no known external financial incentive. The average age was 40.29 ± 14.35 years, and the average educational level of the group was 13.37 ± 2.14 years. The NG contained more males (78%) than females (22%). Diagnoses within the NG were mostly gender identity disorder (33%), followed by MTBI (19%), moderate-to-severe TBI (15%), depression (5%), chronic pain and attention deficit hyperactivity disorder (ADHD 4% each), and anoxia, seizure disorder, Asperger's disorder, and multiple sclerosis (3% each). The remaining 5% were composed of medical diagnoses, including brain tumor, human immunodefieciency virus (HIV), Hepatitis C, and dementia.

A one-way ANOVA showed that LG subjects scored significantly higher on the HHI ($M = 10.13$ [$SD = 3.40$]) compared to the NG subjects ($M = 4.09$ [$SD = 1.86$]). Logistic regression revealed that the HHI was a significant predictor of group membership ($\beta = 0.75$, $SE = 0.12$, $p < .0001$). Classification accuracy was examined with the goal of suggesting cut scores for the HHI that maximized the identification of subjects in the LG while minimizing the number of FP errors. An HHI cut score of ≥ 8 was associated with high classification accuracy (95.2%), good sensitivity (76.9%), and excellent specificity (96.2%). An HHI cut score of ≥ 10 was associated with 100% PPP at base rates from 20% to 40%.

Since the initial publication of the HHI in 2006, only four additional published studies to date have investigated the predictive validity of the scale in clinical and forensic samples. These studies with their associated cut scores and specificity values are depicted in Table 10.1. Cut scores associated with ≥ 0.90 specificity range from a low of ≥ 7 as reported in the most recent 2011 cross-validation study by Henry et al. (2011a) to a high of ≥ 14 noted in the Young et al. 2011 study. Clinicians using the HHI should choose an HHI cut score that most closely matches the context and working diagnosis of the examinee undergoing evaluation while having an aware-

TABLE 10.1 Summary of 15-Item Henry-Heilbronner Index Cut Scores and Specificity Data

First Author (Year)	HHI Cut Score	Specificity
Henry (2006)	≥ 8	0.890
	≥ 9	0.945
Whitney (2008)	≥ 12	0.790
	≥ 13	0.920
Dionysus (2011)	≥ 11	0.881
	≥ 12	0.929
Young (2011)	≥ 13	0.853
	≥ 14	0.940
Henry (2011)	≥ 6	0.785
	≥ 7	0.924

Note. HHI = Henry-Heilbronner Index.

ness of the methodological differences among studies to date that have investigated the HHI as a measure of psychological response validity.

Response Bias Scale

The original version of the RBS, composed of 73 items, was developed to detect negative response bias in forensic neuropsychological or disability settings (Gervais, 2004). The initial 73 items were subsequently reduced to 39 items (Gervais, 2005) and reduced further to the 28-item version, which was published in 2007 (Gervais et al., 2007). The subject sample consisted of 1,212 non–head-injured disability claimants and counseling clients who were administered the MMPI-2 and at least one freestanding SVT. Most subjects had chronic pain (39%), whereas 23% had anxiety-related diagnoses, 15% had orthopedic injuries, and 15% were diagnosed with depression.

A within-study cross-validation of the RBS was also conducted. The cross-validation sample consisted of 317 subjects from the laboratories of Gervais ($n = 209$) and Green ($n = 108$). Gervais' subsample was composed primarily of individuals with anxiety disorders (38%), followed by chronic pain (33%), and depression (25%). Most cases ($n = 191$) had completed the full 567-item MMPI-2, whereas the remaining 18 completed the short 370-item MMPI-2. The other validation subsample provided by Green was composed mostly of persons with mild-to-moderate and severe head injuries (18% and 16%, respectively), whereas 17% were diagnosed with depression, and the remaining 17% with "miscellaneous diagnoses." Most of Wygant's subsample ($n = 89$) completed only the abbreviated 370-item MMPI-2.

Multiple regression analysis using random split halves was used to select MMPI-2 items that predicted failure on ≥ 1 freestanding SVT. This procedure resulted in the 28-item RBS. Cross-validation, carried out via linear regression, supported the incremental validity of the RBS compared to F, Fp, and FBS in discriminating between the subjects who passed versus failed ≥ 1 SVT. An ROC analysis identified RBS cut scores that were most effective in predicting SVT failure in the validation sample. An RBS cutoff of ≥ 17 was associated with high specificity (0.95). The authors concluded, "This provides compelling external validation to support the interpretation of the RBS as an independent index of response bias defined by incomplete effort on cognitive response bias tests" (Gervais et al., p. 204).

A study published later in 2007 (Nelson, Sweet, & Heilbronner, 2007) investigated the relationships between the 39-item RBS and MMPI-2 validity and clinical scales and their ability to discriminate between groups with secondary gain (SG) and no secondary gain (NSG). The SG group ($n = 157$) was composed of litigants and disability claimants with primary diagnoses of mild head injury or toxic exposure. The NSG group ($n = 54$) was composed of "a heterogeneous set of conditions" including mild head injury, anoxia, pain, ADHD, and epilepsy.

Calculation of standardized mean difference effect sizes for all clinical and validity scales revealed the largest effect size (≥ 0.80) for scale 1 (Hs, $d = 0.91$), followed by moderate size effects (0.50–0.79) for scale 3 ($d = 0.70$), RBS ($d = 0.65$), FBS ($d = 0.60$), and the L scale ($d = 0.51$). Increasing RBS scores were associated with an increase in nonspecific symptom reporting as indicated by associated elevations on scales F, Hs, D, Hy, Pa, Pt, Sc, and Si. RBS further demonstrated significant correlations ($p < .001$) with all clinical scales except for Mf. The RBS yielded the greatest between-group difference among all of the validity scales and displayed the highest and significant correlation with the FBS ($r = 0.74$, $p < .001$).

The authors suggested that the RBS and FBS may represent a similar construct of symptom validity and may outperform other MMPI-2 validity scales in discriminating SG and NSG groups. Independent indicators of insufficient cognitive effort were not available for most subjects. The authors opined that no conclusions were possible regarding the ability of the RBS to identify individuals with "known" symptom exaggeration.

Smart et al. (2008) employed a statistical methodology called *classification tree analysis* (CTA) using ODA to generate decision "trees" to identify optimum cut scores for the 39-item RBS and MMPI-2 validity and clinical scales in classifying cognitive effort. A total of 307 adults referred for comprehensive neuropsychological evaluation comprised the initial sample. All subjects were administered the MMPI-2 and SVTs as part of their examination procedures.

The sample of 307 was divided into two groups on the basis of the presence or absence of external incentives (EIs). A secondary gain (SG) group was composed of 198 PI litigants, disability claimants, and individuals with pending workers' compensation claims. Subjects in the SG group mostly had TBI diagnoses (56%), but injury severity level was not reported. Diagnoses for the remaining subjects in the SG group (44%) were not reported. An NSG group was formed with 109 subjects who were not in litigation or being evaluated under a condition of known EIs. This group was composed of 17% patients with TBI, but no information on TBI severity was provided. The NSG group was also composed of "various conditions" (e.g., mild head injury, anoxia, pain, ADHD, and epilepsy). The authors predicted that "somatic/neurotic" scales (e.g., RBS, FBS, and Md) would better discriminate between SG and NSG groups than would the MMPI-2 validity and clinical scales.

Results of the CTA and ODA revealed that the RBS was the best variable in predicting cognitive effort and determining whether a particular subject had given insufficient effort on SVTs. When RBS scores exceeded 16.5, then the MMPI-2 Hysteria (Hy) scale entered the model, with Hy scores > 79.5T associated with insufficient cognitive effort. The FBS failed to enter the model as a significant predictor of effort regardless of whether RBS was included or not. When RBS was removed from the analyses, the Hy was the best predictor of performance on cognitive SVTs. The authors opined that low RBS scores (< 16.5) or low Hy scores (< 79.5T) suggested sufficient effort (SE) on cognitive SVTs, whereas high RBS scores (> 16.5) and high Hy scores (> 79.5T) suggested insufficient effort (IE). Consideration of somatic malingering was suggested when MMPI-2 scales Hs, Hy, and FBS were elevated.

Wygant et al. (2010) investigated the ability of the RBS to identify poor cognitive effort in criminal forensic settings. The criminal forensic group ($n = 127$) was composed of subjects undergoing evaluation for competency to stand trial or sanity (74%) and suitability for a drug diversion program (26%). A comparison group ($n = 141$) was composed of PI litigants and disability claimants. Diagnoses included emotional disability because of work-related stress (42%), MTBI (33%), orthopedic or musculoskeletal injury (16%), and neurologic non-head injury (9%). All subjects were administered a comprehensive battery including the MMPI-2 and the TOMM and/or WMT.

Significant correlations were demonstrated between the RBS and the standard MMPI-2 and MMPI-2-RF validity and most of the RC scales in both groups. The RBS was correlated the highest with Fb, F, Fp, F-r, Fp-r, and RC8 (aberrant experiences) in the criminal sample. *T* tests for the MMPI-2 and MMPI-2-RF validity scales between subjects who passed SVT and subjects who failed SVT were conducted. In the criminal forensic group, scales Fp ($d = 1.65$) and F ($d = 1.61$) showed the greatest effect size in predicting SVT failure, whereas the RBS was associated with the largest effect size ($d = 1.24$) for discriminating pass from fail SVT in the litigant/ disability group. Hierarchical logistic regression showed that RBS added incremental predictive validity to both the MMPI-2 and MMPI-2-RF validity scales in the PI and disability claimant group but not in the criminal forensic group. Classification accuracy of the RBS in identifying SVT failure in the two samples via ROC curves revealed excellent power for both the criminal forensic sample (AUC = 0.85) and PI/disability claimant sample (AUC = 0.81).

The authors concluded that the RBS alone performed approximately as well as other MMPI-2 and MMPI-2-RF validity scales in differentiating SVT performance in the PI litigants and disability claimants, but did not provide additional information to either sets of scales in the criminal forensic sample beyond what was already provided via the standard MMPI-2 or MMPI-2-RF validity scales. The authors suggested that symptom exaggeration in civil litigation is more likely to include overreporting of physical symptoms, contrasted with the overreporting of severe psychopathology or complaints of thought disorder that is more common in criminal settings.

Since the initial publication of the RBS in 2007, there have been only four additional published studies investigating the predictive validity of the scale in clinical and forensic samples. These studies with their associated cut scores and specificity values are depicted in Table 10.2. Cut scores associated with ≥ 0.90 specificity range from a low of ≥ 14 as reported in the Dionysus et al. study (2011) to a high of ≥ 19 noted in the Young et al. (2011) study. Clinicians using the RBS should choose an RBS cut score that most closely matches the context and working diagnosis of the examinee undergoing evaluation while having an awareness of the methodological differences among studies to date that have investigated the RBS as a measure of psychological response validity.

Malingered Mood Disorder Scale

The 15-item MMDS was empirically derived from the MMPI-2 using a known-group design (Henry, Heilbronner, Mittenberg, Enders, & Roberts, 2008). Initial results indicated that a cutoff score of ≥ 7 was associated with 54.8% sensitivity and 93.4% specificity in identifying symptom exaggeration in PI and disability litigants versus nonlitigating patients who are head-injured. A cutoff of ≥ 8 was associated with 100% PPP.

TABLE 10.2 Summary of 28-Item Response Bias Scale Cut Scores and Specificity Data

First Author (Year)	RBS Cut Score	Specificity
Gervais (2007)	≥ 16	0.890
	≥ 17	0.950
Whitney (2008)	≥ 16	0.880
	≥ 17	0.920
Wygant (2010)	≥ 17[a]	0.890
	≥ 19[a]	0.950
	≥ 13[b]	0.840
	> 14[b]	0.910
Dionysus (2011)	≥ 13	0.881
	≥ 14	0.928
Young (2011)	≥ 18	0.850
	≥ 19	0.910

Note. [a]Criminal sample. [b]Disability sample. HHI = Henry-Heilbronner Index.

The only study of the MMDS since then was a 2009 known-group design study (Henry, Heilbronner, Mittenberg, Enders, & Domboski, 2009), which compared the ability of the MMDS, MMPI-2 Restructured Clinical Demoralization Scale (RCd), and MMPI-2 Depression Scale to identify noncredible symptom response sets in 84 PI litigants and disability claimants compared to 77 nonlitigating head-injured controls. All three scales showed large effect sizes (> 0.80). Scale 2 was associated with the largest effect size (d = 2.19), followed by the MMDS (d = 1.65), and the RCd (d = 0.85).

The MMDS was cross-validated in 2011 (Henry et al., 2011b) on a separate sample of 157 subjects who were assigned to one of two groups based on the presence or absence of external financial incentives. Seventy-eight subjects with external financial incentives and who failed at least ≥ 2 freestanding measures of cognitive symptom validity were assigned to the LG. Seventy-eight private clinical patients not in litigation and with no known external financial incentives were assigned to the NG.

The LG was composed of 54 PI litigants and 24 disability claimants with an average age of 44.97 ± 11.66 years. The LG contained more males (57.4%) than females (42.6%), and the average educational level of the group was 14.47 ± 2.94 years. Diagnoses within the LG were mostly MTBI (49%), followed by depression (14%), toxic exposure (9%), anxiety (5%), electrical injury (4%), chronic pain, cancer, and moderate-to-severe TBI (3% each). The remaining 10% were composed of various medical diagnoses including stroke, sleep apnea, multiple sclerosis, cardiac arrest, learning disability, burn injury, and cysticercosis. The NG was composed of 79 private clinical patients with no known EI. The average age was 40.29 ± 14.35 years, and the average educational level of the group was 13.37 ± 2.14 years. The NG contained more males (78%) than females (22%). Diagnoses within the NG were mostly gender identity disorder (33%), followed by MTBI (19%), moderate-to-severe TBI (15%), depression (5%), chronic pain and ADHD (4% each), and anoxia, seizure disorder, Asperger's disorder, and multiple sclerosis (3 % each). The remaining 5% was composed of medical diagnoses, including brain tumor, HIV, Hepatitis C, and dementia.

A one-way ANOVA, showed that subjects in the LG scored significantly higher on the MMDS (M = 8.27 ± 3.18) compared to the NG (M = 4.00 ± 2.18). Logistic regression was used to assess the extent to which the current MMDS predicted group membership and the extent to which the model fit was consistent with that of Henry et al. (2008). The MMDS score was entered into the regression as a predictor of the dichotomous dependent variable group (LG = litigant, NL = nonlitigant). The MMDS score predicted a significant proportion of the variance in group membership (β = 0.75, SE = 0.12, p < .0001). An MMDS cut score of ≥ 8 was associated with good classification accuracy (86.5%), adequate sensitivity (57.7%), and high specificity (92.1%). An MMDS cutoff of ≥ 12 was associated with 100% PPP.

Psychosocial Distress Scale

According to Lamberty (2007), more work is needed to understand the relationship between psychosocial distress and noncredible cognitive performance in clinical disorders seen by clinical neuropsychologists, especially in forensic contexts. Henry, Heilbronner, Mittenberg et al., (2011) empirically derived a 20-item scale from the MMPI-2, which they identified as the PDS. The investigators hypothesized that in addition to symptom exaggeration in the domains of physical, cognitive, and/or emotional complaints, PI litigants and disability claimants involved in a situation of EIs may also overreport complaints relative to psychosocial functioning. Psychosocial distress was broadly defined to include interpersonal, social, and familial factors that influence an individual's response to stress and shape health attitudes.

Review of archival data identified 90 adults (47 PI litigants and 43 disability claimants) who underwent a comprehensive neuropsychological examination, including the MMPI-2, under a condition of known external incentives (EI) and failed $\geq$ 2 freestanding and/or embedded performance-based cognitive effort measures. The EI group was heterogeneous with respect to diagnostic categories. Most of the litigants in the EI group were subjects with a history of mild head injury (60%), whereas the remaining EI litigants presented with diagnoses of toxic exposure (15%), electrical injury (6%), PTSD (6%), moderate head injury (4%), brain tumor (4%), anoxia (3%), and depression (2%). The disability claimants in the incentive group were composed of various psychiatric and medical conditions, including depression (33%), mild head injury (20%), stroke (12%), chronic pain (7%), cardiovascular problems (7%), brain tumor (7%), cancer (5%), seizure disorder (5%), sleep apnea (2%), and brain infection (2%). The average age and education for the EI group was 45.53 years (SD = 10.68) and 14.92 years (SD = 3.06), respectively. The EI group was composed of 44% males and 56% females. A nonincentive (NI) control group composed of 77 private clinical patients, with 85% classified as having sustained MTBIs who were not seeking compensation and were not involved in litigation related to their injuries. The average age and education for the NI group was 38.05 years (SD = 16.48) and 12.64 years (SD = 2.60), respectively, whereas 75% of the NI group was male and 25% female.

Statistical analysis identified 20 items that best predicted group status. A one-way ANOVA showed that the EI group scored significantly higher on the PDS (M = 14.20, SD = 4.34) compared to the NI group (M = 5.70, SD = 2.73) with a large effect size (d = 2.41). Logistic regression was used to identify PDS score thresholds that maximized the identification of individuals in the EI group while minimizing the number of FP classifications. A PDS cut score of $\geq$ 10 or correctly classified 85.7% of the total sample. A PDS score of $\geq$ 12 was associated with 100% specificity and 100% PPP (i.e., no FP errors). Stated in a different manner, a PDS score of $\geq$ 12 correctly classified all subjects in the EI group at base rates of 20%, 30%, and 40%.

To further examine the accuracy of the PDS cutoffs, a cross-validation sample (n = 83, n_{EI} = 46, n_{NI} = 37) was employed to generate a new set of classification statistics. For each individual in the cross-validation sample, group membership was predicted by classifying a case as EI if the PDS value met or exceeded a particular score threshold (e.g., for a cut score of 10, PDS $\geq$ 10 = EI, PDS < 10 = NI). Repeating this process for every discrete PDS value produced cross-validation estimates of classification accuracy. A PDS cut score of $\geq$ 10 was also associated with nearly identical classification accuracy for the total sample (86.5%), with high specificity (91.89%), and adequate sensitivity (82.61%).

Although increasing scores on other validated MMPI-2 symptom validity measures (i.e., Symptom Validity Scale, formerly called the FBS) raises suspicion regarding the validity of an individual's self-report, some (Ben-Porath, Greve, Bianchini, & Kaufman, 2009) have opined that under such clinical circumstances, one should also consider that some psychosocial process, and not neurological injury alone, may be operating to influence symptom reporting. Henry et al. (2011) suggested that when elevated psychosocial symptom reporting occurs in the context of a noncredible cognitive presentation, the examiner should also consider that the examinee has engaged in some degree of negative response bias pertaining to his or her current level of psychosocial functioning, resulting in a co-occurring noncredible psychosocial presentation. Items comprising the 20-item PDS were not reported for test security purposes, but qualified clinicians may obtain the items by contacting the first author.

Conclusions From Studies Comparing the New MMPI-2 Validity Scales

The current review of recent MMPI-2 embedded validity measures has shown that, to date, there have been only nine published studies directly comparing the HHI, RBS, and/or FBS as measures of psychological response validity in forensic contexts with some portion of subjects having MTBI histories. Two studies compared the HHI and FBS (Henry et al., 2006; Henry, Heilbronner, Mittenberg, Enders, & Stanczak, 2008), three studies compared the FBS and RBS (Nelson et al., 2007; Smart et al., 2008; Wygant et al., 2010), and four studies compared the RBS, HHI, and FBS (Dionysus et al., 2011; Jones & Ingram, 2011; Whitney et al., 2008; Young et al., 2011). The Nelson et al. (2007) and Smart et al. (2008) studies used the 39-item RBS and not the current 28-item version. Thus, clinicians should note this methodological difference when considering the predictive validity data.

In the only two studies directly comparing the HHI and FBS to predict symptom exaggeration, the HHI outperformed the FBS. Likewise, the RBS was a better predictor of response bias than the FBS in the three studies directly comparing the two scales. However, in the four studies comparing the ability of all three scales to identify response bias, the RBS was superior to the HHI and FBS in one study (Whitney et al., 2008), whereas the FBS was superior in another study (Dionysus et al., 2011). In the two most recent studies (Jones & Ingram, 2011; Young et al., 2011), the HHI was found to be superior to the RBS and FBS in predicting compensation status and performance on cognitive SVTs.

Methodological differences may explain some of the disparate findings among the few published studies on the HHI to date. The studies by Dionysus et al. (2011) and Young et al. (2011) both used performance on one SVT to classify subjects as credible or noncredible. This practice of forming groups for clinical research is problematic because the sensitivity of any single SVT is rather low, and to base group assignment on one SVT performance increases the probability of underestimating the prevalence of noncredible performance (e.g., FP), which could result in incorrect assignment to the credible group. Thus, specificity would be attenuated to the extent a credible group is contaminated by unknown noncredible subjects. At least for the Young et al.'s VA sample study, this suspicion was confirmed because more subjects in the noncompensation group failed the WMT compared to subjects in the compensation group. Research indicates that a criterion of failure on ≥ 2 SVTs best discriminates credible from noncredible performance profiles with increasing confidence as the number of SVT failures accumulates (Larrabee, 2008b; Victor, Boone, Serpa, Buehler, & Ziegler, 2009). However, two effort test failures are still reported to be associated with a 6% FP error rate (Victor et al., 2009).

In general, the four published studies involving the HHI, FBS, and RBS tend to report a fairly large effect size for all three scales ($d = 0.89$–1.34) in identifying patterns of negative response bias in PI litigants and disability claimants. Although all three embedded measures show moderate-to-strong correlations between scales ($r = 0.51$–0.80), incremental validity data are variable. Given the paucity of published research comparing the HHI, FBS, and RBS as embedded measures of psychological response validity, there is currently no consistent empirical evidence supporting the superiority of one scale over the other. Performance on the three scales appears to fluctuate as a result of methodological differences, but in general, all three scales appear to be offering unique information relevant to psychological response validity independent of scores on performance-based cognitive SVTs. A recent exploratory factor analysis (Hoelzle, Nelson, & Arbisi, 2011) indicated that the HHI and RBS have different factor structures than the FBS. A three-factor structure representing somatic symptoms, cynicism, and cognitive inefficiency/emotional distress was found to be underlying the FBS, whereas the RBS and HHI exhibited good congruency with a factor structure reflecting cognitive inefficiency/emotional distress.

It is recommended that examiners who administer the MMPI-2 (or MMPI-II RF) as part of their forensic evaluation should investigate examinees' scores on the FBS, RBS, and HHI to better clarify issues relative to psychological response validity. Given that the MMDS and PDS also appear to provide unique information relative to overreporting of emotional and psychosocial complaints, respectively, these newly developed measures of psychological response validity should also be considered when investigating the possibility of symptom exaggeration because dissociations may occur both between and within performance-based cognitive SVTs and self-report measures of psychological response validity.

Boone (2007) recommended that the Slick et al.'s (1999) criteria for a determination of "malingered neurocognitive dysfunction" be changed to a determination of "noncredible performance." Specifically, failure on at least two validated and minimally correlated performance-based cognitive effort measures would qualify for consideration of a determination of probable noncredible performance, whereas failure on three or more individual cognitive effort measures sharing minimal variance with specificity set at $\geq 90\%$ would qualify for definite noncredible cognitive performance. However, Boone does not address psychological response validity as depicted in empirically derived MMPI-2 embedded measures for consideration of negative response bias in the psychological domain. We propose that determinations of "probable negative response bias" or symptom exaggeration be made when examinees score above cut scores set at $\geq 90\%$ specificity on two MMPI-2 embedded measures (HHI, RBS, FBS, MMDS, PDS) and "definite negative response bias" be used when examinees score above cut scores set at $\geq 90\%$ specificity on three or more MMPI-2 embedded measures.

CONCLUSIONS

Various measures of emotional state and personality traits are available for use in the neuropsychological evaluation of persons who have sustained MTBIs. Some of these measures have undergone very little symptom validity research with subjects who have MTBI histories and thus have very little, if anything, to contribute to the understanding of symptom validity issues for a given examinee. By far, the most extensively studied measure is the MMPI and its subsequent revisions. Because of its extensive research base, which has included the development of some new symptom validity scales including those with MTBI subjects, the MMPI is the preferred measure with this patient group when a comprehensive understanding of emotional state and personality traits is needed. Clinicians who perform neuropsychological evaluations that are used in forensic contexts (e.g., PI, workers' compensation, disability evaluations, etc.) are well advised to employ personality assessment instruments that have a strong research base and are also clinically relevant for the purpose at hand (e.g., to help the trier of fact understand the facts in evidence). This is particularly important in litigating MTBI cases where symptom complaints may be strongly influenced by psychosocial factors and personality variables and where threats to symptom validity occur with a higher degree of frequency than in a clinical setting.

REFERENCES

Aguerrevere, L. E., Greve, K. W., Bianchini, K. J., & Ord, J. S. (2011). Classification accuracy of the Millon Clinical Multiaxial Inventory-III modifier indices in the detection of malingering in traumatic brain injury. *Journal of Clinical and Experimental Neuropsychology*, 33(5), 497–504.

Ben-Porath, Y. S., Greve, K. W., Bianchini, K. J., & Kaufmann, P. M. (2009). The MMPI-2 Symptom Validity Scale (FBS) is an empirically validated measure of overreporting in personal injury litigant and claimants: Reply to Butcher et al. (2008). *Psychological Injury and Law*, 2(1), 62–85.

Berry, D. T. R., & Schipper, L. J. (2007). Detection of feigned psychiatric symptoms during forensic neuropsychological examinations. In G. J. Larrabee (Ed.), *Assessment of malingered neuropsychological deficits* (pp. 226–263). New York, NY: Oxford University Press.

Berry, D. T. R., Baer, R. A., & Harris, M. J. (1991). Detection of malingering on the MMPI: A meta-analysis. *Clinical Psychology Review*, 11, 585–598.

Boone, K. B. (Ed.). (2007). A reconsideration of the Slick et al. (1999) criteria for malingered neurocognitive dysfunction. In Assessment of feigned cognitive impairment: A neuropsychological perspective (pp. 29–49). New York, NY: Guilford Press.

Breshears, R. E., Brenner, L. A., Harwood, J. E., & Gutierrez, P. M. (2010). Predicting suicidal behavior in veterans with traumatic brain injury: The utility of the personality assessment inventory. *Journal of Personality Assessment*, 92(4), 349–355.

Bury, A. S., & Bagby, R. M. (2002). The detection of feigned uncoached and coached posttraumatic stress disorder with the MMPI-2 in a sample of workplace accident victims. *Psychological Assessment*, 14, 472–484.

Butcher, J. N., Arbisi, P. A., Atlis, M. M., & McNulty J. L. (2003). The construct validity of the Lees-Haley Fake Bad Scale: Does this measure somatic malingering and feigned emotional distress? *Archives of Clinical Neuropsychology*, 18, 473–485.

Butler, M., Retzlaff, P., & Vanderploeg, R. (1991). Neuropsychological test usage. *Professional Psychology: Research and Practice*, 22(6), 510–512.

Cattell, R. B., Cattell, A. K., & Cattell, H. E. P. (1993). *16PF fifth edition questionnaire*. Champaign, IL: Institute for Personality and Ability Testing.

Demakis, G. J., Hammond, F., Knotts, A., Cooper, D. B., Clement, P., Kennedy, J., & Sawyer, T. (2007). The personality assessment inventory in individuals with traumatic brain injury. *Archives of Clinical Neuropsychology*, 22(1), 123–130.

Derogatis, L. R. (1994). *SCL-90-R: Administration, scoring, and procedures manual* (3rd ed.). Minneapolis, MN: National Computer Systems.

Diamond, R., Barth, J. T., & Zillmer, E. A. (1988). An investigation of the psychological component of mild head injury: The role of the MMPI. *International Journal of Clinical Neuropsychology*, 10, 35–40.

Dionysus, K. E., Denney, R. L., & Halfaker, D. A. (2011). Detecting negative response bias with the Fake Bad Scale, Response Bias Scale, and Henry-Heilbronner Index of the Minnesota Multiphasic Personality Inventory-2. *Archives of Clinical Neuropsychology*, 26(2), 81–88.

Elhai, J. D., Ruggiero, K. J., Freuch, B. C., Beckham, J. C., Gold, P. B., & Feldman, M. E. (2002). The Infrequency-Posttraumatic Stress Disorder Scale (Fptsd) for the MMPI-2: Development and initial validation with veterans presenting with combat-related PTSD. *Journal of Personality Assessment*, 79(3), 531–549.

Gervais, R. O., Ben-Porath, Y. S., Wygant, D. B., & Green, P. (2007). Development and validation of a response bias scale (RBS) for the MMPI-2. *Assessment*, 14(2), 196–208.

Gervais, R. O. (2004, November). *A response bias scale for the MMPI-2: Development and preliminary findings*. Paper presented at the annual meeting of the National Academy of Neuropsychology, Seattle, WA.

Gervais, R. O. (2005, April). *Development of an empirically-derived Response Bias Scale for the MMPI-2*. Paper presented at the annual MMPI-2 Symposium and Workshops, Fort Lauderdale, FL.

Goldberg, H. E., Back-Madruga, C., & Boone, K. B. (2007). The impact of psychiatric disorders on cognitive symptom validity test scores. In K. B. Boone (Ed.), *Assessment of feigned cognitive impairment: A neuropsychological perspective* (pp. 281–309). New York, NY:Guilford Press.

Greiffenstein, M.F., Fox, D., & Lees-Haley, P.R. (2007). The MMPI-2 Fake Bad Scale in detection of noncredible brain injury claims. In K. B. Boone (Ed.), *Assessment of feigned cognitive impairment: A neuropsychological perspective* (pp. 210–238). New York, NY: Guilford Press.

Green, P. (2007). Spoiled for choice: Making comparisons between forced-choice effort tests. In K. B. Boone (Ed.), *Assessment of feigned cognitive impairment* (pp. 50–77). New York, NY: Guilford Press.

Henry, G. K., Heilbronner, R. L., King, J., Blackwood, D., Thoma, R., & Lundy, L. (2011a, June). *Cross validation of the MMPI-2 Henry-Heilbronner Index* (HHI). Paper presented at the 9th annual American Academy of Clinical Neuropsychology Conference, Washington, DC.

Henry, G. K., Heilbronner, R. L., King, J., Blackwood, D., Thoma, R., & Lundy, L. (2011b, June). *Cross validation of the MMPI-2 Malingered Mood Disorder Scale* (MMDS). Paper presented at the 9th annual American Academy of Clinical Neuropsychology Conference, Washington, DC.

Henry, G. K., Heilbronner, R. L., Mittenberg, W., & Enders, C. (2006). The Henry-Heilbronner Index: A 15-item empirically derived MMPI-2 subscale for identifying probable malingering in personal injury litigants and disability claimants. *The Clinical Neuropsychologist*, 20(4), 786–797.

Henry, G. K., Heilbronner, R. L., Mittenberg, W., Enders, C., & Domboski, K. (2009). Comparison of the MMPI-2 restructured demoralization scale, depression scale, and malingered mood disorder scale in identifying non-credible symptom reporting in personal injury litigants and disability claimants. *The Clinical Neuropsychologist*, 23(1), 153–166.

Henry, G. K., Heilbronner, R. L., Mittenberg, W., Enders, C., & Roberts, D. (2008). Empirical derivation of a new MMPI-2 scale for identifying probable malingering in personal injury litigants and disability claimants: The 15-item malingered mood disorder scale (MMDS). *The Clinical Neuropsychologist*, 22(1), 158–168.

Henry, G. K., Heilbronner, R. L., Mittenberg, W., Enders, C., & Stanczak, S. R. (2008). Comparison of the Lees-Haley Fake Bad Scale, Henry-Heilbronner Index, and Restructured Clinical Scale 1 identifying noncredible symptom reporting. *The Clinical Neuropsychologist*, 22(5), 919–929.

Henry, G. K., Heilbronner, R. L., Mittenberg, W., Enders, C., Stevens, A., & Dux, M. (2011). Noncredible performance in individuals with external incentives: Empirical derivationand cross-validation of the Psychosocial Distress Scale (PDS). *Applied Neuropsychology*, 18(1), 47–53.

Hoelzle, J. B., Nelson, N. W., & Arbisi, P. A. (2011, June). Exploratory factor analysis of cognitive and somatic MMPI-2-RF validity scales. Paper presented at the 9th annual American Academy of Clinical Neuropsychology Conference, Washington, DC.Jones, A., & Ingram, M. V. (2011). A comparison of selected MMPI-2 and MMPI-2-RF validity scales in assessing effort on cognitive tests in a military sample. *The Clinical Neuropsychologist*, 25 (7), 1207–1227.Kelly & Smith. (1981).

Lamberty, G. (2007). *Understanding somatization in the practice of clinical neuropsychology*. New York, NY: Oxford University Press.

Larrabee, G. J., (1998). Somatic malingering on the MMPI and MMPI-2 in personal injury lititgants. *The Clinical Neuropsychologist*, 12, 179–188

Larrabee, G. J., (2003). Detection of malingering using atypical performance patterns on standard neuropsychological tests. *The Clinical Neuropsychologist*, 17, 410–425

Larrabee, G. J., (2005). Forensic neuropsychology: A scientific approach. *Oxford University Press: New York*.

Larrabee, G. J., (2007). Assessment of malingered neuropsychological deficits. *Oxford University Press: New York*.

Larrabee, G. (2008a). *Evaluation of new MMPI-2 validity scales in malingering civil litigants and non-malingering clinical patients*. Paper presented at the 36th annual International Neuropsychology Conference, Waikoloa, HI.

Larrabee, G. (2008b). Aggregation across multiple indicators improves the detection of malingering: Relationship to likelihood ratios. *The Clinical Neuropsychologist*, 22(4), 666–679.

Lees-Haley, P. R. (1992). Efficacy of MMPI-2 validity scales and MCMI–II modifier scales for detecting spurious PTSD claims: F, F-K, fake bad scale, ego strength, subtle-obvious subscales, DIS, and DEB. *Journal of Clinical Psychology*, 48(5), 681–689.

Lees-Haley, P. R., English, L. T., and Glenn, W. J. (1991). A fake bad scale for the MMPI-2 for personal injury claimants. *Psychological Reports*, 68(1), 203–210.

Lees-Haley, P. R., Smith, H. H., Williams, C. W., & Dunn, J. T. (1996). Forensic neuropsychological test usage: An empirical survey. *Archives of Clinical Neuropsychology*, 11, 45–51.

Leininger, B. E., Kreutzer, J. S., & Hill, M. R. (1991). Comparison of minor and severe head injury emotional sequelae using the MMPI. *Brain Injury*, 5, 199–205.

Lidvall, H. F., Linderoth, B., & Norlin, B. (1974). Causes of the post-concussional syndrome. *Acta Neurologica Scandanavica*, 50, 7–144.

Lishman, W. A. (1988). Physiogenesis and psychogenesis in the 'post-concussion syndrome'. *British Journal of Psychiatry*, 153, 460–469.

McCann, J. T., & Dyer, F. J. (1996). *Forensic assessment with the Millon inventories*. New York, NY: Guilford Press.

McQuire, B. E., & Shores, E. A. (2001). Simulated pain on the Symptom Checklist 90-Revised. *Journal of Clinical Psychology*, 57, 1589–1596.

Middleboe, T., Birket-Smith, M., Anderson, H. S., & Fris, M. L. (1992). Personality traits in patients with postconcussional sequelae. *Journal of Personality Disorders*, 6, 246–255.

Millon, T., Davis, R. D., & Millon, C. (1997). *Manual for the Millon Clinical Multiaxial Inventory—III* (MCMI-III) (2nd ed.). Minneapolis, MN: National Computer Systems.

Millon, T., Green, C. J., & Meagher, R. B. (1982). *Millon Behavioral Health Inventory manual*. Minneapolis, MN: National Computer Systems.

Morey, L. C. (1991). *Personality Assessment Inventory professional manual*. Odessa, FL: Psychological Assessment Resources.

Nelson, N. W., Sweet, J. J., & Heilbronner, R. L. (2007). Examination of the new MMPI-2 response bias scale (Gervais): Relationship with MMPI-2 validity scales. *Journal of Clinical and Experimental Neuropsychology*, 29(1), 67–72.

Rabin, L. A., Barr, W. A., & Burton, L. A. (2005). Assessment practices of clinical neuropsychologists in the United States and Canada: A survey of INS, NAN, and APA Division 40 members. *Archives of Clinical Neuropsychology*, 20(1), 33–65.

Rogers, R., Salekin, R. T., & Sewell, K. W. (1999). Validation of the Millon Clinical Multiaxial Inventory for Axis II disorders: Does it meet the Daubert standard? *Law and Human Behavior*, 23(4), 425–443.

Rogers, R., Sewell, K. W., & Ustad, K. L. (1995). Feigning among chronic outpatients on the MMPI-2: A systematic examination of fake-bad indicators. *Assessment*, 2, 81–89.

Ruocco, A. C., Swirsky-Sacchetti, T., Chute, D. L., Mandel, S., Platek, S. M., & Zillmer, E. A. (2008). Distinguishing between neuropsychological malingering and exaggerated psychiatric symptoms in a neuropsychological setting. *The Clinical Neuropsychologist*, 22(3), 547–564.

Russell, M. T., & Karol, D. (2002). *The 16PF 5th Edition: Administrator's manual*. Champaign, IL: Institute for Personality and Ability Testing.

Schoenberg, M. R., Dorr, D., & Morgan, C. D. (2003). The ability of the Million Clinical Multiaxial Inventory, third edition, to detect malingering. *Psychological Assessment*, 15, 198–204.

Shaw, D. J., & Matthews, C. G. (1965). Differential MMPI performance of brain-damaged vs. pseudo-neurologic groups. *Journal of Clinical Psychology*, 21(4), 405–408.

Slick, D. J., Sherman, E. M., & Iverson, G. L. (1999). Diagnostic criteria for malingered neurocognitive dysfunction: Proposed standards for clinical practice and research. *The Clinical Neuropsychologist*, 13(4), 545–561.

Smart, C. M., Nelson, N. W., Sweet, J. J., Bryant, F. B., Berry, D. T., Granacher, R. P., & Heilbronner, R. L. (2008). Use of MMPI-2 to predict cognitive effort: A hierarchically optimal classification tree analysis. *Journal of the International Neuropsychological Society*, 14(5), 842–852.

Till, C., Christensen, B. K., & Green, R. E. (2009). Use of the personality assessment inventory (PAI) in individuals with traumatic brain injury. *Brain Injury*, 23(7), 655–665.

Victor, T. L., Boone, K. B., Serpa, J. G., Buehler, J., & Ziegler, E. A. (2009). Interpreting the meaning of multiple symptom validity test failure. *The Clinical Neuropsychologist*, 23(3), 297–313.

Wallis, B. J. & Bogduk, N. (1996). Faking a profile: Can naive subjects simulate whiplash responses? *Pain*, 66, 223–227.

Whiteside, D., Clinton, C., Diamonti, C., Stroemel, J., White, C., Zimberoff, A., Waters, D. (2010). Relationship between suboptimal cognitive effort and the clinical scales of the personality assessment inventory. *The Clinical Neuropsychologist*, 24(2), 315–325.

Whiteside, D. M., Dunbar-Mayer, P., & Waters, D. P. (2009). Relationship between TOMM performance and PAI validity scales in a mixed clinical sample. *The Clinical Neuropsychologist*, 23(3), 523–533.

Whiteside, D. M., Galbreath, J., Brown, M., & Turnbull, J. (2012). Differential response patterns on the Personality Assessment Inventory (PAI) in compensation-seeking and non–compensation-seeking mild traumatic brain injury patients. *Journal of Clinical and Experimental Neuropsychology*, 32(2), 172–182.

Whitney, K. A., Davis, J. J., Shepard, P. H., & Herman, S. M. (2008). Utility of the response bias scale and other MMPI-2 validity scales in predicting TOMM performance. *Archives of Clinical Neuropsychology*, 23(7–8), 777–786.

Wygant, D. B., Sellbom, M., Gervais, R. O., Ben-Porath, Y. S., Stafford, K. P., Freeman, D. B., & Heilbronner, R. L. (2010). Further validation of the MMPI-2 and MMPI-2-RF response bias scale: Findings from disability and criminal forensic settings. *Psychological Assessment*, 22(4), 745–756.

Young, J. C., Kearns, L. A., & Roper, B. L. (2011). Validation of the MMPI-2 response bias scale and Henry-Heilbronner index in a U.S. veteran population. *Archives of Clinical Neuropsychology*, 26(3), 194–204.

Strategies for Non-Neuropsychology Clinicians to Detect Noncredible Presentations After Mild Traumatic Brain Injury

11

Dominic A. Carone

The study of malingering has, we fear, been somewhat neglected by the scientific physician, who, more bent on establishing the features of true disease, has instinctively recoiled from the subject of feigned disorders. While such repugnance to dwelling on the seamy side of human nature may do credit to his fastidiousness, it is nevertheless alien to the scientific spirit whose ultima thule is the "vantage ground of truth."—A. Bassett Jones (1917)

Symptom validity assessment is considered an important component of neuropsychological evaluations as indicated by consensus statements from the National Academy of Neuropsychology (NAN; Bush et al., 2005) and the American Academy of Clinical Neuropsychology (AACN, 2007; Heilbronner, Sweet, Morgan, Larrabee, & Millis, 2009). This issue is of particular importance with patients reporting persisting symptoms after known or suspected mild traumatic brain injury (MTBI; also known as concussion) because this is the patient group that has been found to have the highest base rate of symptom exaggeration and/or malingering in clinical neuropsychological evaluations (Mittenberg, Patton, Canyock, & Condit, 2002). As such, clinical neuropsychologists have developed some of the most widely used, well-researched, and psychometrically sound symptom validity tests (SVTs; Lezak, Howieson, & Loring, 2004). For a detailed review of the history of SVTs, see Bianchini, Mathias, and Greve (2001).

Despite the significant increase in symptom validity research in clinical neuropsychology over the past few decades (see Chapter 1), many other health care providers (e.g., physicians, nurse practitioners, therapists, clinical and counseling psychologists) are either unaware of tests or methods to assess symptom validity or do not use them if they have such awareness. The discrepancy between the tendency for neuropsychologists and non-neuropsychologists to assess and comment on symptom validity in clinical settings is problematic because when patients present with persisting symptoms after MTBI, the first health care provider they see is rarely a neuropsychologist. It is typical that if patients with MTBI seek medical care, they will initially present to an emergency room (ER) and follow-up as an outpatient with a primary care physician (PCP) at which point the PCP, nurse practitioner, or physician assistant conducts an evaluation. In some cases, the patient does not present to an ER and goes directly to the PCP's office.

Initial ER and outpatient MTBI evaluations by non-neuropsychologists rely heavily on subjective complaints and often include general symptom checklists to determine a diagnosis and course of treatment. The physical examinations are typically brief (5–10 minutes), general, and limited in scope. Outpatient concussion evaluations may rely heavily on the results of brief computerized cognitive assessments, the most popular of which in nonmilitary contexts is ImPACT (Lovell, Maroon, & Collins, 1990); although similar tests exist such as CogSport (Collie et al., 2003), Automated Neuropsychological Assessment Metrics (ANAM; Reeves, Kane, Winter, Raynsford, & Pancella, 1993), and HeadMinder (Erlanger, Feldman, & Kutner, 2002). Such tests have become widespread and commonplace in concussion assessment despite significant psychometric limitations and clinical risks for incorrect decision making (Randolph, 2011; Randolph & Kirkwood, 2009; Randolph, McCrea, & Barr, 2005).

Depending on the patients' reported symptoms, they may be referred to other medical specialties such as neurology, psychiatry, chiropractic medicine, optometry, or ophthalmology. Expensive chronic treatments may also be initiated such as (a) physical therapy, occupational therapy, speech therapy, massage therapy, and/or acupuncture treatments; (b) medications (e.g., neurostimulants, pain medications); (c) amber-tinted sunglasses to reduce reported photosensitivity; or (d) a transcutaneous electric nerve stimulation (TENS) unit to decrease pain. These treatments are often accompanied by recommendations to rest for extended periods (e.g., weeks to months), restricting most forms of stimulating activities (including sports), written support of total disability, and/or written support for numerous academic accommodations. Although some of these treatments and recommendations may be appropriate in the acute to subacute postinjury phase, efforts are not always made to objectively measure their effectiveness. This neglect of objective indictors of progress can lead to prolonged (i.e., years) use of unnecessary and ineffective "treatment(s)" for patients reporting chronic symptoms after MTBI. Such treatments can unintentionally worsen the patient's symptoms (iatrogenesis) by fostering misattribution bias (Ferguson, Mittenberg, Barone, & Schneider, 1999; Mittenberg, DiGiulio, Perrin, & Bass, 1992) and overdependence, as well as worsening or causing cognitive symptoms with medications such as topiramate to treat headaches (Loring, Williamson, Meador, Wiegand, & Hulihan, 2011; Salinsky et al., 2005; Thompson, Baxendale, Duncan, & Sander, 2000).

Despite the extensive focus on medical issues, there is sometimes minimal-to-no evaluation of confounding psychiatric, psychosocial, and motivational factors that may be contributing to distorted symptom reporting and exaggerated clinical presentation (Department of Veteran Affairs, 2009; Iverson, Lange, Brooks, & Rennison, 2010; Lange, Iverson, & Rose, 2010). As a result, such patients are not always involved in traditional weekly to biweekly psychotherapy to address these factors. Although some patients may be receiving supportive counseling, such treatment is not always performed by a doctoral level psychologist who is knowledgeable about the MTBI scientific literature. This treatment by well meaning but uninformed or misinformed clinicians can lead to a situation in which the patient's misattributions are validated by the provider, resulting in a stronger belief that his or her course of recovery will be long and unpredictable and that chronic symptoms are permanent and a result of brain damage. This same type of message may also be conveyed by other health care providers and may be described as "brain injury education." This so-called education is paradoxical because the actual brain injury education that has been empirically studied to reduce chronic symptoms after MTBI involves de-emphasizing the term "brain injury," normalizing symptoms in the acute to subacute stage after injury, focusing on the nonpermanency of symptoms, and suggesting ways to better cope with the symptoms (Department of Veteran Affairs, 2009; Miller & Mittenberg, 1998; Mittenberg, Canyock, Condit, & Patton, 2001; Mittenberg, Tremont, Zielinski, Fichera, & Rayls, 1996; Ponsford et al., 2002). A major cause of this problem is that some health care providers misapply knowledge about patients with moderate-to-severe TBI to MTBI when these are actually vastly different entities (McCrea, 2008), or they rely on media accounts of the effects of concussion, which can be inaccurate.

When the patient with MTBI fails to improve and the health care provider coordinating care has exhausted expensive diagnostic evaluations (e.g., structural and functional neuroimaging, electroencephalography, brainstem-evoked potentials), a referral for a neuropsychological evaluation may be made to gain a better objective understanding of the patient's presentation. Unfortunately, it can sometimes be more than a year after the initial injury before such a referral is made. For example, over the last 5 years, the average length of time that has elapsed between the initial injury and neuropsychological evaluation in my practice is 18 months. By this time, at least tens of thousands of dollars have probably been spent on medical appointments and various diagnostic tests and treatments, often with no apparent benefit to the patient and self-reported worsening of symptoms.

The neuropsychological evaluation is often the first time since the injury that SVTs have been administered and that psychiatric and psychosocial factors contributing to chronic symptom maintenance have been thoroughly evaluated and commented on. Particularly in cases where symptom exaggeration or malingering is detected for the first time, the patient and the health care system would have been much better served if such an evaluation had taken place within a few months postinjury or if other health care providers routinely used symptom validity techniques in their assessments to detect a possible problem earlier. This early symptom validity assessment is important because proper detection of symptom exaggeration and malingering early in the evaluative process helps to triage patients to more appropriate evaluation and treatment resources (e.g., neuropsychology, psychology), reduces misdiagnosis, limits the use of expensive medications and undesirable side effects, and limits the use of expensive diagnostic tests and associated health risks such as radiation exposure from recurrent brain computerized tomography scans (Sodickson et al., 2009). This avoidance of unneeded procedures, in turn, opens up treatment resources for patients who would more clearly benefit from them. Examples of more appropriate use of resources include electroencephalogram (EEG) for a patient with severe TBI who may be experiencing posttraumatic seizure activity, speech therapy for a patient with aphasic stroke, and physical therapy for the patient with multiple sclerosis along with postural instability.

Despite what would seem to be the common sense approach outlined earlier, there are several reasons why it is not always followed. To begin with, identification of exaggeration and/or malingering can place most health care providers in several undesirable and socially uncomfortable situations. These situations include accepting the possibility that the patient is not being straightforward, the realization that treatment may not be working for reasons other than an external cause beyond the patient's control (e.g., brain injury), the need to address uncovered symptom validity concerns directly with the patient, the possibility that insurance may refuse to pay for further treatment, the possibility that revealing symptom validity failure may have a harmful effect on the patient's financial status (e.g., disability payments, pending litigation), and dealing with angry reactions including formal administrative complaints and physical threats. These potential problems can be threatening to the treating clinician who wants to be perceived as helpful, particularly if he or she views himself or herself as a patient advocate (Waddell, 2004a). Thus, many treatment providers have a tendency to be overly trusting on patient self-report and fear that identification of symptom invalidity can threaten the therapeutic relationship. Although these concerns are certainly understandable, failure to identify symptom exaggeration and malingering is a serious omission in the evaluation process because for treatment to be effective, the health care provider needs to have objective assurances that they are treating a valid condition or set of symptoms and that the patient is motivated to improve. This need for assurance of symptom validity is the reason why the American Medical Association's *Guides to the Evaluation of Permanent Impairment* (6th edition) states that examiners should always be aware of possible malingering, especially when there is the possibility for financial gain or avoidance of perceived unpleasant duties by presenting oneself as more ill than is actually the case (Rondinelli, 2008). If symptom exaggeration is present but not assessed, more time and resources will likely be spent on the case than is necessary. This point is worth bearing in mind for health care providers who are concerned that they will not have enough time to assess symptom validity. If symptom validity problems are identified, systematic techniques can be used to provide feedback about such findings to patients to reduce the chances of damaging the therapeutic relationship (see Chapter 6 and Carone, Iverson, & Bush, 2010).

SPECIFIC SYMPTOM VALIDITY METHODS FOR THE NON-NEUROPSYCHOLOGIST

Specific symptom validity methods for the non-neuropsychologist include clinical reasoning based on the knowledge of the evidence-based literature, behavioral observations, and specific SVTs (see Table 11.1). When evaluating patients with MTBI, it is critically important to have a strong understanding of the evidence-based literature because this understanding provides the clinician with objective scientific information regarding the natural course of the injury and factors that can modify the presentation over time. A review of this extensive literature is beyond the scope of this chapter but is summarized in a text by McCrea (2008). The most helpful studies for evaluating the effects of MTBI are prospective studies that use trauma controls. Using this knowledge, the clinician can begin to assess whether the individual patient's presentation makes conceptual sense. A useful method for doing this is provided through coherence analysis.

Coherence Analysis

Coherence analysis is a method pioneered by Stewart-Patterson (in press) to aid in potential malingering detection during medical records reviews in the context of independent medical evaluations. However, the system can be applied in clinical situations when evaluating patients if the provider is willing and able to take the time to do so. The method incorporates a combination of clinical reasoning and analysis of objective data points. The analysis is designed to determine if the overall data "coheres" or holds together in a manner that makes clinical sense. The system uses a useful mnemonic known as the "Seven Cs" which are summarized subsequently.

Continuity of Clinical Findings

This aspect of coherence analysis involves considering whether the patient's clinical presentation (e.g., symptoms, physical findings) is continuous in a manner that would be expected based on scientific understanding of the clinical condition. For MTBI, this continuity would involve consideration of prospective longitudinal research with comparisons on variables of interest (i.e., cognitive test scores) preferably made against trauma controls (as opposed to healthy controls) to account for the effects of general trauma. If the patient with MTBI significantly varies from the expected continuous trajectory (e.g., reports late onset of cognitive symptoms, significant worsening over time, or significant symptom fluctuation for a year or more), this pattern should raise concerns about symptom exaggeration or malingering if there is no reasonable medical explanation. It is important to clarify that exaggeration does not equate to purposeful distortion. For example, a patient with depression may have exaggerated cognitive complaints because they are overly negativistic in their thinking.

Consistency of Clinical Data

This aspect of coherence analysis examines both intrarater and interrater observations by examining whether there is a reasonable degree of uniformity in the assessment of a clinical parameter (e.g., grip strength, Romberg test, tandem walking, symptom self-report scales). An example of intrarater inconsistency would be if the examinee demonstrates 2/5 strength when the reported dysfunctional limb is examined yet inadvertently demonstrates 5/5 strength (i.e., full strength) with the same limb at a later point in the evaluation (e.g., via distraction technique). An example of interrater inconsistency would be if records review showed that in ten prior evaluations with different providers, the examinee failed the Romberg test six times and passed four times in seemingly random order. Some self-report scales and functional capacity evaluations (see subsequent discussion) include measures of consistency. Genuine impairment should present with a reasonable degree of consistency even with distraction techniques (Demeter & Andersson, 2002). A high frequency of inconsistency that cannot be reasonably and medically explained raises suspicion of symptom exaggeration or malingering.

Congruence

This aspect of coherence analysis examines whether various aspects of the patient's clinical presentation are compatible with each other and whether the presentation matches what one would reasonably expect with the condition. That is, one is forced to think in terms of biological plausibility (Larrabee, 1990, 1997). Thus, if a patient with a history of MTBI reports 18 months later that he or she cannot walk without feeling extremely dizzy and claims to be extremely symptomatic and totally disabled, yet he or she is laughing casually throughout the interview and was unknowingly observed walking for long distances without any apparent difficulty, this is incongruent information that raises concerns about symptom validity. Genuine medical impairment should present with a reasonable degree of congruence over time (Rondinelli, 2008). For a helpful sample checklist guide for the assessment of symptom amplification and malingering after MTBI in civil litigants (which includes two sections on congruence), see Sreenivasan, Eth, Kirkish, and Garrick (2003).

Compliance

This aspect of coherence analysis involves examining patient compliance with the assessment and treatment of reported symptoms. Examples of concerns regarding treatment compliance would include frequent missed appointments (cancellation, no shows, arriving at the wrong time), repeatedly not following through with treatment suggestions, or quick discontinuation of medication trials (e.g., not because of side effects) before the time frame it would normally take for the medication to work.

All of these issues raise concerns about symptom validity because they indicate that the patient may not actually be as symptomatic as indicated because of poor follow-through with treatment. Of course, the clinician needs to consider if there are reasonable explanations for noncompliance (e.g., missing appointments because of transportation problems, death in the family, financial reasons). In the end, failure on objective SVTs can also be viewed as a form of noncompliance with the evaluation.

Causation of Injury or Illness

This aspect of coherence analysis requires consideration of whether the condition is actually caused by the alleged event or whether there is an alternative explanation. This determination is important because one form of malingering is false imputation (Resnick, 1988) in which one falsely attributes symptoms from an unrelated injury (e.g., fall at home) to a compensable event (fall at work).

Comorbidity

This aspect of coherence analysis involves examining for the presence of other diagnoses that may explain the patient's presentation. For example, a patient with persisting symptoms after MTBI may report extreme fatigue, irritability, concentration problems, slowed thinking, and memory difficulties because of major depressive disorder. In other instances, such patients may present with headache, dizziness, and blurry vision because of undiagnosed hypertension. Some older adult patients with concussion who report persisting symptoms may have a coincident dementia. Identification of comorbidities does not mean that the patient is malingering, but it can help explain why the symptomatic presentation may be exacerbated, amplified, or exaggerated, particularly if the comorbidity is psychiatric (Sreenivasan et al., 2003).

Cultural Factors

This last factor of coherence analysis requires the examiner to consider the manner by which cultural factors may impact the patient's presentation. For example, although some cultures may tend to present as more stoic and are thus more likely to minimize symptoms, other cultures may tend to present as more dramatic and are thus more likely to exaggerate symptoms. Before concluding that malingering is present, cultural factors need to be considered.

Cognitive Measures of Effort

Although coherence analysis is primarily a system based on clinical reasoning, there are several objective assessment measures available to non-neuropsychologists to assess symptom validity. These include measures of cognitive performance, measures of physical performance, and self-report scales. A description of some of these techniques follows, beginning with two cognitive effort measures that were specifically designed for use by physicians as well as neuropsychologists.

The Medical Symptom Validity Test

The Medical Symptom Validity Test (MSVT; Green, 2004a) is a brief computerized measure of cognitive effort and memory. According to the test author, the MSVT was designed to shorten the administration of the test's parent version, the Word Memory Test (WMT; Green, 2005) and in response to the increasing demand by physicians for an efficient cognitive effort measure (Green, personal communication, November 15, 2011). The test was initially validated with the assistance of physicians performing independent medical evaluations (Gill, Green, Flaro, & Pucci, 2007; Richman et al., 2006). Thus, the conceptualization and initial validation of this test as being specifically intended for physician use allowed for a psychological test to be used by non-psychologists, although psychologists are obviously encouraged to use the test as well. According to the test author (Green, personal communication, November 15, 2011), nurses are also allowed to administer the test in physicians offices provided that they have been properly trained in test administration by the physician. One of the most significant concerns regarding administration of effort tests is to avoid coaching patients by warning them of the purpose of the tests because doing so would ruin their use and compromise years of test validation studies.

For a detailed review of the MSVT, see Carone (2009). Briefly, the test involves the presentation of common word pairs that represent a single concept (e.g., belly button) over two consecutive trials. The test assesses immediate recognition (IR), delayed recognition (DR), and the consistency (CNS) between IR and DR. The delay between IR and DR is 10 minutes, which is spent by doing other tasks that would not interfere with word recall. Immediately after the DR subtest, the patient is administered the paired associates (PA) and free recall (FR) subtests to measure actual memory ability. Some of these subtests are designed to measure effort, whereas others are designed to measure memory ability. The test includes the option of using a stealth version (which looks similar to the original version but contains different word pairs) if coaching is suspected. The MSVT effort subtests can be passed easily by patients with moderate-to-severe neurological conditions (Carone, 2008; Gill et al., 2007; Green, 2004a; Richman et al., 2006). The MSVT uses an empirical method of profile analysis across the various subtests to reduce false positives in dementia (Howe, Anderson, Kaufman, Sachs, & Loring, 2007; Howe & Loring, 2009).

As an example of the useful data the MSVT can provide in detecting noncredible performance in patients with a history of known or suspected MTBI, I published the aforementioned study in 2008 comparing such patients to children with moderate-to-severe brain damage because of acquired (e.g., TBI, stroke) or developmental (e.g., autism) neurological conditions. The results of the study were striking in that 21% ($n = 14/67$) of the known or suspected MTBI group (referred to below as the MTBI group) failed the MSVT, whereas only 5% ($n = 2/38$) of the children failed. The two children who failed were the only two children who were clearly not cooperating with the exam based on behavioral observations, showing why such tests should also be used in pediatric evaluations. The study also introduced the use of posttest difficulty ratings in which patients were asked to rate how difficult the MSVT effort subtests were on a 10-point scale with 10 indicating the greatest difficulty. The results showed that the MTBI group that failed effort testing rated the easy effort subtests as significantly more difficult (mean rating = 5.6) than the children who were moderately to severely brain-injured (mean rating = 1.3). The results clearly indicated exaggerated cognitive test performance and exaggerated self-reporting by this group of patients with a history of MTBI.

The Nonverbal Medical Symptom Validity Test

The Nonverbal Medical Symptom Validity Test (NV-MSVT; Green, 2008) is a computerized test of effort and cognition that was also initially validated with the assistance of physicians (Henry, Merten, Wolf, & Harth, 2009; Singhal, Green, Ashaye, Shankar, & Gill, 2009). For a detailed review of the NV-MSVT, see Wager and Howe (2010). The NV-MSVT is similar to the MSVT in that 10 semantically associated stimulus pairings (e.g., horse and cart) are presented twice to the patient who is then subsequently tested with IR, DR, PA, and FR subtests. CNS between the IR and DR subtests is automatically calculated. However, there are no words on the screen, and two additional forced-choice effort subtests are used, known as DR archetypes (DRA) and DR variations (DRV). The test is not truly "nonverbal" because patients are required to name the objects presented to them and to recall them later on. The NV-MSVT is failed if the mean of various effort subtest combinations fall at or below a certain level specified in the test manual. In a recent study, Green (2011) showed that no patient with a history of moderate-to-severe TBI failed the NV-MSVT, whereas 26% of patients with MTBI and with disability claims failed the test.

As with the MSVT and WMT, the NV-MSVT also has a validated method to reduce false positives by analyzing the pattern of scores across the effort and ability subtests. Patients with severe cognitive impairment (e.g., advanced dementia) who score below the traditional effort cutoffs yet show a pattern consistent with the severe impairment profile would not be classified as poor effort. As an example, the study by Henry et al. (2009) showed that the NV-MSVT has 98.5% specificity with patients with neurological problems, one-third of whom had dementia. The study by Singhal et al. (2009) showed 100% specificity in a dementia group for the NV-MSVT and MSVT and 80% sensitivity to poor effort in a simulator group.

Because the MSVT is much easier and faster to administer than the NV-MSVT, the MSVT would be the obvious choice for most clinicians. However, non-neuropsychologists must be aware of the possibility of false negatives (i.e., stating effort is good when it is poor) with patients with MTBI if they are only using one validated cognitive effort measure. For example, the MSVT is known to be less sensitive than the WMT, with about 11%–15% of patients who pass the MSVT failing the WMT (Green, 2004a). This difference between measures is why the use of multiple validated effort measures throughout an examination is recommended (Bush et al., 2005; Heilbronner et al., 2009). Both the MSVT and NV-MSVT are commonly used effort measures in neuropsychological test batteries. Although they can be used by other psychologists, physicians, and those directly supervised by physicians, they are generally not open to use by other health care professionals who would need to contact the test publisher to seek a special exemption.

Other Cognitive Effort Measures

Other cognitive effort measures exist, but none was both specifically developed for use by physicians and initially validated (in part) by physicians such as the MSVT and NV-MSVT. These other measures include freestanding tests such as the WMT, Test of Memory Malingering (Tombaugh, 1996), Victoria Symptom Validity Test (Slick, Hopp, Strauss, & Thompson, 1997), and Dot Counting Test (Rey, 1941), as well as measures of effort embedded in cognitive ability tests that were not originally designed to measure effort. Two of the most common embedded effort measures include Reliable Digit Span (Greiffenstein, Baker, & Gola, 1994) and recognition hits on the California Verbal Learning Test (Trueblood & Schmidt, 1993). These measures are primarily used by neuropsychologists but can also be used by other psychologists administering cognitive tests (see Chapters 8 and 9 of this book for a detailed review of freestanding and embedded effort measures.).

Physical Measures of Effort

In addition to measures of cognitive symptom validity, various methods have been developed or adopted to assess physical symptom validity. Some of these methods may be particularly well suited for non-neuropsychologists and non-psychologists.

Although a detailed discussion of all such methods is beyond the scope of this book, many are presented in Table 11.1. Detailed description of some selected methods in the physical realm follows.

TABLE 11.1 Qualitative Variables in Assessing Response Bias

Qualitative Variables in Assessing Response Bias	
Time/Response Latency Comparisons Across Similar Tasks	Inconsistencies across tasks
Performance on easy tasks presented as hard	Low scores or unusual errors
Remote memory report	Difficulties, especially if < recent memory, or severely impaired in absence of gross amnesia
Personal information	Very poor personal information in absence of gross amnesia
Comparison between test performance & behavioral observations	Discrepancies
Inconsistencies in history and/or complaints (performance)	Inconsistencies across time, interviewer, etc.
Comparisons for inconsistencies within testing session (quantitative & qualitative)	A. Within tasks (e.g., easy vs. hard items) B. Between tasks (e.g., easy vs. hard) C. Across repetitions of same/parallel tasks (R/O fatigue) D. Across similar tasks under different motivational sets
Comparisons across testing sessions (qualitative & quantitative)	Poorer/inconsistent performance on retesting
Symptom self-report (complaints)	High frequency of complaints: patient complaints > significant others'
Main & Spanswick indicators • Failure to comply with reasonable treatment • Report of severe pain with no associated psychological effects • Marked inconsistencies in effects of pain on general activities • Poor work record and history of persistent appeals against awards • Previous litigation	
Symptom self-report: early vs. late symptom complaint	Early symptoms reported late
Neuromedical Indicators	
Hoover's test	Test for malingered lower extremity weakness associated with normal crossed extensor response
Astasia-abasia	"Drunken type" gait with near falls, but no actual falls to ground
Nonorganic sensory loss	Patchy sensory loss, midline sensory loss, large scotoma in visual field, tunnel vision
Nonorganic upper extremity drift	Long tract involvement results in pronator type drift. Proximal shoulder girdle weakness and malingering typically present with downward drift while in supination.
Stenger's Test	Test for malingered hearing loss during audiologic evaluation.
Gait discrepancies when observed vs. not observed	If organic should be consistent regardless of whether observed or not.

(Continued)

TABLE 11.1 Qualitative Variables in Assessing Response Bias *(Continued)*

Neuromedical Indicators *(Continued)*	
Gait discrepancies relative to direction of requested ambulation	Gait for a patient with hemiparesis should present similarly in all directions; malingerers do not, as a rule, practice a feigned gait in all directions.
Forearm pronation, hand clasping, and forearm supination test for digit/finger sensory loss	Malingered finger sensory loss is difficult to maintain in this perceptually confusing intertwined hand/finger position
Pain vs. temperature discrepancies	Because of the fact that both sensory modalities run in the spinothalamic tract, they should be found to be commensurately impaired contralateral to the side of the CNS lesion.
Lack of atrophy in a chronically paretic/paralytic limb	Lack of atrophy in a paralyzed/paretic limb suggests the limb is being used or is getting regular electrical stimulation to maintain mass.
Impairment diminishes under influence of sodium amytal, hypnosis, or lack of observation	All these observations are most consistent with nonorganic presentations including consideration of malingering or conversion disorder.
Incongruence between neuroanatomical imaging and neurologic examination	Lack of any static imaging findings on brain CT or MRI in the presence of a dense motor or sensory deficit suggests nonorganicity.
Arm drop test	An aware patient malingering profound alteration in consciousness or significant arm paresis will not let his or her own hand when held over his or her head, drop onto their face.
Presence of ipsilateral findings when implied neuroanatomy would dictate contralateral findings	An examinee claiming severe right brain damage who claims right eye blindness and right-sided weakness and sensory loss.
Tell me "when I'm not touching" responses	An examinee with claimed sensory loss who endorses that he or she does not feel you touch him or her when you ask him or her to tell you "if you do not feel this."
Lack of shoe wear in presence of gait disturbance	An examinee with claimed longer term gait deviation because of orthopedic or neurologic causes should demonstrate commensurate wear on shoes (if worn with any frequency).
Calluses on hands in "totally disabled" examinee	An examinee who is unable to work should not present with signs of ongoing evidence of physical labor.
Assistive device "wear and tear" signs	In any examinee using assistive devices for any time, e.g., cane, crutches, there should be commensurate wear on the device consistent with his or her claimed impairment and disability.
Mankopf's maneuver	Increase in heart rate commensurate with nociceptive stimulation during exam (there is some controversy on whether this always occurs).

(Continued)

TABLE 11.1 Qualitative Variables in Assessing Response Bias (*Continued*)

Neuromedical Indicators (*Continued*)	
Lack of atrophy in a limb that is claimed to be significantly impaired	If side-to-side measurements and/or inspection do not bear out atrophy, consider other causes aside from one being claimed.
Sudden motor give away or ratchitiness on manual strength testing	Considered to normally be a sign of incomplete effort or symptom exaggeration.
Weakness on manual muscle testing without commensurate asymmetry of DTRs or muscle bulk.	Suggests simulated muscle weakness if longstanding.
Toe test for simulated low back pain	Flexion of hip and knee with movement only of toes should not produce an increase in low back pain.
Magnuson's test	Have examinee point to area several times over the period of examination; inconsistencies suggest increased potential for nonorganicity.
Delayed response sign	Pain reaction temporarily delayed relative to application of perceived nociceptive stimulus.
Wrist drop test	In an examinee with claimed wrist extensor loss, have him or her pronate forearm, extend elbow, and flex shoulder. . .if on making a fist in this position he or she also extends wrist, then nonorganicity should be suspected.
Object drop test	Examinee claims inability to bend down yet does so to pick up a light object "inadvertently" dropped by examiner.
Hip adductor test	Test for claimed paralysis of lower extremity, similar to Hoover's test yet looks for crossed adductor response.
Disparity between tested range of motion (ROM) and observed ROM of any joint	When ROM under testing is significantly disparate (e.g. less) from observed spontaneous ROM, suspect functional contributors.
Straight leg raise (SLR) disparities dependent on examinee positioning	Differences in SLR between sitting, standing, and/or bending may suggest a functional overlay to low back complaints.
Grip strength testing via dynamometer	Three repetitions at any given setting should not vary more than 20%, and/or bell-shaped curve should be generated if all 5 positions are tested.
Sensory "flip" test	Sensory findings should be the same if testing upper extremity in supination or pronation of lower extremity in internal vs. external rotation. Differences may suggest a functional overlay.
Pinch test for low back pain	Pinching the lumbar fat pad should not reproduce pain because of axial structure involvement; if test is positive, suspect a functional overlay.

Note. This table is reproduced here with the permission of the copyright holder (Taylor & Francis) and was originally presented as part of Table 16.6 in Martelli, M. F., Zasler, N. D., Bush, S. S., & Pickett, T. C. (2006). Assessment of response bias in impairment and disability examinations. In J. León-Carrión, K. R. H. von Wild, & G. A. Zitnay (Eds.), *Brain injury treatment: Theories and practices* (pp. 354–384). New York, NY: Taylor & Francis. CNS = central nervous system; CT = computed tomography; DTRs = deep tendon reflexes; MRI = magnetic resonance imaging; R/O = ruled out.

Psychogenic Gait and Stance Assessment

Psychogenic disorders of gait and stance have been a known clinical entity for more than a century (Blocq, 1888; Charcot, 1879; Lasegue, 1864; Mesnet, 1852). One of the most widely known systems currently used to assess psychogenic disorders of gait and stance was developed by Lempert, Brandt, Dietrich, and Huppert (1991). The system is based on a study that used video analysis to distinguish six types of psychogenic gait and stance characteristics. These characteristics were present alone or in combination in 97% of patients studied who were known to have psychogenic disorders of gait and stance because there was no known reasonable medical explanation for their presentation. The six characteristics included (a) momentary fluctuations of stance and gait, often in response to suggestion; (b) excessive slowness or hesitation of locomotion incompatible with neurological disease; (c) psychogenic Romberg test with a build up of sway amplitudes after a silent latency or with improvement by distraction; (d) uneconomic postures with wastage of muscular energy; (e) the "walking on ice" gait pattern, which is characterized by small cautious steps with fixed ankle joints; and (f) sudden buckling of the knees, usually without falls. The study also used 13 drama students to simulate gait disturbances, which was less conspicuous and more difficult to detect than the clinical psychogenic disorders. In a later study (Baik & Lang, 2007) that reviewed 279 videotapes, patients with psychogenic movement disorder and gait disturbance were found to present with excessive slowness, buckling of the knees, and astasia-abasia (inability to walk, having to hold onto an examiner or an inanimate object to maintain a standing posture, collapsing to the floor usually without causing harm). The features from these two studies remain the classic signs of psychogenic gait disturbance described today (Peckham & Hallett, 2009).

Analysis of psychogenic gait should be an important aspect of gait assessment in patients complaining of persisting symptoms after MTBI, such as imbalance and dizziness, given that some recent studies have associated chronic MTBI with altered gait and stance (Martini et al., 2011; Sosnoff, Broglio, Shin, & Ferrara, 2011). However, none of these studies applied a formal analysis of psychogenic gait patterns. This omission of formal analysis is important because the presence of an obvious psychiatric disturbance, somatization, or an ongoing or impending compensation claim are evidence of a psychogenic movement disorder, which may or may not be malingered (Peckham & Hallett, 2009). Although there are some genuine neurological conditions that can lead to bizarre and inconsistent gait patterns—such as hyperkinetic disorders (chorea), dystonia, and neuroacanthocytosis—bizarre, inconsistent, and nonstereotypical gaits are often correctly diagnosed as psychogenic gait disorders (Van Gerpen, 2011). Reasonable medical explanations for atypical gait patterns should be ruled out before labeling atypical gait as psychogenic.

Distraction Tests

As implied by the name, distraction tests are examination methods designed to distract the patient from focusing on certain symptoms and their impact on functioning when directly examined. Through indirect observation in the presence of the examiner, the purpose is to test whether the patient is actually capable of performing a specific task of function that was not performed during direct observation. These tests are typically performed when the examiner suspects that a symptom is being embellished. Distraction tests have been described in the literature since at least the early 20th century (Catton, 1917; Jones, 1917).

As more recently described by Waddell, McCulloch, Kummel, and Venner (1980), distraction tests should be nonpainful, nonemotional, and nonsurprising.

Take the case of a patient with a history of an MTBI who reports chronic dizziness and instability with postural changes who begins to sway, shake, and report extreme dizziness when asked to bend over. The distraction technique would involve the examiner dropping a pen in front of the patient later in the examination. If the patient proceeded to quickly bend over, grab the pen, and hand it to the examiner without any reported or observable difficulties, this behavior would be considered a marked inconsistency. The type(s) of distraction test used depend on the patient's symptoms and the creativity of the examiner. As this example indicates, although it is easy to remove pain and emotion from distraction tests, they do involve some degree of surprise because they rely on the patient being unexpectedly and indirectly evaluated, leading to the person doing something unintended. Thus, when they used the term "nonsurprised," Waddell and colleagues (1980) likely meant that the patient should not be startled, particularly because they emphasized that the distraction should be nonemotional. Because distraction tests involve assessing gross discrepancies in behavior, lack of standardization is not a significant concern. There is likely less of a chance that sophisticated exaggerators and malingers will be detected by distraction tests.

Surveillance Methods

Distraction techniques are useful because the patient is unsuspecting of being examined. Behavior under indirect observation that is grossly discrepant from illness behavior produced on direct examination is one of the few ways to make stronger inferences regarding intentionality. Another method that relies on indirect observation is surveillance. Surveillance typically takes the form of video monitoring (known as sub rosa investigations) of the patient by private investigators hired by an insurance company that is later made available for review. For example, one adult patient I evaluated 14 months after an MTBI in the context of a workers' compensation insurance claim arrived to the evaluation ambulating very slowly with a cane. Video surveillance was provided showing the patient slowly walking into medical clinics with the use of a cane, but later that day walking quickly out of a store while carrying a pizza, later nimbly operating a manual car wash hose, and walking around the car many times—all without use of a cane.

Although surveillance video has been described in the medical literature as a tool to detect malingering after many conditions (Kurlan, Brin, & Fahn, 1997; LoPiccolo, Goodkin, & Baldewicz, 1999; Ochoa & Verdugo, 2010) from MTBI (Trueblood & Binder, 1997) to severe TBI (Boone & Lu, 2003), not much has been written in that literature regarding cautions for its use. Before relying on such video to form clinical opinions, it is important that (a) the patient is clearly and unmistakably recognizable; (b) the video does not appear heavily edited; (c) the patient is clearly displaying abilities that are significantly at variance with self-report; (d) the video was taken close to the time period of the patient's complaints (preferably the day of, before, or after a health care visit); (e) the time period is most clearly established with a video of the daily newspaper (because digital recording times can be altered); (f) there was sufficient video recorded before and after the contradictory behavior of interest (e.g., to show that there are no ill effects afterward); and (g) a pattern of contradictory behavior is shown over various time periods (as opposed to a single event).

In most clinical situations, video surveillance will be unavailable. However, there are more informal surveillance methods that can be used if the case warrants it. For example, one method is to observe how patients behave by watching them in the waiting area or observing them through an office window as they enter or leave the building. For example, one patient I previously evaluated 6 months after an MTBI who retained an attorney presented with many bizarre symptoms (e.g., profound retrograde amnesia) that included an unstable and bizarre zigzagging gait. One morning, the patient happened to be walking down a seemingly empty hallway when I coincidentally happened to be coming down a stairway that put her in view. The patient was initially observed to be walking perfectly straight, looked upward, saw that I was present, and instantly began walking in a zigzagging pattern again.

The Pen Test

The pen test is described here for the first time as a method to assess symptom validity of grip strength and upper extremity weakness. I discovered the technique accidentally when trying to informally assess grip strength during the neurobehavioral examination component of the evaluation (prior to beginning formal objective testing). Because my practice involves assessment of children and adults with various neurological conditions (e.g., severe TBI, dementia, neoplasms, stroke, developmental disorders), it eventually became clear that the only patients unable to hold on to the pen were patients who were hemiplegic, hemiparetic, or who had severe peripheral damage to the hand or upper extremity (e.g., arthritis). When these types of patients were excluded from consideration, it was noticed that every patient making a basic effort (including children down to 5 years of age) were able to grip the pen strongly and resist the examiner's efforts to pull it out. The only patients for whom this was not the case were adult patients who reported persisting symptoms after known or suspected MTBI.

The instructions for administering the pen test are as follows. First, be sure to ask the patient if he or she is experiencing any hand pain, and do not administer the test if there is any indication that significant pain is present that may interfere with grip. Do not administer the test to patients with obviously valid explanations for poor grip (as previously described). Next, take a pen (preferably standard size) and tell the patient, "*I am going to place this pen in your hand.*" If a pen is not available, a pencil can be used. Tell the patient to make sure the hands are dry and to dry them off if they are not. Then tell the patient to open the dominant (say "*right*" or "*left*") hand. Place the pen firmly inside (point side up). About 2 inches of the pen should be accessible from the top of the pen for the examiner to grab. Once the pen is firmly in place say, "*I am going to pull on the pen. Grip it as hard as you can, and do not let me pull it out of your hand.*" Pull on the pen with moderate tug. If the patient is making an effort the pen should remain firmly in place. Subtle weakness may allow the pen to move up slightly, but the patient should still be able to grip the pen so that it does not come out quickly or easily. Repeat the process on the other side. There is one trial per hand, making this a test that should only take between 10 and 20 seconds to administer when the patient passes. If there is a concern that the pen may not be in place properly or that the hand(s) are (still) sweaty, the procedure should be repeated until the examiner is confident that no extraneous factors are interfering with performance. Passing the pen test is indicated by the examiner being unable to pull out the pen from either hand.

When patients are *not* making a good effort on the pen test, the pen will quickly and easily slide out of the hand. Moreover, unlike patients who have demonstrable lesions in the frontal motor cortex, which cause a contralateral upper extremity motor paresis (McNeal et al., 2010), my observation has been that all known or suspected patients with MTBI who fail this test allow the pen to slide quickly and easily out of both hands. This is sometimes accompanied by half-hearted attempts to appear that a solid pen grip is attempted, sometimes with the hand(s) partly or fully opening and closing. However, at other times, the patient will not make any detectable attempt to grip the pen strongly. Another point of interest is that unlike cases of genuine arm paresis after moderate-to-severe TBI, which tends to recover in 2–6 months (Katz, Alexander, & Klein, 1998), patients with known or suspected MTBI who fail the pen test tend to be well over 6 months postinjury, often up to several years postinjury.

After the patient fails the pen test, the examinee should not make any attempt to immediately inform the patient that the performance is noncredible. Rather, the examiner should try to repeat the procedure with the following instructions: *"I want you to imagine that I am going to give you a million dollars if I cannot get this pen out of your hand. So be sure to grip it as strong as you can, OK?"* This instruction is provided because it provides a strong imaginary incentive that should encourage any person making a good effort to pass the test. Although my experience has been that this added instruction leads to the same exact performance (i.e., failure), this added step is useful to document because it shows that the examiner did everything possible to motivate the patient. Conclude the pen test by asking the patient in a nonjudgmental tone, *"OK, are you sure that you were gripping the pen as strongly as you could?"* Document the response and move on with other aspects of the evaluation. In my experience, the response to this question has always been *"yes."*

When the entire examination is concluded, I have found it helpful to politely but firmly tell the patient that there are strong indications from the examination that he or she is capable of performing much better. This feedback may be based on the pen test or another SVT. However, it is very important not to reveal the identity or methods behind any of the SVTs so that the security and integrity of the procedures are maintained.

If the clinician decides to take this next step, it is recommended to say the following, *"I have administered this test very many times, and I know that you are capable of gripping the pen much harder than you did. So, let's try it again, shall we?"* Then repeat the original procedure. Often, the patient's performance will drastically change, and it is then impossible to remove the pen from the patient's hand. This change occurs despite the patient previously stating that he or she was squeezing the pen as hard as possible with an imaginary $1 million at stake. This optional procedure provides invaluable information to the clinician because it is typically the first time that the patient is shown to be capable of performing much better in the physical realm than he or she claimed and previously demonstrated. Patients who fail physical effort tests will not always fail cognitive effort tests and vice versa, likely because the patient considers one particular form of limitation to be of primary critical importance to maintaining disability. For example, patients whose jobs heavily rely on hand use (e.g., mechanics) are more likely to fail the pen test in my experience. At present, formal reliability and validity data on the pen test has not been established and is an area in need of future research.

Waddell's Signs and Symptoms

Waddell's signs are a group of physical signs named after the physician (Waddell et al., 1980) who first described them as indicators of nonorganic (psychological) components in patients complaining of chronic back pain. There are a total of eight Waddell's signs in five categories which include (a) distraction techniques (see earlier section); (b) tenderness tests (reported tenderness that is superficial, diffuse, and deviates from what is anatomically possible); (c) simulation tests (patient reports pain in response to a simulated movement that is not actually performed); (d) regional disturbances (reported weakness or sensory changes that deviate from what is neuroanatomically possible); and (e) overreaction (signs that show that the patient is reacting or behaving in a much more dramatic manner during testing than is normal). Any individual sign is considered positive for the category. Positive signs in three or more of the five categories were considered clinically significant. Although some later research indicated that presence of any of these signs is clinically significant (Gaines & Hegmann, 1999; Werneke, Harris, & Lichter, 1993), Waddell (2004a) still argues against interpreting positive single signs.

The use of Waddell's signs has been highly controversial for more than 30 years for two main reasons. The first reason is that they have a history of being inappropriately and overly used as proof of malingering despite evidence to the contrary (Fishbain, Cutler, Rosomoff, & Rosomoff, 2004; Gallagher, 2003; Lechner, Bradbury, & Bradley, 1998) and despite consistent admonitions against using the signs in this way from Waddell (2004a; Waddell et al., 1980; Waddell, Pilowsky, & Bond, 1990). The second source of controversy is that some have concluded that Waddell's signs can occur as a result of genuine physical causes (Centeno, Elkins, & Freeman, 2004; Fishbain et al., 2003; Margoles, 1990). This is a point Waddell has vigorously disputed when the signs form a consistent and clear pattern (Waddell, 2004a, 2004b; Waddell et al., 1990). Waddell (2004a) has also criticized the methodology that was recently used to discredit his signs by Fishbain et al. (2003) as "riddled with fatal methodological flaws" (p. 199), such as incomplete search and retrieval of studies, reference to abstracts or conference proceedings, double and triple counting of studies, misclassification of studies, selective reporting of results, inappropriate quality criteria, and unfounded and mutually contradictory conclusions.

Given the persistent controversy over the use of Waddell's signs, each clinician will need to weigh the evidence and decide whether to incorporate them into the physical examination. Use of the signs should be done with recognition of their strengths, limitations, and the caveats established by Waddell (2004a), which includes not using them with people older than 60 years, non-Caucasian minorities, or patients with serious spinal pathology or widespread neurological damage. Clinicians must remember that Waddell's signs were designed to serve as a screening mechanism for a more comprehensive psychological assessment before rushing into more complex medical care. Provided that the signs are used in the manner described by Waddell, they can provide some of the first clues that may lead to a referral for psychological assessment, which, in turn, can lead to a more detailed symptom validity assessment.

Waddell symptoms are a list of nonanatomic or behavioral descriptions of symptoms, which include pain in the tip of the tailbone, *whole* leg pain, whole leg numbness, whole leg give way, and reporting no time in the past year with very little pain (Waddell, Bircher, Finlayson, & Main, 1984; Waddell, Main, Morris, Di Paola, & Gray, 1984). Much less research has been done on these symptoms, but recent research has indicated that the presence of two or more symptoms indicates the presence of factors beyond tissue pathology that may warrant clinical attention and are indicators of the need for a comprehensive psychological assessment (Carleton, Abrams, Kachur, & Asmundson, 2009a, 2009b). Waddell's signs and symptoms have primarily been studied with patients with back pain and have yet to be scientifically studied with patients with MTBI. However, given the complaints of imbalance, dizziness, postural instability, pain, sensory changes, weakness, and extreme illness behavior that patients with chronic MTBI sometimes present with, this is clearly an area of potential clinical usefulness and future study.

Functional Capacity Evaluations

Functional capacity evaluations (FCEs) are standardized batteries of functional measures commonly used to assess an injured worker's ability to perform work-related activities (Gross & Battié, 2005). They are commonly administered by physical therapists or occupational therapists but are also administered by other health care professionals (King, Tuckwell, & Barrett, 1998). FCEs are often used to make disability determinations for patients reporting disabling symptoms after MTBI. There are a wide variety of FCE systems, which vary in length, variety, and adequacy of assessment methods, degree of standardization, and theoretical foundation (King et al., 1998). Despite their popularity, many FCE systems have been criticized for lacking scientific evidence to support their use (King et al., 1998).

Most FCEs contain measures of physical effort and cooperation such as (a) grip strength consistency; (b) nonorganic signs (e.g., Waddell signs; previously described); (c) comparing heart rate changes with self-reported pain intensity; (d) major discrepancies between self-reported functional limitations and actual test results; and (e) observations of atypical pain behavior. However, some of these techniques have been criticized as not being studied adequately because of methodological flaws, such as having poor reliability, validity, and generalizability and not taking into account cultural and individual variability in pain expression (Lechner et al., 1998; Lechner, Roth, & Straaton, 1991; Lemstra, Olszynski, & Enright, 2004; Westbrook, Tredgett, Davis, & Oni, 2002). Lemstra et al. (2004) studied 17 commonly used measures of physical effort and found that five were able to individually differentiate between maximal and submaximal effort (zero competitive test behaviors, three measures of grip strength consistency, and self-terminating the test). The authors urged caution in labeling patients as exerting submaximal effort on FCEs (particularly with isolated findings) until better tests are developed. See Lemstra et al. (2004) and Roy (2003) for a more detailed review of effort measures used in FCEs.

With the aforementioned cautions in mind, those who have concluded that patients are exerting submaximal effort on FCEs have found that they are more anxious and depressed, have more negative performance expectations, and have higher perceptions of disability than those exerting maximal effort (Kaplan, Wurtele, & Gillis, 1996). Thus, it has been advised that patients experiencing significant psychological distress should not be scheduled for an FCE until psychological treatment has addressed the previously described issues (Kaplan et al., 1996). This need for psychological treatment is particularly relevant in patients complaining of disabling chronic symptoms after MTBI, where significant psychological, psychosocial, and psychiatric problems are often present (Iverson, 2005; Iverson, Zasler, & Lange, 2006) and can potentially confound the results of the assessment. If poor effort is concluded based on the FCE (which is easiest when variability is high and there are obvious indicators present), explanations other than malingering (e.g., pain, fear of pain or reinjury) should be also considered, some of which may be treatable (Geisser, Robinson, Miller, & Bade, 2003; Pransky & Dempsey, 2004; Strong, Baptiste, Clarke, Cole, & Costa, 2004).

Self-Report Scales

The use of self-report scales in symptom validity assessment with patients who have a history of MTBI is covered in detail in Chapter 10. This section provides a brief overview of some methods that non-neuropsychologists can employ for this purpose.

"Concussion" Checklists

There are numerous brief "concussion" symptom checklists available that contain multiple physical, emotional, and cognitive items. These scales are sometimes referred to as concussion checklists despite the fact that none of the symptoms (e.g., headaches, concentration problems, irritability) is specific to concussion (Gunstad & Suhr, 2002; Iverson, 2006; Iverson & Lange, 2003; Iverson et al., 2006; Lees-Haley, Fox, & Courtney, 2001; Suhr & Gunstad, 2002; Wang, Chan, & Deng, 2006). One of the most commonly used scales is the Postconcussion Syndrome Checklist (PCSC; Gouvier, Cubic, Jones, Brantley, & Cutlip, 1992). Developed two decades ago, the questionnaire asks patients to rate the frequency, intensity, and duration of 10 symptoms experienced that day.

A significant limitation with the PCSC and most other concussion checklists (e.g., King, Crawford, Wenden, Moss, & Wade, 1995) is that they do not contain any items to assess for invalid or exaggerated responding. However, these measures can be used in such a manner when used longitudinally. Specifically, I have long been encouraging health care providers to administer this checklist when the patient *first* arrives for outpatient clinical care and at regular intervals (e.g., monthly) to monitor progress. Provided that the patient has not suffered a repeat concussion or some other neurological event between the various assessment periods, reports of increasing symptoms over time or decreased symptoms followed by worsening of symptoms is evidence that there is a nonneurological process contributing to symptom reporting. The same is true when all (or mostly all) symptoms are reported at the most extreme severity from the outset, with no significant improvement over time. This pattern is important because actual neurologically induced concussive symptoms should generally improve over time (Dikmen, Machamer, Fann, & Temkin, 2010). Of course, the clinician needs to rule out the possibility that the increased symptoms were not caused by some isolated stressful event that occurred that day. When monitored over a regular basis, however, a pattern can begin to emerge that does not match with known prospectively studied postconcussive symptom recovery trajectories. The longer this pattern is present and the more extreme the ratings are, the more confident the examiner can be that nonneurological factors are confounding the presentation. These nonneurological factors can be a mood disorder, malingering, interference from comorbid medical conditions, substance abuse, the effects of medications, or other factors and will require a thorough evaluation to be understood more clearly.

For those wishing to use a concussion checklist that contains embedded validity items, the Postconcussion Syndrome Questionnaire (PCSQ) is recommended. Initial data were gathered on the PCSQ by Lees-Haley (1992, 1993), and the test was further developed and refined into a 44- and 45-item version (Axelrod, Fox, Lees-Haley, Earnest, & Dolezal-Wood, 1998; Axelrod et al., 1996; Axelrod & Lees-Haley, 2002). Items are rated on a 0–5 points scale in terms of how much the patient reports being affected by them. The symptoms are then rated in terms of whether they have gotten better, worse, or remained the same. The test contains several validity items, which are implausible or impossible symptoms to experience as a result of concussion (e.g., triple vision, itchy teeth) and provide stronger evidence of symptom exaggeration than traditional concussion checklists. When patients with chronic MTBI report that most of their symptoms have remained the same or worsened since injury, this also provides strong evidence of nonneurological factors contributing to symptom reporting because improvement is expected when the only cause of the symptoms is neurological. Clinicians can also get a sense as to which of these factors (e.g., litigation, depression) may be playing a role by examining which items are reported as most distressing and worsening (e.g., the emotional items). Two 19-item short forms of the PCSQ exist: the PCSQ-19 and the PCSQ Negative Impression Management Scale (PCSQ-NIM; Van Dyke, Axelrod, & Schutte, 2010). The PCSQ-19 does not contain any of the validity items, but scores greater than 11 require examination for aberrant response patterns. The PCSQ-NIM contains one of the validity items but was designed to measure negative impression management by identifying the items that best differentiated between patients with MTBI who failed at least two effort tests and patients with moderate-to-severe TBI.

The Memory Complaints Inventory

The Memory Complaints Inventory (MCI; Green, 2004b) is a 58-item computerized self-report measure that assesses the validity of self-reported memory problems (although some items also address concentration). The measure is appropriate for use by most health care providers and takes about 10 minutes to administer. The inventory items consist of common and implausible memory problems across nine scales: general memory problems (GMP); numeric information problems (NIP); visuospatial memory problems (VSP); verbal memory problems (VMP); pain interferes with memory (PIM); memory interferes with work (MIW); impairment of remote memory (IRM); amnesia for complex behavior (ACB); and amnesia for antisocial behavior (AAB). The first six scales contain the most common memory complaints, whereas the last three scales contain the most implausible memory complaints. Implausible memory complaints are those that are rarely found in patients with genuine neurological disease or severe injury. As such, these implausible memory complaints are likely to be associated with psychological/psychiatric overlay or exaggerated/feigned memory complaints. MCI results can be compared against 56 comparison groups (as of March 16, 2011), which include healthy controls, patients with neurological problems, patients with psychiatric illnesses, and patients with other medical conditions (e.g., orthopedic injuries; Green, 2009). On the MCI, patients with moderate-to-severe TBIs or neurological disorders who pass effort tests generally report significantly fewer memory complaints compared to patients with a history of MTBI, chronic pain, anxiety, or depression who fail effort tests (Gervais, Ben-Porath, Wygant, & Green, 2008; Green, 2004b). However, the MCI's automated interpretation system also shows that even among patients with TBI who pass effort testing, patients with a history of MTBI (especially women) report more memory problems than patients with moderate-to-severe TBI.

Initial studies on the MCI were presented at annual meetings of the National Academy of Neuropsychology (Green & Allen, 2000; Green, Allen, & Iverson, 1999) and showed that MCI scores were differentially elevated in TBI litigants who failed effort testing and were not significantly correlated with objective tests of memory ability or other ability measures. In a later study using a sample that was 2.5 times greater ($n = 1,479$), Green, Gervais, and Merten (2005) found that there were some significant but very low correlations (-0.10–0.26) between MCI scores and memory ability scores and that most of those correlations became nonsignificant when poor effort was controlled for. In general, patients tend to report more problems with verbal memory than visuospatial memory regardless of effort test performance. This difference is likely because most daily memory complaints tend to be in the verbal domain (e.g., forgetting information from conversations or reading materials), given that verbal expression is the primary manner by which people communicate (Green & Allen, 2000).

Patients with high levels of depression who pass effort testing have been found to report much higher memory complaints on the MCI than patients with low levels of depression (Rohling, Green, Allen, & Iverson, 2002). These authors also found that the relationship between the MCI summary score and performance on objective cognitive tests was clinically nonsignificant. Given the MCI's use as a self-report validity scale in neurological and psychiatric groups, the test was used in the development and validation studies of another self-report validity measure, the Response Bias Scale (RBS), which is described in the next section.

The Minnesota Multiphasic Personality Inventory

The Minnesota Multiphasic Personality Inventory (MMPI) is the most popular objective test of personality and psychopathology. The test is currently in its second edition (MMPI-2; Greene, 2000), but more recently a restructured form (MMPI-2-RF; Ben-Porath & Tellegen, 2008) was published that greatly reduced the item content from 567 to 338 and eliminated item overlap between the scales. Although other personality inventories exist, such as the NEO (Costa & McCrae, 2010), the Personality Assessment Inventory (Morey, 1991), and the Millon Clinical Multiaxial Inventory-III (Millon, Davis, & Millon, 1997), there is no personality test that has been used to more extensively to study the reliability and validity of self-reported symptoms than those in the MMPI family.

Initial versions of the MMPI contained validity scales that focused on the overreporting of psychopathology (e.g., infrequency [F] and infrequency psychopatholgy [Fp] scales), underreporting of psychopathology (lie [L] and defensiveness [K] scales), and the internal reliability of self-reporting across the hundreds of items (e.g., variable and true response inconsistency [VRIN and TRIN]). However, in recent years, there has been development of additional scales that have been useful in identifying overreporting of cognitive symptoms, such as the Fake Bad Scale (now known as the Symptom Validity Scale) and the RBS. Although the Fake Bad Scale has been the subject of frequent controversy (Arbisi & Butcher, 2004; Ben-Porath, Greve, Bianchini, & Kaufmann, 2009; Butcher, Arbisi, Atlis, & McNulty, 2003; Butcher, Gass, Cumella, Kally, & Williams, 2008; Greve & Bianchini, 2004; Lees-Haley & Fox, 2004; Williams, Butcher, Gass, Cumella, & Kally, 2009), the RBS has not received such criticism and is reviewed briefly here.

The RBS consists of 28 items from the MMPI-2 and MMPI-2-RF that were best able to differentiate those who failed three well-validated effort tests from those who passed such effort tests in forensic neuropsychological and disability assessment settings (Gervais, Ben-Porath, Wygant, & Green, 2007). Scores are interpreted along a continuum, with higher scores indicating increased probability and magnitude of effort test failure and symptom exaggeration on objective testing and self-reported symptoms (e.g., cognitive, emotional). Because the scale was later validated with the MCI (Gervais et al., 2008; Gervais, Ben-Porath, Wygant, & Sellbom, 2010), it provides predictive statements about how elevated MCI scores are expected to be. Information from the RBS can be very helpful to clinical or counseling psychologists evaluating patients with MTBI to gain a better understanding of the likelihood that exaggeration and response bias is present. High RBS scores should lead the clinician to make more cautionary statements about the degree to which self-reported symptoms accurately reflects the patient's level of functioning and the need for additional symptom validity assessment. The RBS was originally validated in patients without head injury but was also independently validated with patients with MTBI pursuing compensation (Dionysus, Denney, & Halfaker, 2011; Nelson, Sweet, & Heilbronner, 2007; Smart et al., 2008; Whitney, Davis, Shepard, & Herman, 2008).

CONCLUSION

There are several techniques available to non-neuropsychologists to assess symptom validity, the most sophisticated of which are in the psychological realm. Although psychological SVT methods are most appropriate for use by psychologists, some of these techniques are also available to physicians and other health care providers who have the appropriate training, education, and meet qualifications of the test publisher. Unfortunately, many health care providers are unaware that SVTs exist or fail to incorporate them into their exams and case conceptualization if they are aware of them. Some physical therapists (Lechner et al., 1998) have seriously questioned whether it is appropriate for their profession to attempt to detect poor effort because of statistical limitations of their available methods and possible negative effects of incorrect decisions on the patient (e.g., termination of benefits, job loss, low self-esteem). However, to completely ignore effort and symptom validity assessment is to ignore a major variable that can confound the assessment, leading to misdiagnosis, incorrect treatment, incorrect disability determinations (Jahn, Cupon, & Steinbaugh, 2004), harm of other patients through improper and inefficient allocation of health care resources, and harm to society through rising health care costs. Thus, a balance needs to be struck by assessing symptom validity in a comprehensive manner with the best available techniques combined with empirically based clinical reasoning and the proper application of caveats.

If a health care provider does not believe that his or her profession has developed empirically validated tools to assess symptom validity in patients with a history of MTBI, there are several steps that should be taken. The first is to acknowledge in the clinical report that the results of the evaluation may be invalid and unreliable because symptom validity was not assessed. The second is to help contribute to the development of better symptom validity assessment techniques in that specific profession. The third is to develop standards for the use of probabilistic language similar to those developed in neuropsychology (Slick, Sherman, & Iverson, 1999). The fourth is to refer the patient to the profession that has developed the most scientifically rigorous measures of symptom validity—clinical neuropsychology.

Although progress in advancing the science, and use of symptom validity assessment has been made by physicians specializing in independent medical evaluations (IMEs), much more progress is needed for symptom validity assessment to be incorporated into standard routine *clinical* care for non-neuropsychologists. This progress will partly be accomplished via educational methods, such as workshops, journal articles, and books. However, for symptom validity assessment research to gain more attention outside of the psychology and legal/IME/FCE realm, there is a greater need for publications in this area outside of psychology, occupational medicine, and physical therapy journals, which is where much of this research currently resides. In addition, the need for symptom validity assessment should be endorsed by mainstream national organizations run by physicians (e.g., American Medical Association; American College of Environmental and Occupational Medicine), other psychology specialty organizations (National Association of School Psychology), and other professional associations (e.g., American Occupational Therapy Association, American Physical Therapy Association).[1] This broader endorsement of symptom validity assessment would hopefully result in the development of empirically based guidelines similar to those developed by national neuropsychological organizations (i.e., NAN, AACN) encouraging the routine use of symptom validity assessment techniques in clinical and nonclinical evaluations.

---

[1] The American Physical Therapy Association published guidelines in 1997 stating that the consistency of effort should be evaluated in FCEs.

REFERENCES

American Academy of Clinical Neuropsychology. (2007). American Academy of Clinical Neuropsychology (AACN) practice guidelines for neuropsychological assessment and consultation. *The Clinical Neuropsychologist*, 21(2), 209–231.

Arbisi, P. A., & Butcher, J. N. (2004). Failure of the FBS to predict malingering of somatic symptoms: Response to critiques by Greve and Bianchini and Lees Haley and Fox. *Archives of Clinical Neuropsychology*, 19(3), 341–345.

Axelrod, B. N., Fox, D. D., Lees-Haley, P. R., Earnest, K., & Dolezal-Wood, S. (1998). Application of the postconcussive syndrome questionnaire with medical and psychiatric outpatients. *Archives of Clinical Neuropsychology*, 13(6), 543–548.

Axelrod, B. N., Fox, D. D., Lees-Haley, P. R., Earnest, K., Dolezal-Wood, S., & Goldman, R. S. (1996). Latent structure of the postconcussion syndrome questionnaire. *Psychological Assessment*, 8(4), 422–427.

Axelrod, B. N., & Lees-Haley, P. (2002). Construct validity of the PCSQ as related to the MMPI-2. *Archives of Clinical Neuropsychology*, 17(4), 343–350.

Baik, J. S., & Lang, A. E. (2007). Gait abnormalities in psychogenic movement disorders. *Movement Disorders*, 22(3), 395–399.

Ben-Porath, Y. S., Greve, K., Bianchini, K., & Kaufmann, P. M. (2009). The MMPI-2 Symptom Validity Scale (FBS) is an empirically validated measure of overreporting in personal injury litigants and claimants: Reply to Butcher et al. (2008). *Psychological Injury and Law*, 2, 62–85.

Ben-Porath, Y. S., & Tellegen, A. (2008). *MMPI-2-RF manual for administration, scoring, and interpretation.* Minneapolis, MN: University of Minnesota Press.

Bianchini, K. J., Mathias, C. W., & Greve, K. W. (2001). Symptom validity testing: A critical review. *The Clinical Neuropsychologist*, 15(1), 19–45.

Blocq, P. (1888). Sur une affection caractérisée par de l'astasie et de l'abasie. *Archives of Neurology (Paris)*, 15, 24–51.

Boone, K. B., & Lu, P. (2003). Noncredible cognitive performance in the context of severe brain injury. *The Clinical Neuropsychologist*, 17(2), 244–254.

Bush, S. S., Ruff, R. M., Tröster, A. I., Barth, J. T., Koffler, S. P., Pliskin, N. H., . . . Silver, C. H. (2005). Symptom validity assessment: Practice issues and medical necessity NAN policy & planning committee. *Archives of Clinical Neuropsychology*, 20(4), 419–426.

Butcher, J. N., Arbisi, P. A., Atlis, M. M., & McNulty, J. L. (2003). The construct validity of the Lees-Haley Fake Bad Scale. Does this scale measure somatic malingering and feigned emotional distress? *Archives of Clinical Neuropsychology*, 18(5), 473–485.

Butcher, J. N., Gass, C. S., Cumella, E., Kally, Z., & Williams, C. L. (2008). Potential for bias in MMPI-2 assessments using the Fake Bad Scale (FBS). *Psychological Injury and Law*, 1, 191–209.

Carleton, R. N., Abrams, M. P., Kachur, S. S., & Asmundson, G. J. (2009a). Waddell's symptoms as correlates of vulnerabilities associated with fear-anxiety-avoidance models of pain: Pain-related anxiety, catastrophic thinking, perceived disability, and treatment outcome. *Journal of Occupational Rehabilitation*, 19(4), 364–374.

Carleton, R. N., Kachur, S. S., Abrams, M. P., & Asmundson, G. J. (2009b). Waddell's symptoms as indicators of psychological distress, perceived disability, and treatment outcome. *Journal of Occupational Rehabilitation*, 19(1), 41–48.

Carone, D. A. (2008). Children with moderate/severe brain damage/dysfunction outperform adults with mild-to-no brain damage on the Medical Symptom Validity Test. *Brain Injury*, 22(12), 960–971.

Carone, D. A. (2009). Test review of the Medical Symptom Validity Test. *Applied Neuropsychology*, 16(4), 309–311.

Carone, D. A., Iverson, G. L., & Bush, S. S. (2010). A model to approaching and providing feedback to patients regarding invalid test performance in clinical neuropsychological evaluations. *The Clinical Neuropsychologist*, 24(5), 759–778.

Catton, J. H. (1917). Malingering; its diagnosis and clinical significance. *California State Journal of Medicine*, 15(11), 458–461.

Centeno, C. J., Elkins, W. L., & Freeman, M. (2004). Waddell's signs revisited? *Spine (Phila Pa 1976)*, 29(13), 1392–1393.

Charcot, J. M. (1879). *Lectures on the diseases of the nervous system. Delivered at the la Salpêtriére* (G. Sigerson, Trans.). Philadelphia, PA: Henry C Lea.

Collie, A., Maruff, P., Makdissi, M., McCrory, P., McStephen, M., & Darby, D. (2003). CogSport: Reliability and correlation with conventional cognitive tests used in postconcussion medical evaluations. *Clinical Journal of Sport Medicine*, 13(1), 28–32.

Costa, P. T., & McCrae, R. R. (2010). *NEO inventories for the NEO Personality Inventory-3 (NEO-PI-3), NEO Five-Factor Inventory-3 (NEO-FFI-3), NEO Personality Inventory-Revised (NEO PI-R): Professional manual*. Odessa, FL: Psychological Assessment Resources.

Demeter, S. L., & Andersson, G. B. J. (2003). *Disability evaluation* (2nd ed.). St. Louis, MO: Mosby.

Department of Veteran Affairs. (2009). *Va/DoD Clinical Practice Guidelines for Management of Concussion/ Mild Traumatic Brain Injury*. Washington, DC: Department of Defense.

Dikmen, S., Machamer, J., Fann, J. R., & Temkin, N. R. (2010). Rates of symptom reporting following traumatic brain injury. *Journal of the International Neuropsychological Society*, 16(3), 401–411.

Dionysus, K. E., Denney, R. L., & Halfaker, D. A. (2011). Detecting negative response bias with the Fake Bad Scale, Response Bias Scale, and Henry-Heilbronner Index of the Minnesota Multiphasic Personality Inventory-2. *Archives of Clinical Neuropsychology*, 26(2), 81–88.

Erlanger, D. M., Feldman, D. J., & Kutner, K. C. (2002). *HeadMinder: Concussion Resolution Index (CRI): Professional Manual*. New York: HeadMinder.

Ferguson, R. J., Mittenberg, W., Barone, D. F., & Schneider, B. (1999). Postconcussion syndrome following sports-related head injury: Expectation as etiology. *Neuropsychology*, 13(4), 582–589.

Fishbain, D. A., Cole, B., Cutler, R. B., Lewis, J., Rosomoff, H. L., & Rosomoff, R. S. (2003). A structured evidence-based review on the meaning of nonorganic physical signs: Waddell signs. *Pain Medicine*, 4(2), 141–181.

Fishbain, D. A., Cutler, R. B., Rosomoff, H. L., & Rosomoff, R. S. (2004). Is there a relationship between nonorganic physical findings (Waddell signs) and secondary gain/malingering? *The Clinical Journal of Pain*, 20(6), 399–408.

Gaines, W. G. Jr., & Hegmann, K. T. (1999). Effectiveness of Waddell's nonorganic signs in predicting a delayed return to regular work in patients experiencing acute occupational low back pain. *Spine (Phila Pa 1976)*, 24, 396–401.

Gallagher, R. M. (2003). Waddell signs: Objectifying pain and the limits of medical altruism. *Pain Medicine*, 4(2), 113–115.

Geisser, M. E., Robinson, M. E., Miller, Q. L., & Bade, S. M. (2003). Psychosocial factors and functional capacity evaluation among persons with chronic pain. *Journal of Occupational Rehabilitation*, 13(4), 259–276.

Gervais, R. O., Ben-Porath, Y. S., Wygant, D. B., & Green, P. (2007). Development and validation of a Response Bias Scale (RBS) for the MMPI-2. *Assessment*, 14(2), 196–208.

Gervais, R. O., Ben-Porath, Y. S., Wygant, D. B., & Green, P. (2008). Differential sensitivity of the Response Bias Scale (RBS) and MMPI-2 validity scales to memory complaints. *The Clinical Neuropsychologist*, 22(6), 1061–1079.

Gervais, R. O., Ben-Porath, Y. S., Wygant, D. B., & Sellbom, M. (2010). Incremental validity of the MMPI-2-RF over-reporting scales and RBS in assessing the veracity of memory complaints. *Archives of Clinical Neuropsychology*, 25(4), 274–284.

Gill, D., Green, P., Flaro, L., & Pucci, T. (2007). The role of effort testing in independent medical examinations. *The Medico-Legal Journal*, 75(Pt. 2), 64–71.

Gouvier, W. D., Cubic, B., Jones, G., Brantley, P., & Cutlip, Q. (1992). Postconcussion symptoms and daily stress in normal and head-injured college populations. *Archives of Clinical Neuropsychology*, 7(3), 193–211.

Green, P. (2005). *Green's word memory test for Windows: User's manual and program* (Rev. ed.). Edmonton, Canada: Green's Publishing.

Green, P. (2004a). *Green's medical symptom validity test (MSVT) for Microsoft Windows* (user manual). Edmonton, Canada: Green's Publishing.

Green, P. (2004b). *Green's memory complaints inventory (MCI)*. Edmonton, Canada: Green's Publishing.

Green, P. (2008). *Green's non-verbal medical symptom validity test (NV-MSVT) for Microsoft Windows: User's manual 1.0*. Edmonton, Canada: Green's Publishing.

Green, P. (2009). *The advanced interpretation program for the WMT, MSVT, NV-MSVT and MCI*. Edmonton, Canada: Green's Publishing.

Green, P. (2011). Comparison between the Test of Memory Malingering (TOMM) and the Nonverbal Medical Symptom Validity Test (NV-MSVT) in adults with disability claims. *Applied Neuropsychology*, 18(1), 18–26.

Green, P., & Allen, L. M. III. (2000). Patterns of memory complaints in 577 consecutive patients passing or failing symptom validity tests. *Archives of Clinical Neuropsychology*, 15(8), 844–845.

Green, P., Allen, L. M. III & Iverson, G. L. (1999). Utility of the memory complaints inventory for identifying symptom exaggeration in mild to moderate traumatic brain injury. *Archives of Clinical Neuropsychology*, 14(8), 743–744.

Green, P., Gervais, R., & Merten, T. (2005). Das memory complaints inventory (MCI): Gedächtnisstörungen, Beschwerdenschilderung und Leistungsmotivation [The Memory Complaints Inventory (MCI):

Memory impairment, symptom presentation, and test effort.]. *Neurologie and Rehabilitation*, 11, 139–144.

Greene, R. (2000). *The MMPI-2: An interpretive manual* (2nd ed.). Needham Heights, MA: Allyn & Bacon.

Greiffenstein, M. F., Baker, W. J., & Gola, T. (1994). Validation of malingered amnesia measures with a large clinical sample. *Psychological Assessment*, 6, 218–224.

Greve, K. W., & Bianchini, K. J. (2004). Response to Butcher et al., the construct validity of the Lees-Haley Fake-Bad Scale. *Archives of Clinical Neuropsychology*, 19(3), 337–339; author reply 341–345.

Gross, D. P., & Battié, M. C. (2005). Factors influencing results of functional capacity evaluations in workers' compensation claimants with low back pain. *Physical Therapy*, 85(4), 315–322.

Gunstad, J., & Suhr, J. A. (2002). Perception of illness: Nonspecificity of postconcussion syndrome symptom expectation. *Journal of the International Neuropsychological Society*, 8(1), 37–47.

Heilbronner, R. L., Sweet, J. J., Morgan, J. E., Larrabee, G. J., & Millis, S. (2009). American Academy of Clinical Neuropsychology Consensus Conference Statement on the neuropsychological assessment of effort, response bias, and malingering. *The Clinical Neuropsychologist*, 23(7), 1093–1129.

Henry, M., Merten, T., Wolf, S. A., & Harth, S. (2009). Nonverbal Medical Symptom Validity Test performance of elderly healthy adults and clinical neurology patients. *Journal of Clinical and Experimental Neuropsychology*, 32(1), 19–27.

Howe, L. L., Anderson, A. M., Kaufman, D. A., Sachs, B. C., & Loring, D. W. (2007). Characterization of the Medical Symptom Validity Test in evaluation of clinically referred memory disorders clinic patients. *Archives of Clinical Neuropsychology*, 22(6), 753–761.

Howe, L. L., & Loring, D. W. (2009). Classification accuracy and predictive ability of the Medical Symptom Validity Test's dementia profile and general memory impairment profile. *The Clinical Neuropsychologist*, 23(2), 329–342.

Iverson, G. L. (2005). Outcome from mild traumatic brain injury. *Current Opinion in Psychiatry*, 18(3), 301–317.

Iverson, G. L. (2006). Misdiagnosis of the persistent postconcussion syndrome in patients with depression. *Archives of Clinical Neuropsychology*, 21(4), 303–310.

Iverson, G. L., & Lange, R. T. (2003). Examination of "postconcussion-like" symptoms in a healthy sample. *Applied Neuropsychology*, 10(3), 137–144.

Iverson, G. L., Lange, R. T., Brooks, B. L., & Rennison, V. L. (2010). "Good old days" bias following mild traumatic brain injury. *The Clinical Neuropsychologist*, 24(1), 17–37.

Iverson, G. L., Zasler, N. D., & Lange, R. T. (2006). Post-concussive disorder. In N. D. Zasler, D. I. Katz, & R. D. Zafonte (Eds.), *Brain injury medicine: Principles and practice* (pp. 374–385). New York, NY: Demos Medical Publishing.

Jahn, W. T., Cupon, L. N., & Steinbaugh, J. H. (2004). Functional and work capacity evaluation issues. *Journal of Chiropractic Medicine*, 3(1), 1–5.

Jones, B. (1917). *Malingering or the simulation of disease*. London, UK: W. Heinemann.

Kaplan, G. M., Wurtele, S. K., & Gillis, D. (1996). Maximal effort during functional capacity evaluations: An examination of psychological factors. *Archives of Physical Medicine and Rehabilitation*, 77(2), 161–164.

Katz, D. I., Alexander, M. P., & Klein, R. B. (1998). Recovery of arm function in patients with paresis after traumatic brain injury. *Archives of Physical Medicine and Rehabilitation*, 79(5), 488–493.

King, N. S., Crawford, S., Wenden, F. J., Moss, N. E., & Wade, D. T. (1995). The Rivermead Post Concussion Symptoms Questionnaire: A measure of symptoms commonly experienced after head injury and its reliability. *Journal of Neurology*, 242(9), 587–592.

King, P. M., Tuckwell, N., & Barrett, T. E. (1998). A critical review of functional capacity evaluations. *Physical Therapy*, 78(8), 852–866.

Kurlan, R., Brin, M. F., & Fahn, S. (1997). Movement disorder in reflex sympathetic dystrophy: A case proven to be psychogenic by surveillance video monitoring. *Movement Disorders*, 12(2), 243–245.

Lange, R. T., Iverson, G. L., & Rose, A. (2010). Post-concussion symptom reporting and the "good-old-days" bias following mild traumatic brain injury. *Archives of Clinical Neuropsychology*, 25(5), 442–450.

Larrabee, G. J. (1990). Cautions in the use of neuropsychological evaluation in legal settings. *Neuropsychology*, 4(4), 239–247

Larrabee, G. J. (1997). Neuropsychological outcome, post concussion symptoms, and forensic considerations in mild closed head trauma. *Seminars in Clinical Neuropsychiatry*, 2(3), 196–206.

Lasegue, C. (1864). De l'anesthésia et de l'ataxie hystériques. *Archives Generales de Medicine*, 385–402.

Lechner, D. E., Bradbury, S. F., & Bradley, L. A. (1998). Detecting sincerity of effort: A summary of methods and approaches. *Physical Therapy*, 78(8), 867–888.

Lechner, D. E., Roth, D., & Straaton, K. (1991). Functional capacity evaluation in work disability. *Work*, 1, 37–47.

Lees-Haley, P. R. (1992). Neuropsychological complaint base rates of personal injury claimants. *Forensic Reports*, 5, 385–391.

Lees-Haley, P. R., & Brown, R. S. (1993). Neuropsychological complaint base rates of 170 personal injury claimants. *Archives of Clinical Neuropsychology*, 8(3), 203–209

Lees-Haley, P. R., & Fox, D. D. (2004). Commentary on Butcher, Arbisi, Atlis, and McNulty (2003) on the Fake Bad Scale. *Archives of Clinical Neuropsychology*, 19(3), 333–336; author reply 341–335.

Lees-Haley, P. R., Fox, D. D., & Courtney, J. C. (2001). A comparison of complaints by mild brain injury claimants and other claimants describing subjective experiences immediately following their injury. *Archives of Clinical Neuropsychology*, 16(7), 689–695.

Lempert, T., Brandt, T., Dieterich, M., & Huppert, D. (1991). How to identify psychogenic disorders of stance and gait. A video study in 37 patients. *Journal of Neurology*, 238(3), 140–146.

Lemstra, M., Olszynski, W. P., & Enright, W. (2004). The sensitivity and specificity of functional capacity evaluations in determining maximal effort: A randomized trial. *Spine (Phila Pa 1976)*, 29(9), 953–959.

Lezak, M. D., Howieson, D. B., & Loring, D. W. (2004). *Neuropsychological assessment* (4th ed.). New York, NY: Oxford University Press.

LoPiccolo, C. J., Goodkin, K., & Baldewicz, T. T. (1999). Current issues in the diagnosis and management of malingering. *Annals of Medicine*, 31(3), 166–174.

Loring, D. W., Williamson, D. J., Meador, K. J., Wiegand, F., & Hulihan, J. (2011). Topiramate dose effects on cognition: A randomized double-blind study. *Neurology*, 76(2), 131–137.

Lovell, M., Maroon, J., & Collins, M. W. (1990). *ImPACT*. Retrieved from http://www.impacttest.com/

Margoles, M. S. (1990). Clinical assessment and interpretation of abnormal illness behaviour in low back pain, G. Waddell, I. Pilowsky and M. Bond, Pain, 39 (1989) 41–53. *Pain*, 42(2), 258–259.

Martini, D., Sabin, M., Depesa, S., Leal, E., Negrete, T., Sosnoff, J., & Broglio, S. P. (2011). The chronic effects of concussion on gait. *British Journal of Sports Medicine*, 45, 361–362.

McCrea, M. (2008). *Mild traumatic brain injury and postconcussion syndrome: The new evidence base for diagnosis and treatment*. New York, NY: Oxford University Press.

McNeal, D. W., Darling, W. G., Ge, J., Stilwell-Morecraft, K. S., Solon, K. M., Hynes, S. M., . . . Morecraft, R. J. (2010). Selective long-term reorganization of the corticospinal projection from the supplementary motor cortex following recovery from lateral motor cortex injury. *The Journal of Comparative Neurology*, 518(5), 586–621.

Mesnet, E. (1852). Etude des paralysies hysteriques. Paris, France: Rignoux.

Miller, L. J., & Mittenberg W. (1998). Brief cognitive behavioral interventions in mild traumatic brain injury. *Applied Neuropsychology*, 5(4), 172–183.

Millon, T., Davis, R., & Millon, C. (1997). Millon Clinical Multiaxial Inventory-III. Minneapolis, MN: National Computer Systems.

Mittenberg, W., Canyock, E. M., Condit, D., & Patton, C. (2001). Treatment of post-concussion syndrome following mild head injury. *Journal of Clinical and Experimental Neuropsychology*, 23(6), 829–836.

Mittenberg, W., DiGiulio, D. V., Perrin, S., & Bass, A. E. (1992). Symptoms following mild head injury: Expectation as aetiology. *Journal of Neurology, Neurosurgery, and Psychiatry*, 55(3), 200–204.

Mittenberg, W., Patton, C., Canyock, E. M., & Condit, D. C. (2002). Base rates of malingering and symptom exaggeration. *Journal of Clinical and Experimental Neuropsychology*, 24(8), 1094–1102.

Mittenberg, W., Tremont, G., Zielinski, R. E., Fichera, S., & Rayls, K. R. (1996). Cognitive-behavioral prevention of postconcussion syndrome. *Archives of Clinical Neuropsychology*, 11(2), 139–145.

Morey, L. C. (1991). *Personality assessment inventory professional manual*. Odessa, FL: Psychological Assessment Resources.

Nelson, N. W., Sweet, J. J., & Heilbronner, R. L. (2007). Examination of the new MMPI-2 response bias scale (Gervais): Relationship with MMPI-2 validity scales. *Journal of Clinical and Experimental Neuropsychology*, 29(1), 67–72.

Ochoa, J. L., & Verdugo, R. J. (2010). Neuropathic pain syndrome displayed by malingerers. *The Journal of Neuropsychiatry and Clinical Neurosciences*, 22(3), 278–286.

Peckham, E. L., & Hallett, M. (2009). Psychogenic movement disorders. *Neurologic Clinics*, 27(3), 801–819, vii.

Ponsford, J., Willmott, C., Rothwell, A., Cameron, P., Kelly, A. M., Nelms, R., & Curran, C. (2002). Impact of early intervention on outcome following mild head injury in adults. *Journal of Neurology, Neurosurgery, and Psychiatry*, 73(3), 330–332.

Pransky, G. S., & Dempsey, P. G. (2004). Practical aspects of functional capacity evaluations. *Journal of Occupational Rehabilitation*, 14(3), 217–229.

Randolph, C. (2011). Baseline neuropsychological testing in managing sport-related concussion: Does it modify risk? *Current Sports Medicine Reports*, 10(1), 21–26.

Randolph, C., & Kirkwood, M. W. (2009). What are the real risks of sport-related concussion, and are they modifiable? *Journal of the International Neuropsychological Society*, 15(4), 512–520.

Randolph, C., McCrea, M., & Barr, W. B. (2005). Is neuropsychological testing useful in the management of sport-related concussion? *Journal of Athletic Training*, 40(3), 139–152.

Reeves, D., Kane, R., Winter, K., Raynsford, K., & Pancella, T. (1993). *Automated neuropsychological assessment metrics (ANAM): Test administrator's guide, version 1.0.* St. Louis, MO: Missouri Institute of Health.

Resnick, P. (1988). Malingering of posttraumatic disorders. In R. Rogers (Ed.), *Clinical assessment of malingering and deception* (pp. 84–103). New York, NY: Guilford Press.

Rey, A. (1941). L'examen psychologique dans les cas d'encephalopathie traumatique. *Archives de Psychologie*, 28, 286–340.

Richman, J., Green, P., Gervais, R., Flaro, L., Merten, T., Brockhaus, R., & Ranks, D. (2006). Objective tests of symptom exaggeration in independent medical examinations. *Journal of Occupational and Environmental Medicine*, 48(3), 303–311.

Rohling, M. L., Green, P., Allen, L. M. III & Iverson, G. L. (2002). Depressive symptoms and neurocognitive test scores in patients passing symptom validity tests. *Archives of Clinical Neuropsychology*, 17(3), 205–222.

Rondinelli, R. (Ed.). (2007). *Guides to the evaluation of permanent impairment* (6th ed.). Chicago, IL: American Medical Association.

Roy, E. (2003). Functional capacity evaluations and the use of validity testing: What does the evidence tell us? *The Case Manager*, 14(2), 64–69.

Salinsky, M. C., Storzbach, D., Spencer, D. C., Oken, B. S., Landry, T., & Dodrill, C. B. (2005). Effects of topiramate and gabapentin on cognitive abilities in healthy volunteers. *Neurology*, 64(5), 792–798.

Singhal, A., Green, P., Ashaye, K., Shankar, K., & Gill, D. (2009). High specificity of the medical symptom validity test in patients with very severe memory impairment. *Archives of Clinical Neuropsychology*, 24(8), 721–728.

Slick, D., Hopp, G., Strauss, E., & Thompson, G. B. (1997). *Victoria symptom validity test.* Odessa, FL: Psychological Assessment Resources.

Slick, D. J., Sherman, E. M., & Iverson, G. L. (1999). Diagnostic criteria for malingered neurocognitive dysfunction: Proposed standards for clinical practice and research. *The Clinical Neuropsychologist*, 13(4), 545–561.

Smart, C. M., Nelson, N. W., Sweet, J. J., Bryant, F. B., Berry, D. T., Granacher, R. P., & Heilbronner, R. L. (2008). Use of MMPI-2 to predict cognitive effort: A hierarchically optimal classification tree analysis. *Journal of the International Neuropsychological Society*, 14(5), 842–852.

Sodickson, A., Baeyens, P. F., Andriole, K. P., Prevedello, L. M., Nawfel, R. D., Hanson, R., & Khorasani, R. (2009). Recurrent CT, cumulative radiation exposure, and associated radiation-induced cancer risks from CT of adults. *Radiology*, 251(1), 175–184.

Sosnoff, J. J., Broglio, S. P., Shin, S., & Ferrara, M. S. (2011). Previous mild traumatic brain injury and postural-control dynamics. *Journal of Athletic Training*, 46(1), 85–91.

Sreenivasan, S., Eth, S., Kirkish, P., & Garrick, T. (2003). A practical method for the evaluation of symptom exaggeration in minor head trauma among civil litigants. *The Journal of the American Academy of Psychiatry and the Law*, 31(2), 220–231.

Stewart-Patterson, C. (in press). Detection of potential malingering indicators through document review. *IAIABC Journal.*

Strong, S., Baptiste, S., Clarke, J., Cole, D., & Costa, M. (2004). Use of functional capacity evaluations in workplaces and the compensation system: A report on workers' and report users' perceptions. *Work*, 23(1), 67–77.

Suhr, J. A., & Gunstad, J. (2002). Postconcussive symptom report: The relative influence of head injury and depression. *Journal of Clinical and Experimental Neuropsychology*, 24(8), 981–993.

Thompson, P. J., Baxendale, S. A., Duncan, J. S., & Sander, J. W. (2000). Effects of topiramate on cognitive function. *Journal of Neurology, Neurosurgery, and Psychiatry*, 69(5), 636–641.

Tombaugh, T. (1996). *Test of memory malingering.* Los Angeles, CA: Western Psychological Services.

Trueblood, W., & Binder, L. M. (1997). Psychologists' accuracy in identifying neuropsychological test protocols of clinical malingerers. *Archives of Clinical Neuropsychology*, 12(1), 13–27.

Trueblood, W., & Schmidt, M. (1993). Malingering and other validity considerations in the neuropsychological evaluation of mild head injury. *Journal of Clinical and Experimental Neuropsychology*, 15(4), 578–590.

Van Dyke, S. A., Axelrod, B. N., & Schutte, C. (2010). The utility of the post-concussive symptom questionnaire. *Archives of Clinical Neuropsychology*, 25(7), 634–639.

Van Gerpen, J. A. (2011). Office assessment of gait and station. *Seminars in Neurology*, 31(1), 78–84.

Waddell, G. (2004a). *The back pain revolution* (2nd ed.). Edinburgh, UK: Churchill Livingstone.

Waddell, G. (2004b). Nonorganic signs. *Spine (Phila Pa 1976)*, 29, 1393.

Waddell, G., Bircher, M., Finlayson, D., & Main, C. J. (1984). Symptoms and signs: physical disease or illness behaviour? *British Medical Journal (Clinical Research Edition)*, 289(6447), 739–741.

Waddell, G., Main, C. J., Morris, E. W., Di Paola, M., & Gray, I. C. (1984). Chronic low-back pain, psychologic distress, and illness behavior. *Spine (Phila Pa 1976)*, 9(2), 209–213.

Waddell, G., McCulloch, J. A., Kummel, E., & Venner, R. M. (1980). Nonorganic physical signs in low-back pain. *Spine (Phila Pa 1976)*, 5(2), 117–125.

Waddell, G., Pilowsky, I., & Bond, M. (1990). Non-anatomical symptoms and signs: A response to critics. *Pain*, 42(2), 260–261.

Wager, J. G., & Howe, L. L. (2010). Nonverbal medical symptom validity test: Try faking now! *Applied Neuropsychology*, 17(4), 305–309.

Wang, Y., Chan, R. C., & Deng, Y. (2006). Examination of postconcussion-like symptoms in healthy university students: Relationships to subjective and objective neuropsychological function performance. *Archives of Clinical Neuropsychology*, 21(4), 339–347.

Werneke, M. W., Harris, D. E., & Lichter, R. L. (1993). Clinical effectiveness of behavioral signs for screening chronic low-back pain patients in a work-oriented physical rehabilitation program. *Spine (Phila Pa 1976)*, 18(16), 2412–2418.

Westbrook, A. P., Tredgett, M. W., Davis, T. R., & Oni, J. A. (2002). The rapid exchange grip strength test and the detection of submaximal grip effort. *The Journal of Hand Surgery*, 27(2), 329–333.

Whitney, K. A., Davis, J. J., Shepard, P. H., & Herman, S. M. (2008). Utility of the response bias scale (RBS) and other MMPI-2 validity scales in predicting TOMM performance. *Archives of Clinical Neuropsychology*, 23(7–8), 777–786.

Williams, C. L., Butcher, J. N., Gass, C. S., Cumella, E., & Kally, Z. (2009). Inaccuracies about the MMPI-2 fake bad scale in the reply by Ben-Porath, Greve, Bianchini, and Kaufman (2009). *Psychological Injury and Law*, 2, 181–197.

Assessing Noncredible Attention, Processing Speed, Language, and Visuospatial/Perceptual Function in Mild Traumatic Brain Injury Cases

12

Tara L. Victor, Alexis D. Kulick, & Kyle Brauer Boone

Traumatic brain injury (TBI) is highly prevalent, and most of these injuries are considered mild TBIs (MTBIs; Bazarian, McClung, Shah, Cheng, Flesher, & Kraus, 2005; Lezak, Howeison & Loring, 2004; Sosin, Sniezek, & Thurman, 1996). Approximately 5% of these patients continue to complain of persisting postconcussive symptoms (Greiffenstein, 2009; Iverson, 2005; McCrea, 2008). Although the exact number of combat-related TBIs is unknown (see Chapter 18), the U.S. military involvement in Iraq and Afghanistan has further increased rates of MTBI.

Although TBI has long been known to cause functional damage that is proportional to the severity of the injury and inversely proportional to the amount of time elapsed since the injury, meta-analytic research has repeatedly shown that individuals with a single-event uncomplicated MTBI do not exhibit chronic cognitive changes on formal testing (e.g., 133 studies, *n* = 1,463 [Belanger, Curtiss, Demery, Lebowitz, & Vanderploeg, 2005]; 21 studies, *n* = 790 [Belanger & Vanderploeg, 2005]; 120 studies [Carroll et al., 2004]; 17 studies, *n* = 634 [Frencham, Fox, & Maybery, 2005]; 39 studies, *n* = 1,716 [Schretlen & Shapiro, 2003]) unless there is some other comorbid neurological event (e.g., multiple sclerosis; see Meyers, 2007). In fact, resolution of symptoms typically occurs between 1 week and 3 months in most people and even faster in young healthy athletes (McCrea, 2008).

There are a myriad of other social-cognitive (e.g., the "good old days" bias; Iverson, Lange, Brooks, & Rennison, 2010) and psychological factors (e.g., somatization; Lamberty, 2007) in addition to other complicating factors (e.g., secondary gain; Belanger et al., 2005; Bianchini, Curtis & Greve, 2006; Binder & Rohling, 1996; Binder, Rohling, & Larrabee, 1997) associated with these injuries that can influence both symptom reporting and the level of effort individuals put forth during evaluations. Binder and Rohling clarified the role of secondary gain on symptom reporting, concluding "complaints associated with closed-head injury would decrease by 23%" if secondary gain was eliminated (p. 9). Likewise, Belanger and colleagues (2005) identified litigation and malingering as the strongest factors associated with persisting cognitive complaints by patients with a history of MTBI. Indeed, the highest base rate of malingering is in personal injury litigants alleging MTBI (approximately 40%; Larrabee, 2007). Further, there is ample evidence that normal community-dwelling individuals have knowledge of the impairments associated with head injury (Suhr & Gunstad, 2000) and can "fake" a pattern of scores characteristic of brain injury (albeit often more extensive than expected for the severity of injury; Meyers, 2007). When an individual with a history of MTBI exhibits performance dispro-portionately deficient to the level of injury, neuropsychologists must attempt to de-termine what factors (cognitive, psychological, secondary gain, or otherwise) are underlying the discrepancy. Thorough assessment of such factors is critical to inform accurate diagnosis and guide treatment.

Approximately 50% of the variance in neuropsychological test performance is accounted for by motivation or effort (Green, Rohling, Lees-Haley, & Allen, 2001; Meyers, Volbrecht, Axelrod, & Reinsch-Boothby, 2011; Rohling & Demakis, 2010). The validity and reliability of the initial neuropsychological assessment, therefore, depends greatly on the inclusion of effort testing (i.e., "symptom validity tests" [SVTs]; Boone, 2007) to minimize diagnostic errors. If neuropsychologists cannot ensure the veracity of the test results, then appropriate diagnostic decisions or mean-ingful treatment recommendations cannot be made. Tests specifically designed to identify faking or exaggeration of cognitive symptoms have primarily focused on documenting feigned impairments in short-term memory (e.g., Iverson, 1995; Levin, 1990; Niogi et al., 2008; Sim, Terryberry-Spohr, & Wilson, 2008), as effort was histori-cally viewed as a unitary construct that could be adequately sampled by inserting one or two memory-based measures of response bias during a neuropsychological exam. Although memory-based SVT failures are, indeed, the most frequent failures made by individuals attempting to feign cognitive deficits (e.g., Meyers et al., 2011), other non–memory-based SVTs are often failed as well or instead of memory effort measures.

Failure on tests that appear to measure different cognitive abilities than memory is consistent with emerging data that show test takers motivated to underperform on exams and may adopt differing strategies (Boone, 2009; Larrabee, 2004; Nitch, Boone, Wen, Arnold, & Alfano, 2006; Tan, Slick, Strauss, & Hultsch, 2002; see Meyers, 2007 for a review), with only 16% failing in all measures of response bias adminis-tered (Boone, 2009). In particular, some individuals exaggerate or feign deficits only in one or two specific cognitive domains, and it is usually the domains within which they are reporting symptoms (Boone, 2009). For example, Osmon, Plambeck, Klein, and Mano (2006) observed that simulators feigning reading impairment were better detected by a test specifically developed to identify feigned reading deficits than by a commonly used verbal memory effort indicator (i.e., Word Memory Test). Additional cases have been reported showing that individuals feigning verbal memory impair-ment may not be detected by visual memory effort measures (e.g., Test of Memory Malingering [TOMM], Rey 15-item), and individuals feigning visuoperceptual, spa-tial, and memory deficits are not necessarily captured by some verbal memory effort indicators (e.g., Rey Word Recognition Test; Boone, 2009). Analogue studies suggest that feigning attention deficits and processing delays are the two most common types of faking strategies after feigned amnesia (Tan et al., 2002). In combination with the fact that a patient's effort can fluctuate significantly over the course of an evaluation for a host of reasons (Boone, 2009), several SVTs within various cognitive domains should be included in a given neuropsychological battery.

Techniques have been validated to identify feigned cognitive symptoms in do-mains other than memory including, but not limited to, tests of simple attention (e.g., digit span [DSp]; Babikian, Boone, Lu, & Arnold, 2006; Iverson & Franzen, 1994, 1996), mental speed or calculation ability (e.g., Dot Counting Test [DCT]; Boone, Lu & Herzberg, 2002b), and recognition of overlearned and highly familiar informa-tion (e.g., b Test; Boone, Lu & Herzberg, 2002a). Although other chapters in this edition have addressed both freestanding and embedded methods for assessing non-credible presentations of memory dysfunction in MTBI cases, in the next two chapters, we review several methods for assessing noncredible presentations in domains *other than* memory, that is, from the domains of attention, processing speed, language, visuoperceptual/spatial, motor, sensory, and executive functioning. In fact, it is with our strongest recommendation that clinicians routinely use nonmemory measures of effort dispersed throughout a test battery to ensure adequate and thorough sampling of effort in the testing situation (Boone, 2009; Larrabee, 2004; Rohling & Boone, 2007). This broad sampling allows neuropsychologists to assess for a wider range of approaches that an individual might use when attempting to perform poorly on a neuropsychological evaluation.

In this chapter, we organize our review of the extant literature regarding use of these methods by the cognitive domains of attention, processing speed, language, and visuospatial/perceptual function, reviewing in detail only those studies that include at least a subsample of patients with MTBI. Chapter 13 reviews methods in the cognitive domains of motor, sensory, and executive function, as well as those derived from full test batteries. In both chapters, we review simulation (i.e., studies employing analogue designs where there is one noninjured normal group of subjects who are instructed to feign a head injury or cognitive impairment without detection), "known groups" (i.e., studies employing knowledge of incentive and independent measures of effort as criteria for assigning subjects to groups), specificity (i.e., studies examining the false positive rate associated with various cut scores in different clinical groups), and mixed, or hybrid, study designs where appropriate and when data are available. It is obvious that the extent to which authors adequately described their TBI samples, how they defined MTBI, and the extent to which they analyzed MTBI subjects separately are of critical importance as to the conclusions that can be drawn from this review.

ATTENTION

Attention refers to many different, but related, aspects of what it means to become aware of, and process, internal and external stimuli (Lezak et al., 2004). Although selective, sustained, divided, and alternating types of attention are more vulnerable to brain injury, simple immediate attention "is a relatively effortless process that tends to be resistant to the effects of aging and of many brain disorders" (Lezak et al., 2004, p. 34). Thus, tasks of simple attention such as the Digit Span (DSp) subtest from the Wechsler scales—Wechsler Adult Intelligence Scale-Revised (WAIS-R; Wechsler, 1981), WAIS-III (Wechsler, 1997a), WAIS-IV (Wechsler, 2008a), Wechsler Memory Scale-Revised (WMS-R; Wechsler, 1987), WMS-III (Wechsler, 1997b), and WMS-IV (Wechsler, 2008b)—have proven helpful in assessing symptom validity within the context of neuropsychological evaluation.

DSp is a measure of attention and concentration in which the respondent is asked to immediately repeat increasingly longer strings of numbers read aloud in the same order in which they are presented (digits forward) and in the reverse order (digits backward). Research has indicated that individuals who have brain damage resulting from multiple etiologies, including moderate and severe TBIs, demonstrate relatively normal scores on this subtest (Black, 1986; Capruso & Levin, 1992). Therefore, this subtest has been found to be one of the most widely used embedded measure of response bias. Several scores from the DSp subtest have been identified as effective indices of noncredible performance. These scores include age-corrected scaled score (ACSS; Iverson & Franzen, 1994, 1996; Suhr, Tranel, Wefel, & Barrash, 1997); reliable digit span (RDS; Greiffenstein, Baker, & Gola, 1994); and vocabulary minus DSp difference scores (Millis, Ross, & Ricker, 1998; Mittenberg et al., 2001).

Other aspects of performance on DSp performance have also been investigated such as timed scores on digits forward (Babikian et al., 2006) and combined maximum forward and backward span (Heinly, Greve, Bianchini, Love, & Brennan, 2005). In the following section, we review each one in turn.

Digit Span: Age-Corrected Scaled Score

The DSp ACSS has been shown to be useful in identifying persons who may be demonstrating noncredible performance. Babikian and Boone (2007) and Suhr and Barrash (2007) reviewed all studies investigating DSp ACSS as an SVT up to 2006. These authors reviewed WAIS-R DSp ACSS including both simulation (Bernard, 1990; Demakis, 2004; Heaton, Smith, Lehman, & Vogt, 1978; Iverson & Franzen, 1994, 1996; Klimczak, Donovick, & Burright, 1997; Mittenberg, Theroux-Fichera, Zielinski, & Heilbronner, 1995; Shum, O'Gorman, & Alpar, 2004, for WMS-R) and known groups (Rawlings & Brooks, 1990; Suhr et al., 1997; Trueblood & Schmidt, 1993; Trueblood, 1994) designs, as well as WAIS-III DSp ACSS simulation (Mittenberg et al., 2001; Schwarz, Gfeller, & Oliveri, 2006), known groups (Axelrod, Fichtenberg, Millis, & Wertheimer, 2006; Babikian et al., 2006; Heinly et al., 2005; Youngjohn, Burrows, & Erdal, 1995), and specificity (Iverson & Tulsky, 2003) study designs. The known groups studies, cut scores, and associated classification accuracy data, where available for MTBI specifically, are summarized in Table 12.1.

The authors of these reviews concluded that DSp ACSS can be useful in screening for noncredible performance in patients presenting with MTBI; however, the sensitivity values associated with established cutoffs from simulation studies appear to be higher than those seen in real clinical samples. For example, for a cut score of ACSS < 4, Iverson and Franzen (1994, 1996) obtained sensitivity estimates ranging from 78% to 83% in simulators, whereas that cutoff produced sensitivity values less than 30% in real MTBI samples (i.e., 25%, Axelrod et al., 2006; 28%, Heinly et al., 2005). Fortunately, higher cutoffs that maintain adequate specificity can be employed with actual MTBI patients. For ACSS as an example, a cutoff of ≤ 6 was associated with sensitivity values from 50% to 80% and specificity values from 83% to 90% (Axelrod et al., 2006; Heinly et al., 2005; Trueblood, 1994; Trueblood & Schmidt, 1993). The same cut score (≤ 6) resulted in ≥ 90% specificity in all of the Iverson and Tulsky (2003) clinical groups except left temporal lobectomy (12.5% false positive rate).

Reliable Digit Span

Greiffenstein and colleagues (1994) introduced the notion of using RDS as a measure of poor effort. RDS is calculated by adding the longest string of digits forward and digits backward in which both trials are passed. Babikian and Boone (2007) and Suhr and Barrash (2007) reviewed all studies investigating RDS as a SVT up to 2006. They summarized WAIS-R RDS including both simulation (Inman & Berry, 2002) and known groups (Greiffenstein et al., 1994; Greiffenstein, Gola, & Baker, 1995; Meyers & Volbrecht, 1998) designs, as well as WAIS-III RDS simulation (Schwarz et al., 2006; Strauss et al., 1999; Strauss et al., 2002) and known groups (Babikian et al., 2006; Larrabee, 2003; Mathias, Greve, Bianchini, Houston, & Crouch, 2002; Meyers & Volbrecht, 2003) designs. The known groups studies that included at least a subsample of MTBI are summarized in Table 12.1; cut scores and associated classification accuracy data are provided where available.

Since the publication of the aforementioned reviews, the WAIS-III RDS was reexamined by Larrabee (2008) in his paper on aggregation of effort indicators. In

TABLE 12.1 Known Groups Studies of Symptom Validity Test Effectiveness Within the Domain of Attention in Mild Traumatic Brain Injury

Study	Sample	Test/Score	Cut Score	Sensitivity	Specificity		
		DSp ACSS					
Trueblood & Schmidt (1993)	Patients with definite MND MTBI (n = 8) Patients with probable MND MTBI (n = 8) Demographically matched controls (n = 16)	WAIS-R DSp ACSS	< 7	63% (definite) 75% (probable)	93.8% (matched MTBI controls) 85% (larger sample of credible MTBI)		
Trueblood (1994)	Patients with definite MTBI (n = 12) Patients with MND (n = 10) Demographically matched controls (n = 22)	WAIS-R DSp ACSS	< 7	75% (definite) 80% (probable)	86%		
Suhr et al. (1997)	Probable malingering (PM) patients with MTBI (n = 31) Litigating patients with MTBI (n = 31) Nonlitigating mild/ moderate TBI (n = 20) Nonlitigating severe TBI (n = 15) Patients with somatization disorder (n = 29) Patients who are depressed (n = 30)	WAIS-R DSp ACSS	< 5	"modest sensitivity"; no value provided	85%–100%		
Heinly et al. (2005)	Patients with MND MTBI (n = 48) Credible patients with MTBI (n = 77) Credible patients with moderate-to-severe TBI (n = 69) General clinical patients (n = 1063)	WAIS-III DSp ACSS	≤ 7 ≤ 6 ≤ 5 ≤ 4	80% 62% 41% 28%	MTBI 74% 90% 94% 100%	Mod/sev 79% 89% 92% 100%	Clin 71% 85% 90% 96%
Axelrod et al. (2006)	Patients with MND MTBI (n = 36) Credible litigating patients with MTBI (n = 22) Credible nonlitigating patients with moderate-to-severe TBI (n = 29)	WAIS-III DSp ACSS	≤ 7 ≤ 6 ≤ 5 ≤ 4 ≤ 3	75% 50% 36% 25% 8%	MTBI 77%	All TBI 69% 83% 97% 97% 100%	

(Continued)

TABLE 12.1 Known Groups Studies of Symptom Validity Test Effectiveness Within the Domain of Attention in Mild Traumatic Brain Injury (Continued)

Study	Sample	Test/Score	Cut Score	Sensitivity	Specificity		
		RDS					
Greiffenstein et al. (1994)	PM (n = 43) Patients with PPCS (n = 30) Credible patients with moderate-to-severe TBI (n = 33)	WAIS-R RDS	≤ 8 ≤ 7	82% 68%–70%	PPCS 69% 89%	Mod/sev 54% 73%	
Greiffenstein et al. (1995)	PM (n = 68) Patients with PPCS (n = 53) Credible patients with moderate-to-severe TBI (n = 56)	WAIS-R RDS	≤ 7	86–89%	PPCS 68%	Mod/sev 57%	
Meyers & Volbrecht (1998)	Litigating patients with MTBI (n = 47) Nonlitigating patients with MTBI (n = 49)	WAIS-R RDS	≤ 7	49%	96%		
Mathias et al. (2002)	Patients with MND TBI (75% of whom were classified as MTBI; n = 24) Credible patients with TBI (34% of whom were classified as MTBI; n = 30)	WAIS-R and WAIS-III RDS	≤ 5 ≤ 6 ≤ 7 ≤ 8	21% 38% 67% 88%	100% 97% 93% 80%		
Larrabee (2003)	Patients with MND (79% of whom were MTBI; n = 24) Credible patients[a] with moderate-to-severe TBI (n = 31)	WAIS-R RDS	≤ 7	50%	94%		
Heinly et al. (2005)	Patients with MND MTBI (n = 48) Credible patients with MTBI (n = 77) Credible patients with moderate-to-severe TBI (n = 69) General clinical patients (n = 1,063)	WAIS-III RDS	≤ 7 ≤ 6 ≤ 5 ≤ 4	71% 46% 27% 15%	MTBI 83% 93% 100% 100%	Mod/sev 91% 99% 100% 100%	Clin 58% 74% 89% 93%
Larrabee (2008)	Patients with MND (n = 26; 81% of whom were MTBI) Credible patients with moderate-to-severe TBI (n = 31)	WAIS-III RDS	≤ 7	50%	93.5%		

(Continued)

TABLE 12.1 Known Groups Studies of Symptom Validity Test Effectiveness Within the Domain of Attention in Mild Traumatic Brain Injury (*Continued*)

Study	Sample	Test/Score	Cut Score	Sensitivity	Specificity		
		V-DS					
Millis et al. (1998)	PM patients with MTBI (*n* = 50) Credible patients with moderate-to-severe TBI (*n* = 50)	WAIS-R V-DS	≥ 2	72%	86%		
Mittenberg et al. (2001)	PM (*n* = 36) Nonlitigating patients with TBI (19% of whom were mild; *n* = 36) Noninjured simulators (*n* = 36)	WAIS-III V-DS	≥ 2	55.6 (simulators) 25% (PM)	86%		
Greve et al. (2003)	Patients with MND TBI (*n* = 28; 79% of whom were MTBI) Credible, non-litigating patients with TBI (*n* = 37; 43% of whom were MTBI)	WAIS-R V-DS WAIS-III V-DS Across both versions	≥ 2 ≥ 3 ≥ 4 ≥ 2 ≥ 3 ≥ 4 ≥ 2 ≥ 3 ≥ 4	MTBI only 13% 0% 0% 36% 29% 21% 27% 18% 14%	MTBI 82% 82% 82% 80% 80% 100% 81% 81% 88%	Mod/sev 100% 100% 100% 69% 77% 77% 81% 86% 86%	
Mittenberg et al. (2005)	PM patients with MTBI (*n* = 59) Credible patients with moderate-to-severe TBI (*n* = 59)	WAIS-III V-DS DFA	> 0	76%	75%		
Curtis et al. (2009)	Patients with MND MTBI (*n* = 31) Credible patients with MTBI (*n*=26) Credible patients with moderate/severe TBI (*n* = 26) General clinical patients (*n* = 80)	V-DS	No significant group differences				
		Other DSp variables					
Heinly et al. (2005)	Patients with MND MTBI (*n* = 48) Credible patients with MTBI (*n* = 77) Credible patients with moderate-to-severe TBI (*n* = 69)	WAIS-III MSF2 MSF1	≤ 2 ≤ 3 ≤ 4 ≤ 3 ≤ 4 ≤ 5	4% 29% 67% 6% 35% 67%	MTBI 100% 96% 83% 100% 96% 80%	Mod/sev 100% 100% 94% 100% 99% 81%	Clin 98% 92% 67% 98% 87% 63%

(*Continued*)

TABLE 12.1 Known Groups Studies of Symptom Validity Test Effectiveness Within the Domain of Attention in Mild Traumatic Brain Injury *(Continued)*

Study	Sample	Test/Score	Cut Score	Sensitivity	Specificity		
		Other DSp variables					
Heinly et al. (2005)	General clinical patients (*n* = 1,063)	MFB	≤ 6	17%	MTBI	Mod/sev	Clin
					100%	100%	90%
			≤ 7	35%	97%	97%	81%
			≤ 8	54%	88%	90%	66%
		MSB2	0	10%	100%	100%	90%
			≤ 2	46%	92%	91%	59%
			≤ 3	83%	61%	61%	28%
		MSB1	0	4%	100%	100%	94%
			≤ 2	21%	99%	94%	79%
			≤ 3	58%	83%	81%	47%
		Working Memory Index					
Curtis et al. (2009)	Patients with MND MTBI (*n* = 31)	Standard score	< 65	19%	MTBI	Mod/sev	Clin
					100%	100%	92%
	Credible patients with MTBI (*n* = 26)		< 70	26%	96%	96%	90%
			< 75	48%	88%	88%	77%
	Credible patients with moderate-to-severe TBI (*n* = 26)		< 80	61%	85%	81%	67%
			< 85	77%	77%	77%	57%
	General clinical patients (*n* = 80)						
		TOVA					
Henry (2005)	Patients with MND MTBI (*n* = 26)	Omission errors	≥ 3	89%	81%		
			≥ 4	81%	85%		
	Credible patients with MTBI (*n* = 26)		≥ 5	81%	85%		
			≥ 6	81%	85%		
			≥ 7	77%	89%		
			≥ 8	69%	92%		
			≥ 9	65%	96%		
		CPT-II					
Ord et al. (2010)	Patients with MND MTBI (*n* = 27)	Omission errors	> 45	26%	MTBI	Mod/sev	
					100%	100%	
	Credible patients with MTBI (*n* = 31)		> 40	26%	97%	100%	
			> 35	30%	97%	100%	
	Credible patients with moderate-to-severe TBI (*n* = 24)		> 30	33%	94%	96%	
			> 25	41%	90%	96%	
			> 20	41%	90%	96%	
			> 15	56%	87%	96%	
		Hit reaction time SE	> 28	11%	100%	100%	
			> 24	22%	97%	100%	
			> 20	33%	97%	100%	
			> 16	41%	97%	96%	
			> 14	52%	90%	92%	
			> 12	59%	84%	87%	

(Continued)

TABLE 12.1 Known Groups Studies of Symptom Validity Test Effectiveness Within the Domain of Attention in Mild Traumatic Brain Injury *(Continued)*

Study	Sample	Test/Score	Cut Score	Sensitivity	Specificity
		SRT			
Trueblood & Schmidt (1993)	Patients with definite MND MTBI (*n* = 8) Patients with probable MND MTBI (*n* = 8) Demographically matched controls (*n* = 16)	Total errors	≥ 9	63% (definite) 50% (probable)	100% (matched MTBI controls) 80% (larger sample of credible MTBI)
Ross et al. (2006)	PM patients with MTBI (*n* = 46) Credible patients with TBI (*n* = 49; 62% mild, 38% moderate-to-severe)	Total errors	≥ 8 ≥ 9 ≥ 10 ≥ 13	76% 70% 59% 30%	74% 86% 92% 98%
Curtis et al. (2010)	Patients with MND MTBI (*n* = 27) Credible patients with MTBI (*n* = 24) Credible patients with moderate-to-severe TBI (*n* = 23) General clinical patients (*n* = 90)	Total errors	≥ 7 ≥ 8 ≥ 9 ≥ 10 ≥ 15	52% 44% 41% 37% 11%	MTBI Mod/sev Clin 79% 65% 61% 87% 74% 69% 87% 83% 73% 96% 83% 76% 100% 91% 89%
		SSPT			
Trueblood & Schmidt (1993)	Patients with definite MND MTBI (*n* = 8) Patients with probable MND MTBI (*n* = 8) Demographically matched controls (*n* = 16)	Total errors	≥ 17	88% (Definite) 38% (probable)	94% (matched MTBI controls) 96% (larger sample of credible MTBI)
Ross et al. (2006)	PM patients with MTBI (*n* = 46) Credible patients with moderate/severe TBI (*n* = 49; 62% mild, 38% moderate/severe)	Total errors	≥ 17 ≥ 13	63% 70%	98% 90%

(Continued)

particular, his sample consisted of 26 individuals diagnosed with malingered neuro-cognitive dysfunction (MND; i.e., they performed below chance on the Portland Digit Recognition Test [PDRT] and had an identifiable external incentive to perform poorly on exam), 21 of whom had alleged MTBI (defined as no documented loss of consciousness [LOC] or posttraumatic amnesia [PTA], and negative neuroimaging). This sample was compared to 31 credible subjects with moderate-to-severe TBI. With respect to their performance on the RDS, a cutoff score of ≤ 7 maintained adequate specificity (i.e., 93.5%) with sensitivity at 50%.

Suhr and Barrash (2007) concluded that RDS "has been well validated in many diverse samples and across different research designs" (p. 136). Babikian and Boone

TABLE 12.1 Known Groups Studies of Symptom Validity Test Effectiveness Within the Domain of Attention in Mild Traumatic Brain Injury (*Continued*)

Study	Sample	Test/Score	Cut Score	Sensitivity	Specificity		
		SSPT					
Curtis et al. (2010)	Patients with MND MTBI (*n* = 27)	Total errors			MTBI	Mod/Sev	Clin
			≥ 17	44%	100%	78%	84%
	Credible patients with MTBI (*n* = 24)		≥ 15	55%	96%	74%	77%
			≥ 13	59%	96%	74%	
	Credible patients with moderate/severe TBI (*n* = 23)		≥ 12	59%	92%	74%	63%
			≥ 11	67%	77%	65%	57%
	Credible general patients (*n* = 90)						

Note. ACSS = age-corrected scale score; Clin = credible clinical group; CPT-II = Conners' Continuous Performance Test-2nd edition; DFA = discriminant function analysis; DSp = digit span; MND = malingered neurocognitive dysfunction; MFB = combined maximum forward and backward span; MSB1 = maximum span backward; MSB2 = maximum span backward both trials correct; MSF1 = maximum span forward; MSF2 = maximum span forward both trials correct; MTBI = mild traumatic brain injury; Mod/sev = credible moderate-to-severe TBI; PM = probable malingerers; PPCS = persistent postconcussive syndrome; RDS = reliable digit span; SE = standard error; SRT = Seashore Rhythm Test; SSPT = Speech-Sounds Perception Test; SVT = Symptom Validity Test; TBI = traumatic brain injury; TOVA = Test of Variable Attention; V-DS = vocabulary minus DSp; WAIS-R = Wechsler Adult Intelligence Scale-Revised; WAIS-III = Wechsler Adult Intelligence Scale-3rd edition.

[a] Some of the credible moderate-to-severe TBI group were in litigation; however, litigants and nonlitigants did not differ on standard cognitive tests so they were collapsed into one group.

(2007) concurred, explaining that a cutoff of ≤ 7 would indicate symptom invalidity in patients with MTBI, especially in the presence of other supporting evidence. However, in light of relatively poor specificity rates in general clinical patient samples, consideration of comorbid medical and/or psychiatric factors must be made. Babikian and Boone (ibid) stated that an RDS cutoff of ≤ 7 may only have adequate specificity in nonlitigating patients with MTBI without comorbid illness (89%–96%; Greiffenstein et al., 1995; Meyers & Volbrecht, 1998). Lowering the cutoff decreases sensitivity (Heinly et al., 2005; Mathias et al., 2002) but assures adequate specificity depending on the clinical situation.

Vocabulary Minus Digit Span

Similar to the DSp subtest, the vocabulary subtest from the WAIS-R and WAIS-III has been shown to be relatively resistant to decline in central nervous system (CNS) dysfunction and normal aging (Lezak et al., 2004; Mitrushina, Boone, Razani & D'Elia, 2005). Mittenberg, Theroux-Fichera, Zielinski, & Heilbronner (1995) discovered that suppressed DSp performance relative to vocabulary subtest performance on the WAIS-R could be used to identify biased responding. They calculated a difference score by subtracting DSp ACSS from vocabulary ACSS (V-DS).

Babikian and Boone (2007) and Larrabee (2007) reviewed all studies investigating V-DS as a SVT up to 2006. The authors reviewed simulation (Demakis, 2004; Mittenberg et al., 1995 [WAIS-R]; Schwarz et al., 2006; Strauss et al., 2002), known groups (Babikian et al., 2006; Greve, Bianchini, Mathias, Houston, & Crouch, 2003; Millis et al., 1998; Mittenberg, Roberts, Patton, & Legler, 2005), mixed (Mittenberg et al., 2001; WAIS-III), and specificity (Axelrod & Rawlings, 1999; Miller, Ryan, Carruthers, & Cluff, 2004) study designs. Limitations of some of these studies included failing to present classification accuracy rates by severity in their TBI samples and including samples of veterans reportedly without incentive to feign (e.g., Miller et al., 2004), which is typically not the case, given the Veterans Affairs (VA) context has inherent incentives to present as impaired (e.g., securing treatment, establishing service connection; Vanderploeg & Belanger, 2009). For the known groups and mixed studies with at least a subsample of patients with MTBI, cut scores and associated classification accuracy data are summarized in Table 12.1.

Since the review chapters referenced previously, Curtis, Greve, and Bianchini (2009) investigated the classification accuracy of V-DSp and other WAIS-III variables in a known groups design with MTBI subjects. In particular, these authors compared (a) credible patients with MTBI ($n = 26$); (b) patients with MTBI who met Slick, Sherman, and Iverson's (1999) criteria for MND ($n = 31$); (c) credible patients with moderate-to-severe TBI ($n = 26$); and (d) a general clinical, noncompensation-seeking, patient comparison group ($n = 80$). MTBI was defined as PTA $<$ 24 hrs, Glasgow Coma Scale [GCS] $\geq$ 13, LOC $\leq$ 30 min, negative neuroimaging, and no focal neurological signs. The V-DSp failed to differentiate malingering from nonmalingering patients with MTBI in this study.

In summary, a V-DSp cutoff of $\geq$ 2 has been associated with sensitivity values ranging from 63% to 86% and low specificity values from 63% to 79% in simulation studies (Mittenberg et al., 2001; Schwarz et al., 2006). In known groups studies evaluating litigating patients with MTBI suspected of malingering, a cutoff of $\geq$ 2 yields sensitivity values ranging from 36% to 72%, specificity values ranged from 80% to 86% in credible patients with TBI of all severities (Millis et al., 1998; Mittenberg et al., 2001; Greve et al., 2003), and from 80% to 82% in credible MTBI populations specifically (Greve et al., 2003). However, specificity rates for this cutoff are lower in patients with acute TBI who exhibit a higher false positive rate (i.e., 30%; Axelrod & Rawlings, 1999).

Consistent with this high rate of false positives, Iverson and Tulsky (2003) examined the standardization and clinical samples of the WAIS-III and found that a V-DSp difference score of $>$ 2 occurred in 21% of the former and in 14% of the moderate-to-severe TBI clinical sample ($n = 22$). More recent data suggest that V-DSp is unable to effectively distinguish MND from non-MND in MTBI cases specifically (Curtis et al., 2009), which leads to questions about the use of this particular SVT. This finding is consistent with data from our group, suggesting that V-DSp is relatively insensitive to MND in a general clinical population, and that the sensitivity of this score appears to depend too heavily on education. That is, V-DSp is only sensitive to MND in individuals of higher education (i.e., individuals of more education will have higher vocabulary scores and, therefore, likely higher discrepancies between vocabulary and DSp performance compared to their lower education counterparts; Victor, Boone, Dean, Zeller, & Hess, 2007), although this pattern is difficult to interpret because overall IQ is suppressed as well when the individual is feigning on WAIS subtests. Nevertheless, Greve and colleagues (2003) found that V-DSp was much more sensitive in their higher IQ group (high IQ sensitivity = 50%, specificity = 84%; low IQ sensitivity = 5%, specificity = 92%), which is also consistent with this hypothesis.

Additional Digit Span Indicators

In addition to ACSS, RDS, and V-DSp, other elements of DSp performance have been the focus of research. Babikian and Boone (2007) and Suhr and Barrash (2007) reviewed the available literature up to 2006 summarizing simulation (DSp forward and backward; Iverson & Franzen, 1994, 1996), DSp total raw score (Martin, Hayes, &

Gouvier, 1996), DSp forward and backward (Schwarz et al., 2006), known groups (DSp forward, longest digits forward and backward, average time for three- and four-digit strings; Babikian et al., 2006; longest digits forward and backward: Binder & Willis, 1991), and specificity study designs (Axelrod & Rawlings, 1999; Iverson & Tulsky, 2003). The Heinly and colleagues (2005) study provides the most extensive data because it relates to using other DSp variables as SVTs in MTBI specifically. The DSp indices, cut scores, and associated classification accuracy data are presented in Table 12.1. Results are consistent with those of Iverson and Tulsky's (2003) specificity study; a longest span forward score of ≤ 4 was associated with ≥ 90% specificity in all of their clinical comparison groups, including patients with Alzheimer's disease. This cut score also appears to best classify credible and noncredible MTBI groups in the Heinly and colleagues study. Likewise, longest span backward of ≤ 2 best classifies both credible and noncredible MTBI groups in the Heinly and colleagues (ibid) study and also occurred in approximately 5% or less in Iverson and Tulsky's (ibid) normal and clinical groups. However, notably, this cut score was associated with only 79% specificity in Heinly and colleagues general clinical comparison group.

Finally, a study of particular note is that of Babikian and colleagues (2006) who observed that noncredible patients often paused to demonstrate effortful retrieval of digits; they examined the time it took for respondents to recite digits forward as a possible indicator of suboptimal effort. Three samples were investigated: (a) 66 litigating patients demonstrating noncredible performance (according to Slick et al., 1999 criteria), 28 of whom were diagnosed with TBI (the large majority were MTBI); (b) 56 nonlitigating patients, 13 of whom were diagnosed with TBIs (all were moderate-to-severe TBI); and (c) 32 controls. Forward span time cut scores (average time for completing a three-digit string is > 2 min, average time for completing a four-digit string is > 4 min, and average time per digit for all items attempted is > 1 min) were associated with respective sensitivity rates in 66 noncredibles of 38% (39% in TBI), 37% (28% in TBI), and 50% (50% in TBI) at specificity ≥ 89%.

In summary, the various effort indices derived from the DSp subtests appear to have moderate sensitivity when cutoffs are set to levels that minimize false positive rates (~10%), with perhaps the exception of V-DSp, which most recently was found to be ineffective in distinguishing credible from noncredible MTBI groups (Curtis et al., 2009). Performance that exceeds cutoffs can be used to support the notion of noncredible performance. However, given the moderate sensitivity of these indicators, normal performance cannot be used to "rule out" malingering (i.e., a passing performance is not confirmatory of adequate effort). It is also important to note that DSp performance is impacted by cultural and linguistic factors requiring some adjustment of cutoffs in ethnic minorities and in patients for whom English is a second language (Salazar, Lu, Wen, & Boone, 2007).

Working Memory Index

The Working Memory Index (WMI) of the WAIS-III has shown promise in detecting malingering in chronic pain (Etherton, Bianchini, Ciota, Heinly, & Greve, 2006) and more recently in MTBI samples. More specifically, in the study by Curtis and colleagues (2009) described earlier, the classification accuracy of WMI was evaluated, among other WAIS-III variables. The authors compared the following groups: (a) credible patients with MTBI ($n = 26$); (b) patients with MTBI meeting Slick et al. (1999) criteria for MND ($n = 31$); (c) credible patients with moderate-to-severe TBI ($n = 26$); and (d) a general clinical, non–compensation-seeking, patient comparison group ($n = 80$). Results indicated that the MTBI MND group had significantly lower WMI scores than non-MND patients with MTBI and the patients with moderate-to-severe TBI. A WMI cutoff of ≤ 70 resulted in 26% sensitivity with 6% false positives in non-MND MTBI subjects. At this cutoff, specificity was lower for patients with memory disorders (11% false positive rate), indicating that this validity indicator should be used cautiously in patients with objective evidence of neurological dysfunction. Ord, Greve, and Bianchini (2008) also obtained similar results. Thus, the WMI has shown promise in identifying symptom invalidity for uncomplicated cases of MTBI.

Test of Variables of Attention

The test of variables of attention (TOVA; Greenberg, Kindschi, Dupuy, & Corman, 1996; Lezak et al., 2004; Mitrushina et al., 2005) is a non–language-based continuous performance test that requires the examinee to press a button when a target stimulus appears on a screen. The test lasts for 21.6 minutes. The target stimulus appears infrequently (3.5:1 nontarget-to-target ratio) in the first half of the test and frequently (3.5:1 target-to-nontarget ratio) during the second half of the test. Performance is quantified in four ways: errors of omission, errors of commission, mean response time, and variability of response time. These scores are provided for each quarter, both halves, and for the entire test. As reviewed in Alfano and Boone (2007), there is only one simulation (Leark, Dixon, Hoffmann, & Huynh, 2002) and one known groups (Henry, 2005) study investigating the TOVA as an SVT.

Although Leark and colleagues (2002) instructed their simulators to feign attention deficit disorder, Henry (2005) examined the TOVA as an SVT using a known groups design. The Henry sample included 52 litigating/disability-seeking patients with MTBI divided into two groups based on independent SVT performance: patients with MTBI meeting Slick and colleagues' (1999) criteria for MND ($n = 26$) and credible patients with MTBI ($n = 26$). The MND group performed significantly worse than the non-MND group on all TOVA variables. Discriminant function analysis suggested that a cutoff of ≥ 3 TOVA omission errors was the most accurate predictor with sensitivity of 88.5% and specificity of 80.8%. Raising the cutoff to ≥ 7 reduced false positives to 8% while still achieving an impressive 77% sensitivity. These findings differed from Leark and colleagues' simulation study in that the simulators in that study produced significantly more omission and commission errors as well as slower response time and greater response time variability. These findings underscore the notion that it can be difficult to extrapolate findings of simulation studies to real clinical populations. Henry's study supported the use of TOVA omission errors in discriminating probable malingerers from nonmalingerers in a litigating MTBI population.

Conners' Continuous Performance Test-II

Similar to the TOVA described previously, Conners' Continuous Performance Test-II (CPT-II; Conners, 2000) is a computerized continuous performance measure that requires the respondent to press the space bar when letters, except an "X", appear on the screen. Several scores are derived that include omissions, commissions, hit reaction time, hit reaction time standard error, variability, and perseverations. Although the CPT-II was developed as a measure of sustained attention and concentration, recent research suggests that it may have use in the detection of symptom invalidity (see review in Alfano & Boone, 2007 for a review of CPTs used to detect feigned attention deficit hyperactivity disorder [ADHD]). We were unable to locate any MTBI simulation studies examining the CPT-II. However, Ord, Boettcher, Greve, and Bianchini (2010) used a known groups design to examine the classification accuracy of the CPT-II omissions (missed targets) and hit reaction time standard error (reaction time variability) in (a) 27 MND patients with MTBI, (b) 31 credible patients with MTBI, and (c) 24 credible patients with moderate-to-severe TBI. MTBI was defined as PTA < 24 hr, GCS ≥ 13, LOC < 30 min, and negative neuroimaging. The authors found that the malingering group scored significantly worse than the other groups on all CPT-II variables with the exception of hit reaction time. An omission cutoff of > 30 yielded 33% sensitivity and 94% specificity (MTBI non-MND group). A reaction time standard error score of > 16 was associated with 41% sensitivity and 97% specificity (MTBI non-MND group). This study provides evidence that the CPT-II can be used as an effort indicator with MTBI cases, but the authors advised that "suspicious scores" should be interpreted in the context of the patient's history (i.e., ADHD should be ruled out) and other tests of neuropsychological function.

Seashore Rhythm Test

The seashore rhythm test (SRT), one of the subtests from the Halstead-Reitan Neuropsychological Battery (HRNB), involves the presentation of 30 pairs of tape-recorded rhythm patterns. For each pair, the respondent is asked to decide if the two sounds are the same or different. The responses are dichotomously scored as correct or incorrect (Lezak et al., 2004; Mitrushina et al., 2005). Although the test was designed to evaluate sustained auditory attention and concentration, studies examining insufficient effort suggest it is useful in the detection of malingering.

Suhr and Barrash (2007) and Alfano and Boone (2007) reviewed all studies investigating the SRT as a SVT up to 2006. The authors reviewed both simulation (Gfeller & Cradock, 1998; Inman & Berry, 2002; Mittenberg et al., 1996) and known groups (Ross, Putnam, Millis, Adams, & Krukowski, 2006; Spector, Lewandowski, Kelly, & Kaylor, 1994; Trueblood & Schmidt, 1993) designs, the latter of which are summarized in Table 12.1.

Since that time, Curtis, Greve, Brasseux, and Bianchini (2010) investigated the SRT (total score correct) using a known groups design to detect MND, stratifying classification accuracy data by injury severity. In particular, the following groups were compared: (a) 24 MTBI non-MND, (b) 27 MTBI MND, (c) 23 moderate-to-severe TBI non-MND, and (d) 90 heterogeneous clinical patients. MTBI was defined as PTA < 24 hr, GCS ≥ 13, LOC ≤ 30 min, negative neuroimaging, and no focal neurological signs. Overall, the MTBI MND group scored significantly worse on the SRT than the other groups. Cut scores and classification accuracy data are presented in Table 12.1.

In sum, the data from simulation and known groups studies have generally supported the use of the SRT in identifying noncredible performance in MTBI samples. The cutoff score established by Trueblood and Schmidt (1993) of > 8 errors has not yielded consistently high specificity rates in more recent studies of symptom invalidity in MTBI cases, however. Those studies suggest that the cutoff score should be raised to > 10 to minimize false positives, with sensitivity ranging from 37% to 59% (Curtis et al., 2010; Ross et al., 2006).

Speech Sounds Perception Test

Another subtest from the HRNB, the speech sounds perception test (SSPT) consists of 60 nonsense words that have the "ee" sound in the middle of the word. The words are spoken on a tape recorder, and the respondent has to choose one of four written responses to match the word to the sound. Responses are scored dichotomously as correct or incorrect (Lezak et al., 2004; Mitrushina et al., 2005). Studies examining insufficient effort suggest that it is also useful in the detection of malingering.

Suhr and Barrash (2007) and Alfano and Boone (2007) reviewed all studies investigating the SSPT as a SVT up to 2006. The authors reviewed both simulation (Heaton et al., 1978; Mittenberg et al., 1996) and known groups (Ross et al., 2006; Trueblood & Schmidt, 1993) designs, the latter of which are summarized in Table 12.1. Since that time, Curtis and colleagues (2010; study described previously), investigated the SSPT (total errors) to detect MND, stratifying classification accuracy data by injury severity. In particular, the following groups were compared: (a) 24 non-MND patients with MTBI, (b) 27 MND patients with MTBI, (c) 23 non-MND patients with moderate-to-severe TBI, and (d) 90 heterogeneous clinical patients. Overall, the MTBI MND group scored significantly worse on the SSPT than the other groups, and the SSPT was more effective than the SRT in terms of classification accuracy. Cut scores and classification accuracy data for the SSPT are presented in Table 12.1.

Overall, the SSPT has been shown to be effective in discriminating malingerers from nonmalingerers, although the recommended cutoffs have varied across studies, ranging from ≥ 12 (sensitivity = 59%, specificity = 92%; Curtis et al., 2010) to ≥ 17 total errors (sensitivity = 88%, specificity = 96%; Trueblood & Schmidt, 1993). Additional research is warranted to determine the most accurate cut scores for patients with MTBI.

Summary of Attention-Based Symptom Validity Tests

DSp ACSS and RDS have been well validated in both simulation and large clinical samples with well-defined malingering groups and a wide various clinical comparison groups for establishing specificity. Although lower cut scores for ACSS and RDS are necessary to maintain adequate specificity in moderate-to-severe TBI and general neuropsychology clinic samples (≤ 5 and ≤ 6, respectively), cutoffs can be raised to ≤ 6 and ≤ 7, respectively, when it is clear that a patient has sustained an uncomplicated MTBI. Several other DSp and WAIS-III indicators (longest forward span, timed scores, WMI, etc.) show promise but require cross validation in MTBI samples. Taken together, the data suggest that V-DSp is likely unable to effectively distinguish MND from non-MND in MTBI cases specifically. This is especially true for individuals of low education. V-DSp is also associated with a relatively high false positive rate in more severely impaired populations. Likewise, as Curtis and colleagues (2010) pointed out, examining the false positive error rates in the credible moderate/severe TBI and clinical comparison samples for the SRT and SSPT clarifies how these tests are sensitive to bonafide neurological impairment. The SSPT had a higher false positive rate compared to the SRT. Joint classification criterion for failure decreased the overall false positive rate and it is, therefore, a recommended practice (we describe joint classification and aggregating across tests in the next chapter). Finally, there is also certainly some evidence that CPT measures have use in the detection of feigned cognitive impairment in MTBI populations. This finding is not unexpected, given that they measure both performance inconsistency (hit reaction time standard error [SE]) and magnitude of errors—two types of responses that are established methods for detecting symptom invalidity (Rogers, 1997).

PROCESSING SPEED

Processing speed refers to the rate at which an individual processes perceived stimuli. Slowing of mental activity can be most clearly observed in delayed reaction times and in taking longer than average to perform mental tasks (Lezak et al., 2004; Mitrushina et al., 2005). It has been argued that malingerers may try to exaggerate their impairment by slowing their performance (e.g., Osimani, Alon, Berger, & Abarbanel, 1997; Tan et al., 2002; van Gorp et al., 1999). Here, we review the Dot Counting Test (DCT), various subtests and indices from the WAIS, and the symbol digit modalities test (SDMT) to the extent they hold promise or have been previously investigated as SVTs in MTBI samples.

Dot Counting Test

Originally developed by André Rey (1941) and reviewed by Lezak and colleagues (2004), the DCT has been used to assess noncredible cognitive presentations (Boone, Lu, Back, et al., 2002). It consists of 12 cards with a varying number of printed black dots on each card. Examinees are asked to count the dots as quickly as they can and verbalize their answers aloud. The first six cards have dots randomly arranged, and a pattern of longer counting times is expected on cards with greater numbers of dots. The second six cards have dots grouped in ways that facilitate the use of multiplication, which should take less time. Both errors and response times are recorded for each card.

Boone and Lu (2007) and Nitch and Glassmire (2007) reviewed the DCT as a method of detecting symptom invalidity, and the readers are referred to their chapters for a summary of the literature up to 2006. The reviews covered both simulation (Beetar & Williams, 1995; Binks, Gouvier, & Waters, 1997; Erdal, 2004; Hiscock, Branham, & Hiscock, 1994; Martin et al., 1996; Paul, Franzen, Cohen, & Fremouw, 1992; Rose, Hall, Szalda-Petree, & Bach, 1998) and known groups (Boone, Lu, Back, et al., 2002; Greiffenstein et al., 1994; Youngjohn et al., 1995) studies. The authors noted in their reviews the paucity of studies available, even though the test has been in existence for more than 60 years, and the large majority of studies that do exist are simulation studies. It is unfortunate that many of the studies did not include a real-world MTBI subsample or, when they did, classification data for the MTBI subsample was not provided separately (e.g., Strauss et al., 2002).

Of particular note, however, is the work of Boone, Lu, Back, and colleagues (2002) who formally standardized the test and developed an E score formula that combined multiple DCT scores given earlier research suggesting that individual scores were relatively insensitive (Greiffenstein et al., 1994, Rose et al., 1998, Vickery, Berry, Inman, Harris, & Orey, 2001). The following E score formula increased sensitivity of this test for the detection of feigned cognitive impairment:

E score = mean ungrouped time + mean grouped time + total number of errors

In particular, Boone, Lu, Back, and colleagues (ibid) compared the DCT performance of 85 noncredible patients (42% of whom claimed TBI, severity not reported, but the large majority were MTBI), 14 noncredible inpatient prisoners (based on staff consensus), and 9 credible clinical groups, including 20 individuals with moderate-to-severe brain injury (confirmed by positive neuroimaging) still in rehabilitation. Using an E score cutoff of ≥ 17 across clinical groups led to an overall high classification rate (sensitivity = 79%, specificity = 90%). An E score cutoff of ≥ 19 for the TBI comparison group in particular was more accurate for this group (sensitivity = 72%, specificity = 90%). Cross validation (Boone & Lu, 2007) comparing 91 noncredible patients (many of whom claimed TBI, severity not reported, but a sizeable percentage were MTBI) and 111 credible heterogeneous patients using a cutoff of ≥ 17 resulted in sensitivity of 73% and specificity of 89%. In the original validation study, none of the patients with moderate-to-severe TBI made > 4 errors on the test, and none averaged > 7 sec to count grouped dots, thus suggesting that scores beyond these cutoffs are likely characteristic of noncredible performance.

The authors of the two recent reviews of the DCT concluded that initial negative findings regarding test effectiveness were "likely an artifact of the choice of scores studied and the use of simulating rather than 'real-world' noncredible subjects" (Nitch & Glassmire, 2007, p. 91). In other words, although simulation studies suggest that using individual scores from the DCT are insensitive, the use of several DCT scores (i.e., total errors and response times) in combination is adequately sensitive in a heterogeneous noncredible neuropsychological population (Boone et al., 2002). However, examination of a DCT database available at the time of this writing (Boone, Victor, Cottingham, Ziegler, & Zeller, in progress) shows that in MTBI subjects performing in a noncredible manner (n = 101; compensation-seeking failed at least 2 independent SVTs not including DCT with low cognitive scores inconsistent with normal activities of daily living), use of an E score cutoff of ≥ 17 was associated with sensitivity of 45%, whereas a mean grouped time score of > 7 sec was associated with 35% sensitivity, and > 4 errors identified only 11% of noncredible performance in patients with MTBI. These data suggest that the DCT identifies noncredible performance in only about half of individuals feigning symptoms of MTBI.

Wechsler Adult Intelligence Scale Revised/Third Edition Digit Symbol

Babikian and Boone (2007) and Suhr and Barrash (2007) reviewed all WAIS-R/WAIS-III indices that had been investigated as SVTs up to 2006. The authors reviewed both simulation (e.g., Inman & Berry, 2002) and known groups (e.g., Trueblood, 1994; Youngjohn et al., 1995) designs, the latter of which are summarized in Table 12.2 of this chapter. Trueblood (1994) was the first to investigate the use of WAIS-R digit symbol (DSym) in MTBI samples using a known groups design. In particular, he divided his sample into four groups: (a) 12 malingerers (identified based on forced-choice testing); (b) 10 individuals with "questionable validity" (QV) who produced profiles that did not make neuropsychological "sense"; however, they were not clearly malingering; (c) 12 controls demographically matched to Group a; and (d) 10 controls demographically matched to Group b. Groups a and b performed worse than their control comparison groups on WAIS-R DSym. An ACSS cutoff < 5 correctly classified four malingerers (sensitivity = 33%) and two individuals with QV (20%) with zero false positive errors (100% specificity). Qualitatively, multiple errors and reversals were noted in the invalid groups' performance. Further, Babikian and Boone (2007) suggested that "drawing of Digit Symbol codes upside down is pathognomonic for malingering, albeit this is very rare" (p. 123).

Given other reports that DSym rotational errors may be associated with feigning (Binder, 1992) and our previous work suggesting memory-based effort measures (e.g., Kim, Boone, Victor, Marion, et al., 2010) and timed scores (e.g., Babikian et al., 2006) are useful as embedded SVTs, our group (Kim, Boone, Victor, Marion, et al.) added a timed recognition trial to the standard administration of the WAIS-III DSym to investigate it as a SVT. We used a known groups design using a large sample of "real-world" noncredible patients (n = 82; defined by presence of incentive to perform poorly and failure on two or more independent SVTs not because of other psychiatric, neurologic, or developmental disorders), and credible patients (n = 89; defined by absence of incentive to perform poorly, failure on less than 2 independent SVTs, full scale IQ [FSIQ] > 70, and no evidence of dementia). The recognition trial included foils (rotations of the correct answer) for five of the items. Subjects were

TABLE 12.2 Known Group Studies of Symptom Validity Test Effectiveness Within the Domain of Processing Speed in Mild Traumatic Brain Injury

Study	Sample	Test/Score	Cut Score	Sensitivity	Specificity		
		SDMT					
Backhaus et al. (2004)	Litigants with MND MTBI (n = 25)	Written	< 38 < 30 < 24	56% 36% 20%	100% 100% 100%		
	Credible patients with MTBI (n = 25)	Oral	< 43 < 35 < 28	64% 40% 20%	96% 100% 100%		
		WAIS indices					
Trueblood (1994)	Patients with definite MND MTBI (n = 12) Patients with probable MND MTBI (n = 10) Demographically matched credible patients with MTBI (n = 22)	WAIS-R DSym	< 5	33% (definite) 20% (probable)	100%		
Curtis et al. (2009)	Patients with MND MTBI (n = 31) Credible patients with MTBI (n = 26) Patients with moderate-to-severe TBI (n = 26) General clinical patients (n = 80)	WAIS-III Processing Speed Index	< 60 < 65 < 70 < 75 < 80	10% 16% 36% 55% 68%	MTBI 100% 96% 92% 85% 73%	Mod/sev 92% 88% 80% 64% 48%	Clin 95% 92% 81% 74% 55%
Kim et al. (2010)	General clinical patients with MND (n = 82), including subset of MTBI (n = 28) Credible general clinical patients (n = 89)	WAIS-III DSym Recognition Equation	≤ 57	74% (MTBI only)	89% (general clinical)		

Note. Clin = credible clinical group; DSym = digit symbol subtest; MND = malingered neurocognitive dysfunction; Mod/Sev = credible moderate-to-severe TBI; SDMT = Symbol Digit Modalities Test; SVT = Symptom Validity Test; TBI = traumatic brain injury; WAIS-R = Wechsler Adult Intelligence Scale-Revised; WAIS-III = Wechsler Adult Intelligence Scale-3rd edition.

asked to circle the symbol that went with each number in the task they just completed. Five scores were examined for their ability to differentiate credible versus noncredible effort: DSym ACSS, raw score, and three variables from the recognition trial (recognition correct, recognition time [in seconds], and recognition rotations [i.e., false positive errors]). Results suggested that the recognition trial (which did not include the false positive error score) was more sensitive in identifying poor effort than other standard DSym scores, and that an equation incorporating several scores and a cutoff of ≤ 57 led to 80% sensitivity at 89% specificity:

$$[(DSym\ ACSS + recognition\ correct) \times 10] - recognition\ time$$

We investigated accuracy rates associated with the ≤ 57 cutoff in a subset of noncredible patients with MTBI ($n = 28$) and found 74% sensitivity. We concluded that although standard DSym scores may be inadequately sensitive, the equation combining ACSS with scores from the newly added recognition trial holds promise in both general clinical and MTBI populations.

Wechsler Adult Intelligence Scale-III Processing Speed Index

The WAIS-III processing speed index (PSI; Wechsler, 1997a), onto which DSym loads, has also been investigated as a potential SVT. After finding that the PSI had some clinical use in identifying symptom invalidity in a noncredible pain population (Etherton, Bianchini, Greve, & Heinly, 2005), Curtis and colleagues (2009; described earlier) investigated the PSI using a known groups design based on diagnosis of MND (Slick et al., 1999). They investigated several WAIS-III subtests and indices as SVTs in a clinical sample that included separate analysis of individuals with a history of MTBI (defined by PTA < 24 hr, initial GCS $= 13$–15, and LOC ≤ 30 min) in addition to the absence of positive neuroradiological findings or focal neurological signs ($n = 57$). Comparison groups included moderate-to-severe TBI and general clinical patients. For the PSI in particular, these authors found that a cutoff score of < 70 was associated with sensitivity of 36% and specificity of 92%. See Table 12.2 for a range of cut scores and associated classification accuracy statistics. It is important to note the higher false positive rate in the credible moderate-to-severe TBI group, suggesting the PSI is not an appropriate SVT (or a higher cutoff is needed) in the context of anything more severe than an uncomplicated MTBI.

Symbol Digit Modalities Test

Finally, the symbol digit modalities test (SDMT; Smith, 1973) was one of 11 different validity indicators evaluated by Backhaus, Fichentenberg, and Hanks (2004) using a normative floor effect. In particular, they used cutoffs on standard cognitive tests that were set at or below the 50th percentile of performance displayed by credible patients with moderate-to-severe TBI in their sample ($n = 70$) to detect symptom invalidity in a sample of MND MTBI litigants ($n = 25$). These authors also included a sample of nonlitigating patients with MTBI for clinical comparison ($n = 25$). Using this approach, the authors found that cutoffs on the SDMT of < 38 (written) and < 43 (oral) were associated with 56% 64% sensitivity while maintaining specificity more than 96%.

Summary of Processing Speed-Based Symptom Validity Tests

Preliminary evidence indicates that WAIS-III DSym is particularly effective at discriminating credible and noncredible MTBI groups, especially with the inclusion of the recognition paradigm (Kim, Boone, Victor, Lu, et al., 2010). Furthermore, the DCT, SDMT, and WAIS-III PSI have shown modest-to-moderate sensitivity in identifying noncredible patients with MTBI.

LANGUAGE

Relative to the abundance of literature regarding noncredible memory performance, there is very little information available regarding patterns of noncredible language symptoms. The few empirical reports of language deficits (primarily verbal fluency) persisting past 1 year in MTBI samples (Hannay, Howieson, Loring, Fischer, & Lezak, 2004; Mathias & Coats, 1999; Raskin & Rearick, 1996; Whelan, Murdoch, & Bellamy, 2007) failed to assess for response bias and/or somatoform symptomatology. Further, although there are some reports of "foreign accent syndrome" (FAS) presenting after MTBI (Laures-Gore, Henson, Weismer, & Rambow, 2006; Lippert-Gruener, Weinert, Greisback, & Wedekind, 2005), the possibility of a somatoform disorder and the potential impact of secondary gain were not considered in these cases, even when obvious signs of somatoform symptomatology were present (long histories of unexplained illnesses, etc.). Heinly (2008) found that, after controlling for effort, there was no evidence of language impairment related to MTBI. Indeed, poor effort/ response bias has been found to have seven times the effect on language performances (including verbal comprehension, confrontation naming, verbal fluency, and reading recognition) in comparison to the impact of moderate or severe TBI on those skills.

A review of the extant literature on feigned language symptoms revealed only a handful of published articles on this topic, and these were confined to case reports involving verbal dysfluency (Tsuruga, Kobayashi, Hirai, & Kato, 2008; van Borsel, Janssens, & Santens, 2005), atypical dysarthria (Kallen, Marshall, & Casey, 1986), stuttering (Mahr & Leith, 1992; Roth, Aronson, & Davis, 1989; Seery, 2005), and severe expressive aphasia as a part of a feigned dementia presentation (Abudarham & White, 2001).

More recently, Cottingham and Boone (2010) presented the first published case of feigned language impairment after MTBI that included comprehensive neuropsychological test data, various response bias indicators, and objective personality testing. In particular, they presented a case of a 36-year-old female civil litigant who complained of primary difficulties with expressive language following MTBI. GCS was 15 at the scene of the accident, and all neuroimaging was normal. However, medical records indicated she was diagnosed as having dysarthria and severe apraxia of speech. On neuropsychological evaluation 3 years after the injury, in addition to her expressive deficits, she presented with a "vague foreign accent." The litigant's presentation was fraught with behavioral inconsistencies, atypical errors, and an atypical course (i.e., initial speech difficulties beginning 3 days postaccident, notable worsening 1 week later, improvement during hospitalization, and subsequent worsening of symptoms on discharge, with exacerbation at the time of depositions). However, on effort testing, the patient passed 10 indicators, including those appearing to be tests of verbal memory, that is, Rey Word Recognition Test (Nitch et al., 2006), Warrington Recognition Memory Test for words (Kim, Boone, Victor, Marion, et al., 2010), Rey Auditory Verbal Learning Test equation (Boone, Lu, & Wen, 2005), and Rey Auditory Verbal Learning Test/Rey Figure discriminant function (Sherman, Boone, Lu, & Razani, 2002). Other effort measures used included those in the areas of visuoconstructional ability/visual memory (Rey Complex Figure Test [RCFT] effort equation; Lu, Boone, Cozolino, & Mitchell, 2003), math/number skills

(DCT; Boone, Lu, & Herzberg, 2002b), DSp accuracy scores (Babikian et al., 2006), motor speed (Finger Tapping Test, dominant hand; Arnold et al., 2005), and attention (DSp ACSS and RDS; Babikian et al., 2006). In particular, she failed effort indicators requiring letter discrimination and processing speed (i.e., b Test), rapid verbal repetition (i.e., timed forward DSp), and sensory function (i.e., finger agnosia errors). These effort test failures were within the same domains in which she exhibited poor cognitive performance, including speech and language (i.e., the Wide Range Achievement Test 4 [WRAT 4] word reading, Stroop Color-Word Test word reading and color naming, Multilingual Aphasia Examination [MAE] sentence repetition (SR), verbal fluency–FAS), auditory discrimination (Wepman Auditory Discrimination Test), processing speed (Trail Making Test, parts A and B), and motor speed (Finger Tapping Test, nondominant hand). Her WAIS-III verbal IQ (VIQ) was 13 points lower than her PIQ. Other language skills were within normal limits, such as reading and aural comprehension (MAE reading comprehension and aural comprehension), word retrieval (Boston Naming Test), and spelling (WRAT 4).

Although the relative contributions of "unconscious" and conscious factors for feigning were difficult to determine in this case (and, of course, the two are not mutually exclusive), the authors pointed out that had there been only more traditional or well-known effort indicators within the domain of memory administered, the noncredible nature of this litigant's language, processing speed, and motor/sensory performances would not have been documented through objective SVTs. Although the noncredible presentation of language deficits may be less common than exaggerated deficits involving other neuropsychological abilities, the authors concluded that there is a need for validation of additional measures to detect feigned language impairment. Here, we review the b Test, various subtests and indices from the WAIS, Meyers Neuropsychological Battery, SR, and the Token Test (TT) to the extent they hold promise or have been previously investigated as SVTs in MTBI samples.

The b Test

The genesis of the b Test (Boone, Lu, & Herzberg, 2002a; Boone et al., 2000) resulted from observations that noncredible patients with MTBI reported they had become "dyslexic" (i.e., now saw letters "upside down and backward"), even though individuals with significant brain injury did not report this phenomenon. Thus, the test was designed to detect noncredible test-taking performance by using recognition of overlearned information (i.e., rapid letter identification/discrimination). Several studies indicate that overlearned skills, such as sight reading, are spared in patients with brain injuries (Crawford, Besson, & Parker, 1988). In the b Test, respondents are asked to circle all the lower case b's interspersed with similar looking letters (lower case d's, p's, and q's) in a 15-page booklet. The stimuli on successive pages gets progressively smaller, and on some pages, the similar-looking letters have diagonal or additional stems. The scores that are derived include total number of commission errors (circling figures other than b's), omission errors (not circling b's), and total time to complete the task.

There are no identified simulation studies of the b Test. However, the validation sample (Boone et al., 2000) was composed of 34 real-world suspected malingerers and several clinical comparison groups, including 20 patients who had moderate-to-severe brain injuries. The authors found that suspected malingerers performed significantly worse on the b Test than patients with TBI and most other comparison groups. More specifically, they committed significantly more commission and omission errors and required significantly more time to complete the task than the moderate-to-severe TBI group. A cutoff of > 2 commission errors correctly classified 76.5% of the malingerers, with specificity of $> 82\%$ for all other comparison groups and 100% for the TBI sample. A cutoff of > 40 omission errors yielded a sensitivity rate of 58.8% for the malingerers, and a specificity of $> 85.1\%$ for the comparison groups and 95% for the TBI subjects. A cutoff of > 12 min also correctly classified 57.6% of suspected malingerers, with a specificity of $> 83.9\%$ for comparison groups and 85% for TBI subjects.

Boone and colleagues (2002a) generated the following equation, incorporating mean time per page, number of omissions errors, and number of commission errors, which was the most sensitive measure of detecting suspect effort.

$$E \text{ score} = [(\text{number of commission errors} + \text{number of d commission errors}) \times 10] + \text{number of omission errors} + \text{mean time per page}$$

Boone and colleagues (2002a) compared 91 litigants/compensation-seeking patients who failed at least two independent effort indices and demonstrated at least one behavioral criterion for feigning with six credible, nonlitigating, and non–compensation-seeking clinical groups, including a group of patients with moderate-to-severe brain injury ($n = 20$). A cutoff score of ≥ 90 using the aforementioned equation resulted in 77% sensitivity and 90% specificity in this latter group.

More recent cross-validation data from our laboratory (Boone, Cottingham, Victor, Zeller, & Ziegler, in progress), comparing 293 general clinical patients meeting MND criteria with 108 credible, nonlitigating, and non–compensation-seeking general clinical patients, demonstrated that the E score can be lowered to > 88 while still maintaining $\geq 90\%$ specificity, resulting in 68.3% sensitivity. In the subsample of 98 noncredible patients with MTBI, application of this cutoff resulted in 58.2% sensitivity, indicating that the b Test is less sensitive to the types of neurocognitive deficits feigned in MTBI as compared to other claimed conditions but still detects a moderate number of noncredible MTBI subjects.

Wechsler Adult Intelligence Scale-III Verbal Intelligence Quotient/Verbal Comprehension Index

In the known groups study by Curtis and colleagues (2009) described earlier, various verbal indices from the WAIS-III were examined as SVTs in patients with MTBI (including both credible and noncredible patients with MTBI). Comparison groups included moderate-to-severe TBI and general clinical patients. The WAIS-III VIQ and verbal comprehension index (VCI) were successful in discriminating credible and noncredible MTBI groups, although sensitivity was modest (i.e., 26%–29%) at cut scores (i.e., < 70 for both) that maintained $< 10\%$ false positive error rate in credible MTBI subjects. (see Table 12.3 for a range of cut scores and associated classification accuracy statistics).

Sentence Repetition

SR (Meyers, Volkert, & Diep, 2000; Strauss, Sherman, & Spreen, 2006) is a test of auditory attention span and language abilities (Lezak et al., 2004; Mitrushina et al., 2005) scored as the total number of sentences correctly repeated out of 22 possible sentences. The sentences are read aloud by the examiner or played on a cassette tape. The patient is asked to repeat each sentence verbatim, and each sentence increases in length as the test progresses. Poor performance has been associated with left hemisphere brain damage (Lezak et al., 2004; Mitrushina et al., 2005).

TABLE 12.3 Known Group Studies of Symptom Validity Test Effectiveness Within the Domain of Language in Mild Traumatic Brain Injury

Study	Sample	Test/Score	Cut Score	Sensitivity	Specificity		
		WAIS-III Indices					
Curtis et al. (2009)	Patients with MND MTBI (n = 31) Credible patients with MTBI (n = 26) Credible patients with moderate/ severe TBI (n = 26) General clinical patients (n = 80)	WAIS-III Verbal IQ			MTBI	Mod/sev	Clin
			< 65	13%	100%	96%	99%
			< 70	26%	96%	96%	92%
			< 75	42%	85%	96%	84%
			< 80	58%	69%	88%	72%
		Verbal Comprehension Index			MTBI	Mod/sev	Clin
			< 65	19%	100%	100%	97%
			< 70	29%	92%	96%	92%
			< 75	45%	81%	96%	87%
			< 80	58%	65%	88%	79%
		Sentence repetition					
Backhaus et al. (2004)	Litigants with MND MTBI (n = 25) Credible patients with MTBI (n = 25)	Total correct score[a]	< 11	76%	84%		
			< 10	64%	88%		
			< 9	56%	100%		
		Token Test					
Backhaus et al. (2004)	Litigants with MND MTBI (n = 25) Credible patients with MTBI (n = 25)	Total correct score	< 43	68%	80%		
			< 40	36%	96%		
			< 38	24%	96%		

Note. Clin = credible clinical group; MND = malingered neurocognitive dysfunction; MTBI = mild traumatic brain injury; Mod/sev = credible moderate-to-severe TBI; SVT = Symptom Validity Test; TBI = traumatic brain injury; WAIS-III = Wechsler Adult Intelligence Scale–3rd edition.
[a]Adjusted scores.

SR has also been examined as a measure of effort in simulation (Meyers, Morrison, & Miller, 2001), known groups (Backhaus et al., 2004; Meyers & Volbrecht, 2003; Schroeder & Marshall, 2010), and specificity (Meyers et al., 2000) study designs. It is calculated as the total number of sentences correctly repeated, and a score of ≤ 9 indicates failure when used as a SVT (Meyers, Galinsky, & Volbrecht, 1999; Meyers & Volbrecht, 2003).

Schroeder and Marshall (2010) recently investigated the use of SR in a sample of 1,031 patients with a wide range of clinical diagnoses, identifying sensitivity and specificity rates by diagnostic group. Nearly half of the subjects (44%) had a reported history of head injury in addition to multiple medical and psychiatric comorbidities. More than half of these subjects reported either no LOC or LOC less than 5 min. Although the authors reported excellent specificity rates for these patients with TBI at both a cutoff of ≤ 9 (99.2%) and ≤ 10 (91.3%), sensitivity rates specific to the patients with TBI were not reported. A cutoff score of ≤ 10 reached sensitivity of 56.8% while maintaining adequate specificity of 95.8%.

Token Test

In the TT (Lezak et al., 2004; Strauss et al., 2006), subjects are instructed to follow simple instructions (e.g., "Move the red circle away from the green square.") that progressively become more grammatically complex. The test consists of 62 commands nested in five sections of increasing complexity (full credit is given to responses correct on first presentation). A score of ≤ 150 was associated with 45% sensitivity in simulators while maintaining 100% specificity in control comparison groups, including a group of patients with MTBI with no incentive to perform poorly (Meyers et al., 1999). Meyers and his colleagues found that it is helpful to reverse the order of item presentation, that is, to start with the more difficult items and progress to the easier ones. Subjects who do well on the more difficult items and then fail some of the simpler ones are judged to have performed in an improbable manner that does not make neuropsychological "sense." The only other study identified that investigated the TT in an MTBI sample was Backhaus and colleagues (2004; study described earlier). In particular, using their normative floor effect approach, a cut score of < 40 was associated with 36% sensitivity and 96% specificity.

Summary of Language-Based Symptom Validity Tests

Although there are promising language-based SVTs, more research is needed in MTBI samples. Much of the existing research has been in the context of simulation studies and/or primarily concerned with feigned learning disability rather than head injury (i.e., the word reading test; Osmon et al., 2006). With respect to the development of new language-based SVTs, close collaboration between neuropsychologists and speech/language pathologists, who have in-depth knowledge of speech/language disorders as well as tests to identify them, may be fruitful.

VISUOSPATIAL/PERCEPTUAL

Visuospatial/perceptual functions are those involved in tasks such as assembling, building, constructing, and drawing in which the end product is dependent on successful representation of objects in space (Lezak et al., 2004; Mitrushina et al., 2005). Greiffenstein (2007) provided a summary of the literature investigating feigned visuospatial deficits up to 2006, reviewing simulation (Bernard, 1990; Chouinard & Rouleau, 1997), known groups (Lu et al., 2003), and mixed (Iverson & Franzen, 1994; Meyers & Volbrecht, 1998, 1999) designs, as well as case studies (Khan, Fayaz, Ridgley, & Wennberg, 2000). Greiffenstein (2007) argued that individual visuospatial measures may be less sensitive to biased responding compared to SVTs derived from tests assessing other domains. However, others (e.g., Boone, 2007, 2009; Larrabee, 2007) suggested that it is an area worthy of further study. Here, we review various WAIS-III indices, judgment of line orientation (JOLO), the Knox Cube Test (KCT), and other measures of visuospatial/perceptual function to the extent they have been investigated as SVTs in MTBI. Note that the RCFT is only briefly reviewed here because a review exists in Chapter 9 of this volume. Relevant cut scores and classification accuracy statistics for the SVTs reviewed here can be found in Table 12.4.

Wechsler Adult Intelligence Scale-III Performance Intelligence Quotient/Perceptual Organization Index

In the known groups study by Curtis and colleagues (2009; described earlier), several WAIS-III indices including PIQ and perceptual organization index (POI) were exam-

TABLE 12.4 Known Group Studies of Symptom Validity Test Effectiveness Within the Domain of Visual Perceptual/Spatial Functioning in Mild Traumatic Brain Injury

Study	Sample	Test/Score	Cut Score	Sensitivity	Specificity		
		WAIS-III indices					
Curtis et al. (2009)	Patients with MND MTBI (n = 31)	Performance IQ			MTBI	Mod/sev	Clin
			< 65	10%	100%	92%	95%
			< 70	23%	100%	88%	89%
	Credible patients with MTBI (n = 26)		< 75	39%	96%	77%	82%
			< 80	71%	81%	69%	69%
			< 85	81%	61%	54%	54%
	Credible patients with moderate-to-severe TBI (n = 26)	Perceptual Organization Index	< 70	20%	MTBI	Mod/sev	Clin
			< 75	33%	100%	92%	90%
			< 80	50%	100%	92%	85%
			< 85	67%	88%	80%	74%
	General clinical patients (n = 80)				77%	76%	64%
		Picture completion					
Trueblood (1994)	Patients with definite MND MTBI (n = 12)	WAIS-R PC ACSS	< 7	50% (definite) 30% (probable)	96%		
	Patients with probable MND MTBI (n = 10)	Total errors on items 1–5	≥ 2	42% (definite) 20% (probable)	100%		
	Demographically matched credible patients with MTBI (n = 22)						
Solomon et al. (2010)	General clinical patients with MND (n = 195), including subset of MTBI (n = 51)	"Most discrepant" index[a]	≤ 2	56% (MTBI only)	93% (general clinical)		
	Credible general clinical patients (n = 172)						

(Continued)

ined as SVTs in a sample of patients with MTBI (both credible and noncredible) and clinical comparison groups. See Table 12.4 for a range of cut scores and associated classification accuracy statistics. Selection of cutoffs (i.e., < 75 for both) to maintain adequate specificity (≥ 90%) resulted in only modest sensitivity (≤ 39%).

Picture Completion Subtest

The picture completion (PC) subtest is a measure of alertness to visual detail. Examinees are asked to identify the parts of pictures that are missing. Because it is "relatively" resistant to the effects of brain damage compared to some of the other subtests (Reitan & Wolfson, 1992), it has appeared promising as a potential SVT.

TABLE 12.4 Known Group Studies of Symptom Validity Test Effectiveness Within the Domain of Visual Perceptual/Spatial Functioning in Mild Traumatic Brain Injury (*Continued*)

Study	Sample	Test/Score	Cut Score	Sensitivity	Specificity	
		JOLO				
Iverson (2001)	Credible litigants (*n* = 203)	Total correct score		MTBI only	MTBI	Mod/sev
			≤ 12	11%	98%	99%
	Noncredible litigants (*n* = 91)		≤ 13	14%	98%	99%
			≤ 14	16%	98%	99%
	Credible litigants with MTBI (*n* = 89)		≤ 15	18%	98%	99%
			≤ 16	19%	95%	97%
			≤ 17	25%	93%	96%
	Noncredible litigants with MTBI (*n* = 57)		≤ 18	30%	92%	91%
			≤ 19	33%	91%	88%
			≤ 20	44%	90%	85%
			≤ 21	44%	85%	82%
			≤ 22	47%	81%	73%
Iverson (2001)	Credible litigants with moderate-to-severe TBI (*n* = 78) Noncredible litigants with moderate-to-severe TBI (*n* = 24)					
Backhaus et al. (2004)	Litigants with MND MTBI (*n* = 25) Credible patients with MTBI (*n* = 25)	Total correct score	< 23	80%	84%	
			< 20	60%	92%	
			< 14.6	32%	100%	
		RCFT				
Whiteside et al. (2011)	Credible general clinical patients (*n* = 415) Noncredible patients (*n* = 30), 40% of which were MTBI	Copy score	≤ 22.5	27%	92%	
			≤ 23	27%	90%	
			≤ 23.5	27%	90%	
			≤ 24	30%	89%	
			≤ 24.5	32%	89%	
			≤ 25	32%	86%	
			≤ 25.5	32%	85%	
		BFRT				
		Total score	≤ 36	17%	96%	
			≤ 37	26%	94%	
			≤ 38	29%	92%	
			≤ 39	40%	90%	
			≤ 40	40%	89%	
			≤ 41	46%	84%	
		HVOT				
		Total score	≤ 20	27%	92%	
			≤ 20.5	27%	92%	
			≤ 21	45%	88%	
			≤ 21.5	46%	88%	
			≤ 22	52%	83%	
			≤ 22.5	52%	82%	

(*Continued*)

TABLE 12.4 Known Group Studies of Symptom Validity Test Effectiveness Within the Domain of Visual Perceptual/Spatial Functioning in Mild Traumatic Brain Injury (*Continued*)

Study	Sample	Test/Score	Cut Score	Sensitivity	Specificity
		JOLO			
		Total score	≤ 15	23%	95%
			≤ 16	23%	94%
			≤ 17	28%	92%
			≤ 18	31%	90%
			≤ 19	31%	87%
			≤ 20	40%	85%
		Combined Visual Spatial Measures[b]	≤ 130	40%	90%
			≤ 132	50%	88%
			≤ 133	50%	88%
			≤ 134	57%	87%
			≤ 135	58%	85%
		VFT			
Larrabee (2008)	Patients with MND TBI (*n* = 26), 21 of whom alleged MTBI Credible patients with moderate-to-severe TBI (*n* = 31)	Total score	< 26	48%	93%

Note. ACSS = age-corrected scaled score; BFRT = Benton Facial Recognition Test; Clin = credible clinical group; HVOT = Hooper Visual Organization Test; JOLO = judgment of line orientation; MND = malingered neurocognitive dysfunction; MTBI= mild traumatic brain injury; Mod/sev = credible moderate-to-severe TBI; PC = picture completion; RCFT = Rey Complex Figure Test; SVT = Symptom Validity Test; TBI = traumatic brain injury; VFT = Benton Visual Form Discrimination Test; WAIS-R = Wechsler Adult Intelligence Scale-Revised; WAIS-III = Wechsler Adult Intelligence Scale-3rd edition.
[a]The "most discrepant" index consists of six items that showed at least a 40-point difference in correct endorsement between credible and noncredible groups: items 8, 9, 10, 13, 14, and 21 (Solomon et al., 2010).
[b]The combined visual spatial measures included five scores summed together: RCFT copy score, RCFT recognition score, BFRT total score, HVOT total score, and JOLO total score.

Most studies that used the WAIS and WAIS-R versions of PC had small samples, and/or only used moderate-to-severe TBI comparison subjects (e.g., Heaton et al., 1978). Rawlings and Brooks (1990) demonstrated that their 16 MTBI litigants actually obtained somewhat higher WAIS-R PC ACSS than their 16 severe TBI litigant controls, in contrast to findings by Trueblood (1994; study described earlier). The malingering and QV groups performed worse than their control comparison groups on WAIS-R PC ACSS. A cutoff < 7 correctly classified six malingerers (sensitivity = 50%) and three individuals with QV (30%) with only one false positive error (96% specificity). Qualitatively, significant "scatter" (i.e., early errors) was noticed in the malingerers' performances (i.e., ≥ 2 errors on PC items from one to five correctly identified five malingerers (42%) and two individuals with QV (20%) with no false positive errors). Likewise, Larrabee (2003) demonstrated that 26 compensation-seeking patients identified as malingerers scored significantly worse than a group of 31 patients with moderate-to-severe TBI on WAIS-R PC, but PC was not retained as a predictor in a discriminant function analysis. Finally, PC has also been investigated as a SVT as a contributor to discriminant function analysis (e.g., Millis et al., 1998, reviewed later in this chapter).

Solomon and colleagues (2010) are the only ones to have investigated use of several scores from the WAIS-III PC subtest as an SVT in a large clinical sample using a known groups design (i.e., PC age-adjusted scaled score, raw score, most discrepant index [6- and 10-item], rarely correct index, and rarely missed index). They found that the "most discrepant" index (i.e., the six items that were the most discrepant in correct endorsement between groups) was the most accurate at correctly classifying the 167 noncredible subjects (identified by the presence of incentive and failure $\geq$ 2 independent SVTs) and the 175 credible patients (sensitivity = 65%, specificity = 93%). The index was also more effective in identifying noncredible individuals with less than 12 years of education (76.7% vs. 58.3%). When the authors examined a subsample of only noncredible MTBI subjects (n = 43), sensitivity was 56%. Index specificity declined to unacceptable levels in patients with low intelligence, but the authors reasoned that it is because patients with MTBI demonstrate normal IQ scores 1 year postinjury (Dikmen, Machamer, Winn, & Temkin, 1995).

> . . . if the available data suggest that a mild traumatic brain injury patient had low average or higher intelligence preaccident, it would be reasonable to use picture completion scores as a measure of effort, even if postaccident IQ scores are borderline or lower. (Dikmen et al., p. 1254).

Judgment of Line Orientation

JOLO (Benton, Sivan, Hamsher, Varney, & Spreen, 1994) is a motor-free test that requires the individual to correctly match the angles of two black lines per trial with numbered black lines shown at different angles in a half circle pattern. The test has two forms with good reliability and is sensitive to brain injury (Benton, Hamsher, Varney, & Spreen, 1983). JOLO has also been examined as a measure of effort in both simulation (Meyers et al., 1999) and known groups (Iverson, 2001; Meyers & Rohling, 2004; Meyers & Volbrecht, 2003; Whiteside, Wald, & Busse, 2011) study designs. Correct numbers of $\leq$ 12 are considered a failure when used as a SVT (Meyers et al., 1999; Meyers & Volbrecht, 2003).

Two additional studies have investigated JOLO as a SVT, both suggesting that although Meyers' cut score of $\leq$ 12 minimizes false positive errors, it is too low to have clinical use in detection of MND. In particular, Iverson (2001) examined the classification accuracy of JOLO in a large sample of head injury litigants (most of whom were classified as having suffered MTBI characterized by LOC < 5 min, PTA < 5 min, GCS = 15, and no positive neuroimaging findings). There were also patients with "complicated mild," moderate, and severe TBI collectively characterized by either GCS < 13, LOC > 20 min, PTA > 24 hr, or positive neuroimaging findings. Results were presented for three groups including (a) MTBI litigants (n = 146); (b) definite TBI litigants (i.e., the patients with complicated mild, moderate, and severe TBI described previously; n = 102); and the (c) entire sample of TBI litigants (Groups a and b combined). These groups were further subdivided based on their performance on two independent SVTs leading to nested credible and noncredible subgroups, specifically (a) 203 credible TBI (mild and definite combined) litigants, (b) 91 noncredible TBI (mild and definite combined) litigants, (c) 89 credible MTBI litigants, (d) 57 noncredible MTBI litigants, (e) 78 credible definite TBI litigants, and (f) 24 noncredible definite TBI litigants. Using a cut score from Meyers and colleagues (1999) of $\leq$ 12, specificity was 98%, but sensitivity was only 10.5%. Raising the cutoff to $\leq$ 18 increased sensitivity to 29.8% while maintaining specificity of 92%.

In the study by Whiteside and colleagues (2011, described previously), use of a $\leq$ 18 cutoff score resulted in a sensitivity rate of 31% while maintaining a 90%

specificity rate. The Meyers and colleagues (1999) cutoff of ≤ 12 resulted in an essentially useless rate of sensitivity (7%). Thus, both independent investigations suggest the JOLO cutoff can be raised to maximize sensitivity to MND in a MTBI population while still maintaining adequate specificity.

Knox Cube Test

The KCT is a measure of immediate visual attention span and has been described as a "visual-spatial analog to the digit span procedure" (Iverson & Franzen, 1994, p. 325). In the only identified study of this test as an SVT, Iverson and Franzen (1994) used a mixed-simulator/clinical-specificity design, comparing 20 nonlitigating patients with TBI (severe = 80%, moderate = 15%, and mild = 5%) with memory impairment to 40 male inmates and 40 undergraduate students with no neurological conditions or impairment. The inmate and undergraduate groups were randomly assigned as controls or to a group in which they were instructed to simulate malingering in the context of a lawsuit. The simulators scored significantly lower on the KCT total score than nonlitigating patients with TBI with documented memory impairments. A cutoff of < 3 cubes performed in correct sequence correctly identified 72% of simulators while maintaining 100% specificity. However, as Grieffenstein (2007) pointed out, the KCT needs to be validated in a "natural litigating group" and in real clinical samples of patients with TBI.

Rey Complex Figure Test

The RCFT (Rey, 1941; Meyers & Meyers, 1995) is a commonly used measure of visuospatial skills and perceptual organization as well as immediate and delayed visual memory. With the recognition portion of the test, the RCFT has demonstrated sensitivity to brain injury (Meyers & Lange, 1994). The RCFT has been investigated as an embedded effort indicator using information from both copy (visuospatial portion of the test) and recognition (memory portion of the test; Lu et al., 2003; Meyers, Bayless, & Meyers, 1996; Meyers & Volbrecht, 1999; Sherman et al., 2002) and is, therefore, also reviewed in Chapter 9 of this book.

A recent investigation of the RCFT copy score, alone, as an SVT was undertaken by Whiteside and colleagues (2011; study described earlier) who compared two groups defined by their performance on two independent memory-based SVTs: credibles (passed both SVTs; $n = 415$) and noncredibles (failed both SVTs; $n = 30$). The most common diagnosis in the sample was MTBI (total MTBI = 101; noncredible MTBI = 12). However, subjects in both groups carried other neuropsychiatric diagnoses. Subjects with known right cerebral lesions or with previous diagnoses of mental retardation were excluded. Results indicated that a RCFT copy cutoff score of < 25 maximized sensitivity (32%) while maintaining adequate specificity (89%). One major limitation of this study is that not all subjects in the noncredible group had incentive to feign cognitive deficit, raising questions as to whether they were in fact noncredible or if their SVT failures represented false positive identifications. However, noncredible test performance can occur without incentive to perform poorly.

Benton Facial Recognition Test

The Benton Facial Recognition Test (BFRT: Benton, Hamsher, & Sivan, 1994) is a test of visual recognition and discrimination requiring examinees to match pictures of unfamiliar faces and to discriminate familiar from unfamiliar faces. Arguing the BFRT is a relatively easy test that may appear challenging to examinees. Whiteside and colleagues (2011, described previously) conducted the only study known to us that investigated use of the BFRT as a SVT. Recall that the most common diagnosis in the sample was MTBI, and a good portion of the noncredible group (n = 12) was referred secondary to suspected MTBI. A cutoff score of ≤ 39 maximized sensitivity at 40% while maintaining a 90% specificity rate.

Hooper Visual Organization Test

The Hooper Visual Organization Test (HVOT; Hooper, 1958) is a test of visual integration that requires examinees to mentally combine individual pieces of disconnected drawings of common objects to discern their identity. Such as the BFRT, Whiteside and colleagues (2011; study described earlier) argued that this test is relatively easy, yet might appear challenging, therefore potentially serving as a useful SVT. A cutoff score of ≤ 22 maximized sensitivity at 46% while maintaining borderline adequate specificity (88%).

Visual Form Discrimination Test

The Visual Form Discrimination Test (VFD; Benton, Sivan, Hamsher, et al., 1994) was originally investigated as an SVT in Larrabee's (2003) atypical performance pattern paper. In particular, he compared 24 litigants (including 19 alleging MTBI) who met criteria for definite MND (Slick et al., 1999) and 27 credible patients with moderate-to-severe TBI. The VFD total raw score was also reexamined in Larrabee's (2008) paper using much of the same sample from 2003 on the clinical use of aggregating across multiple effort indicators. In particular, his sample consisted of 26 individuals meeting MND criteria (21 of whom had alleged MTBI), and this sample was compared to 31 credible subjects with moderate-to-severe TBI. With respect to their performance on the VFD, a cutoff score of < 26 maintained adequate specificity (i.e., 93%) with sensitivity at 48%

Summary of Visuospatial/Perceptual-Based Symptom Validity Tests

Several visuospatial/perceptual-based SVTs appear to be useful for detecting symptom invalidity. However, sensitivity is relatively low compared to other memory-based SVTs (see Chapters 8 and 9 in this volume). Thus, a negative finding does not rule out poor effort, but a positive finding does provide useful information regarding performance credibility. In addition, most of the SVTs reviewed here require validation in an MTBI sample specifically. It may be helpful to aggregate across several scores to increase sensitivity of measures in this domain and perhaps others. For example, in the study by Whiteside and colleagues (2011), when all visuospatial measures were summed into a single score, there was improved classification accuracy compared to any visuopatial measure alone (cutoff < 134, sensitivity = 52%, specificity = 88%).

CONCLUSION

Previous work has focused mostly on assessing feigned memory deficits with dedicated SVTs, but it is important to recognize that people fake or exaggerate symptoms in various cognitive domains other than memory. Although there is some evidence indicating that individuals feigning in the context of MTBI do so by targeting their poor performance on perceived measures of memory (e.g., Nitch et al., 2006), not all do, and effort needs to be assessed *throughout* the evaluation and across several cognitive domains (Boone, 2009). The nature of the strategy or approach to feigning will vary; as Meyers and colleagues (2011) pointed out,

> . . . individuals do not fail all SVTs equally, but instead are more selective of their SVT performance. . . . the approach to malingering varies based on the nature of the task and the "perception" of the individual as to what cognitive deficits he/she is trying to portray. (p. 14)

In this chapter, we attempted to provide a concise review of SVTs in domains other than memory that hold promise for detecting MND in MTBI populations specifically. We focused on the domains of attention, processing speed, language and visuospatial/perceptual function. In the next chapter, we review SVTs in the domains of motor/sensory and executive function, as well as those SVTs derived from discriminant functions and embedded in the context of comprehensive test batteries. Overall conclusions and clinical implications are presented at the end of the next chapter.

REFERENCES

Abudarham, S., & White, A. (2001). "Insuring" a correct differential diagnosis—a "forensic" collaborative experience. *International Journal of Language and Communication Disorder*, (Suppl. 36), 58–63.

Alfano, K., & Boone, K. B. (2007). The use of effort tests in the context of actual versus feigned attention-deficit/hyperactivity disorder and learning disability. In Boone, K. B. (Ed.), *Assessment of Feigned Cognitive Impairment: A Neuropsychological Perspective* (pp. 366–383). New York, NY: Guilford Press.

Arnold, G., Boone, K., Lu, P., Dean, A., Wen, J., Nitch, S., McPherson, S. (2005). Sensitivity and specificity of finger tapping test scores for the detection of suspect effort. *The Clinical Neuropsychologist*, 19(1), 105–120.

Axelrod, B. N., Fichtenberg, N. L., Millis, S. R., & Wertheimer, J. C. (2006). Detecting incomplete effort with digit span from the Wechsler Adult Intelligence Scale–Third Edition. *The Clinical Neuropsychologist*, 20(3), 513–523.

Axelrod, B. N., & Rawlings, D. B. (1999). Clinical utility of incomplete effort WAIS-R formulas: A longitudinal examination of individuals with traumatic brain injuries. *Journal of Forensic Neuropsychology*, 1(2), 15–27.

Babikian, T., & Boone, K. B. (2007). Intelligence tests as measures of effort. In K. B. Boone (Ed.), *Assessment of feigned cognitive impairment: A neuropsychological perspective* (pp. 103–127), New York, NY: Guilford Press.

Babikian, T., Boone, K. B., Lu, P., & Arnold, G. (2006). Sensitivity and specificity of various digit span scores in the detection of suspect effort. *The Clinical Neuropsychologist*, 20(1), 145–159.

Backhaus, S. L., Fichtenberg, N. L., & Hanks, R. A. (2004). Detection of sub-optimal performance using a floor-effect strategy in patients with traumatic brain injury. *The Clinical Neuropsychologist*, 18(4), 591–603.

Bazarian, J., McClung, J., Shah, M. N., Cheng, Y. T., Flesher, W., & Kraus, J. (2005). Mild traumatic brain injury in the United States, 1998–2000. *Brain Injury*, 19(2), 85–91.

Beetar, J. T., & Williams, J. M. (1995). Malingering response styles on the memory assessment scales and symptom validity tests. *Archives of Clinical Neuropsychology*, 10(1), 57–72.

Belanger, H. G., Curtiss, G., Demery, J. A., Lebowitz, B. K., & Vanderploeg, R. D. (2005). Factors moderating neuropsychological outcomes following mild traumatic brain injury: A meta-analysis. *Journal of the International Neuropsychological Society*, 11(3), 215–227.

Belanger, H. G., & Vanderploeg, R. D. (2005). The neuropsychological impact of sports-related concussion: A meta-analysis. *Journal of the International Neuropsychological Society*, 11(4), 345–357.

Benton, A. L., Hamsher, K. de S., & Sivan, A. B. (1994). *Multilingual aphasia examination: Manual of instructions* (3rd ed.). Iowa City, IA: AJA Associates.

Benton, A. L., Hamsher, K., Varney, N., & Spreen, O. (1983). *Contributions to neuropsychological assessment: A clinical manual.* New York, NY: Oxford University Press.

Benton, A. L., Sivan, A. B., Hamsher, K. de S., Varney, N. R., & Spreen, O. (1994). *Contributions to neuropsychological assessment, a clinical manual* (2nd ed.). New York, NY: Oxford University Press.

Bernard, L. C. (1990). Prospects for faking believable memory deficits on neuropsychological tests and the use of incentives in simulation research. *Journal of Clinical and Experimental Neuropsychology*, 12(5), 715–728.

Bianchini, K. J., Curtis, K. L., & Greve, K. W. (2006). Compensation and malingering in traumatic brain injury: A dose-response relationship? *The Clinical Neuropsychologist*, 20(4), 831–847.

Binder, L. M. (1992). Deception and malingering. In A. Puente & R. McCaffrey (Eds.), *Handbook of neuro-psychological assessment: A biopsychosocial perspective* (pp. 353–372). New York, NY: Springer Publishing.

Binder, L. M., & Rohling, M. L. (1996). Money matters: A meta-analytic review of the effects of financial incentives on recovery after closed-head injury. *American Journal of Psychiatry*, 153(1), 7–10.

Binder, L. M., Rohling, M. L., & Larrabee, G. (1997). A review of mild head trauma Part I: Meta-analytic review of neuropsychological studies. *Journal of Clinical and Experimental Neuropsychology*, 19(3), 421–431.

Binder, L. M., & Willis, S. C. (1991). Assessment of motivation after financially compensable minor head trauma. *Psychological Assessment*, 3, 175–181.

Binks, P. G., Gouvier, W. D., & Waters, W. F. (1997). Malingering detection with the Dot Counting Test. *Archives of Clinical Neuropsychology*, 12(1), 41–46.

Black, F. W. (1986). Digit repetition in brain-damaged adults: Clinical and theoretical implications. *Journal of Clinical Psychology*, 42(5), 770–782.

Boone, K. B. (2007). *Assessment of feigned cognitive impairement: A neuropsychological Perspective.* New York, NY: The Guilford Press.

Boone, K. B. (2009). The need for continuous and comprehensive sampling of effort/response bias during neuropsychological examinations. *The Clinical Neuropsychologist*, 23(4), 729–741.

Boone, K. B., & Lu, P. (2007). Non-forced-choice effort measures. In G. J. Larrabee (Ed.), *Assessment of malingered neuropsychological deficits*, (pp. 27–43). New York, NY: Oxford University Press.

Boone, K. B., Lu, P., Back, C., King, C., Lee, A., Philpott, L., . . . Warner-Chacon, K. (2002). Sensitivity and specificity of the Rey Dot Counting Test in patients with suspect effort and various clinical samples. *Archives of Clinical Neuropsychology*, 17(7), 625–642.

Boone, K., Lu, P., & Herzberg, D. S. (2002a). *The b test manual.* Los Angeles, CA: Western Psychological Services.

Boone, K. B., Lu, P., & Herzberg, D. S. (2002b). *The Dot Counting Test manual.* Los Angeles, CA: Western Psychological Services.

Boone, K. B., Lu, P., Sherman, D., Palmer, B., Back, C. Shamieh, E., . . . Berman, N. G. (2000). Validation of a new technique to detect malingering of cognitive symptoms: The b test. *Archives of Clinical Neuropsychology*, 15(3), 227–241.

Boone, K. B., Lu, P., & Wen, J. (2005). Comparison of various RAVLT scores in the detection of non-credible memory performance. *Archives of Clinical Neuropsychology*, 20(3), 301–319.

Capruso, D. X., & Levin, H. S. (1992). Cognitive impairment following closed head injury. *Neurologic Clinics*, 10(4), 879–893.

Carroll, L. J., Cassidy, J. D., Peloso, P. M., Borg, J., von Holst, H., Holm, L., . . . Pépin, M. (2004). Prognosis for mild traumatic brain injury: Results of the WHO Collaborating Center Task Force on mild traumatic brain injury. *Journal of Rehabilitation Medicine*, 36(Suppl. 43), 84–105.

Chouinard, M. J., & Rouleau, I. (1997). The 48-picture test: A two-alternative forced-choice recognition test for the detection of malingering. *Journal of the International Neuropschological Society*, 3, 545–552.

Conners, C. K. (2000). *Conners' Continuous Performance Test-II.* Toronto, ON: Multi Health Systems.

Cottingham, M. E., & Boone, K. B. (2010). Non-credible language deficits following mild traumatic brain injury. *The Clinical Neuropsychologist*, 24(6), 1006–1025.

Curtis, K. L., Greve, K. W., & Bianchini, K. J. (2009). The Wechsler Adult Intelligence Scale-III and malingering in traumatic brain injury: Classification accuracy in known groups. *Assessment*, 16(4), 401–414.

Curtis, K. L., Greve, K. W., Brasseux, R., & Bianchini, K. J. (2010). Criterion groups validation of the seashore rhythm test and speech sounds perception test for the detection of malingering in traumatic brain injury. *The Clinical Neuropsychologist*, 24(5), 882–897.

Crawford, J. R., Besson, J. A., & Parker, D. M. (1988). Estimation of premorbid intelligence in organic conditions. *British Journal of Psychiatry*, 153, 178–181.

Demakis, G. J. (2004). Application of clinically-derived malingering cutoffs on the California Verbal Learning Test and the Wechsler Adult Intelligence Test-Revised to an analog malingering study. *Applied Neuropsychology*, 11(4), 222–228.

Dikmen, S., Machamer, J. E., Winn, H. R., & Temkin, N. R. (1995). Neuropsychological outcome at 1-year post head injury. *Neuropsychology, 9*(1), 80–90.

Erdal, K. (2004). The effects of motivation, coaching, and knowledge of neuropsychology on the simulated malingering of head injury. *Archives of Clinical Neuropsychology, 19*(1), 73–88.

Etherton, J. L., Bianchini, K. J., Ciota, M. A., Heinly, M. T., & Greve, K. W. (2006). Pain, malingering, and the WAIS-III Working Memory Index. *Spine Journal, 6*(1), 61–67.

Etherton, J. L., Bianchini, K. J., Greve, K. W., & Heinly, M. T. (2005). Sensitivity and specificity of reliable digit span in malingered pain-related disability. *Assessment, 12*(2), 130–136.

Etherton, J. L., Bianchini, K. J., Heinly, M. T., & Greve, K. W. (2006). Pain, malingering, and performance on the WAIS-III Processing Speed Index. *Journal of Clinical and Experimental Neuropsychology, 28*(7), 1218–1237.

Frencham, K. A., Fox, A. M., & Maybery, M. T. (2005). Neuropsychological studies of mild traumatic brain injury: A meta-analytic review of research since 1995. *Journal of Clinical and Experimental Neuropsychology, 27*(3), 334–351.

Gfeller, J. D., & Cradock, M. M. (1998). Detecting feigned neuropsychological impairment with the Seashore Rhythm Test. *Journal of Clinical Psychology, 54*(4), 431–438.

Green, P., Rohling, M. L., Lees-Haley, P. R., & Allen, L. M. III. (2001). Effort has a greater effect on test scores than severe brain injury in compensation claimants. *Brain Injury, 15*(12), 1045–1060.

Greenberg, L., Kindschi, C., Dupuy, T., & Corman, C. (1996). *Test of variables of attention.* Los Alamitos, CA: Universal Attention Disorders.

Greiffenstein, M. F. (2007). Motor, sensory, and perceptual-motor pseudoabnormalities. In G. Larrabee (Ed.), *Assessment of malingered neuropsychological deficits* (pp. 100–130). New York, NY: Oxford University Press.

Greiffenstein, M. F. (2009). Clinical myths of forensic neuropsychology. *The Clinical Neuropsychologist, 23*(2), 286–296.

Greiffenstein, M. F., Baker, W. J., & Gola, T. (1994). Validation of malingered amnesia measures with a large clinical sample. *Psychological Assessment, 6,* 218–224.

Greiffenstein, M. F., Gola, T., & Baker, W. J. (1995). MMPI-2 validity scales versus domain specific measures in detection of factitious traumatic brain injury. *Clinical Neuropsychologist, 9,* 230–240.

Greve, K. W., Bianchini, K. J., Mathias, C. W., Houston, R. J., & Crouch, J. A. (2003). Detecting malingered performance on the Wechsler Adult Intelligence Scale: Validation of Mittenberg's approach in traumatic brain injury. *Archives of Clinical Neuropsychology, 18*(3), 245–260.

Hannay, H. J., Howieson, D. B., Loring, D. W., Fischer, J. S., & Lezak, M. D. (2004). Neuropathology for neuropsychologists. In M. D. Lezak, D. B. Howieson, & D. W. Loring (Eds.), *Neuropsychological assessment* (pp. 157–285). New York, NY: Oxford University Press.

Heaton, R. K., Smith, H. H. Jr., Lehman, R. A. W., & Vogt, A. T. (1978). Prospects for faking believable deficits on neuropsychological testing. *Journal of Consulting and Clinical Psychology, 46*(5), 892–900.

Heinly, M. T. (2008). Language dysfunction in traumatic brain injury while controlling for effort. *Dissertation Abstracts International, 68* (12), 534B. (UMI No. 3292293).

Heinly, M. T., Greve, K. W., Bianchini, K. J., Love, J. M., & Brennan, A. (2005). WAIS digit span-based indicators of malingered neurocognitive dysfunction: Classification accuracy in traumatic brain injury. *Assessment, 12*(4), 429–444.

Henry, G. K. (2005). Probable malingering and performance on the test of variables of attention. *The Clinical Neuropsychologist, 19*(1), 121–129.

Hiscock, C. K., Branham, J. D., & Hiscock, M. (1994). Detection of feigned cognitive impairment: The two-alternative forced-choice method compared with selected conventional tests. *Journal of Psychopathology and Behavioral Assessment, 16,* 95–110.

Hooper, H. E. (1958). *The Hooper visual organization test: Manual.* Los Angeles, CA: Western Psychological Services.

Inman, T. H., & Berry, D. T. R. (2002). Cross-validation of indicators of malingering: A comparison of nine neuropsychological tests, four tests of malingering, and behavioral observations. *Archives of Clinical Neuropsychology, 17*(1), 1–23.

Iverson, G. L. (1995). Qualitative aspects of malingered memory deficits. *Brain Injury, 9*(1), 35–40.

Iverson, G. L. (2001). Can malingering be identified with the judgment of line orientation test? *Applied Neuropsychology, 8*(3), 167–173.

Iverson, G. L. (2005). Outcome from mild traumatic brain injury. *Current Opinion in Psychiatry, 18*(3), 301–317.

Iverson, G. L., & Franzen, M. D. (1994). The Recognition Memory Test, digit span, and Knox Cube Test as markers of malingered memory impairment. *Assessment, 1*(4), 323–334.

Iverson, G. L., & Franzen, M. D. (1996). Using multiple objective memory procedures to detect simulated malingering. *Journal of Clinical and Experimental Neuropsychology, 18*(1), 38–51.

Iverson, G. L., Lange, R. T., Brooks, B. L., & Rennison, V. L. (2010). "Good old days" bias following mild traumatic brain injury. *The Clinical Neuropsychologist*, 24(1), 17–37.

Iverson, G. L., & Tulsky, D. S. (2003). Detecting malingering on the WAIS-III. Unusual digit span performance patterns in the normal population and in clinical groups. *Archives of Clinical Psychology*, 18(1), 1–9.

Kallen, D., Marshall, R. C., & Casey, D. E. (1986). Atypical dysarthria in Munchausen syndrome. *British Journal of Disorders of Communication*, 21(3), 377–380.

Khan, I., Fayaz, I., Ridgley, J., & Wennberg, R. (2000). Factitious clock drawing and constructional apraxia. *Journal of Neurology, Neurosurgery, and Psychiatry*, 68(1), 106–107.

Kim, N., Boone, K. B., Victor, T., Lu, P., Keatinge, C., & Mitchell, C. (2010). Sensitivity and specificity of digit symbol recognition trial in the identification of response bias. *Archives of Clinical Neuropsychology*, 25(5), 420–428.

Kim, M. S., Boone, K. B., Victor, T., Marion, S. D., Amano, S., Cottingham, M. E., . . . Zeller, M. A. (2010). The Warrington recognition memory test for words as a measure of response bias: Total score and response time cutoffs developed on "real world" credible and non-credible subjects. *Archives of Clinical Neuropsychology*, 25(1), 60–70.

Klimczak, N. J., Donovick, P. J., & Burright, R. (1997). The malingering of multiple sclerosis and mild traumatic brain injury. *Brain Injury*, 11(5), 343–352.

Lamberty, G. J. (2007). *Understanding somatization in the practice of clinical neuropsychology*. Oxford, UK: Oxford University Press.

Larrabee, G. J. (2003). Detection of malingering using atypical performance patterns on standard neuropsychological tests. *The Clinical Neuropsychologist*, 17(3), 410–424.

Larrabee, G. J. (2004). *Identification of subtypes of malingered neurocognitive dysfunction*. Presented at the 32nd Annual Meeting of the International Neuropsychological Society, Baltimore, MA.

Larrabee, G. J. (2007). Identification of malingering by pattern analysis on neuropsychological tests. In G. J. Larrabee (Ed.), *Assessment of malingered neuropsychological deficits* (pp. 80–99). New York, NY: Oxford University Press.

Larrabee, G. J. (2008). Aggregation across multiple indicators improves the detection of malingering: Relationship to likelihood ratios. *The Clinical Neuropsychologist*, 22(4), 666–679.

Laures-Gore, J., Henson, J. C., Weismer, G., Rambow, M. (2006). Two cases of foreign accent syndrome: An acoustic-phonetic description. *Clinical Linguistics & Phonetics*, 20(10), 781–790.

Leark, R. A., Dixon, D., Hoffman, T., & Huynh, D. (2002). Fake bad test response bias effects on the test of variables of attention. *Archives of Clinical Neuropsychology*, 17(4), 335–342.

Levin, H. (1990). Memory deficit after closed head injury. *Journal of Clinical and Experimental Neuropsychology*, 12(1), 129–153.

Lezak, M., Howeison, D. B., & Loring, D. W. (2004). *Neuropsychological assessment* (4th ed.). New York, NY: Oxford University Press.

Lippert-Gruener, M., Weinert, U., Greisbach, T., & Wedekind, C. (2005). Foreign accent syndrome following traumatic brain injury. *Brain Injury*, 19(11), 955–958.

Lu, P. H., Boone, K. B., Cozolino, L., & Mitchell, C. (2003). Effectiveness of the Rey-Osterrieth complex figure test and the Meyers and Meyers recognition trial in the detection of suspect effort. *The Clinical Neuropsychologist*, 17(3), 426–440.

Mahr, G., & Leith, W. (1992). Psychogenic stuttering of adult onset. *Journal of Speech and Hearing Research*, 35(2), 283–286.

Martin, R. C., Hayes, J. S., & Gouvier, W. D. (1996). Differential vulnerability between postconcussion self-report and objective malingering tests in identifying simulated mild head injury. *Journal of Clinical and Experimental Neuropsychology*, 18(2), 265–275.

Mathias, J. L., & Coats, J. L. (1999). Emotional and cognitive sequelae to mild traumatic brain injury. *Journal of Clinical and Experimental Neuropsychology*, 21(2), 200–215.

Mathias, C. W., Greve, K. W., Bianchini, K. J., Houston, R. J., & Crouch, J. A. (2002). Detecting malingered neurocognitive dysfunction using the reliable digit span in traumatic brain injury. *Assessment*, 9(3), 301–308.

McCrea, M. A. (2008). *Mild traumatic brain injury and postconcussion syndrome: The new evidence base for diagnosis and treatment* (AACN Workshop Series). New York, NY: Oxford University Press.

Meyers, J. E. (2007). Malingering mild traumatic brain injury: Behavioral approaches used by both malingering actors and probable malingerers. In K. B. Boone (Ed.), *Assessment of Feigned Cognitive Impairment: A Neuropsychological Perspective* (pp. 239–258). New York, NY: Guilford Press.

Meyers, J. E., Bayless, J., & Meyers, K. R. (1996). The Rey complex figure: Memory error patterns and functional abilities. *Applied Neuropsychology*, 3, 89–92.

Meyers, J. E., Galinsky, A., & Volbrecht, M. (1999). Malingering and mild brain injury: How low is too low. *Applied Neuropsychology*, 6(4), 208–216.

Meyers, J. E., & Lange, D. (1994). Recognition subtest for the complex figure. *The Clinical Neuropsychologist*, 8, 153–166.

Meyers, J. E., & Meyers, K. (1995). *Rey complex figure and the recognition trial: Professional manual*. Odessa, FL: Psychological Assessment Resources.

Meyers, J. E., Morrison, A. L., & Miller, J. C. (2001). How low is too low, revisited: Sentence repetition and AVLT-recognition in the detection of malingering. *Applied Neuropsychology*, 8(4), 234–241.

Meyers, J. E., & Rohling, M. L. (2004). Validation of the Meyers short battery on mild TBI patients. *Archives of Clinical Neuropsychology*, 19(5), 637–651.

Meyers, J. E., & Volbrecht, M. (1998). Validation of reliable digits for detection of malingering. *Assessment*, 5(3), 303–307.

Meyers, J. E., & Volbrecht, M. (1999). Detection of malingerers using the Rey complex figure and recognition trial. *Applied Neuropsychology*, 6(4), 201–207.

Meyers, J. E., & Volbrecht, M. E. (2003). A validation of multiple malingering detection methods in a large clinical sample. *Archives of Clinical Neuropsychology*, 18(3), 261–276.

Meyers, J. E., Volbrecht, M., Axelrod, B. N., & Reinsch-Boothby, L. (2011). Embedded symptom validity tests and overall neuropsychological test performance. *Archives of Clinical Neuropsychology*, 26(1), 8–15.

Meyers, J. E., Volkert, K., & Diep, A. (2000). Sentence repetition test: Updated norms and clinical utility. *Applied Neuropsychology*, 7(3), 154–159.

Miller, L. J., Ryan, J. J., Carruthers, C. A., & Cluff, R. B. (2004). Brief screening indexes for malingering: A confirmation of vocabulary minus digit span from the WAIS-III and the rarely missed index from the WMS-III. *Clinical Neuropsychologist*, 18(2), 327–333.

Millis, S. R., Ross, S. R., & Ricker, J. H. (1998). Detection of incomplete effort on the Wechsler Adult Intelligence Scale-Revised: A cross-validation. *Journal of Clinical and Experimental Neuropsychology*, 20(2), 167–173.

Mitrushina, M., Boone, K. B., Razani, J., & D'Elia, L. F. (2005). *Handbook of normative data for neuropsychological assessment* (2nd ed.)..New York, NY: Oxford University Press.

Mittenberg, W., Roberts, D. M., Patton, C., & Legler, W. (2005, October). *Identification of malingered head injury with WAIS-3 Vocabulary and Digit Span*. Paper presented at the 25th annual meeting of the National Academy of Neuropsychology, Tampa, FL.

Mittenberg, W., Rotholc, A., Russel, E., & Heilbronner, R. (1996). Identification of malingered head injury of the Halstead-Reitan battery. *Archives of Clinical Neuropsychology*, 11(4), 271–281.

Mittenberg, W., Theroux, S., Aguila-Puentes, G., Bianchini, K., Greve, K., & Rayls, K. (2001). Identification of malingered head injury on the Wechsler adult intelligence scale (3rd ed.). *The Clinical Neuropsychologist*, 15(4), 440–445.

Mittenberg, W., Theroux-Fichera, S., Zielinski, R. E., & Heilbronner, R. L. (1995). Identification of malingered head injury on the Wechsler Adult Intelligence Scale (Rev. ed.). *Professional Psychology: Research and Practice*, 26, 491–498.

Niogi, S. N., Mukherjee, P., Ghajar, J., Johnson, C. E., Kolster, R., Lee, H., . . . McCandliss, B. D. (2008). Structural dissociation of attentional control and memory in adults with and without mild traumatic brain injury. *Brain*, 131(Pt. 12), 3209–3221.

Nitch, S., Boone, K. B., Wen, J., Arnold, G., & Alfano, K. (2006). The utility of the Rey word recognition test in the detection of suspect effort. *The Clinical Neuropsychologist*, 20(4), 873–887.

Nitch, S. R., & Glassmire, D. M. (2007). Non-forced-choice measures to detect noncredible cognitive performance. In K. B. Boone (Ed.), *Assessment of feigned cognitive impairment: A neuropsychological perspective* (pp. 78–102). New York, NY: Guilford Press.

Ord, J. L., Greve, K. W., & Bianchini, K. J. (2008). Using the Wechsler memory scale-III to detect malingering in mild traumatic brain injury. *The Clinical Neuropsychologist*, 22(4), 689–704.

Ord, J. S., Boettcher, A. C., Greve, K. W., & Bianchini, K. J. (2010). Detection of malingering in mild traumatic brain injury with the Conners' continuous performance test-II. *Journal of Clinical and Experimental Neuropsychology*, 32(4), 380–387.

Osimani, A., Alon, A., Berger, J., & Abarbanel, A. (1997). Use of the Stroop phenomenon as a diagnostic tool for malingering. *Journal of Neurology, Neurosurgery, and Psychiatry*, 62(6), 617–621.

Osmon, D. C., Plambeck, E., Klein, L., & Mano, Q. (2006). The word reading test of effort in adult learning disability: A simulation study. *The Clinical Neuropsychologist*, 20(2), 315–324.

Paul, D. S., Franzen, M. D., Cohen, S. H., & Fremouw, W. (1992). An investigation into the reliability and validity of two tests used in the detection of dissimulation. *International Journal of Clinical Neuropsychology*, 14, 1–9.

Raskin, S. A., & Rearick, E. (1996). Verbal fluency in individuals with mild traumatic brain injury. *Neuropsychology*, 10, 416–422.

Rawlings, P., & Brooks, N. (1990). Simulation index: A method for detecting factitious errors on the WAIS-R and WMS. *Neuropsychology*, 4, 223–238.

Reitan, R. M., & Wolfson, D. (1992). *Neuropsychological evaluation of older children*.Tucson AZ: Neuropsychology Press.

Rey, A. (1941). L'examen psychologie dans las cas d'encephalopathie traumatique. *Archives de Psychologie*, 28, 286–340.

Rogers, R. (Ed.). (1997). *Current status of clinical methods*. In *Clinical assessment of malingering and deception* (2nd ed., pp. 373–397). New York, NY: Guilford Press.

Rohling, M. L., & Boone, K. B. (2007). Future directions in effort assessment. In K. B. Boone (Ed.), *Assessment of feigned cognitive impairment: A neuropsychological perspective* (pp. 453–470). New York, NY: Guilford Press.

Rohling, M. L., & Demakis, G. J. (2010). Bowden, Shores, & Mathias (2006): Failure to replicate or just failure to notice. Does effort still account for more variance in neuropsychological test scores than TBI severity? *The Clinical Neuropsychologist*, 24(1), 119–136.

Rose, F. E., Hall, S., Szalda-Petree, A. D., & Bach, P. J. (1998). A comparison of four tests of malingering and the effects of coaching. *Archives of Clinical Neuropsychology*, 13, 349–363.

Ross, S. R., Putnam, S. H., Millis, S. R., Adams, K. M., & Krukowski, R. A. (2006). Detecting insufficient effort using the Seashore Rhythm and Speech Sounds Perception Test in head injury. *The Clinical Neuropsychologist*, 20(4), 798–815.

Roth, C., Aronson, A. E., & Davis, L. J. Jr. (1989). Clinical studies in psychogenic stuttering of adult onset. *Journal of Speech and Hearing Disorders*, 54(4), 634–646.

Salazar, X., Lu, P. H., Wen, J., & Boone, K. B. (2007). The use of effort tests in ethnic minorities and in non-English-speaking and English as a second language populations. In K. B. Boone (Ed.), *Assessment of feigned cognitive impairment: A neuropsychological perspective* (pp. 405–427). New York, NY: Guilford Press.

Schretlen, D. J., & Shapiro, A. M. (2003). A quantitative review of the effects of traumatic brain injury on cognitive functioning. *International Review of Psychiatry*, 15(4), 341–349.

Schroeder, R. W., & Marshall, P. S. (2010). Validation of the Sentence Repetition Test as measure of suspect effort. *The Clinical Neuropsychologist*, 24(2), 326–343.

Schwarz, L. R., Gfeller, J. D., & Oliveri, M. V. (2006). Detecting feigned impairment with the digit span and vocabulary subtests of the Wechsler Adult Intelligence Scale–Third Edition.). *The Clinical Neuropsychologist*, 20(4), 741–753.

Seery, C. H. (2005). Differential diagnosis of stuttering for forensic purposes. *American Journal of Speech-Language Pathology*, 14(4), 284–297.

Sherman, D. S., Boone, K. B., Lu, P., & Razani, J. (2002). Re-examination of a Rey Auditory Verbal Learning Test/Rey Complex Figure discriminant function to detect suspect effort. *The Clinical Neuropsychologist*, 16(3), 242–250.

Shum, D. H., O'Gorman, J. G., & Alpar, A. (2004). Effects of incentive and preparation time on performance and classification accuracy of standard and malingering-specific memory tests. *Archives of Clinical Neuropsychology*, 19(6), 817–823.

Sim, A., Terryberry-Spohr, L., & Wilson, K. R. (2008). Prolonged recovery of memory functioning after mild traumatic brain injury in adolescent athletes. *Journal of Neurosurgery*, 108(3), 511–516.

Slick, D. J., Sherman, E. M., & Iverson, G. L. (1999). Diagnostic criteria for malingering neurocognitive dysfunction: Proposed standards for clinical practice and research. *Clinical Neuropsychologist*, 13(4), 545–561.

Smith, A. (1973). *Symbol Digit Modalities Test Manual*. Los Angeles, CA: Western Psychological Services.

Solomon, R., Boone, K. B., Miora, D., Skidmore, S., Cottingham, M., Victor, T. L., . . . Zeller, M. (2010). Use of the WAIS-III Picture Completion subtest as an embedded measure of response bias. *The Clinical Neuropsychologist*, 24(7), 1243–1256.

Sosin, D. M., Sniezek, J. E., & Thurman, D. J. (1996). Incidence of mild and moderate brain injury in the United Stated. *Brain Injury*, 10, 47–57.

Spector, J., Lewandowski, A. G., Kelly, M. P., & Kaylor, J. A. (1994, November). *The use of the Seashore Rhythm test as a forced-choice measure to detect malingering in a compensation-seeking mildly head-injured sample*. Paper presented at the 14th annual conference of the National Academy of Neuropsychology, Orlando, FL.

Strauss, E., Hultsch, D. F., Hunter, M., Slick, D. J., Patry, B., & Levy-Bencheton, J. (1999). Using intraindividual variability to detect malingering in cognitive performance. *The Clinical Neuropsychologist*, 13(4), 420–432.

Strauss, E., Sherman, E. M., & Spreen, O. (2006). *A compendium of neuropsychological tests: Administration, norms, and commentary* (3rd ed.). New York, NY: Oxford University Press.

Strauss, E., Slick, D. J., Levy-Bencheton, J., Hunter, M., MacDonald, S. W., & Hultsch, D. F. (2002). Intraindividual variability as an indicator of malingering in head injury. *Archives of Clinical Neuropsychology*, 17(5), 423–444.

Suhr, J. A., & Barrash, J. (2007) Performance on standard attention, memory and psychomotor speed tasks as indicators of malingering. In G. J. Larrabee (Ed.), *Assessment of malingered neuropsychological deficits* (pp. 131–170). New York, NY: Oxford University Press.

Suhr, J. A., & Gunstad, J. (2000). The effect of coaching on the sensitivity and specificity of malingering measures. *Archives of Clinical Neuropsychology, 15*(5), 415–424.

Suhr, J., Tranel, D., Wefel, J., & Barrash, J. (1997). Memory performance after head injury: Contributions of malingering, litigation status, psychological factors, and medication use. *Journal of Clinical and Experimental Neuropsychology, 19*(4), 500–514.

Tan, J. E., Slick, D. J., Strauss, E., & Hultsch, D. F. (2002). How'd they do it? Malingering strategies on symptom validity tests. *The Clinical Neuropsychologist, 16*(4), 495–505.

Trueblood, W. (1994). Qualitative and quantitative characteristics of malingered and other invalid WAIS-R and clinical memory data. *Journal of Clinical and Experimental Neuropsychology, 16*(4), 597–607.

Trueblood, W., & Schmidt, M. (1993). Malingering and other validity considerations in the neuropsychological evaluation of mild head injury. *Journal of Clinical and Experimental Neuropsychology, 15*(4), 578–590.

Tsuruga, K., Kobayashi, T., Hirai, N., & Kato, S. (2008). Foreign accent syndrome in a case of dissociative (conversion) disorder. *Seishin Shinkeigaku Zasshi, 110*(2), 79–87.

Van Borsel, J., Janssens, L., & Santens, P. (2005). Foreign accent syndrome: An organic disorder? *Journal of Communication Disorders, 38*(6), 421–429.

Vanderploeg, R. D., & Belanger, H. G. (2009). Multifactorial contributions to questionable effort and test performance within a military context. In J. E. Morgan & J. J. Sweet (Eds.), *Neuropsychology of Malingering Casebook* (pp. 41–52). New York, NY: Psychology Press.

Van Gorp, W. G., Humphrey, L., Kalechstein, A., Brumm, V., McMullen, W. J., Stoddard, M., & Pachana, N. A. (1999). How well do standard clinical neuropsychological tests identify malingering? A preliminary analysis. *Journal of Clinical and Experimental Neuropsychology, 21*(2), 245–250.

Vickery, C. D., Berry, D. T. R., Inman, T. H., Harris, M. J., & Orey, S. A. (2001). Detection of inadequate effort in neuropsychological testing. *Archives of Clinical Neuropsychology, 16*(1), 45–73.

Victor, T. L., Boone, K. B., Dean, A., Zeller, M., & Hess, R. (2007, February). *Vocabulary minus digit span as a function of education*. Poster presented at the 35th Annual International Neuropsychological Society Conference, Portland, OR.

Wechsler, D. A. (1981). *Wechsler Adult Intelligence Scale* (Rev. ed.). San Antonio, TX: The Psychological Corporation.

Wechsler, D. (1987). *Wechsler Memory Scale* Rev. ed., San Antonio, TX: The Psychological Corporation.

Wechsler, D. A. (1997a). *Wechsler Adult Intelligence Scale: Administration and scoring manual* (3rd ed.). San Antonio, TX: The Psychological Corporation.

Wechsler, D. A. (1997b). *Wechsler Memory Scale* (3rd ed .). San Antonio, TX: The Psychological Corporation.

Wechsler, D. A. (2008a). *Wechsler Adult Intelligence Scale: Administration and scoring manual* (4th ed.). San Antonio, TX: The Psychological Corporation.

Wechsler, D. A. (2008b). *Wechsler Memory Scale* (4th ed.). San Antonio, TX: The Psychological Corporation.

Whelan, B. M., Murdoch, B. E., & Bellamy, N. (2007). Delineating communication impairments associated with mild traumatic brain injury: A case report. *The Journal of Head Trauma Rehabilitation, 22*(3), 192–197.

Whiteside, D., Wald, D., & Busse, M. (2011). Classification accuracy of multiple visual spatial measures in the detection of suspect effort. *The Clinical Neuropsychologist, 25*(2), 287–301.

Youngjohn, J. R., Burrows, L., & Erdal, K. (1995). Brain damage or compensation neurosis? The controversial post-concussion syndrome. *The Clinical Neuropsychologist, 9*, 112–123.

Assessing Noncredible Sensory, Motor, and Executive Function, and Test Battery Performance in Mild Traumatic Brain Injury Cases

13

Tara L. Victor, Kyle Brauer Boone, & Alexis D. Kulick

In the previous chapter, we reviewed symptom validity tests (SVTs) used to identify feigned cognitive symptoms in domains *other than* memory. In particular, we reviewed those indicators that fell within the domains of attention, processing speed, language, and visuospatial/perceptual function. In this chapter, we examine SVTs within the domains of motor/sensory and executive function, as well as those derived from discriminant functions and neuropsychological test batteries. As stated in the previous chapter, it is with our strongest recommendation that clinicians routinely use nonmemory measures of effort dispersed throughout a test battery to ensure adequate and thorough sampling of effort in the testing situation (Boone, 2009; Larrabee, 2004; Rohling & Boone, 2007). This broad sampling allows neuropsychologists to assess for a wider range of approaches that an individual might use when attempting to perform poorly on neuropsychological evaluation.

We once again organize our review of the extant literature regarding use of these methods by cognitive domain, reviewing in detail only those studies that include at least a subsample of patients with mild traumatic brain injury (MTBI). We then turn to discriminant functions and SVTs derived from comprehensive neuropsychological test batteries. Further, we review simulation (i.e., studies employing analogue designs where there is one noninjured, normal group of subjects who are instructed to feign a head injury, or cognitive impairment without detection), "known groups" (i.e., studies employing knowledge of incentive and independent measures of effort as criteria for assigning subjects to groups), specificity (i.e., studies examining the false positive rate associated with various cut scores in different clinical groups), and mixed or hybrid study designs where appropriate and when data are available. It is obvious that the extent to which authors adequately described their TBI samples, how they defined MTBI, and the extent to which they analyzed MTBI subjects separately are of critical importance to the conclusions that can be drawn from this review. Finally, in this chapter, we outline our preliminary conclusions regarding the use of particular SVTs in TBI populations specifically, concluding with a discussion of both clinical implications and suggestions for future research.

MOTOR/SENSORY

Successful completion of a motor response (assuming no peripheral damage is present) depends on neuroanatomical "pathways at different stages (initiation, positioning, coordination, and/or sequencing of motor components) . . . " (Lezak, Howeison, & Loring, 2004, p. 31). Related is the speed of motor responses. Sensory perception involves "an arousal process that triggers central registration leading to analysis, encoding, and integrative activities" associated with sight, hearing, touch, taste, and smell (p. 23). Tests assessing both motor and sensory function have been examined as SVTs. As Arnold and Boone (2007) explained, "Individuals feigning brain injury are often under the misconception that any type of brain injury inevitably causes impairments in motor speed/coordination/strength and sensation . . . such measures (therefore) have the potential to be particularly effective effort measures" (p. 178). Both Arnold and Boone (2007) and Greiffenstein (2007) provided reviews of the literature up to 2006 for motor and sensory-based SVTs, and the readers are referred to both for a detailed description. Here, we review those studies relevant to MTBI. Known groups studies in MTBI subjects with classification accuracy statistics are summarized in Table 13.1.

Finger Tapping

Finger tapping (FT; Heaton, Grant, & Matthews, 1991; Reitan & Wolfson, 1993) is a measure of pure motor speed and control and can be assessed manually or electronically (Lezak et al., 2004; Mitrushina, Boone, Razani, & D'Elia, 2005). Arnold and Boone (2007) and Greiffenstein (2007) provided reviews of publications on FT as a SVT up to 2006, including both simulation (Heaton, Smith, Lehman, & Vogt, 1978; Mittenberg, Rotholc, Russell, & Heilbronner, 1996; Orey, Cragar, & Berry, 2000; Rapport, Farchione, Coleman, & Axelrod, 1998; Reitan & Wolfson, 2000; Tanner, Bowles, & Tanner, 2003; Vickery et al., 2004) and known groups (Arnold et al., 2005; Backhaus, Fichtenberg, & Hanks, 2004; Binder, Kelly, Villanueva, & Winslow, 2003; Binder & Willis, 1991; Greiffenstein, Baker, & Gola, 1996; Larrabee, 2003; Trueblood & Schmidt, 1993) study designs. Although simulation studies consistently demonstrate worse performance in simulators compared to their credible counterparts, the results of known groups studies have been less consistent.

Overall, Arnold and Boone (2007) concluded that FT holds promise as an SVT in MTBI cases. They pointed out limiting factors in the known groups studies that found nonsignificant results, including small sample size (Trueblood & Schmidt, 1993), failure to report litigation status of comparison groups (Greiffenstein et al., 1996), and the inclusion of litigants in clinical comparison groups in combination with other problems in group assignment that may have led to a significant number of noncredible patients in the credible groups (e.g., Binder et al., 2003; Trueblood & Schmidt, 1993). Those studies that did find use of FT as an SVT in MTBI populations did not suffer from these methodological limitations and, in fact, suggest that stringent cut scores may be warranted in this population (Arnold et al., 2005). More specifically, in Arnold and colleagues' (2005) gender-stratified comparison of 77 heterogeneous patients meeting criteria for malingered neurocognitive dysfunction (MND; Slick, Sherman, & Iverson, 1999) and six credible diagnostic groups of patients, including 24 patients with moderate-to-severe TBI, a dominant hand FT cut score of ≤ 35 for men was associated with 50% sensitivity and 90% specificity. A dominant hand FT cut score of ≤ 28 for women was associated with 61% sensitivity and 92% specificity. However, in a subsample of patients with MND MTBI, sensitivity at these cutoffs was lower (i.e., 41% for males and 50% for females).

Although it could be argued that in combination with the inconsistent findings of known groups studies, perhaps FT is not a particularly useful SVT in MTBI compared to other presenting diagnoses, simply raising the cut scores for MTBI cases appears to be an alternative. In particular, raising the dominant hand FT cut score

TABLE 13.1 Known Groups Studies of Symptom Validity Test Effectiveness Within the Domain of Motor and Sensory Function in Mild Traumatic Brain Injury

Study	Sample	Test/Score	Cut Score	Sensitivity	Specificity
		Finger Tapping			
Larrabee (2003)	MND patients with TBI (n=24), 19 of whom alleged MTBI Credible patients with moderate-to-severe TBI (n=27)	Sum of the average for dominant and nondominant hands	< 63	40%	93.5%
Backhaus et al. (2004)	MND MTBI litigants (n=25) Credible patients with MTBI (n=25)	Average dominant hand	< 43.6 < 37.7 < 29.6	48% 32% 16%	84% 100% 100%
		Average nondominant hand	< 38.9 < 32.9 < 23.5	56% 28% 16%	87.5% 100% 100%
Arnold et al. (2005)	Subsample of MND patients with MTBI Comparison groups of credible patients with moderate-to-severe TBI	Average number of taps for three 10-second trials of dominant hand	Women ≤ 15 ≤ 28 ≤ 32 ≤ 35 ≤ 38 Men ≤ 21 ≤ 33 ≤ 35 ≤ 38 ≤ 40	(n = 12) 17% 50% 67% 67% 67% (n = 22) 18% 32% 41% 46% 46%	(n = 7) 100% 100% 100% 86% 57% (n = 16) 100% 94% 87% 87% 81%
Larrabee (2008)	MND patients with TBI (n=26), 21 of whom alleged MTBI Credible patients with moderate-to-severe TBI (n= 31)	Sum of the average for dominant and nondominant hands	< 63	40%	94%
		TFR and FTNW			
Trueblood & Schmidt (1993)	Definite MND patients with MTBI (n=8) Probable MND patients with MTBI (n=8) Matched controls (n=16)	TFR total errors both hands	> 3	50% (definite) 75% (probable)	94% 80%
		FTNW total errors	> 5	63% (definite) 63% (probable)	94% 85%
Binder et al. (2003)	MND patients with MTBI (n=34) Credible patients with MTBI (n=22) Credible patients with moderate-to-severe TBI (n=60)	TFR total errors both hands	> 4	56%	MTBI Mod/Sev 82% 93%
		FTNW total errors both hands	> 17	18%	MTBI Mod/Sev 100% 95%
Backhaus et al. (2004)	MND MTBI litigants (n=25) Credible patients with MTBI (n=25)	Finger localization	< 56 < 53 < 49	80% 56% 36%	80% 92% 100%

Note. FTNW = Finger Tip Number Writing; MND = malingered neurocognitive dysfunction; Mod/Sev = credible moderate-to-severe TBI; MTBI = mild traumatic brain injury; SVT = Symptom Validity Test; TBI = traumatic brain injury; TFR = Tactile Finger Recognition (a test of finger agnosia).

to ≤ 38 in men was associated with 46% sensitivity in the MND MTBI subsample while still maintaining 87% specificity in the credible moderate-to-severe TBI comparison group. In the same manner, raising the cut score to ≤ 32 in women was associated with 67% sensitivity and 100% specificity in the credible moderate-to-severe TBI comparison group. Limitations of this study include the small subsamples and associated instability of specificity values that resulted from dividing the sample by gender; therefore, replication is recommended (Arnold et al., 2005).

In Greiffenstein's (2007) review, he likewise concluded that FT is an effective SVT in MTBI cases. In particular, although he did not provide information on cut scores, he integrated the data on FT by calculating the mean of the combined (dominant plus nondominant hand) scores obtained in three groups: (a) volunteer simulators (mean score = 60), (b) known noncredibles (most of whom were MTBI litigants; mean score = 70), and (c) patients with genuine brain disease (including some movement disorders such as Huntington's disease) across several studies (mean score = 81), arguing that FT combined scores less than the clinical benchmark of 81 in minor or MTBI could be considered noncredible.

Dikmen, Machamer, Winn, and Temkin (1995) found their credible 161 patients with MTBI to demonstrate a mean FT combined score of 98. Reitan and Wolfson (2000) reported that their 18 credible patients suffering acute concussion (only 14 days postinjury) achieved FT combined scores in the low 90s, which was comparable to normal controls. Butters, Goldstein, Allen, and Shemansky (1998) published FT scores for various movement disorder groups who achieved mean FT combined scores between 45 and 60. Therefore, the implication is that no patient with MTBI should be performing well below these rates (assuming no other medical or psychiatric complications). Perhaps, it would be accurate to conclude that FT combined scores less than 81 suggest probable symptom invalidity, whereas scores less than 60 suggest definite symptom invalidity; although given the well-documented superiority of men in FT speed, these cutoffs may have problematic specificity in female populations. Known groups studies for which classification accuracy statistics could be determined in MTBI samples are shown in Table 13.1.

Examination of our clinical database at the time of this writing (Boone, Victor, Cottingham, Ziegler, & Zeller, in progress) shows that for males, using a dominant hand cutoff of ≤ 37 (90% specificity) yielded 51% sensitivity in noncredible patients without MTBI (n = 109; compensation seeking, failed at least two independent SVTs not including FT, and low cognitive scores were inconsistent with normal function in activities of daily living [ADLs]), but only 31% sensitivity in noncredible patients without MTBI (n = 93). For women, a dominant hand cut score of ≤ 25 (≥ 90% specificity) was associated with 36% sensitivity in the noncredible non-MTBI group (n = 77), but only 24% sensitivity in the noncredible MTBI cases (n = 33). Thus, it would appear that FT is less useful in detecting noncredible MTBI presentations than for detecting noncredible presentations in other clinical groups.

Estimated Finger Tapping

Meyers and Volbrecht (2003) developed an equation to provide an *estimated* FT (EFT) score (based on tests that require use of the dominant hand fingers) to compare with actual finger tapping performance.

EFT = [(block design scale score × 0.361) + (digit symbol scale score × 0.491) + (RCFT raw score × 0.185)] + 31.34

Difference = actual mean FT score for the dominant hand − EFT

The formula was calculated using linear regression of scores of 650 heterogeneous patients with neuropsychological problems, and it was found that individuals with a history of MTBI were not expected to score less than a -10 difference.

Recent cross-validation data from our laboratory (Curiel, 2011) involving 101 noncredible subjects (motive to feign, failure on at least two SVTs, and low neurocognitive scores inconsistent with normal function in ADLs; 14 MTBI cases) and 180 credible patients (no motive to feign, failure on $\leq$ 1 SVT, no full scale IQ [FSIQ] < 70, and no diagnoses of dementia) showed that when an actual minus EFT score cutoff of < -10 was employed, sensitivity was only 38.6% (at 85.6% specificity). All of the individual scores that comprise the equation, with the exception of FT, outperformed the full Meyers and Volbrecht (2003) formula (i.e., led to better classification accuracy rates). Given concerns that the poor sensitivity rate for FT was suppressing the effectiveness of the Meyers and Volbrecht formula, the FT component was removed and the sensitivity rate for the remaining portion of the equation using Rey Complex Figure Test and Recognition Trial (RCFT) copy, block design, and digit symbol was calculated. The use of a cutoff of < 10.3 for this shortened equation yielded the highest sensitivity (70.3% at > 90% specificity), which outperformed all individual subtests and the whole formula by a large margin. However, the small number of noncredible subjects with MTBI ($n = 14$) precluded examination of the effectiveness of this partial formula in identification of feigned MTBI symptoms.

Grip Strength

Grip strength (GS) is frequently part of a neuropsychological exam and typically assessed with either the Smedley (Reitan & Wolfson, 1993) or the Jamar dynamometer (Lezak et al., 2004; Mitrushina et al., 2005). The typical score is the highest average score obtained (i.e., "peak strength") and is expressed in pounds or kilograms. Arnold and Boone (2007) and Grieffenstein (2007) reviewed the literature on GS as a SVT up until 2006, summarizing both simulation (Fairfax, Balnave, & Adams, 1995; Gilbert & Knowlton, 1983; Hamilton, Balnave, & Adams, 1994; Heaton et al., 1978; Lechner, Bradbury, & Bradley, 1998; Mittenberg et al., 1996; Niebuhr & Marion, 1987) and known groups (Greiffenstein et al., 1996; Hagström & Carlsson, 1996; Olivegren, Jerkvall, Hagström, & Carlsson, 1999; Peterson, 1998) designs. Most of the known groups studies included patients with MTBI. Grieffenstein (2007) concluded that GS shows robust effect sizes (ES) associated with group means across both types of study designs (mean ES all simulators = -1; mean ES all known groups = -0.92), and therefore, "GS should provide excellent positive predictive power" (p. 114).

Greiffenstein and Baker (2006) compared 607 litigating patients with MTBI and persistent postconcussive symptoms with 159 patients with moderate-to-severe MTBI. There were substantial gender differences noted, requiring gender-stratified group comparisons. The patients with MTBI produced overall lower GS scores compared to the patient who are more severely injured, and about 40% of the MTBI group produced suspiciously poor GS performances, defined as performance < -1 standard deviation (SD) of the moderate-to-severe TBI reference group mean. However, as Arnold and Boone (2007) pointed out, "no data on sensitivity/specificity values have been published, thus limiting the clinical application of this measure . . ." (p. 188).

Grooved Pegboard

The Grooved Pegboard Test (GP; Lewis & Kupke, 1977) is a measure of fine motor dexterity (Lezak et al., 2004; Mitrushina et al., 2005) that has been investigated as an

SVT. Arnold and Boone (2007) and Grieffenstein (2007) provided complete reviews of the test across clinical populations, which summarized both simulation (Heaton et al., 1978; Inman & Berry, 2002; Johnson & Lesniak-Karpiak, 1997; Rapport et al., 1998; Vickery et al., 2004; Wong, Lerner-Poppen, & Durham, 1998) and known groups (Binder & Willis, 1991; Greiffenstein et al., 1996; van Gorp et al., 1999) studies up to 2006. The reviews noted that student simulators appear not to behave in the same manner as actual clinical patients on this test. The few studies in real-world patients either show no group effects or even better performance in probable malingerers. None of the studies reviewed provided cutoff scores with associated sensitivity and specificity. The reviewers concluded that given the lack of significant group differences between simulators/real-world patients with suspect effort and moderate-to-severe TBI comparison groups, the test does not appear appropriate for use as an SVT in general, let alone with an MTBI population in particular. However, there were several limitations of the aforementioned studies that could have obscured the potential of GP as an SVT (e.g., failure to stratify groups by gender; see Arnold & Boone, 2007 for additional detail). Performance trends in the data suggest that future research might focus on suppression of dominant hand performance, in particular, as an indicator of poor effort.

Hand Movements Subtest of Kaufman Assessment Battery for Children

Arnold and Boone (2007) reviewed one study (i.e., Bowen & Littell, 1997) on the hand movements subtest of the Kaufman Assessment Battery for Children (KABC), which compared 21 litigating/compensation-seeking patients with TBI (most of whom were patients with MTBI) with 25 non–compensation-seeking general clinical patients and an archival database of 80 healthy controls. The mean score on the test for the litigant group was equivalent to that of a 4-year-old child. A cutoff of ≥ 10 was associated with 66% sensitivity and 90% specificity in the credible patient comparison group. The authors concluded that the test holds promise as a SVT but requires additional validation in larger samples of patients with MTBI.

Dichotic Listening Test

The dichotic listening test (DLT; Meyers, Roberts, Bayless, Volkert, & Evitts, 2002) presents words via audiotape and headphones (Auditec of St. Louis, 1991) to both the left and right ear simultaneously, which subjects are to identify. DLT performance has been found to be sensitive to brain injury and disease (Damasio & Damasio, 1979; Levin et al., 1989; Risse, Gates, Lund, Maxwell, & Rubens, 1989; Roberts et al., 1994). DLT-both (DLB) is the score obtained for all trials in which the words presented to both ears are correctly identified. Assuming an individual passes the general hearing test (which precedes the actual test), a score of ≤ 9 indicates noncredible performance (by virtue of no credible MTBI subjects or normal controls performing below this criterion; Meyers & Volbrecht, 1999; 2003).

Somatosensory Tests

Arnold and Boone (2007) and Greiffenstein (2007) reviewed several tests of somatosensory function that have been investigated as SVTs. They described case studies: (a) two-choice tactile sensation test (Binder, 1992), (b) two-point tactile discrimination test (Greve, Bianchini, & Ameduri, 2003), and (c) two-choice discrimination test (Pankratz, 1979); simulation studies: (a) tactile discrimination (Greve et al., 2005), (b) bilateral hearing loss (Haughton, Lewsley, Wilson, & Williams, 1979), and (c) finger agnosia errors (Heaton et al., 1978; Mittenberg et al., 1996); and known groups designs: (a) finger localization (Backhaus et al., 2004), (b) finger agnosia/fingertip number writing (FTNW) combined errors (Binder & Willis, 1991; Binder et al., 2003), and (c) finger agnosia and FTNW errors (Trueblood & Schmidt, 1993), as well as a further study (Youngjohn, Burrows, & Erdal, 1995), which documented finger agnosia and FTNW errors in the 55 compensation-seeking persistent postconcussive syndrome subjects, half of whom displayed evidence of symptom invalidity.

As an example of a known groups design study that included a litigating but credible MTBI comparison group, Trueblood and Schmidt (1993; study described earlier) examined finger agnosia total errors in a litigating MTBI sample. A finger agnosia total error cutoff of > 3 correctly identified four malingerers (50%) and six individuals with questionable credibility (75%) with specificity maintained at 80.3% to 90%. In the same manner, a total errors > 5 cutoff for FTNW correctly identified five malingerers (63%) and five individuals with questionable credibility (63%) with specificity maintained between 84.5% and 95%.

Arnold and Boone (2007) concluded that both tactile finger recognition (TFR; the measure of finger agnosia) and FTNW (from the Klove-Reitan Sensory-Perceptual Examination; Reitan & Wolfson, 1993) appear to hold promise in detecting symptom invalidity in MTBI cases, but that the measures have been understudied and underused in clinical practice. Recent data from our laboratory (Taylor, 2011) on 67 noncredible subjects (as defined by motive to feign, failure on at least 2 of 11 separate neurocognitive SVTs, and low neurocognitive scores at variance with evidence as to normal function in ADLs) revealed that they averaged 6.3 finger agnosia errors, and that 61% of the sample exceeded the cutoff of > 3 errors. Examination of the subset of 44 noncredible subjects claiming problems from MTBI showed that they averaged 5.57 errors, and employing the cutoff of > 3 errors, sensitivity was 66%.

Summary of Motor/Sensory-Based Symptom Validity Tests

FT (average for dominant hand), GS, TFR, and FTNW appear to be valid and reliable SVTs in MTBI cases, but research sample sizes have generally been small. In addition, gender needs to be considered when selecting cut scores for some measures, and there is some suggestion that other demographic factors may be relevant to feigning strategies on these tests (socioeconomic status [SES], intelligence, educational, and/or occupational level; Arnold & Boone, 2007). GP does not appear to be adequately validated for use as an SVT in MTBI cases at the present time. FT, in particular, is the most thoroughly researched of the motor/sensory SVTs, but sensitivity is moderately relative to other nonmotor SVTs. Recent data suggest that finger agnosia errors may be more sensitive than FT in identifying negative response bias in MTBI cases.

One important point that has since gone unmentioned as it relates to motor tests as SVTs is pattern of performance analysis. As Arnold and Boone (2007) and Greiffenstein (2007) explained, moderate-to-severe TBI samples produce a characteristic pattern of motor performance consistent with greater impairment as task complexity increases (i.e., GP < FT < GS). In contrast, patients with MTBI with persisting postconcussive symptoms tend to produce the opposite pattern (GP > FT > GS). Therefore, the presence of such a pattern suggests the possibility of symptom invalidity (Greiffenstein et al., 1996), although this observation has not been replicated in simulation designs (Rapport et al., 1998). Arnold and Boone (2007) speculated as to whether sample-specific factors (i.e., SES and IQ) influence the occurrence of the nonphysiologic motor pattern, specifically that it appears in low SES samples but not in simulators of higher education, suggesting that lower SES individuals may perceive motor weakness as a particularly salient characteristic to feign. These authors concluded that the motor pattern analysis requires further investigation with attention to demographic moderators.

EXECUTIVE FUNCTIONS

Executive functions refer to those "capacities that enable a person to engage successfully in independent, purposive, self-serving behavior" (Lezak et al., 2004, p. 35). Examples of such functions include planning ahead, inhibiting behavior, problem solving, and multitasking. Impaired executive functioning is often highly associated with disability. Given that disability, or loss of function, is often the determinant of compensable injuries in the United States, it is reasonable to assume that there is motivation to feign or exaggerate deficits in this domain. In this vein, Meyers (2007) found that at approximately 1-year postinjury, simulators and probable malingerers showed a pattern of performance most similar to patients with bifrontal injuries.

Wisconsin Card Sorting Test

The Wisconsin Card Sorting Test (WCST; Heaton, Chelune, Talley, Kay, & Curtiss, 1993) is a widely used measure of executive function from which measures of symptom invalidity have been derived (Bernard, McGrath, & Houston, 1996; Suhr & Boyer, 1999). Although the test is highly sensitive to brain injury, effort also explains a significant portion of variance in performance and has been found to have a larger impact on WCST performance than mild or moderate-to-severe TBI (Ord, Greve, Bianchini, & Aguerrevere, 2010).

Greve and Bianchini (2007) and Sweet and Nelson (2007) provided excellent reviews of the WCST as a method for detecting symptom invalidity, and the readers are referred to their chapters for a summary of the literature up to 2006. The reviews cover simulation (Bernard et al., 1996; Suhr & Boyer, 1999), known groups (Greve, Bianchini, Mathias, Houston, & Crouch, 2002; Heinly, Greve, Love, & Bianchini, 2006; King, Sweet, Sherer, Curtiss, & Vanderploeg, 2002; Larrabee, 2003; Miller, Donders, & Suhr, 2000), and specificity (Donders, 1999; Greve & Bianchini, 2002; King et al., 2002) studies. The known groups studies are summarized in Table 13.2. The authors concluded from their extensive review that three WCST indicators have some effectiveness in detecting poor effort in MTBI specifically, including the Bernard discriminant function (which is generally based on the assumption that noncredible examinees would perform more poorly on the "obvious" categories completed score compared to the more "subtle" scores of perseverative errors/responses; Bernard et al., 1996), the Suhr and Boyer formula (which was based on the assumption that noncredible examinees would performance more poorly on the obvious categories completed score compared to the more subtle score of failure to maintain set [FMS]; Suhr & Boyer, 1999), and finally, the FMS score itself (Greve et al., 2002). However, the authors caution the use of these indicators with individuals who have sustained moderate-to-severe TBI, given high false positive rates, and it is explicitly recommended that the indices not be used at all in cases of more severe TBI. Further, it is recommended that additional known groups studies be conducted to verify appropriate cutoffs for various clinical groups.

TABLE 13.2 Known Groups Studies of SVT Effectiveness Within the Domain of Executive Function in Mild TBI

Study	Sample	Test/Score	Cut Score	Sensitivity	Specificity
		WCST			
Miller, Donders & Suhr (2000)	Severe TBI no incentive (n=30)	Bernard DFA	—[a]	0%	95%
	MTBI without incentive (n=30)	Suhr formula	≥ 3.16	0%	95%
	MTBI with incentive (n=30), 13 of which were "likely malingerers"				
King et al. (2002) Study 1	Probable malingerers (n=27)	Bernard DFA	—[a]	63%	94%
	Credible patients with moderate-to-severe TBI (n=33)	King formula	≥ 2.13	70%	82%
		Suhr formula	≥ 3.16	59%	88%
Greve et al. (2002)	89 patients with TBI (majority MTBI) divided into four groups: • no incentive control (n=17) • probable MND (n=32) • suspect (n=30) • incentive only (n=10)	Bernard DFA	> −3 > 0	38% 16%	89% 94%
		Suhr formula	> 1.90 > 3.68	47% 34%	89% 94%
		Unique responses	≤ 1 > 1	35% 22%	94% 100%
		Perfect matches missed	> 0 > 1	9% 0%	100% 100%
Larrabee (2003)	Definite MND (n=26) Derivation: moderate-to-severe TBI (n=31) Cross-validation: TBI and mixed neurological/ psychiatric (n=27)	Suhr formula	> 0 > 2.41	64% 40%	52% 87%
		FMS	> 1 > 2	48%	87% 96%
Heinly et al. (2006)[b]	Patients with MTBI (MND n=47; nonmalingering, n=90) Patients with moderate-to-severe TBI (MND n=21; nonmalingering n=118) Patients with chronic severe TBI (n=101) General clinical patients (n>1,000)	Bernard DFA	> 3 > 0	32% 24%	87% 91%
		Suhr formula	> 0 > 1.90 > 2.41 > 3.16 > 3.68 ≥ 4.00 ≥ 4.50	57% 37% 33% 29% 22% 22% 9%	60% 88% 88% 90% 93% 94% 98%
		FMS	> 1 > 2 > 3	35% 24% 16%	85% 92% 100%
Larrabee (2008)	MND patients (n=24; 21 of whom alleged MTBI) Credible patients with moderate-to-severe TBI (n=31)	FMS	> 1	48%	87%
Greve et al. (2009)[b]	Credible patients with MTBI n=55 Credible patients with moderate-to-severe TBI (n=92) MND patients with MTBI (n=38) Credible patients with severe TBI (n=91)	Bernard DFA Suhr formula	≥ −1 ≥ 3	26% 32%	89% 89%
		King formula FMS	> 0 ≥ 3	32% 29%	94% 89%

(Continued)

TABLE 13.2 Known Groups Studies of SVT Effectiveness Within the Domain of Executive Function in Mild TBI (Continued)

Study	Sample	Test/Score	Cut Score	Sensitivity	Specificity
		WCST			
Greve et al. (2009)[b]	General clinical patients (n=766)	Perseverative Responses	≥ 45	16%	89%
		Categories Completed	≤ 2	26%	87%
		Unique Responses	≤ 2	34%	87%
		CT			
Greve et al. (2007)	Patients with MTBI (MND n=43; credible n=43)	Total errors	≥ 80	51%	84%
			≥ 85	47%	91%
	Patients with moderate-to-severe TBI (MND n=16; credible=34)		≥ 90	47%	91%
			≥ 95	30%	93%
		Bolter items[c]	≥ 2	33%	95%
	General clinical patients (MND n=60; credible n=137)	Easy items	≥ 3	37%	91%
		Forrest DFA[d]	≥ 60	44%	88%
			≥ 65	37%	93%
		COWAT			
Backhaus et al. (2004)	MND MTBI litigants (n=25)	Total correct word score	< 29	48%	88%
	Credible patients with MTBI (n=25)		< 22	12%	100%
			< 19.1	12%	100%
Silverberg et al. (2008)	Healthy controls (n=28)	Silverberg formula	> .45	59%	86%
	Simulators (n=24)		> .50	59%	89%
	Moderate-to-severe TBI (n=35)		> .55	47%	91%
	MND MTBI (n=15)		> .60	41%	94%
Curtis et al. (2008)	Patients with MTBI (MND n=44; credible=152)	FAS total correct word T-score[e]	< 31	21%	97%
			< 32	27%	94%
	Patients with moderate-to-severe TBI (MND n=21; credible=75)		< 33	34%	92%
			< 34	36%	89%
			< 35	43%	87%
	General clinical patients (n=488)		< 36	48%	88%
		Stroop			
Backhaus et al. (2004)	MND MTBI litigants (n=25)	Total words	< 89	88%	92%
	Credible patients with MTBI (n=25)		< 75.2	52%	96%
			< 52.2	32%	100%
		TMT			
Backhaus et al. (2004)	MND MTBI litigants (n=25)	Part A Total Time	> 37	40%	92%
	Credible patients MTBI (n=25)		> 49.3	24%	96%
			> 63.3	8%	100%
		Part B Total Time	> 96.5	56%	80%
			> 147	32%	96%
			> 192.6	24%	100%

Note. CT = Category Test; COWAT = Controlled Oral Word Association Test; DFA = Discriminant Function Analysis; FMS = failure to maintain set; MND = malingered neurocognitive dysfunction; Mod/sev = credible moderate-to-severe TBI; MTBI = mild traumatic brain injury; SVT = Symptom Validity Test; TBI = traumatic brain injury; TMT = Trail Making Test; WCST = Wisconsin Card Sorting Test.

[a]Any score that exceeded that of the brain injury formula (see Table 6 on page 241 of the original article for details).
[b]Sensitivity/specificity data are provided for MTBI only.
[c]Bolter items are 18 items that were rarely missed by individuals with bona fide brain damage (Bolter, Picano, & Zych, 1985, as described by Sweet & King, 2002).
[d]Forrest, T. J., Allen, D. N., & Goldstein, G. (2004). Malingering indexes for the Halstead Category Test. The Clinical Neuropsychologist, 18(2), 334–347.
[e]The T score is adjusted for education using metanorms by Loonstra et al. (2001) in Table 11-12 on page 457 of Spreen & Strauss (1991).

Since the publication of the aforementioned 2007 reviews (note that these studies are also included in Table 13.2), FMS was reexamined by Larrabee (2008) in his paper on aggregation of effort indicators. In particular, his sample consisted of 26 individuals diagnosed with MND, 21 (i.e., 81%) of whom had alleged MTBI. This sample was compared to 31 credible subjects with moderate-to-severe TBI. With respect to their performance on the FMS, a cutoff score of > 1 maintained borderline adequate specificity (i.e., 87%) with sensitivity at 48%.

More recently, Greve, Heinly, Bianchini, and Love (2009) published some of their previously presented data (i.e., Heinly et al., 2006) on the WCST as a SVT in MTBI cases specifically using a known groups design defined by the Slick and colleagues' (1999) criteria for MND. Three hundred and seventy-three patients with TBI (146 or 39% of whom were MTBI; defined by posttraumatic amnesia [PTA] < 24 hr, Glasgow Coma Scale [GCS] 30-min postinjury = 13–15, loss of consciousness [LOC] < 30 min, and no positive neuroimaging findings) were compared to 766 general clinical patients on all three aforementioned formulas in addition to several other WCST scores. Classification accuracy for seven of the indicators was inadequately sensitive for distinguishing malingerers from nonmalingerers. Thus, only the remaining scores were compared among the following groups: (a) 55 nonmalingering patients with MTBI, (b) 92 nonmalingering patients with moderate-to-severe TBI, (c) 38 malingering patients with MTBI, and (d) 91 nonmalingering patients with severe TBI.

Results revealed that the malingering MTBI group (Group C) performed significantly worse than the nonmalingering MTBI group (Group A), and Group C also performed at a level commensurate with the nonmalingering moderate-to-severe and the severe TBI groups (Groups B and D). Regarding accuracy rates for specific indicators, perseverative responses, categories completed, and unique responses all performed rather poorly at discriminating malingerer from nonmalingerer patients with MTBI. Consistent with the findings of Greve and colleagues (2002), perfect matches missed (i.e., the number of times an examinee fails to match a response card to its identically matched key card) also failed to discriminate among groups in this sample. FMS was the best with a cutoff of ≥ 3 associated with 29% sensitivity and 89% specificity; an FMS of > 3 was rare in the heterogeneous nonmalingering general clinical population comparison group. With respect to the malingering equations, the authors found that the Suhr and Boyer (1999) formula and the King et al. (2002) formula were associated with 32% sensitivity at 89% (Suhr & Boyer, 1999) to 94% (King et al., 2002) specificity. In contrast, the Bernard formula did not perform as well in the MTBI population (sensitivity = 26%; specificity = 89%). See Table 13.2 for a list of cut scores and associated accuracy data for all WCST indicators examined in this study.

In summary, although there are high false positive rates associated with use of the Bernard et al. (1996), Suhr and Boyer (1999), and King et al. (2002) formulae in patients with more severe pathology (e.g., severe TBI, stroke, comorbid posttraumatic stress disorder [PTSD], and other psychiatric difficulties), they appear appropriate for use in uncomplicated MTBI cases (i.e., simple concussions) with perhaps the Suhr and Boyer and King et al. formulae performing slightly better. In addition, FMS also appears to be of some value in identifying poor effort in an MTBI population. As the scores on these indicators increase, so does the likelihood of symptom invalidity. That said, sensitivity of these WCST indicators is relatively low compared to other SVTs (when setting cutoffs at adequate specificity), and such a negative finding does not rule out malingering.

Category Test

The Category Test (CT; Strauss, Sherman, & Spreen, 2006) is a widely used measure of executive function that assesses abstract thinking and problem-solving ability (Rabin, Barr, & Burton, 2005). Greve and Bianchini (2007) and Sweet and Nelson (2007) also included a review of this test in their chapters because it relates to the detection of symptom invalidity, and the readers are once again referred to these chapters for a summary of the literature up to 2006. The reviews covered simulation (e.g., DiCarlo, Gfeller, & Oliveri, 2000; Ellwanger, Tenhula, Rosenfeld, & Sweet, 1999; Forrest, Allen, & Goldstein, 2004; Goebel, 1983; Heaton et al., 1978; Mittenberg et al., 1996; Tenhula & Sweet, 1996; Williamson, Green, Allen, & Rohling, 2003) and known groups (e.g., Greve, Bianchini, & Roberson, 2007; Trueblood & Schmidt, 1993) studies. As the authors pointed out, although many of the simulator studies included moderate-to-severe TBI clinical comparison groups to determine specificity, the cut-offs are likely less applicable to MTBI cases because they would result in too many false negative errors (i.e., would be too insensitive). Further, in the first known groups study (Trueblood & Schmidt, 1993), the sample sizes were very small, and no classification accuracy data were provided.

The known groups studies are summarized in Table 13.2. The study by Greve and colleagues (2007) is worth particular mention because it provided data by injury severity (i.e., for MTBI alone, defined as PTA < 24 hr, GCS = 13–15 after 30 min, LOC < 30 min, and negative neuroimaging). Data on 12 CT variables are reported for four groups: (a) 77 nonmalingering patients with TBI, (b) 70 suspect malingering patients with TBI, (c) 59 patients with TBI meeting Slick and colleagues' (1999) criteria for MND, and (d) 60 nonlitigating and non–compensation-seeking general clinical patients on 12 CT variables. Examining only the MTBI subsample, the total errors raw score was the most accurate indicator, correctly detecting 47% of malingering patients with MTBI with 91% specificity. The results of the other CT indices that appeared to hold some promise as applied to MTBI samples can be found in Table 13.2.

The authors concluded from their extensive review that there were much higher rates of false positive errors in known groups studies when using cutoffs identified in simulator studies. Altering cutoffs in the real-world samples to maintain adequate specificity lowered sensitivity of the indicators. Greve and Bianchini (2007), therefore, suggested caution when using these indicators with individuals who sustained a moderate or severe TBI given the higher false positive rates (i.e., different cutoffs may be required). The authors suggested that several CT indicators show promise for use in uncomplicated MTBI cases; however, sensitivity of these CT indicators is relatively low compared to other SVTs (when setting cutoffs at adequate specificity), and a negative finding does not rule out malingering.

Verbal and Visual Fluency

The Controlled Oral Word Association Test (COWAT; Benton, Hamsher, & Sivan, 1994) is a well-known and widely used measure of phonemic fluency that is sensitive to brain dysfunction (Strauss et al., 2006). At least a couple versions of the COWAT consist of three 60-second trials during which the examinee is asked to generate as many different words as possible that begin with a particular letter (i.e., one letter per trial; Benton et al., 1994; Lezak et al., 2004; Mitrushina et al., 2005; Strauss et al., 2006). Commonly used letters are F, A, and S. Animal naming test is a semantic fluency task that requires the examinee to generate as many animal names as possible in a single 60-second trial (Lezak et al., 2004; Mitrushina et al., 2005; Strauss et al.,

2006). In combination, these tests are the most frequently used versions of verbal fluency tests (Strauss et al., 2006). The visual analogue to these tests is the Ruff Figural Fluency Test (RFFT; Ruff, Light, & Evans, 1987) requiring an examinee to draw as many unique designs as possible on a five-dot stimuli within five 60-second trials.

A review of the few studies investigating the use of verbal and visual fluency tasks as SVTs can be found in Sweet and Nelson's (2007) chapter, which covers both simulator (Demakis, 1999; Vickery et al., 2004) and known groups (Backhaus et al., 2004; van Gorp et al., 1999) study designs up to 2006. The reviewers noted that no classification accuracy data were provided in the studies, and they concluded that there is no adequate evidence indicating these tests have use as SVTs. However, Backhaus and colleagues (2004) did provide accuracy data, which are reproduced here in Table 13.2.

Since that time, two additional studies have been conducted attempting to fill in this gap in the literature. First, Silverberg, Hanks, Buchanan, Fichtenberg, and Millis (2008) used a combined simulation and known groups design in which they compared 28 healthy controls, 35 credible patients with moderate-to-severe TBI, 24 simulators, and 17 probable/definite malingering patients with MTBI (defined as GCS = 15, only brief alterations of consciousness, if any, and no PTA) on an expanded version of the COWAT (that included the letter cues "J" and "W" after C, T, and L). Three patterns of performance found in healthy controls (and found to be unaltered in credible patients with TBI) were combined into a logistic regression equation that was derived from their simulation comparisons (cut scores and associated classification data are presented in Table 13.2). In particular, it was found that low phonemic clustering, stable production of words over time, and similar performance across letter trials were characteristic of response bias and not related to the presence of TBI. The formula was found to correctly classify 59% of the probable/definite patients with MTBI while maintaining adequate specificity (89%). The procedure for deriving the expanded COWAT response bias index can be found in the Appendix of the original article. It is unfortunate that the authors did not specify the type of external incentive associated with their probable and definite malingering groups.

Recognizing the limitations of external validity associated with an analogue design, Curtis, Thompson, Greve, and Bianchini (2008) used a known groups design (Greve & Bianchini, 2004) based on diagnosis of MND to investigate verbal fluency measures as SVTs in a clinical sample that included separate analysis of individuals with a history of MTBI (defined by PTA < 24 hr, initial GCS = 13–15, and LOC < 30 min) who also had no positive neuroradiological findings or focal neurological signs (n = 108). Recall that comparison groups included moderate-to-severe TBI and general clinical patients. These authors found that FAS total correct word T score (adjusted for education using meta-norms by Loonstra, Tarlow, & Sellers, 2001) provided the best accuracy rates of all 11 verbal fluency indicators (from the COWAT and animals list generation tests) examined for identifying poor effort in patients with MTBI. In particular, maintaining specificity > 90%, a cutoff T score of ≤ 33 was associated with a sensitivity rate of 36% within the MTBI group (additional classification accuracy data are presented in Table 13.2). Notably, none of the 11 indicators effectively identified symptom invalidity in the moderate-to-severe TBI group. Thus, this cutoff is not appropriate for identifying MND in more severe TBI populations.

In sum, although sensitivity is relatively low compared to SVTs from other domains, the expanded COWAT (Silverberg et al., 2008) and FAS total correct word (educationally adjusted) T score (Curtis et al., 2008) holds some promise in detecting symptom validity in MTBI cases.

Stroop Color Word Test

The Stroop Color Word Test (SCWT; Lezak et al., 2004; Mitrushina et al., 2005; Strauss et al., 2006) Part C is a primary measure of response inhibition (i.e., to inhibit one's overlearned reading response). Parts A and B involve simple word and color naming and therefore require the recognition (and verbalization) of overlearned and highly familiar information. This latter type of knowledge is particularly resistant to brain injury as reflected by the fact that highly practiced skills, such as word reading, are relatively spared in acquired brain impairment, and in fact, this is the rationale behind the use of word-reading tasks to assess premorbid level of function (Nelson & McKenna, 1975). In particular, the presence of relatively spared sight reading skills has been confirmed in patients with TBI (Crawford, Parker, & Besson 1988), dementia (Crawford et al., 1988; Nelson & McKenna, 1975), cortical disease (Ruddle & Bradshaw, 1982), schizophrenia (Crawford et al., 1992), and depression (Crawford, Besson, Parker, Sutherland, & Keen, 1987). Thus, an SVT requiring this skill should have a relatively low false positive rate in patients with actual cerebral dysfunction.

Lu, Boone, Jimenez, and Razani (2004) administered the SCWT to six patients claiming total inability to read (most secondary to TBI) and who met criteria (Slick et al., 1999) for probable malingering. The patients indicated that they could not read the words on the word reading section of the SCWT, but when administered Part C, they demonstrated difficulty inhibiting a reading response, thus providing incontrovertible evidence of malingering (i.e., they were captured doing what they claimed complete inability to do). The authors concluded that the SCWT can function as a "pathognomonic indicator" of feigned inability to read as documented by presence of errors of reading under instructions to name colors on the interference section of the SCWT.

A full review of the few studies investigating the SCWT as an SVT is provided by Nelson and Sweet (2007), with the authors concluding that the instrument had minimal use in the detection of negative response bias. However, more recently, Arentsen and colleagues (in progress) found, in examining a large sample of noncredible patients ($n = 129$; motive to feign, failed at least two out of 10 SVTs, normal ADLs) and a heterogeneous credible clinical sample ($n = 371$; no motive to feign, failed one or fewer SVTs, no FSIQ < 70, or dementia diagnoses), moderate sensitivity for word reading and color naming trials of the Comalli version of the SCWT, but that use of the test as an SVT was problematic in individuals with histories of reading difficulties. In particular, for SCWT A, although a cutoff score of ≥ 64 s could be employed in the nonlearning challenged group (associated with sensitivity of 55.8%), it had to be raised to ≥ 76 s for the group with a history of learning difficulties (resulting in a drop in sensitivity to 37.2%). In the same manner, for SCWT B, a cutoff score of > 91 s could be employed for the credible group with no learning problems (55.1% sensitivity) but had to be increased to ≥ 99 s in the learning difficulties group (40.2% sensitivity). Finally, the cutoff for SCWT C associated with $\geq 90\%$ specificity in the nonlearning disabled group was ≥ 181 s (sensitivity of 37.8%), but a cutoff score of ≥ 207 s was required for the learning challenged group (sensitivity of 23.5%). No data were available regarding noncredible MTBI subjects in isolation.

Trail Making Test

The Trail Making Test (TMT; Reitan, 1992) is a very commonly used neuropsychological test that measures a combination of visuomotor speed, sequencing, and set-shifting abilities (Lezak et al., 2004; Mitrushina et al., 2005; Strauss et al., 2006). The test is valid, reliable, and has demonstrated sensitivity to brain injury. Performance on this test is also influenced by age, education, and IQ (Lezak et al., 2004; Mitrushina et al., 2005).

Suhr and Barrash (2007) and Sweet and Nelson (2007) provided reviews of the TMT because it relates to the detection of symptom invalidity, and the readers are referred to their chapters for a summary of the literature up to 2006. The reviews cover simulation (e.g., Goebel, 1983; Haines & Norris, 2001; Heaton et al., 1978; Ruffolo, Guilmette, & Willis, 2000) and known groups (e.g., Backhaus et al., 2004; Iverson, Lange, Green, & Franzen, 2002; Martin, Hoffman, & Donders, 2003; O'Bryant, Hilsabeck, Fisher, & McCaffrey, 2003; Trueblood & Schmidt, 1993; van Gorp et al., 1999) study designs. Early results suggested a ratio score of TMT B to TMT A completion times may be a potential indicator of response bias (e.g., Goebel, 1983; Lamberty, Putnam, Chatel, Bieliauskas, & Adams, 1994). The ratio between Part A and Part B would be expected to be smaller for malingerers than bona fide patients presenting in a valid manner who often take much longer to complete Part B compared to Part A. However, later studies did not replicate this finding and instead found total errors (i.e., ≥ 4 errors on either Part A or B) and completion times on TMT A or TMT B more helpful in discriminating groups (e.g., Iverson et al., 2002; O'Bryant et al., 2003; Ruffolo et al., 2000; Trueblood & Schmidt, 1993). Yet, as the authors pointed out, no classification accuracy data (Ruffolo et al., 2000) or range of cutoff scores (e.g., O'Bryant et al., 2003) were reported in several of the studies. Further, in the first known groups design (Trueblood & Schmidt, 1993), sample sizes were very small, and no classification accuracy data were provided. Both sets of reviewers concluded that the existing literature is too limited and inconclusive to reliably or validly use the TMT as an indicator of poor effort at this time.

The Iverson and colleagues' (2002) study is worthy of specific mention, however, because of its very large sample of MTBI subjects. The authors investigated the TMT ratio, total errors, and time to complete scores as SVTs in a large sample of patients with TBI presenting to a trauma service, including (a) 328 uncomplicated patients with MTBI (GCS = 13–15 and no evidence of skull fracture or positive neuroimaging findings); (b) 86 patients with MTBI with skull fracture (GCS = 13–15 and skull fracture on x-ray but no computed tomography [CT] abnormality); (c) 117 complicated patients with MTBI (GCS = 13–15 and abnormal neuroimaging); and (d) 40 patients with moderate-to-severe TBI (GCS < 13 and positive neuroimaging). The sample represented acute injury; most patients were tested within the first week of presenting to the service and all within 1 month of injury.

Another group of 228 patients seeking disability was also examined in this study by Iverson and colleagues (2002) including (a) 77 credible patients with MTBI (defined by LOC < 10 min and PTA < 1 hr); (b) 42 malingerers with suspected MTBI; (c) 83 credible patients with "well-defined head injury" (WDHI; characterized by LOC > 30 min and PTA > 24 hr); and (d) 27 malingerers with suspected WDHI. Cutoff scores at the 5th percentile on the TMT for the total clinical non–compensation-seeking sample with acute TBI were used to classify TBI compensation seekers as credible or noncredible (i.e., TMT Part A time to complete ≥ 63 s, TMT Part B time to complete ≥ 200 s, TMT ratio ≤ 1.49). In the MTBI group, the TMT Part A time cutoff was associated with 16.7% sensitivity and 100% specificity, the TMT Part B time cutoff resulted in 7.1% sensitivity and 100% specificity, and the TMT ratio had only 2.4% sensitivity and 87% specificity. Overall, the authors concluded the TMT provided little benefit for identifying poor effort, but their cutoffs may have been too conservative, given that most resulted in 100% specificity and were derived on patients who are acutely injured; less conservative cutoffs set to 90% specificity in patients with remote MTBI histories would have greater sensitivity and be more appropriate to the typical litigation exam context in which injuries occurred years earlier.

Arguing that Iverson and colleagues (2002) may have erred too strongly on the side of reducing Type II error rates given their choice of cut scores (and resulting low sensitivities), Powell, Locke, Smigielski, and McCrea (2011) recently attempted reinvestigation of TMT indices in an acquired brain injury rehabilitation population (n = 76) and found promising results (i.e., TMT Part A time to complete cutoff of ≥ 48 s was associated with 72% sensitivity and 82% specificity; TMT Part B time to complete cutoff of ≥ 125 s was associated with 50% sensitivity and 80% specificity); however, the sample was mixed (79% TBI; 28% of whom were MTBI), and the TBI subsample was not examined separately by severity. Thus, generalizability of these more recent results to the present examination of non–memory-based SVTs in MTBI populations, specifically, is limited. However, the case could be made that because more patients with severe TBI were included, a specificity of ≥ 80% would be an underestimate in MTBI samples. Notably, neither total errors nor Part B/A ratio scores were successful at distinguishing optimal and suboptimal effort groups. The results of this study suggested that additional research may be warranted to investigate the use of TMT Part A and B completion time scores in MTBI cases.

Summary of Executive-Based Symptom Validity Tests

In summary, sensitivity of executive-based SVTs in MTBI samples is relatively low compared to other SVTs (see Table 8.8 on p. 212 of Greve & Bianchini, 2007, for a comparison of WCST and CT indicators with well-known freestanding and embedded validity indicators in MTBI samples). Thus, although a negative finding does not rule out poor effort, a positive finding can provide information regarding presence of response bias.

Greve and Bianchini (2007) and Greve and colleagues (2009) discussed why there may be low sensitivity associated with executive functioning based SVTs. In particular, they suggested that large individual difference variables (independent of acquired brain injury) play a role (e.g., 20% of the variance in WCST performance is associated with demographics such as age and education). In addition, they suggested that measures of executive function are very sensitive to brain damage, so when studies use patients with bona fide brain injury as a control comparison group, they are likely to score in the range of malingering. In this vein, the most compelling reason why executive measures have limited use in identification of response bias is that the most effective effort indicators are those that appear difficult but are, in fact, easy. In contrast, executive tasks are among the most genuinely difficult cognitive tasks in a neuropsychological battery. As a result, lower cutoffs set to protect credible patients will result in inadequate sensitivity.

NEUROPSYCHOLOGICAL TEST BATTERIES AND DISCRIMINANT FUNCTIONS

Whereas the aforementioned literature addressed SVTs derived as a single score from a single test (e.g., b Test), another approach to the detection of symptom invalidity through the use of embedded tests is through examining atypical patterns of performance across a test battery. In the case of MTBI, investigations of non–memory-based symptom invalidity testing have been undertaken for the Halstead-Reitan Battery (HRB; Reitan & Wolfson, 1993), the Luria-Nebraska Neuropsychological Battery (LNNB; Golden, Purisch, & Hammeke, 1985), the Meyers Neuropsychological Battery (MNB; Meyers & Rohling, 2004; Volbrecht, Meyers, & Kaster-Bundgaard, 2000), as well as the Wechsler Adult Intelligence Scale-Revised (WAIS-R; Wechsler, 1981) and the Wechsler Adult Intelligence Scale-Third Edition (WAIS-III; Wechsler, 1997). Usually, atypical patterns of performance within these batteries of tests have been demonstrated through the use of discriminant function analysis, comparing noninjured simulators of brain injury with real nonlitigating, non–compensation-seeking patients with neurological problems (most often with moderate-to-severe brain injury). Individuals are identified as putting forth variable levels of motivation or effort when they produce a pattern of results that does not make neuropsychological "sense" in that it does not conform to known patterns of performance in genuine neurological conditions.

Larrabee (2007) provided an excellent summary of this work, reviewing data on atypical patterns of performance on the HRB, LNNB, WAIS-R, and WAIS-III. Meyers (2007) provided an excellent summary of his own work specific to the MNB. The readers are referred to these chapters for detailed reviews of the literature up to 2006. A summary is provided here in addition to MTBI-relevant cut scores and classification accuracy statistics in Table 13.3. Here, we also review the literature relevant to this discussion that has emerged since the publication of these reviews.

The Halstead-Reitan Neuropsychological Battery

Larrabee (2007) reviewed simulation (Goebel, 1983; Heaton et al., 1978; Mittenberg et al., 1996), known groups (Thompson & Cullum, 1991), and specificity (McKinzey & Russell, 1997) studies investigating the classification accuracy of the HRB discriminant function analysis (DFA) to distinguish noncredible from credible groups of subjects. Although the original classic study by Heaton and colleagues (1978) led to fairly impressive rates of classification, this was a simulation study, and the patients with TBI comparison in this study were classified as predominantly severe. The DFA was not supported on cross-validation attempt in a litigating and/or compensation-seeking MTBI sample (Thompson & Cullum, 1991).

A second simulation study employing mild, moderate, and severe TBI clinical comparison groups (Mittenberg et al., 1996) led to the derivation of additional DFA equations that, once again, led to impressive classification rates (combining derivation and cross-validation samples led to sensitivity = 84%, specificity = 94%). In terms of performance on specific tests, the simulators performed worse than the TBI groups on the CT, Speech-Sounds Perception Test, Seashore Rhythm Test, FT, GS, FTNW, and finger agnosia, suggesting these tests may be particularly sensitive (note that these tests are reviewed individually in this chapter). Notably, this particular DFA has been applied successfully to a MTBI sample (i.e., to definite patients with MND from the Trueblood & Schmidt [1993] study and to three patients with MTBI in Cullum, Heaton, & Grant [1991]). However, later research questioned the specificity of the DFA, finding unacceptable rates of false positive error when examined in a large general clinical sample (i.e., specificity = 73%, $n = 796$) and in a subgroup of individuals with TBI in particular (specificity = 77.5%; McKinzey & Russell, 1997). Larrabee (2007) pointed out that the McKinzey and Russell (1997) sample was likely contaminated because no validity checks were used to exclude malingerers.

The HRB General Neuropsychological Deficit Scale (GNDS; Reitan & Wolfson, 1985), a summary indicator of performance across the entire battery, has also been investigated as an SVT. Trueblood and Schmidt (1993; study described earlier) reported that a GNDS > 44 cutoff correctly identified six malingerers (75%) and four

TABLE 13.3 Known Groups Studies of SVT Effectiveness From Test Batteries in Mild TBI

Study	Sample	Test/Score	Cut Score	Sensitivity	Specificity		
		HRNB					
Trueblood & Schmidt (1993)	Definite MND patients with MTBI (*n*=8) Probable MND patients with MTBI (*n*=8) Matched controls (*n*=16)	GNDS	> 44	75% (Definite) 50% (Probable)	100% (matched MTBI controls) 94.3% (larger sample of MTBI credibles)		
		WAIS-R/III Indices					
Millis et al. (1998)	Probable malingering patients with MTBI (*n*=50) Credible patients with moderate-to-severe TBI (*n*=50)	WAIS-R Mittenberg DFA	> 0 > 0.10536	88% 88%	86% 92%		
Mittenberg et al. (2001)	Probable malingerers (PM; *n*=36) Non-litigating patients with TBI (19% of whom were mild; *n*=36) Non-injured simulators (*n*=36)	WAIS-III Mittenberg DFA	> 0	72% (simulators) 44% (PM)	83%		
Greve et al. (2003)	MND patients with TBI (*n*=28; 79% of which were mild) Credible, nonlitigating patients with TBI (*n*=37; 43% of which were mild)	WAIS-R Mittenberg DFA WAIS-III Mittenberg DFA Across both versions	> 0 > .212 > 0 > .212 > 0 > .212	MTBI only 50% 38% 57% 57% 54% 50%	MTBI 72% 73% 100% 100% 81% 81%	Mod/sev 88% 100% 85% 92% 86% 95%	
Curtis et al. (2009)	MND patients with MTBI (*n*=31) Credible patients with MTBI (*n*=26) Credible patients with moderate-to-severe TBI (*n*=26) General clinical patients (*n*=80)	WAIS-III Verbal IQ	< 65 < 70 < 75 < 80	13% 26% 42% 58%	MTBI 100% 96% 85% 69%	Mod/sev 96% 96% 96% 88%	Clin 99% 92% 84% 72%
		WAIS-III Performance IQ	< 65 < 70 < 75 < 80 < 85	10% 23% 39% 71% 81%	MTBI 100% 100% 96% 81% 61%	Mod/sev 92% 88% 77% 69% 54%	Clin 95% 89% 82% 69% 54%

(Continued)

TABLE 13.3 Known Groups Studies of SVT Effectiveness From Test Batteries in Mild TBI (*Continued*)

Study	Sample	Test/Score	Cut Score	Sensitivity	Specificity		
		WAIS-R/III Indices					
Curtis et al. (2009) (*Continued*)		WAIS-III Full Scale IQ			MTBI	Mod/sev	Clin
			< 65	13%	100%	96%	94%
			< 70	26%	100%	88%	90%
			< 75	48%	88%	81%	82%
			< 80	74%	65%	73%	67%
		Verbal Comprehension Index			MTBI	Mod/sev	Clin
			< 65	19%	100%	100%	97%
			< 70	29%	92%	96%	92%
			< 75	45%	81%	96%	87%
			< 80	58%	65%	88%	79%
		Perceptual Organization Index			MTBI	Mod/sev	Clin
			< 70	20%	100%	92%	90%
			< 75	33%	100%	92%	85%
			< 80	50%	88%	80%	74%
			< 85	67%	77%	76%	64%
		Working Memory Index			MTBI	Mod/sev	Clin
			< 65	19%	100%	100%	92%
			< 70	26%	96%	96%	90%
			< 75	48%	88%	88%	77%
			< 80	61%	85%	81%	67%
			< 85	77%	77%	77%	57%
		Processing Speed Index			MTBI	Mod/sev	Clin
			< 60	10%	100%	92%	95%
			< 65	16%	96%	88%	92%
			< 70	36%	92%	80%	81%
			< 75	55%	85%	64%	74%
			< 80	68%	73%	48%	55%
		Total failures (≤ 75) on any one Index score			MTBI	Mod/sev	Clin
			≥ 1	73%	73%	60%	61%
			≥ 2	47%	81%	88%	82%
			≥ 3	37%	100%	96%	90%
		Estimated-Obtained IQ discrepancy scores					
Trueblood (1994)	Definite MND patients MTBI (*n*=12) Probable MND patients with MTBI (*n*=10) Demographically-matched credible patients with MTBI (*n*=22)	Barona – WAIS-R FSIQ	> 18	33% (Definite) 60% (Probable)	100% (Definite) 100% (Probable)		
Demakis et al. (2001)	Predominantly patients with MTBI – insufficient effort (*n*=27) Credible patients with moderate-to-severe TBI (*n*=48)	Barona – WAIS-R VIQ	Unavailable from author	59%	79%		
		Barona – WAIS-R PIQ	Unavailable from author	63%	83%		
		Barona – WAIS-R FSIQ	Unavailable from author	59%	81%		

(*Continued*)

TABLE 13.3 Known Groups Studies of SVT Effectiveness From Test Batteries in Mild TBI (*Continued*)

Study	Sample	Test/Score	Cut Score	Sensitivity	Specificity		
		Estimated-Obtained IQ discrepancy scores					
Greve et al. (2008)	MND patients with MTBI (*n*=38)	Barona – VIQ			MTBI	Mod/sev	Clin
			≥ 50	0%	100%	98%	98%
	Credible patients with MTBI (*n*=44)		≥ 45	3%	100%	98%	98%
			≥ 35	11%	100%	98%	92%
	Credible patients with moderate-to-severe TBI (*n*=43)		≥ 26	32%	98%		
			≥ 25	34%	98%	93%	80%
			≥ 24	40%	93%		
			≥ 23	45%	89%		
	Credible general clinical patients (not TBI; *n*=93)	Barona – PIQ			MTBI	Mod/sev	Clin
			≥ 50	0%	100%	100%	100%
			≥ 45	0%	100%	98%	99%
			≥ 40	0%	100%	98%	98%
			≥ 35	5%	98%	95%	93%
			≥ 31	11%	98%		
			≥ 30	13%	95%	86%	87%
			≥ 25	29%	95%	79%	76%
			≥ 24	29%	95%		
			≥ 22	34%	91%		
			≥ 20	50%	86%	67%	58%
		Barona – FSIQ			MTBI	Mod/sev	Clin
			≥ 50	0%	100%	100%	99%
			≥ 45	3%	100%	98%	99%
			≥ 40	5%	100%	98%	96%
			≥ 35	11%	100%	98%	92%
			≥ 30	16%	98%	86%	88%
			≥ 27	29%	98%		
			≥ 25	34%	93%	86%	76%
			≥ 24	40%	89%		
			≥ 20	63%	84%	72%	60%

Note. Clin = credible clinical group; DFA = Discriminant Function Analysis; FSIQ = full scale intelligence quotient; GNDS = General Neuropsychological Deficit Scale; HNRB = Halstead Reitan Neuropsychological Battery; IQ = intelligence quotient; MNB = Meyers Neuropsychological Battery; MND = malingered neurocognitive dysfunction; Mod/sev = credible moderate-to-severe TBI; MTBI = mild traumatic brain injury; PIQ = performance intelligence quotient; SVT = Symptom Validity Test; TBI = traumatic brain injury; VIQ = verbal intelligence quotient; WAIS-R/III = Wechsler Adult Intelligence Scale, Revised/Third Edition.

individuals with questionable credibility (50%) while maintaining specificity of 94.3%–100%.

The Luria-Nebraska Neuropsychological Battery

As Larrabee (2007) pointed out, there has been one derivation and cross-validation attempt to validate a formula for the detection of malingering using the LNNB (McKinzey, Podd, Krehbiel, Mensch, & Trombka, 1997). Although the sample contained individuals with histories of TBI, the sample was neurologically heterogeneous, and we are not aware of any studies that have examined the effectiveness of the LNNB in identifying noncredible performance in MTBI populations.

Meyers Neuropsychological Battery

The Meyers Neuropsychological Battery (MNB; Meyers & Rohling, 2004; Volbrecht et al., 2000), an established battery of well-validated tests, contains nine embedded

SVTs, many of which are in domains other than memory (including language), that have been validated individually (Meyers, Bayless, & Meyers, 1996; Meyers, Galinsky, & Volbrecht, 1999; Meyers, Morrison, & Miller, 2001; Meyers & Volbrecht, 1998, 1999; Rohling, Meyers, & Millis, 2003) and when used in combination (Meyers & Volbrecht, 2003) for discriminating patients with normal controls, depression, chronic pain, and with moderate-to-severe TBI, from individuals with history of MTBI. Meyers (2007) provided an excellent review of all studies investigating the nine embedded SVTs up to 2006, concluding that they are well validated and most effective when used together to monitor effort through the evaluation. The nine internal effort indicators (explained in detail in Meyers, Volbrecht, Axelrod, & Reinsch-Boothby, 2011, p. 11) that sample from several different cognitive domains include (a) reliable digit span (RDS); (b) Judgment of Line Orientation (JOLO) raw uncorrected number correct score; (c) DLB ears score; (d) Token Test (TT) number of correct score; (e) sentence repetition (SR) total correct score; (f) Auditory Verbal Learning Test-Recognition (AVLT-R) true positive; (g) memory error pattern (MEP) score; (h) forced-choice (FC) recognition task total correct score; and (i) EFT score. The original cut scores (set to 0% false positive rate) for each test were established and then cross validated in Meyers and Volbrecht (2003). The reader should note that RDS, JOLO, TT, and SR are reviewed in the previous chapter. DLB and EFT are reviewed in this chapter. Finally, the memory-based embedded indicators (i.e., AVLT-R, MEP, and FC) are reviewed in Chapter 9 of this volume.

Wechsler Adult Intelligence Scales

The Wechsler intelligence scales are the most commonly used tests of intelligence (Lezak et al., 2004; Mitrushina et al., 2005) and currently in the fourth edition (Wechsler, 2008). MTBI has been demonstrated to exert little effect on intelligence test performance (Dikmen et al., 1995). Patterns of improbable relationships between scores in earlier editions of the WAIS in patients with a history of MTBI have been investigated. Babikian and Boone (2007) and Larrabee (2007) provided reviews of the WAIS-R and WAIS-III DFAs and other simulation indices for all studies up to 2006. They reviewed WAIS-R simulation (Mittenberg, Theroux-Fichera, Zielinski, & Heilbronner, 1995), known groups (Milanovich, Axelrod, & Millis, 1996; Millis, Ross, & Ricker, 1998; Rawlings & Brooks, 1990; Trueblood, 1994), and specificity (Axelrod & Rawlings, 1999) studies, as well as studies of WAIS-III mixed simulation/known groups (Mittenberg et al., 2001) and known groups (Greve, Bianchini, Mathias, Houston, & Crouch, 2003) designs.

Babikian and Boone (2007) suggested that sensitivity rates appear to be much higher in simulation studies and may therefore be overestimated (Mittenberg et al., 2001 DFA sensitivity = 72%, compared to Greve et al., 2003 DFA sensitivity = 50%–53%). Further, these authors noted that although specificity rates are comparable across studies, sensitivity rates of the DFA in known group studies vary widely (Millis et al., 1998 DFA sensitivity = 88%; Greve et al., 2003 DFA sensitivity = 53%). Larrabee (2007) concurred with this assertion, stating that additional validation of the DFAs in real-world samples was necessary. Mixed and known groups study cut scores and associated classification rates are displayed in Table 13.3.

More recently, Curtis, Greve, and Bianchini (2009) found that the Mittenberg formula failed to differentiate malingerers from nonmalingerers in their MTBI sample. Although the Mittenberg formula was poor at differentiating patients with MND MTBI from patients with non-MND MTBI, WAIS-III IQ and index scores performed relatively well (see Table 13.3 for a replication of their classification rates at a range of cut scores). When scores were aggregated and joint classification accuracy was determined (a universal cut score of ≤ 75 across all four index scores was used), ≥ 2 index failures was associated with improved sensitivity relative to most individual index scores (sensitivity = 47%, specificity = 81%). In addition, no one in the credible MTBI group demonstrated ≥ 3 failures (specificity = 100%), although this cutoff was associated with a slight drop in sensitivity (i.e., 37%). These data are also shown in Table 13.3. It is important to note that this study's sample excluded people with less than 9 years of education. Therefore, the data cannot be applied to individuals with low levels of education. In fact, the only false positive in the credible MTBI group was a patient with 9 years of education.

Discrepancy Between Estimated Premorbid IQ and Obtained IQ

Lower FSIQ scores have been noted for poorly motivated patients with MTBI compared to credible clinical comparison groups (Binder & Willis, 1991; Trueblood & Schmidt, 1993). Further, a study by Demakis and colleagues (2001) investigated estimated and obtained IQ discrepancy in two groups: 27 litigating/compensation-seeking patients with TBI who failed at least one independent SVT (most of whom would be classified as MTBI) and 48 credible patients with moderate-to-severe TBI. Whereas both groups obtained WAIS-R IQ scores below their estimated premorbid IQ (using Barona Index, Oklahoma Premorbid Intelligence Estimate [OPIE], and Best 3 Methods), the poor effort group demonstrated a significantly larger discrepancy than the credible group. The Barona-based discrepancy score demonstrated higher sensitivity compared to the other methods of estimation (for performance IQ [PIQ] in particular). Likewise, Trueblood (1994) investigated Barona-estimated premorbid and obtained WAIS-R FSIQ scores in their known groups study of patients with MTBI (described earlier). Their noncredible groups (definite and questionable) scored 16–18 points below their estimated premorbid IQs in contrast to their credible MTBI counterparts who scored 3–5 points below their estimated premorbid IQs. Classification accuracy statistics are displayed in Table 13.3.

Babikian and Boone (2007) suggested this particular method of determining symptom validity in MTBI might be fruitful to pursue, and in fact, since the publication of their review, Greve, Lotz, and Bianchini (2008) investigated the classification accuracy of observed WAIS-III verbal IQ [VIQ], PIQ, and FSIQ minus Barona-estimated differential scores in the detection of MND in patients with TBI using a known groups design. In the MTBI subsample (MTBI defined as PTA < 24 hr, initial GCS = 13–15, LOC ≤ 30 min, and negative neuroimaging), 38 patients met criteria for MND (Slick et al., 1999), and 44 were judged to be credible. The MND MTBI group scored lower than the credible MTBI group in all scores, and these indicators successfully distinguished the two groups (a range of cut scores and associated classification accuracy information for clinical use is displayed in Table 13.3). In general, as the authors pointed out, observed IQ scores of ≥ 25 points below estimated IQ score in MTBI cases likely reflects intentional suppression of test performance. In addition, in their analysis of joint classification accuracy, the authors concluded that PIQ did not substantially add value to prediction when combined with VIQ in MTBI cases, suggesting the latter is of greater clinical use.

CLINICAL AND RESEARCH IMPLICATIONS

It has long been established that clinical judgment, alone, is ineffective for detecting individuals who may be "faking" deficits from a brain injury (e.g., Heaton et al.,

1978). The explosion of research in this area of study has clarified how assessment of effort must be a routine part of any neuropsychological evaluation. Recommendations by the National Academy of Neuropsychology (NAN) Policy and Planning Committee (Bush et al., 2005) and the American Academy of Clinical Neuropsychology (AACN, 2007; Heilbronner, Sweet, Morgan, Larrabee, & Millis, 2009) reflect the importance of this process to ensuring the veracity of results and establishing the validity of one's interpretations.

Previous work has focused mostly on assessing feigned memory deficits with dedicated SVTs, but it is important to recognize that people fake or exaggerate symptoms in a variety of cognitive domains other than memory. Although there is some evidence indicating that individuals feigning in the context of MTBI do so by targeting their poor performance on perceived measures of memory (e.g., Nitch, Boone, Wen, Arnold, & Alfano, 2006), not all do, and effort needs to be assessed *throughout* the evaluation and across several cognitive domains (Boone, 2009). The nature of the strategy or approach to feigning will vary, as Meyers and colleagues (2011) pointed out,

> . . . individuals do not fail all SVTs equally, but instead are more selective of their SVT performance . . . the approach to malingering varies based on the nature of the task and the 'perception' of the individual as to what cognitive deficits he/she is trying to portray. (p. 14)

In the last two chapters, we attempted to provide a concise review of SVTs in domains other than memory that hold promise for detecting MND in MTBI populations specifically. Most are "embedded" measures derived from standard neurocognitive tests.

Advantages of Embedded Symptom Validity Tests

Many clinicians have assumed that embedded SVTs are "second-class" measures of response bias because they have not been specifically developed to assess for effort. However, the relative value of SVTs should be based on sensitivity rates (with cutoffs set to $\geq$ 90% specificity). Whether they have a single purpose in evaluating effort is of less relevance. In tracing historical developments in psychometric testing, it is unclear why personality inventories, such as the Minnesota Multiphasic Personality Inventory (MMPI) instruments, were early adopters of symptom validity indices, whereas the WAIS and neuropsychological batteries were not. André Rey, who published in the 1940s, appears to have placed neuropsychology on the path of freestanding effort measures with development of tests such as the Rey 15-item Recognition Test, Rey Dot Counting Test, and Rey Word Recognition Test, with his work followed by Pankratz's refinement of forced choice paradigms as SVTs (Pankratz, 1979; Pankratz, Binder, & Wilcox, 1987; Pankratz, Fausti, & Peed, 1975). But there were investigators, such as Bernard, publishing in the 1990s, who worked to refine embedded neurocognitive indices (e.g., Rey-Osterrith/Rey Auditory Verbal Learning Test (RAVLT) discriminant function; Bernard, 1990; Bernard, Houston, & Natoli, 1993). The fact that initial SVT research in neuropsychology was dominated by freestanding measures appears to have been arbitrary.

Embedded measures have several advantages compared to freestanding methods. First, embedded SVTs do not require additional test administration time. Thus, embedded SVTs are the most efficient method to achieve the recommended goal of repeatedly testing for effort during an exam. Second, they serve as "double duty," measuring both effort and the cognitive ability they were designed to measure (e.g., attention, processing speed, executive function). Third, embedded SVTs measure response bias in "real time," in contrast to the results of freestanding SVTs, which are used to describe quality of effort on standard cognitive tasks before or after the SVT (e.g., "The patient passed the Test of Memory Malingering (TOMM) at 9:30 a.m., therefore, performance on the WCST 2 hours later is valid"). In this example, the results of the TOMM, arguably a measure of immediate visual memory recognition, are being used to comment on effort at a different point in time and on a different type of skill, a rather questionable practice. Relatively few noncredible individuals fail all SVTs (about 17%; Boone, 2009), likely because they perceive that inability to perform on any task would be nonplausible. Rather, the typical noncredible patient is likely to spontaneously "pick and choose" measures during the exam on which to underperform. Examining effort in vivo on each task best allows the examiner to identify when and in which skills the patient is not performing to true ability. As Kim and colleagues (2010) explained, "Ideally, every standard cognitive measure should have an embedded effort indicator" (p. 420). In this way, the examiner can assess the validity of an examinee's performance on each test rather than inserting one or two validity indicators arbitrarily into a large battery and then making general conclusions about malingering or symptom invalidity.

Finally, embedded SVTs are less susceptible to coaching in that searches on the test names will reveal their traditional purpose in measuring neurocognitive skills. In contrast, freestanding SVTs (e.g., TOMM) are more likely to be known to attorneys and accessible on the internet (Bauer & McCaffrey, 2006; Ruiz, Drake, Marcotte, Glass, & van Gorp, 2000), and therefore are more likely to be recognized and manipulated by examinees (Suhr & Gunstad, 2000, 2007).

However, as a whole, nonmemory SVTs generally have sensitivity rates below freestanding memory SVTs. If sensitivity rates are only modest-to-moderate (e.g., 30%–60%), the measures can be used to "rule in" but not "rule out" malingering. That is, a negative finding is not particularly informative in that a large percentage of noncredible patients pass the cutoffs. However, a positive finding provides critical information in that failure is relatively rare in credible populations. Although it may be hard to make the case for administration of freestanding SVTs with modest sensitivity (e.g., minimal "bang for the buck"), embedded SVTs with comparable sensitivity are valuable because they are "free information" (i.e., already available from standard tests), with positive findings contributing to converging evidence of response bias.

Aggregation Across Symptom Validity Tests

With the validation of more and more SVTs, the clinician is faced with the dilemma of how to interpret the various indicators in concert. The task may initially appear overwhelming, but availability of data from multiple indicators actually increases confidence in conclusions.

Many authors have found that failure on two SVTs out of several is associated with virtually 100% specificity in all but the most impaired patients. In the same manner, Larrabee (2003) noted that failure on two out of three embedded indicators (visual form discrimination [VFD], combined FT, RDS, WCST FMS, and the Fake Bad Scale of the MMPI-2) was associated with 87.5% sensitivity and 88.9% specificity, with specificity reaching 100% at three failures. This finding is consistent with the analogue study results of Vickery and colleagues (2004) and Sollman, Ranseen, and Berry (2010), the known groups results of Larrabee (2008), and Victor, Boone, Serpa,

Buehler, and Ziegler (2009), and the hybrid study of Meyers and Volbrecht (2003), which found that a failure rate of two or more internal SVTs correctly classified 83% of their sophisticated simulator sample while maintaining 100% specificity in nonlitigating control and clinical (i.e., patients with depression, chronic pain, and moderate-to-severe TBI) comparison groups. Notably, although Meyers and Volbrecht (2003) suggested the use of the MNB SVTs in MTBI cases, the specific populations with whom these indicators would *not* be appropriately applied are also indicated, including patients who are institutionalized, patients who suffered severe stroke, patients with dementia, and individuals with moderate-to-severe mental retardation.

Alternatively, in a rather novel and effective approach taken by Backhaus and colleagues (2004), cutoffs on standard cognitive tests were set at the 50th percentile of performance of credible moderate-to-severe TBI samples. Using this approach, the authors found that if more than one third of test scores fell at or below this level, sensitivity in noncredible MTBI litigants was 96% with associated specificity in nonlitigant credible MTBI of 92%. Thus, it was very unlikely for credible patients with MTBI to fail (i.e., to obtain a score below a floor set at the 50th percentile) more than one third of the validity checks. The measures providing the best overall classification rate (out of the 11 examined) were the Stroop Neuropsychological Screening Test (SNST), JOLO, SR, SDMT, and finger localization. Of note, when interpreting the results of multiple SVTs in concert, the presence of "passed" indicators does not "erase" or counterbalance documented SVT failures.

Common questions encountered in clinical neuropsychological practice regarding SVTs are "how many" and "which ones" should be administered. A more appropriate question would be, "Have I attempted to repeatedly check for response bias throughout the exam by giving preference to standard cognitive tests that include embedded effort indicators?"

Methodological Issues in Research on SVTs for MTBI Assessments

Some studies validating the effectiveness of SVTs in MTBI cases have relied on simulation designs in which participants are requested to feign deficits. However, many authors have commented on problems with external generalizability from these data. Perusal of simulation studies shows that many obtained sensitivity rates vastly higher than those found in known groups designs (e.g., Iverson & Franzen, 1994, 1996), whereas others find reduced sensitivity (e.g., Rose, Hall, Szalda-Petree, & Bach, 1998). We take the position that techniques should not be employed in the clinical setting until they are validated in known groups.

That said, known groups studies have methodological limitations as well. The astute reader has observed that specificity rates in "credible" compensation-seeking MTBI subjects for some SVTs (e.g., Greve, Bianchini, & Mathias et al., 2003; Heinly, Greve, Bianchini, Love, & Brennan, 2005) are frequently lower than for general clinical patients and patients with moderate-to-severe TBI—a nonsensical finding. In these studies, patients with MTBI were assigned to the credible group because they passed the few SVT(s) used to assign subjects to groups. But SVTs do not have perfect sensitivity, meaning that some noncredible patients will pass them and be inaccurately assigned to the credible group. The result of this error is that performance of the credible group will be lowered, and cutoffs will result in lowered specificity rates. Greve and Bianchini (2006) argued that the mildly lowered neurocognitive scores in "credible" litigants are caused by the stress associated with litigation, but a more likely explanation is that some in this group were in fact feigning or exaggerating but were not detected by the SVTs employed, causing group means to be lowered. The only way the impact of litigation "stress" on cognitive scores can be evaluated is if litigants motivated to *overperform* are studied (i.e., individuals involved in child custody disputes).

The reader might suggest that the best solution in known groups designs is to use patients with MTBI not in litigation as the comparison group. However, the problem with this recommendation is that non–compensation-seeking patients with MTBI do not typically present for evaluation remote from the injury because they have, in fact, recovered. As discussed in the previous chapter, the results of meta-analyses involving dozens of studies and thousands of patients have now shown that there are no long-term cognitive abnormalities associated with a single MTBI (Belanger, Curtiss, Demery, Lebowitz, & Vanderploeg, 2005; Belanger & Vander-ploeg, 2005; Binder, Rohling, & Larrabee, 1997; Carroll et al., 2004; Frencham, Fox, & Maybery, 2005; Rohling et al., 2011; Schretlen & Shapiro, 2003), leading McCrea (2008) in a book summarizing research on MTBI to conclude that there is "no indication of permanent impairment on neuropsychological testing by three months postinjury" (p. 117).

In our data set derived from an outpatient neuropsychology clinic on a county hospital campus, only one non–compensation-seeking patient with MTBI presented for evaluation in more than 20 years of data collection. The dearth of non–compensation-seeking patients with a history of MTBI presenting for clinical evaluation has also been reported by other authors (Lees-Haley & Brown, 1993; Suhr, Tranel, Wefel, & Barrash, 1997). Given that patients with MTBI recover cognitive function, and given the absence of non–compensation-seeking patients with MTBI in clinical data sets, it can be argued that the most appropriate comparison group for research validating SVTs for use in patients with MTBI, is normal controls or orthopedic trauma controls to account for the effect of experiencing a traumatic injury.

The fact that individuals with remote MTBI histories should be performing normally on cognitive testing indicates that SVT cutoffs can be higher in the identification of faking in the context of MTBI. In particular, cutoffs are selected to protect credible patient groups (Heilbronner et al., 2009), and when cutoffs are chosen to produce high specificity rates in patients with significant cognitive abnormalities (e.g., moderate-to-severe TBI, some types of seizure presentations, stroke, learning disabilities), they will be less stringent than cutoffs that allow few false positives in normal individuals. For example, as discussed in the previous chapter, Greiffenstein, Baker, and Gola (1994) found an RDS cutoff of ≤ 7 yielded sensitivity values from 50% to 87% with adequate specificity for nonlitigating patients with MTBI (89%–96%). However, Babikian, Boone, Lu, and Arnold (2006) had to use a cutoff of ≤ 6 to maintain adequate specificity in their sample of general neuropsychology clinic patients. Although in the last two chapters we have focused on SVTs that have been specifically researched in MTBI samples, it should not be concluded that SVTs not specifically validated in MTBI cannot be used in clinical practice with these patients. Rather, these SVTs will have lowered sensitivity in MTBI because of the more lenient cutoffs, but if a patient with MTBI, in fact, fails such indicators, they provide compelling evidence for negative response bias.

A question that arises is whether SVTs should be "cross validated" before clinical use, that is, that the results of initial validation studies be replicated prior to recommendations for clinical use. Psychology graduate students are taught the importance of cross validation as a method to ensure that initial studies of psychometric techniques have not capitalized on unidentified error. However, SVT research is unique in terms of the very large ES documented between credible and noncredible groups. With large ES, cross validation becomes less important. That is, the effect of effort obliterates the impact of contamination from typical sources of error.

A bigger problem would be small sample size, and unfortunately, several of the studies described in this review have employed sample sizes of less than 30. Findings, including cutoffs, from such studies may be less reliable, and more credence should be given to SVT validation studies that have employed relatively large samples. Future research should continue to pursue validation of embedded SVTs for virtually every neuropsychological task administered, with the goal of measuring response bias in "real time."

REFERENCES

American Academy of Clinical Neuropsychology. (2007). American Academy of Clinical Neuropsychology (AACN) Practice Guidelines for Neuropsychological Assessment and Consultation. *The Clinical Neuropsychologist*, 21(2), 209–231

Arnold, G., & Boone, K. B. (2007). Use of motor and sensory test as measures of effort. In K. B. Boone (Ed.), *Assessment of feigned cognitive impairment: A neuropsychological perspective*. (pp. 178–209). New York, NY: Guilford Press.

Arnold, G., Boone, K. B., Lu, P., Dean, A., Wen, J., Nitch, S., & McPherson, S. (2005). Sensitivity and specificity of finger tapping test scores for the detection of suspect effort. *The Clinical Neuropsychologist*, 19(1), 105–120.

Auditec of St. Louis. (1991). *Dichotic word listening test (DWLT)*. St. Louis, MO: Auditec.

Axelrod, B. N., & Rawlings, D. B. (1999). Clinical utility of incomplete effort WAIS-R formulas: A longitudinal examination of individuals with traumatic brain injuries. *Journal of Forensic Neuropsychology*, 1(2), 15–27.

Babikian, T., & Boone, K. B. (2007). Intelligence tests as measures of effort. In K. B. Boone (Ed.), *Assessment of feigned cognitive impairment: A neuropsychological perspective* (pp. 128–151). New York, NY: Guilford Press.

Babikian, T., Boone, K. B., Lu, P., & Arnold, G. (2006). Sensitivity and specificity of various digit span scores in the detection of suspect effort. *The Clinical Neuropsychologist*, 20(1), 145–159.

Backhaus, S. L., Fichtenberg, N. L., & Hanks, R. A. (2004). Detection of sub-optimal performance using a floor effect strategy in patients with traumatic brain injury. *The Clinical Neuropsychologist*, 18(4), 591–603.

Bauer, L., & McCaffrey, R. J. (2006). Coverage of the test of memory malingering, Victoria symptom validity test, and word memory test on the Internet: Is test security threatened? *Archives of Clinical Neuropsychology*, 21(1), 121–126.

Belanger, H. G., Curtiss, G., Demery, J. A., Lebowitz, B. K., & Vanderploeg, R. D. (2005). Factors moderating neuropsychological outcomes following mild traumatic brain injury: A meta-analysis. *Journal of the International Neuropsychological Society*, 11(3), 215–227.

Belanger, H. G., & Vanderploeg, R. D. (2005). The neuropsychological impact of sports-related concussion: A meta-analysis. *Journal of the International Neuropsychological Society*, 11(45), 345–357.

Benton, A. L., Hamsher, K. de S., & Sivan, A. B. (1994). *Multilingual aphasia examination* (3rd ed.). Iowa City, IA: AJA Associates.

Bernard, L. C. (1990). Prospects for faking believable memory deficits on neuropsychological tests and the use of incentives in simulation research. *Journal of Clinical and Experimental Neuropsychology*, 12(5), 715–728.

Bernard, L. C., Houston, W., & Natoli, L. (1993). Malingering on neuropsychological memory tests: Potential objective indicators. *Journal of Clinical Psychology*, 49(1), 45–53.

Bernard, L. C., McGrath, M. J., & Houston, W. (1996). The differential effects of simulating malingering, closed head injury, and other CNS pathology on the Wisconsin Card Sorting Test: Support for the "pattern of performance" hypothesis. *Archives of Clinical Neuropsychology*, 11(3), 231–245.

Binder, L. M. (1992). Deception and malingering. In A. Puente & R. McCaffrey (Eds.), *Handbook of neuropsychological assessment: A biopsychosocial approach* (pp. 353–372). New York, NY: Plenum Press.

Binder, L. M., Kelly, M. P., Villanueva, M. R., & Winslow, M. M. (2003). Motivation and neuropsychological test performance following mild head injury. *Journal of Clinical and Experimental Neuropsychology*, 25(3), 420–430.

Binder, L. M., Rohling, M. L., & Larrabee, G. J. (1997). A review of mild head trauma. Part I: Meta-analytic review of neuropsychological studies. *Journal of Clinical and Experimental Neuropsychology*, 19(3), 421–431.

Binder, L. M., & Willis, S. C. (1991). Assessment of motivation after financially compensable minor head trauma. *Psychological Assessment*, 3(2), 175–181.

Boone, K. B. (2009). The need for continuous and comprehensive sampling of effort/response bias during neuropsychological examinations. *The Clinical Neuropsychologist*, 23(4), 729–741.

Bowen, M., & Littell, C. (1997). Discriminating adult normals, patients, and claimants with a pediatric test: A brief report. *The Clinical Neuropsychologist*, 11, 433–435.

Bush, S. S., Ruff, R. M., Tröster, A. I., Barth, J. T., Koffler, S. P., Pliskin, N. H., . . . Silver, C. H. (2005). Symptom validity assessment: Practice issues and medical necessity NAN policy & planning committee. *Archives of Clinical Neuropsychology*, 20(4), 419–426.

Butters, M. A., Goldstein, G., Allen, D. N., & Shemansky, W. J. (1998). Neuropsychological similarities and differences among Huntington's disease, multiple sclerosis, and cortical dementia. *Archives of Clinical Neuropsychology*, 13(8), 721–735.

Carroll, L. J., Cassidy, J. D., Peloso, P. M., Borg, J., von Holst, H., Holm, L., . . . Pépin, M. (2004). Prognosis for mild traumatic brain injury: Results of the WHO Collaborating Centre Task Force on Mild Traumatic Brain Injury. *Journal of Rehabilitation Medicine*, 36(Suppl. 43), 84–105.

Crawford, J. R., Besson, J. A., Bremner, M., Ebmeier, K. P., Cochrane, R. H., & Kirkwood, K. (1992). Estimation of premorbid intelligence in schizophrenia. *The British Journal of Psychiatry*, 161, 69–74.

Crawford, J. R., Besson, J. A., Parker, D. M., Sutherland, K. M., & Keen, P. L. (1987). Estimation of premorbid intellectual status in depression. *The British Journal of Clinical Psychology*, 26(Pt. 4), 313–314.

Crawford, J. R., Parker, D. M., & Besson, J. A. (1988). Estimation of premorbid intelligence in organic conditions. *The British Journal of Psychiatry*, 153, 178–181.

Cullum, C. M., Heaton, R. K., & Grant, I. (1991). Psychogenic factors influencing neuropsychological performance: Somatoform disorders, factitious disorders, and malingering. In H. O. Doerr & A. S. Carlin (Eds.), *Forensic neuropsychology: Legal and scientific bases* (pp. 141–171). New York, NY: Guilford Press.

Curiel, A. (2011). *A re-examination of the Meyers and Volbrecht motor equation for the identification of suspect effort*. Unpublished doctoral dissertation, Pepperdine University.

Curtis, K. L., Greve, K. W., & Bianchini, K. J. (2009). The Wechsler Adult Intelligence Scale-III and malingering in traumatic brain injury: Classification accuracy in known groups. *Assessment*, 16(4), 401–414.

Curtis, K. L., Thompson, L. K., Greve, K. W., & Bianchini, K. J. (2008). Verbal fluency indicators of malingering in traumatic brain injury: Classification accuracy in known groups. *The Clinical Neuropsychologist*, 22(5), 930–945.

Damasio, H., & Damasio, A. (1979). "Paradoxic" ear extinction in dichotic listening: Possible anatomic significance. *Neurology*, 29(5), 644–653.

Demakis, G. J. (1999). Serial malingering on verbal and nonverbal fluency and memory measures: An analog investigation. *Archives of Clinical Neuropsychology*, 14(4), 401–410.

Demakis, G. J., Sweet, J. J., Sawyer, T. P., Moulthrop, M., Nies, K., & Clingerman, S. (2001). Discrepancy between predicted and obtained WAIS-R IQ scores discriminates between traumatic brain injury and insufficient effort. *Psychological Assessment*, 13(2), 240–248.

DiCarlo, M. A., Gfeller, J. D., & Oliveri, M. V. (2000). Effects of coaching on detecting feigned cognitive impairment with the category test. *Archives of Clinical Neuropsychology*, 15(5), 399–413.

Dikmen, S. S., Machamer, J. E., Winn, H. R., & Temkin, N. R. (1995). Neuropsychological outcome at 1-year post head injury. *Neuropsychology*, 9(1), 80–90.

Donders, J. (1999). Brief report: Specificity of a malingering formula for the Wisconsin Card Sorting Test. *Journal of Forensic Neuropsychology*, 1, 35–42.

Ellwanger, J., Tenhula, W. N., Rosenfeld, J. P., & Sweet, J. J. (1999). Identifying simulators of cognitive deficit through combined use of neuropsychological test performance and event-related potentials. *Journal of Clinical and Experimental Neuropsychology*, 21(6), 866–879.

Fairfax, A. H., Balnave, R., & Adams, R. D. (1995). Variability of grip strength during isometric contraction. *Ergonomics*, 38(9), 1819–1830.

Forrest, T. J., Allen, D. N., & Goldstein, G. (2004). Malingering indexes for the Halstead category test. *The Clinical Neuropsychologist*, 18(2), 334–347.

Frencham, K. A., Fox, A. M., & Maybery, M. T. (2005). Neuropsychological studies of mild traumatic brain injury: A meta-analytic review of research since 1995. *Journal of Clinical and Experimental Neuropsychology*, 27(3), 334–351.

Gilbert, J. C., & Knowlton, R. G. (1983). Simple method to determine sincerity of effort during a maximal isometric test of grip strength. *American Journal of Physician Medicine*, 62(3), 135–144.

Goebel, R. A. (1983). Detection of faking on the Halstead-Reitan Neuropsychological Test Battery. *Journal of Clinical Psychology*, 39(5), 731–742.

Golden, C. J., Purisch, A. D., & Hammeke, T. A. (1985). *Luria-Nebraska Neuropsychological Battery: Forms I and II* (manual). Los Angeles, CA: Western Psychological Services.

Greiffenstein, M. F. (2007). Motor, sensory, and perceptual-motor pseudoabnormalities. In G. J. Larrabee (Ed.), *Assessment of malingered neuropsychological deficits* (pp. 100–130). New York, NY: Oxford University Press.

Greiffenstein, M. F., & Baker, W. J. (2006). Miller was (mostly) right: Head injury severity inversely related to simulation. *Legal and Criminal Psychology*, 11, 131–145.

Greiffenstein, M. F., Baker, W. J., & Gola, T. (1994). Validation of malingered amnesia measures with a large clinical sample. *Psychological Assessment*, 6, 218–224.

Greiffenstein, M. F., Baker, W. J., & Gola, T. (1996). Motor dysfunction profiles in traumatic brain injury and postconcussion syndrome. *Journal of the International Neuropsychology Society*, 2(6), 477–485.

Greve, K. W., & Bianchini, K. J. (2002). Using the Wisconsin Card Sorting Test to detect malingering: An analysis of the specificity of two methods in nonmalingering normal and patient samples. *Journal of Clinical and Experimental Neuropsychology*, 24(1), 48–54.

Greve, K. W., & Bianchini, K. J. (2004). Setting empirical cut-offs on psychometric indicators of negative response bias: A methodological commentary with recommendations. *Archives of Clinical Neuropsychology*, 19(4), 533–541.

Greve, K. W., & Bianchini, K. J. (2006). Classification accuracy of the Portland Digit Recognition Test in traumatic brain injury: Results of a known-groups analysis. *The Clinical Neuropsychologist*, 20(4), 816–830.

Greve, K. W., & Bianchini, K. J. (2007). Detection of cognitive malingering with tests of executive function. In G. J. Larabee (Ed.), *Assessment of malingered neuropsychological deficits.* (pp. 171–225). New York, NY: Oxford University Press.

Greve, K. W., Bianchini, K. J., & Ameduri, C. J. (2003). Use of a forced-choice test of tactile discrimination in the evaluation of functional sensory loss: A report of 3 cases. *Archives of Physical Medicine and Rehabilitation*, 84(8), 1233–1236.

Greve, K. W., Bianchini, K. J., Mathias, C. W., Houston, R. J., & Crouch, J. A. (2002). Detecting malingered performance with the Wisconsin Card Sorting Test: A preliminary investigation in traumatic brain injury. *The Clinical Neuropsychologist*, 16(2), 179–191.

Greve, K. W., Bianchini, K. J., Mathias, C. W., Houston, R. J., & Crouch, J. A. (2003). Detecting malingered performance on the Wechsler Adult Intelligence Scale: Validation of Mittenberg's approach in traumatic brain injury. *Archives of Clinical Neuropsychology*, 18(3), 245–260.

Greve, K. W., Bianchini, K. J., & Roberson, T. (2007). The booklet category test and malingering in traumatic brain injury: Classification accuracy in known groups. *The Clinical Neuropsychologist*, 21(2), 318–337.

Greve, K. W., Heinly, M. T., Bianchini, K. J., & Love, J. M. (2009). Malingering detection with the Wisconsin Card Sorting Test in mild traumatic brain injury. *The Clinical Neuropsychologist*, 23(2), 343–362.

Greve, K. W., Lotz, K. L., & Bianchini, K. J. (2008). Observed versus estimated IQ as an index of malingering in traumatic brain injury: Classification accuracy in known groups. *Applied Neuropsychology*, 15(3), 161–169.

Greve, K. W. Love, J. M., Heinly, M. T., Doane, B. M., Uribe, E., Joffe, C. L., & Bianchini, K. J. (2005). Detection of feigned tactile sensory loss using a forced-choice test of tactile discrimination and other measure of tactile sensation. *Journal of Occupational and Environmental Medicine*, 47(7), 718–727.

Hagström, Y., & Carlsson, J. (1996). Prolonged functional impairments after whiplash injury. *Scandinavian Journal of Rehabilitation Medicine*, 28(3), 139–146.

Haines, M. E., & Norris, M. P. (2001). Comparing student and patient simulated malingerers' performance on standard neuropsychological measure to detect feigned cognitive deficits. *The Clinical Neuropsychologist*, 15(2), 171–182.

Hamilton, A., Balnave, R., & Adams, R. (1994). Grip strength testing reliability. *Journal of Hand Therapy*, 7(3), 163–170.

Haughton, P. M., Lewsley, A., Wilson, M., & Williams, R. G. (1979). A forced-choice procedure to detect feigned or exaggerated hearing loss. *British Journal of Audiology*, 13(4), 135–138.

Heaton, R. K., Chelune, G. J., Talley, J. L., Kay, G. G., & Curtiss, G. (1993). *Wisconsin Card Sorting Test manual: Revised and expanded.* Odessa, FL: Psychological Assessment Resources.

Heaton, R. K., Grant, I. & Matthews, C. G. (1991). *Comprehensive norms for an expanded Halstead-Reitan battery: Demographics corrections, research, and clinical applications.* Odessa, FL: Psychological Assessment Resources.

Heaton, R. K., Smith, H. H. Jr., Lehman, R. A. W., & Vogt, A. T. (1978). Prospects for faking believable deficits on neuropsychological testing. *Journal of Consulting and Clinical Psychology*, 46(5), 892–900.

Heilbronner, R. L., Sweet, J. J., Morgan, J. E., Larrabee, G. J., & Millis, S. R. (2009). American Academy of Clinical Neuropsychology Consensus Conference Statement on the neuropsychological assessment of effort, response bias, and malingering. *The Clinical Neuropsychologist*, 23(7), 1093–1129.

Heinly, M. T., Greve, K. W., Bianchini, K. J., Love, J. M., & Brennan, A. (2005). WAIS digit span-based indicators of malingered neurocognitive dysfunction: Classification accuracy in traumatic brain injury. *Assessment*, 12(4), 429–444.

Heinly, M. T., Greve, K. W., Love, J. M., & Bianchini, K. J. (2006, February). *Sensitivity and specificity of Wisconsin Card Sorting Test indicators of potential malingered neurocognitive dysfunction in traumatic brain injury*. Poster session presented at the 34th Annual Meeting of the International Neuropsychological Society, Boston, MA.

Inman, T. H., & Berry, D. T. R. (2002). Cross-validation of indicators of malingering: A comparison of nine neuropsychological tests, four tests of malingering, and behavioral observations. *Archives of Clinical Neuropsychology*, 17(1), 1–23.

Iverson, G. L., & Franzen, M. D. (1994). The Recognition Memory Test, Digit Span, and Knox Cube Test as markers of malingered memory impairments. *Assessment*, 1(4), 323–334.

Iverson, G. L., & Franzen, M. D. (1996). Using multiple objective memory procedures to detect simulated malingering. *Journal of Clinical and Experimental Neuropsychology*, 18(1), 38–51.

Iverson, G. L., Lange, R. T., Green, P., & Franzen, M. D. (2002). Detecting exaggeration and malingering with the Trail Making Test. *The Clinical Neuropsychologist*, 16(3), 398–406.

Johnson, J. L., & Lesniak-Karpiak, K. (1997). The effect of warning on malingering on memory and motor tasks in college samples. *Archives of Clinical Neuropsychology*, 12(3), 231–238.

Kim, N., Boone, K. B., Victor, T., Lu, P., Keatinge, C., & Mitchell, C. (2010). Sensitivity and specificity of a digit symbol recognition trial in the identification of response bias. *Archives of Clinical Neuropsychology*, 25(5), 420–428.

King, J. H., Sweet, J. J., Sherer, M., Curtiss, G., & Vanderploeg, R. D. (2002). Validity indicators within the Wisconsin Card Sorting Test: Application of new and previously researched multivariate procedures in multiple traumatic brain injury samples. *The Clinical Neuropsychologist*, 16(4), 506–523.

Lamberty, G. J., Putnam, S. H., Chatel, D. M., Bieliauskas, L. A., & Adams, K. M. (1994). Derived Trailing Making Test indices: A preliminary report. *Neuropsychiatry, Neuropsychology, & Behavioral Neurology*, 7, 230–234.

Larrabee, G. J. (2003). Detection of malingering using atypical performance patterns on standard neuropsychological tests. *The Clinical Neuropsychologist*, 17(3), 410–425.

Larrabee, G. J. (2004, February). *Identification of subtypes of malingered neurocognitive dysfunction*. Paper presented at the 32nd Annual Meeting of the International Neuropsychological Society, Baltimore, MD.

Larrabee, G. J. (Ed.). (2007) *Identification of malingering by pattern analysis on neuropsychological tests*. In *Assessment of malingered neuropsychological deficits*. (pp. 80–99). New York, NY: Oxford University Press.

Larrabee, G. J. (2008). Aggregation across multiple indicators improves the detection of malingering: Relationship to likelihood ratios. *The Clinical Neuropsychologist*, 22(4), 666–679.

Lechner, D. E., Bradbury, S. F., & Bradley, L. A. (1998). Detecting sincerity of effort: A summary of methods and approaches. *Physical Therapy*, 78(8), 867–888.

Lees-Haley, P. R., & Brown, R. S. (1993). Neuropsychological complaint base rates of 170 personal injury claimants. *Archives of Clinical Neuropsychology*, 8(3), 203–209.

Levin, H. S., High, W. M. Jr., Williams, D. H., Eisenberg, H. M., Amparo, E. G., Guinto, F. C. Jr., & Ewert, J. (1989). Dichotic listening and manual performance in relation to magnetic resonance imaging after closed head injury. *Journal of Neurology, Neurosurgery, and Psychiatry*, 52(10), 1162–1169.

Lewis, R., & Kupke, T. (1977, May). *The Lafayette Clinic repeatable neuropsychological test battery: It's development and research applications*. Paper presented at the Annual Meeting of the South-Eastern Psychological Association, Hollywood, FL.

Lezak, M. D., Howeison, D. B., & Loring, D. W. (2004). *Neuropsychological assessment* (4th ed.). New York, NY: Oxford University Press.

Loonstra, A. S., Tarlow, A. R., & Sellers, A. H. (2001). COWAT metanorms across age, education, and gender. *Applied Neuropsychology*, 8(3), 161–166.

Lu, P. H., Boone, K. B., Jimenez, N., & Razani, J. (2004). Failure to inhibit the reading response on the Stroop Test: A pathognomonic indicator of suspect effort. *Journal of Clinical and Experimental Neuropsychology*, 26(2), 180–189.

Martin, T. A., Hoffman, N. M., & Donders, J. (2003). Clinical utility of the trail making test ratio score. *Applied Neuropsychology*, 10(3), 163–169.

McCrea, M. A. (2008). *Mild traumatic brain injury and postconcussion syndrome: The new evidence base for diagnosis and treatment* (AACN workshop series). New York, NY: Oxford University Press.

McKinzey, R. K., Podd, M. H., Krehbiel, M. A., Mensch, A. J., & Trombka, C. C. (1997). Detection of malingering on the Luria-Nebraska Neuropsychological Battery: An initial and cross-validation. *Archives of Clinical Neuropsychology*, 12(5), 505–512.

McKinzey, R. K., & Russell, E. W. (1997). Detection of malingering on the Halstead-Reitan battery: A cross-validation. *Archives of Clinical Neuropsychology*, 12(6), 585–589.

Meyers, J. E. (2007). Malingering mild traumatic brain injury: Behavioral approaches used by both malingering actors and probable malingerers. In K. B. Boone (Ed.), *Assessment of feigned cognitive impairment: A neuropsychological perspective*. (pp. 239–258). New York, NY: Guilford Press.

Meyers, J. E., Bayless, J. D., & Meyers, K. R. (1996). Rey complex figure: Memory error patterns and functional abilities. *Applied Neuropsychology*, 3(2), 89–92.

Meyers, J. E., Galinsky, A. M., & Volbrecht, M. (1999). Malingering and mild brain injury: How low is too low. *Applied Neuropsychology*, 6(4), 208–216.

Meyers, J. E., Morrison, A. L., & Miller, J. C. (2001). How low is too low, revisited: Sentence repetition and AVLT-recognition in the detection of malingering. *Applied Neuropsychology*, 8(4), 234–241.

Meyers, J. E., Roberts, R. J., Bayless, J. D., Volkert, K. T., & Evitts, P. E. (2002). Dichotic listening: Expanded norms and clinical application. *Archives of Clinical Neuropsychology*, 17(1), 79–90.

Meyers, J. E., & Rohling, M. L. (2004). Validation of the Meyers short battery on mild TBI patients. *Archives of Clinical Neuropsychology*, 19(5), 637–651.

Meyers, J. E., & Volbrecht, M. E. (1998). Validation of reliable digits for detection of malingering. *Assessment*, 5(3), 303–307.

Meyers, J. E., & Volbrecht, M. E. (1999). Detection of malingerers using the Rey complex figure and recognition trial. *Applied Neuropsychology*, 6(4), 201–207.

Meyers, J. E., & Volbrecht, M. E. (2003). A validation of multiple malingering detection methods in a large clinical sample. *Archives of Clinical Neuropsychology*, 18(3), 261–276.

Meyers, J. E., Volbrecht, M. E., Axelrod, B. N., & Reinsch-Boothby, L. (2011). Embedded symptom validity tests and overall neuropsychological test performance. *Archives of Clinical Neuropsychology*, 26(1), 8–15.

Milanovich, J. R., Axelrod, B. N., & Millis, S. R. (1996). Validation of the simulation index revised with a mixed clinical population. *Archives of Clinical Neuropsychology*, 11(1), 53–59.

Miller, A., Donders, J., & Suhr, J. (2000). Evaluation of malingering with the Wisconsin Card Sorting Test: A cross-validation. *Clinical Neuropsychological Assessment*, 2, 141–149.

Millis, S. R., Ross, S. R., & Ricker, J. H. (1998). Detection of incomplete effort on the Wechsler Adult Intelligence Scale-Revised: A cross-validation. *Journal of Clinical and Experimental Neuropsychology*, 20(2), 167–173.

Mitrushina, M., Boone, K. B., Razani, J., & D'Elia, L. F. (2005). *Handbook of normative data for neuropsychological assessment* (2nd ed.). New York, NY: Oxford University Press.

Mittenberg, W., Rotholc, A., Russel, E., & Heilbronner, R. (1996). Identification of malingered head injury of the Halstead-Reitan battery. *Archives of Clinical Neuropsychology*, 11(4), 271–281.

Mittenberg, W., Theroux, S., Aguila-Puentes, G., Bianchini, K., Greve, K., & Rayls, K. (2001). Identification of malingered head injury on the Wechsler Adult Intelligence Scale-3rd edition. *The Clinical Neuropsychologist*, 15(4), 440–445.

Mittenberg, W., Theroux-Fichera, S., Zielinski, R. E., & Heilbronner, R. L. (1995). Identification of malingered head injury on the Wechsler Adult Intelligence Scale-Revised. *Professional Psychology: Research and Practice*, 26, 491–498.

Nelson, H. E., & McKenna, P. (1975). The use of current reading ability in the assessment of dementia. *The British Journal of Social and Clinical Psychology*, 14(3), 259–267.

Niebuhr, B. R., & Marion, R. (1987). Detecting sincerity of effort when measuring grip strength. *American Journal of Physical Medicine*, 66(1), 16–24.

Nitch, S., Boone, K. B., Wen, J., Arnold, G., & Alfano, K. (2006). The utility of the Rey Word Recognition Test in the detection of suspect effort. *The Clinical Neuropsychologist*, 20(4), 873–887.

O'Bryant, S. E., Hilsabeck, R. C., Fisher, J. M., & McCaffrey, R. J. (2003). Utility of the trail making test in the assessment of malingering in a sample of mild traumatic brain injury litigants. *The Clinical Neuropsychologist*, 17(1), 69–74.

Olivegren, H., Jerkvall, N., Hagström, Y., & Carlsson, J. (1999). The long-term prognosis of whiplash-associated disorders. *European Spine Journal*, 8(5), 366–370.

Ord, J. S., Greve, K. W., Bianchini, K. J., & Aguerrevere, L. E. (2010). Executive dysfunction in traumatic brain injury: The effects of injury severity and effort on the Wisconsin Card Sorting Test. *Journal of Clinical and Experimental Neuropsychology*, 32(2), 132–140.

Orey, S. A., Cragar, D. E., & Berry, D. T. R. (2000). The effects of two motivational manipulations on the neuropsychological performance of mildly head-injured college students. *Archives of Clinical Neuropsychology*, 15(4), 335–348.

Pankratz, L. (1979). Symptom validity testing and symptom retraining: Procedures for the assessment and treatment of functional sensory deficits. *Journal of Consulting and Clinical Psychology*, 47(2), 409–410.

Pankratz, L., Binder, L. M., & Wilcox, L. (1987). Evaluation of an exaggerated somatosensory deficit with symptom validity testing. *Archives of Neurology*, 44(8), 798.

Pankratz, L., Fausti, A., & Peed, S. (1975). A forced-choice technique to evaluate deafness in the hysterical or malingering patient. *Journal of Consulting and Clinical Psychology*, 43(3), 421–422.

Peterson, D. I. (1998). A study of 249 patients with litigated claims of injury. *The Neurologist*, 4(3), 131–137.

Powell, M. R., Locke, D. E., Smigielski, J. S., & McCrea, M. (2011). Estimating the diagnostic value of the trail making test for suboptimal effort in acquired brain injury rehabilitation patients. *The Clinical Neuropsychologist*, 25(1), 108–118.

Rabin, L. A., Barr, W. B., & Burton, L. A. (2005). Assessment practices of clinical neuropsychologists in the United States and Canada: A survey of INS, NAN, and APA division 40 members. *Archives of Clinical Neuropsychology*, 20(1), 33–65.

Rapport, L. J., Farchione, T. J., Coleman, R. D., & Axelrod, B. N. (1998). Effects of coaching on malingered motor function profiles. *Journal of Clinical and Experimental Neuropsychology*, 20(1), 89–97.

Rawling, P. J., & Brooks, D. N. (1990). Simulation index: A method for detecting factitious errors on the WAIS-R and WMS. *Neuropsychology*, 4, 223–238.

Reitan, R. M. (1992). *Trail making test: Manual for administration and scoring.* South Tucson, AZ: Reitan Neuropsychology Laboratory.

Reitan, R. M., & Wolfson, D. (1985). *The Halstead-Reitan neuropsychological test battery: Theory and clinical interpretation.* Tucson, AZ: Neuropsychology Press.

Reitan, R. M., & Wolfson, D. (1993). *The Halstead-Reitan neuropsychological test battery: Theory and clinical applications* (2nd ed.). Tucson, AZ: Neuropsychological Press.

Reitan, R. M., & Wolfson, D. (2000). The neuropsychological similarities of mild and more severe head injury. *Archives of Clinical Neuropsychology*, 15(5), 433–442.

Rey, A. (1941). L'examen psychologique dans les cas d'encephalopathie traumatique. *Archives de Psychologie*, 28, 286–340.

Risse, G. L., Gates, J., Lund, G., Maxwell, R., & Rubens, A. (1989). Interhemispheric transfer in patients with incomplete section of the corpus callosum. Anatomic verification with magnetic resonance imaging. *Archives of Neurology*, 46(4), 437–443.

Roberts, M. A., Persinger, M. A., Grote, C., Evertowski, L. M., Springer, J. A., Tuten, T., . . . Baglio, C. S. (1994). The dichotic word listening test: Preliminary observations in American and Canadian samples. *Applied Neuropsychology*, 1(1–2), 45–56.

Rohling, M. L., Binder, L. M., Demakis, G. J., Larrabee, G. J., Ploetz, D. M., & Langhinrichsen-Rohling, J. (2011). A meta-analysis of neuropsychological outcome after mild traumatic brain injury: Re-analyses and reconsiderations of Binder et al. (1997), Frencham et al. (2005), and Pertab et al. (2009). *The Clinical Neuropsychologist*, 25(4), 608–623.

Rohling, M. L., & Boone, K. B. (2007). Future directions in effort assessment. In K. B. Boone (Ed.), *Assessment of feigned cognitive impairment: A neuropsychological perspective* (pp. 453–470). New York, NY: Guilford Press.

Rohling, M. L., Meyers, J. E., & Millis, S. R. (2003). Neuropsychological impairment following traumatic brain injury: A dose-response analysis. *The Clinical Neuropsychologist*, 17(3), 289–302.

Rose, F. E., Hall, S., & Szalda-Petree, A. D., & Bach, P. J. (1998). A comparison of four tests of malingering and the effects of coaching. *Archives of Clinical Neuropsychology*, 13(4), 349–363.

Ruddle, H. V., & Bradshaw, C. M. (1982). On the estimation of premorbid intellectual functioning: Validation of Nelson & McKenna's formula, and some new normative data. *The British Journal of Clinical Psychology*, 21(Pt. 3), 159–165.

Ruff, R. M., Light, R. H. & Evans, R. W. (1987). The Ruff figural fluency test: A normative study with adults. *Developmental Neuropsychology*, 3, 37–51.

Ruffolo, L. F., Guilmette, T. J., & Willis, W. J. (2000). Comparison of time and error rates on the trail making test among patients with head injuries, experimental malingerers, patients with suspected effort on testing, and normal controls. *The Clinical Neuropsychologist*, 14(2), 223–230.

Ruiz, M. A., Drake, E. B., Marcotte, D., Glass, A., & van Gorp, W. G. (2000, November). *Trying to beat the system: Misuse of the Internet to assist in avoiding the detection of neuropsychological symptom dissimulation.* Poster session presented at the Annual Conference of the National Academy of Neuropsychology, Orlando, FL.

Schretlen, D. J., & Shapiro, A. M. (2003). A quantitative review of the effects of traumatic brain injury on cognitive functioning. *International Review of Psychiatry*, 15(4), 341–349.

Silverberg, N. D., Hanks, R. A., Buchanan, L., Fichtenberg, N., & Millis, S. R. (2008). Detecting response bias with performance patterns on an expanded version of the controlled oral word association test. *The Clinical Neuropsychologist*, 22(1), 140–157.

Slick, D. J., Sherman, E. M. S., & Iverson, G. L. (1999). Diagnostic criteria for malingering neurocognitive dysfunction: Proposed standards for clinical practice and research. *The Clinical Neuropsychologist*, 13(4), 545–561.

Sollman, M. J., Ranseen, J. D., & Berry, D. T. R. (2010). Detection of feigned ADHD in college students. *Psychological Assessment*, 22(2), 325–335.

Spreen, O., & Strauss, E. (1991). *A Compendium of Neuropsychological Tests*. New York: Oxford University Press.

Strauss, E., Sherman, E. M., & Spreen, O. (2006). *A compendium of neuropsychological tests: Administration, norms and commentary* (3rd ed.). New York, NY: Oxford University Press.

Suhr, J. A., & Barrash, J. (2007). Performance on standard attention, memory, and psychomotor speed tasks as indicators of malingering. In G. J. Larrabee (Ed.), *Assessment of malingered neuropsychological deficits* (pp. 131–170). New York, NY: Oxford University Press.

Suhr, J. A., & Boyer, D. (1999). Uses of the Wisconsin Card Sorting Test in the detection of malingering in student simulator and patient samples. *Journal of Clinical and Experimental Neuropsychology*, 21(5), 701–708.

Suhr, J. A., & Gunstad, J. (2000). The effects of coaching on the sensitivity and specificity of malingering measures. *Archives of Clinical Neuropsychology*, 15(5), 415–424.

Suhr, J. A., & Gunstad, J. (2007). Coaching and malingering: A review. In G. J. Larrabee (Ed.), *Assessment of malingered neuropsychological deficits* (pp. 287–310). New York, NY: Oxford University Press.

Suhr, J., Tranel, D., Wefel, J., & Barrash, J. (1997). Memory performance after head injury: Contributions of malingering, litigation status, psychological factors, and medication use. *Journal of Clinical and Experimental Neuropsychology*, 19(4), 500–514.

Sweet, J. J., & Nelson, N. W. (2007). Validity indicators within executive function measures: Use and limits in the detection of malingering. In K. B. Boone (Ed.), *Assessment of feigned cognitive impairment: A neuropsychological perspective* (pp. 152–177). New York, NY: Guilford Press.

Tanner, B. A., Bowles, R. L., & Tanner, E. L. (2003). Detection of intentional sub-optimal performance on a computerized finger-tapping task. *Journal of Clinical Psychology*, 59(1), 123–131.

Taylor, T. (2011). *Sensitivity of finger agnosia as a measure of response bias*. Unpublished doctoral dissertation. Alliant International University.

Tenhula, W. N., & Sweet, J. J. (1996). Double cross-validation of the booklet category test in detecting malingered traumatic brain injury. *The Clinical Neuropsychologist*, 10(1), 104–116.

Thompson, L. L., & Cullum, C. M. (1991). Pattern of performance on neuropsychological tests in relation to effort in mild head injury patients. *Archives of Clinical Neuropsychology*, 6, 231.

Trueblood, W. (1994). Qualitative and quantitative characteristics of malingered and other invalid WAIS-R and clinical memory data. *Journal of Clinical and Experimental Neuropsychology*, 16(4), 597–607.

Trueblood, W., & Schmidt, M. (1993). Malingering and other validity considerations in the neuropsychological evaluation of mild head injury. *Journal of Clinical and Experimental Neuropsychology*, 15(4), 578–590.

Van Gorp, W. G., Humphrey, L. A., Kalechstein, A. L., Brumm, V. L., McMullen, W. J., Stoddard, M. A., & Pachana, N. A. (1999). How well do standard clinical neuropsychological tests identify malingering? A preliminary analysis. *Journal of Clinical and Experimental Neuropsychology*, 21(2), 245–250.

Vickery, C. D., Berry, D. T. R., Dearth, C. S., Vagnini, V. L., Baser, R. E., Crager, D. E., & Orey, S. A. (2004). Head injury and the ability to feign neuropsychological deficits. *Archives of Clinical Neuropsychology*, 19(1), 37–48.

Victor, T. L., Boone, K. B., Serpa, J. G., Buehler, J., & Ziegler, E. A. (2009). Interpreting the meaning of multiple symptom validity test failure. *The Clinical Neuropsychologist*, 23(2), 297–313.

Volbrecht, M., Meyers, J. E., & Kaster-Bundgaard, J. (2000). Neuropsychology outcome of head injury using a short battery. *Archives of Clinical Neuropsychology*, 15(3), 251–265.

Wechsler, D. A. (1981). *Wechsler Adult Intelligence Scale- Revised*. San Antonio, TX: The Psychological Corporation.

Wechsler, D. A. (1997). *Wechsler Adult Intelligence Scale: Administration and scoring manual* (3rd ed.). San Antonio, TX: The Psychological Corporation.

Wechsler, D. A. (2008). *Wechsler Adult Intelligence Scale: Administration and scoring manual* (4th ed.). San Antonio, TX: The Psychological Corporation.

Williamson, D. J. G., Green, P., Allen, L., & Rohling, M. L. (2003). Evaluating effort with the word memory test and category test—Or not: Inconsistencies in a compensation-seeking sample. *Journal of Forensic Neuropsychology*, 3(3), 19–44.

Wong, J. L., Lerner-Poppen, L., & Durham, J. (1998). Does warning reduce obvious malingering on memory and motor tasks in college samples? *International Journal of Rehabilitation and Health*, 4(3), 153.

Youngjohn, J. R., Burrows, L., & Erdal, K. (1995). Brain damage or compensation neurosis? The controversial post-concussion syndrome. *The Clinical Neuropsychologist*, 9(2), 112–123.

Functional Neuroanatomical Bases of Deceptive Behavior and Malingering

14

Jeffrey N. Browndyke

Deceptive behavior ranges from benign "white lies" to malicious lies or malingering. Benign untruthfulness is ubiquitous to all neurologically normal adolescents and adults and arguably holds redeeming value in the initiation and maintenance of interpersonal relations (e.g., "Don't worry about that haircut . . . you look great!"), as well as social cohesion. The general absence of benign untruthfulness can be observed in toddlers and individuals who are neurologically compromised, either from selective brain injury or genetic/developmental conditions where typical social cues and behavior are difficult (Abe et al., 2009; Stuss, Gallup, & Alexander, 2001; Winner, Brownell, Happé, Blum, & Pincus, 1998; Yang et al., 2005). In both the very young and neurologically compromised, the common denominator underlying the tendency toward socially awkward or painful truthfulness is an underdevelopment or impairment of prefrontal lobe function (Anderson, Bechara, Damasio, Tranel, & Damasio, 1999; Byrne & Corp, 2004; Stuss, et al., 2001).

Deceptive behavior can also hide, from oneself and others, those things that may be latent and psychologically painful. Jung and Wertheimer recognized more than 100 years ago that "hidden truth" may be amenable to investigation if one only measured response time differences associated with innocuous versus emotional stimuli of personal importance (Wertheimer, King, Peckler, Raney, & Schaef, 1992). These word association findings led to the appreciation that psychological "complexes" required higher order cognitive processing to maintain the self-deceptive repression of prepotent emotions or thoughts.

These seemingly disparate examples illustrate what has long been suspected—that the frontal lobes are critical to the production and maintenance of deceptive behavior, whether that behavior be benign, malicious, or hidden from consciousness. The "window into the mind" afforded by functional neuroimaging techniques and advanced neuromodulatory devices have largely confirmed this suspicion but often with surprising results.

FUNCTIONAL IMAGING STUDIES OF DECEPTION AND MALINGERING

Prior to the polygraph, the scientific measurement of deception was largely limited to behavioral observation of individuals under direct interrogation and guilt inferences drawn from reaction time response delays (Goldstein, 1923). Reaction time as a reliable index of deception detection began to fall into disfavor in the early 1930s, partly because of a rising appreciation of the measurable autonomic arousal associated with deceptive behavior. Undervalued as it may be then and now, reaction time measurement of deception has since experienced a resurgence with computerized cognitive testing (Schatz & Browndyke, 2002; Vendemia, Buzan, & Simon-Dack, 2005; Willison & Tombaugh, 2006), and almost to a lawful degree, more delayed reaction times during deception are the behavioral common denominator among all the deception studies discussed in this chapter. These subtle, but consistent, reaction time increases during deceptive cognitive performance may eventually lead to useful clinical practice applications, but they inform little about the neural substrates behind the deceptive behavior associated with the response delays (Browndyke et al., 2008). The same fundamental limitation can be said of polygraphic measurement of deception inferred from autonomic arousal, which is additionally known to be fraught with the problems of high false positive detection rates and susceptibility to simple countermeasures (Lykken, 1974).

The first scientifically satisfying peek into the internal cognitive processes governing deception was found in the application of event-related potential (ERP) techniques during the late 1980s (Farwell & Donchin, 1986; Rosenfeld, Nasman, Whalen, Cantwell, & Mazzeri, 1987). Rather than just rely on peripheral measurement of deception-related autonomic arousal, ERP affords direct measurement of electrophysiological characteristics and gross topographical location of information processing events associated with deceptive behavior. ERP components, such as the N400 (Boaz, Perry, Raney, Fischler, & Shuman, 1991), late positive parietal P300 (Farwell & Donchin, 1986; Farwell & Donchin, 1991; Mertens & Allen, 2008; Rosenfeld et al., 1987; Rosenfeld et al., 1998; Rosenfeld, Soskins, Bosh, & Ryan, 2004), and early medial frontal negativities (MFN; Johnson, Henkell, Simon, & Zhu, 2008) have all demonstrated with some degree of success the ability to distinguish deceptive from truthful responding and the suppression of concealed knowledge. But, it is the regional cortical distribution of these electrophysiological characteristics that provided the first in vivo clues of the functional neuroanatomy of deception. Late positive parietal P300 and N400 activity are posited to be associated with visual recognition of previously presented or personally salient stimuli, which should be present in a situation where an individual is actively trying to conceal his or her familiarity with specific crime-related materials (e.g., pictures of murder weapon or unique crime details; Rosenfeld et al., 1998) . Likewise, larger MFN components have been linked to increased need for response monitoring and inhibition during deceptive behavior attempts (Johnson et al., 2008). The relative spatial insensitivity of ERP and limitation of measurement to cortical activity renders these initial in vivo findings of deceptive mental processes intriguing but unsatisfying.

The functional neuroanatomical correlates of deception, as detected by functional magnetic resonance imaging (fMRI) techniques, were first reported by Spence et al. (2001) who were intent on capturing neural activity specific to deception, thereby addressing the persistent confounds of traditional polygraphy and simultaneously providing greater spatial resolution and localization data than what ERP can afford (Browndyke et al., 2008). Spence and colleagues discovered activation in ventrolateral, dorsomedial, and dorsolateral prefrontal cortices (VLPFC, DMPFC, and DLPFC, respectively), as well as the inferior parietal lobule (IPL), during deception, relative to normal responding for both auditory and visual stimuli. These regions have been commonly associated with deceptive responding in functional imaging studies that have followed, and appeared to reflect the generation and inhibition of responses, increased working memory load, metacognition of task performance, and monitoring of social cues necessary to deceive others (Abe, 2011; Abe et al., 2006;

Allen, Bigler, Larsen, Goodrich-Hunsaker, & Hopkins, 2007; Bles & Haynes, 2008; Browndyke et al., 2008; Johnson et al., 2008; Karim et al., 2010; Kozel et al., 2005; Kozel, Padgett, & George, 2004; Langleben et al., 2005; Langleben et al., 2002; Lee et al., 2005; Lee et al., 2002; Phan et al., 2005; Spence et al., 2001; Spence et al., 2004; Spence, Kaylor-Hughes, Farrow, & Wilkinson, 2008; Tian, Sharma, Kozel, & Liu, 2009; Wu, Allen, Goodrich-Hunsaker, Hopkins, & Bigler, 2010).

To date, most deception functional neuroimaging study results show consistencies in regional activation patterns with those also seen in paradigms assessing increased working memory load (Cohen et al., 1997). Bilateral inferior parietal/supramarginal gyrus and bifrontal middle frontal/DLPFC activity are robust to both deception and prototypical "N-back" working memory load fMRI studies (Christ, Van Essen, Watson, Brubaker, & McDermott, 2009). Whether some of these regional activity commonalities between deception and working memory load are primarily a by-product of the increased external or internal task demands of common deception task paradigms or both is unknown. It could be reasonably hypothesized that both the external and internal deception task demands would be salient factors in increasing working memory load. External demands provided by typical "lie/truth" control cues add a layer of task complexity to often simple recognition memory paradigms, whereas internal demands of deceptive behavior maintenance and the tracking of prior responses by individuals to gauge the magnitude of malingered/deceptive behavior almost certainly call on working memory function. Determining the contribution of the former is a simple matter of controlled examination of deceptive brain activity during graded levels of task demand, whereas the latter may require more refined experimental control to ferret out the contribution of behavioral maintenance. In either case, increased working memory load during deceptive behavior or malingering is the likely by-product, which in turn may help account for some of the consistent response time increases associated with deceptive responding (Abe, 2009; Browndyke et al., 2008; Kozel, Padgett, et al., 2004; Lee et al., 2009; Lee et al., 2002; Nuñez, Casey, Egner, Hare, & Hirsch, 2005; Spence et al., 2001).

Ito and colleagues (2011) hypothesized that the functional neuroanatomical correlates of deception for neutral and emotionally charged memories may differ. They reasoned that many deceptive situations in real life carry emotional valence secondary to associated aspects of risk and reward (e.g., deception over criminal acts). A fairly standard recognition memory deception fMRI task paradigm was constructed in which subjects were instructed to either respond truthfully or falsely to neutral and emotionally charged pictures. This paradigm yielded four conditions: (a) truthful and (b) untruthful responses of neutral pictures, and (c) truthful and (d) untruthful responses to emotionally charged stimuli. The main effect of deceptive responses on their pictorial recognition memory task yielded significant activity in regions common to other deception studies (i.e., bilateral supramarginal gyrus, supplementary motor area, and bilateral DLPFC), but activity in these regions did not vary as a function of the emotional valence of presented stimuli. The primary regions that Ito and colleagues found common to both neutral and emotional deceptive responding are commonly observed in fMRI task paradigms assessing for increased working memory load (Christ et al., 2009; Johnson et al., 2008; Larsen, Allen, Bigler, Goodrich-Hunsaker, & Hopkins, 2010). Not common to working memory load, however, were activations in the left ventrolateral, prefrontal, and orbitofrontal cortices, but again, there were no differences as a function of the emotional valence of presented stimuli. The Ito et al. study results suggest that in normal adults, deceptive behavior may be emotionally arousing regardless of stimulus content (possibly because of learned consequences associated with deception detection), but more research is necessary on this front, particularly in the combination of stimulus emotional valence and risk and reward as they apply to deception.

An important, but wholly underexamined, factor inherent to "real-world" malingering and deception is the neuroeconomics of deceptive behavior choices. In clinical and criminal justice settings, deceptive behavior is often motivated by the prospects of secondary gains and/or risk reduction. Prospective monetary reward combined with greed form the basis for most malingering behavior in medicolegal settings (Mittenberg, Patton, Canyock, & Condit, 2002), although there may be other more internal gains to be obtained in a smaller number of malingering cases (e.g., factitious disorders). The reward for deceptive behavior in a criminal justice setting may be monetary as well, but often it is the avoidance of criminal consequences associated with legal behavior (Ardolf, Denney, & Houston, 2007). Secondary gains, whether monetary or associated with consequence avoidance, are not without significant cost. In medicolegal or criminal justice situations, the risk of malingering or deception detection is associated with serious criminal consequences (e.g., fraud, incarceration). The neuroeconomics of risk and reward behavior provides some clues as to the brain regions and circuits that should be involved in an individual's weighing of the relative risk and reward associated with malingering and deception, but to date, direct research examination has not been performed. This is yet another area where our general understanding is lacking. It may be that the results from deception and malingering neuroimaging research have been insensitive to the detection of risk or reward circuitry regions because the motivating factors and risks associated with deception and malingering task paradigms, if present, are only hypothetical and often lack ecological validity. The Guilty Knowledge Test (GKT) is one such task (Langleben et al., 2005; Lykken, 1959).

Because it is typical of almost all fMRI paradigms to detect deceptive behavior (Abe et al., 2008; Kozel, Revell, et al., 2004; Langleben et al., 2002; Mohamed et al., 2006; Spence et al., 2001; Spence et al., 2004), cues under which subjects are to respond truthfully or falsely to presented stimuli are often preestablished. For instance, Ito et al. (2011) instructed subjects to make "old" and "new" recognition memory judgments, but to only respond truthfully when pictorial stimuli were copresented with a blue circle and falsely when presented with a red circle. The same sort of imposed decision demand is present in the GKT (Ganis, Kosslyn, Stose, Thompson, & Yurgelun-Todd, 2003; Langleben et al., 2002; Lykken, 1959) and other various deception paradigms (Kozel et al., 2005; Lee et al., 2005; Mohamed et al., 2006; Phan et al., 2005). This task demand is needed to maintain experimental control and to ensure that a requisite number of events are captured to allow for comparison of fMRI blood oxygen level-dependent (BOLD) signal by condition. However, the introduction of a decision cue transfers the deceptive behavior from personal control to that of the examiner and increases the likelihood that the functional neuroanatomical correlates of task complexity and working memory demands are comingled with those subserving basic deception.

To date, Browndyke et al. (2008) published the only fMRI study of deceptive behavior (more specifically, recognition memory malingering) to leave deceptive response decisions up to the whims of the individual subject. By selecting a simple visual recognition task with a high likelihood of task accuracy, confirmed during normal stimulus encoding and recognition trials, they reasoned that most errors during the malingered recognition trial were intentional. Inadvertently, true memory errors may have been present during the malingered condition, but these were hypothesized to only "dilute" the aggregate BOLD signal strength associated with most intentional memory errors. The experimental advantages of the typical high-control external decision cue (Ganis et al., 2003; Kozel et al., 2005; Langleben et al., 2002; Mohamed et al., 2006; Spence et al., 2004) over the low-control individual decision (Browndyke et al., 2008; Karton & Bachmann, 2011) approaches in deception/malingering task paradigm construction are in natural tension with the desirability for more ecological validity and in capturing brain activity associated with internally driven deception decisions versus those imposed by external task demands.

Meta-analysis of Regional Activation Commonalities in Memory Deception

Now that the broad regional commonalities and cognitive mechanisms generally associated with deception (and their limitations) have been reviewed, focus turns to the functional neuroanatomical correlates of deceptive behavior more akin to what is observed during clinical neuropsychological assessment—malingering of memory deficit.

The first fMRI study of malingered cognitive deficit was conducted by Lee et al. (2005), who discovered that feigned memory impairment on a simple forced-choice task was associated with increased activity in regions commonly associated with the working memory network, that is, bilateral prefrontal Brodmann area (BA) 9, 10, 46; premotor BA 6; parietal BA 7, 40; and anterior cingulate BA 23, 32 areas. But rather than present a literature review of the remaining handful of studies in this area (Abe et al., 2008; Abe, Suzuki, Mori, Itoh, & Fujii, 2007; Abe et al., 2006; Bhatt et al., 2009; Browndyke et al., 2008; Kozel et al., 2005; Kozel, Padgett, et al., 2004; Kozel, Revell, et al., 2004; Lee et al., 2009; Lee et al., 2005), presented here is an empirical examination of statistically significant regional activation commonalities among the aforementioned studies because they relate to the malingering of memory deficit. As a point of comparison, Figure 14.1 presents regional activation commonalities associated with nonpurposeful memory errors (for methods, see Appendix 14.1 at the end of this chapter). Figure 14.1 illustrates the statistically significant regional activation commonalities associated with deceptive memory performance and those common to unintentional memory errors.

It can be observed from the results in Figure 14.1 that feigned memory impairment is consistently associated with large regions of common activity in the right inferior frontal gyrus (4,664 mm^3) and the middle frontal gyrus (1,624 mm^3). These prefrontal lobe activation commonalities were much larger than other significant clusters, with the next largest cluster residing in the superior temporal gyrus region. Activity in the right inferior frontal gyrus has been implicated in several variations of response inhibition (Chikazoe, Konishi, Asari, Jimura, & Miyashita, 2007), and as reviewed earlier, response inhibition processes are consistently implicated as central to deception, particularly if the assumption holds that the tendency toward truthfulness is prepotent (Abe 2011; Spence et al., 2001). The prominent common middle frontal activity during memory performance deception is consistent with prior deception studies (not included in these analyses) and has tantalizingly been associated with confabulatory behavior and pathological lying (Harada et al., 2009; Turner, Cipolotti, Yousry, & Shallice, 2008; Yang et al., 2007; Zannino, Barban, Caltagirone, & Carlesimo, 2008). Additional common regional activity in the anterior medial temporal lobe, particularly the uncus/amygdalar region, and superior parietal cortex (BA 7) may be related to the medial temporal lobe memory function, emotional valence associated with conscious deception, and/or self-referential processing (Abe et al., 2007). As a point of comparison, there were no regions common to both conscious memory performance deception and unintentional errors (see Figure 14.1). The largest common regions associated with nonpurposeful memory errors were

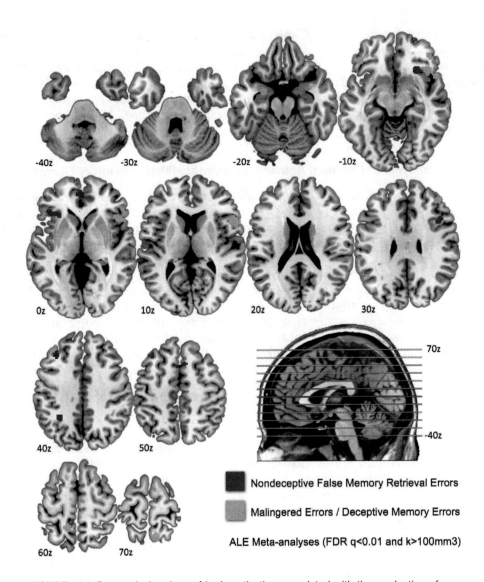

FIGURE 14.1 Prototypical regions of brain activation associated with the production of purposefully deceptive and unintentional false responses (see chapter Appendix 14.1 for methods & results). ALE = activation likelihood estimation; FDR = false discovery rate.

found in the left anterior cingulate (520 mm^3, BA 32), right medial frontal gyrus (872 mm^3, BA 6), and bilaterally in the claustrum.

The multiple significant activation cluster commonalities highlighted in memory deception and unintentional memory error studies, although regionally adjacent, show little direct overlap and emphasize the complexity of latent processes that seem to have qualitative behavioral similarity in clinical practice. In addition, although both study types involve memory processing, it appears from these meta-analytic results that activity in the mesial temporal lobe is neither reliable nor significant enough across studies to differentiate purposeful from unintentional memory errors. Although the deceptive memory meta-analysis yielded one significant cluster in the uncus/amygdalar region (see chapter Appendix 14.1, which includes Tables 14.1 and 14.2), this activity may be more reasonably tied to the emotional valence or potential negative consequences associated with conscious deception.

Functional Neuroanatomical Correlates of Symptom Validity Test Performance

What do common symptom validity test (SVT) procedures that rely on forced-choice recognition memory actually measure in terms of brain function? One would assume that these SVTs routinely rely on mesial temporal lobe function to allow for the proper discrimination of novel foil and familiar target stimuli, but as was seen in the memory deception meta-analysis results earlier, this is not the case (at least in individuals who are cognitively normal).

Allen and colleagues (2007) have conducted the only studies to date that directly address this SVT/memory function conundrum (Allen et al., 2007; Wu et al., 2010). In their assessment of the functional neuroanatomical correlates of the Word Memory Test (WMT; Green, 2003), Allen et al. found that delayed recognition on the WMT relative to a low-effort motor condition was associated with brain activity in the now familiar regions involved in working memory processing (i.e., bifrontal/biparietal and supplementary motor area activity). This finding of predominant working memory network activation during WMT delayed recognition performance is counter to the notion that this SVT or others relying on similar forced-choice recognition memory, such as the Test of Memory Malingering (TOMM; Tombaugh, 1996), are essentially "effortless." In addition, the general lack of mesial temporal lobe activity during WMT delayed recognition memory performance highlights that, although this sort of forced-choice recognition memory procedure is by definition a declarative memory task, it is not likely to be an index of memory capacity in healthy adults.

A subsequent study by Allen's group (Wu et al., 2010) reinforced the likelihood that the brain activity necessary for proper SVT performance differs between individuals with normal cognition and individuals with brain injury. Working memory network activity was once again predominant during WMT delayed recognition performance in both normal control and traumatic brain injury (TBI) cases, but additional mesial temporal lobe activity was only observed in two moderate-to-severe TBI cases, one of whom had predominant temporal lobe sclerosis. The preliminary results carried out to date highlight the importance of working memory network engagement for proper SVT performance, disabusing the notion that effort tests are essentially "effortless" and that the cognitive processes necessary for proper SVT performance are likely to vary as a function of brain pathology or patient type. To this latter point, only SVT-associated brain activity in healthy controls and patients with TBI has been directly investigated, but these initial differences hint that the use of SVT "cut scores" across groups may need reconsideration.

Detection of Deception

Collateral, but no less important, to the neural mechanisms of lie generation and malingering behavior are those governing the detection of deception. What brain regions are involved in our perception of deceptive behavior? Problems with deception detection have been reported in individuals with right hemispheric damage, particularly in attempts to distinguish lies from jokes (Winner et al., 1998), but the lesion location varied widely in the study. Supporting evidence pointing toward the importance of the right hemisphere in deception detection was reported by Etcoff, Ekman, Magee, and Frank (2000), who found that deception detection was superior in patients with aphasia and left middle cerebral artery infarct relative to controls. The findings of Stuss et al. (2001), based on careful lesion location observation, further reinforce the importance of the right hemisphere in deception detection. Stuss and colleagues described more deception detection problems in patients with lesions in the right orbitofrontal region, although some of the patients in question had bilateral orbitofrontal damage.

Grèzes, Frith, and Passingham (2004) were the first to address the question in vivo by measuring fMRI activity associated with the observation of nonverbal deception cues. In their study, the perception of deceptive behavior cues was associated with increased activity in the amygdalae and rostral anterior cingulate. A subsequent study by Grèzes, Berthoz, and Passingham (2006) found that the amygdalae were also active when observers realized that they were the target of deceitful behavior. Lissek and colleagues (2008) demonstrated that the orbitofrontal and medial prefrontal regions are active when individuals are asked to gauge the deceptive intentions of protagonists in controlled scenarios. The functional neural correlates of the perceived morality of deceptive behavior was addressed by Harada and colleagues (2009) who showed that fMRI activity in the left temporoparietal junction is associated with detected deception of antisocial purpose versus deception considered to be of neutral or prosocial intent. General activity associated with the moral judgment of other's behavior was also reported by Harada et al. to be in the medial prefrontal and lateral orbitofrontal cortices, as well as the caudate nucleus and right cerebellum.

The neural correlates of deception detection cannot be adequately captured in these four functional neuroimaging studies existent to date, but it certainly can be inferred from the available data and results from loss-of-function studies (Etcoff et al., 2000; Stuss et al., 2001; Winner et al., 1998) that limbic and higher order prefrontal regions (i.e., medial and orbitofrontal cortices) are involved in the social perception, intention, and appraisal of deceptive behavior.

"Virtual Lesion" Studies of Deception

As with all functional neuroimaging studies of cognition and behavior, the brain regions revealed as potentially significant to deception may not be necessary for deceptive behavior generation or maintenance. Only correlation, not causality, is revealed by traditional functional neuroimaging techniques, that is, fMRI and near-infrared spectroscopy (NIRS); magnetoencephalography (MEG); and positron emission tomography (PET). Model case reports of selective brain damage or disease states, as well as loss-of-function studies using recent direct current stimulation technologies, for example, transcranial direct current stimulation (tDCS) and repetitive transcranial magnetic stimulation (rTMS), bring the neural causality of deceptive behavior and deception detection into better view.

Focused electromagnetic brain stimulation technologies, such as tDCS and rTMS, provide a unique opportunity to examine the causal relations governing deception by observing the behavioral consequences of "virtual lesions/ablation" (Abe, 2009). Of the few deception studies that have employed these methods, results have been surprising and carry wider societal implications that will be addressed later in this chapter. The most significant of the reversible lesion models of deception was conducted by Karim et al. (2010), who recently discovered that tDCS-mediated suppression of anterior prefrontal cortex (aPFC, BA region 10) excitability did not impair deception abilities but actually improved them. This improvement in deceptive behavior was not only manifested in quicker reaction times while lying but also in decreased sympathetic physiological response and lowered self-reported feelings of guilt when subjects were actively deceiving the study investigators. The Karim et al. results reinforce the findings of numerous fMRI studies that the aPFC (BA 10) is a region integral to deception behavior (but certainly not the only region involved in deceptive behavior). As with the true lesion studies of Stuss and colleagues (2001), there is a moderate weight of evidence to suggest that somatic marker (Damasio, 1996) and moral conflict aspects of deception are contributors to the greater aPFC activation seen in fMRI deception studies. By damaging or "turning off" portions of this region, moral conflict or valuation may be minimized, which in turn facilitates deceptive responding and makes it harder to detect by both reaction time and physiological means. Elegantly, Karim et al. reinforced the likelihood that their aPFC suppression results were specific to the reduction of moral conflict by demonstrating that suppression in the same region had no effect on Stroop inhibition trial performance, indicating that the tDCS results were not simply a function of general executive functioning or prepotent (truth) response inhibition.

Priori et al. (2008) applied tDCS to the bilateral DLPFC (BA regions 9 & 46) and then asked the subjects to engage in truthful or deceptive responding for the memory of previously presented pictures. Rather than simply examining the main difference between truth and deception, the investigators examined the influence of tDCS cortical excitability in the DLPFC on deception for different memory response types (i.e., deceptive errors of omission [intentional hit misses] and deceptive errors of commission [intentional false alarm errors]). They found that tDCS application in the DLPFC had no effect on reaction times for intentional false alarms but significantly lengthened the response times for deceptive omission errors. Although the magnitude of the response time increase for these intentional omission errors was relatively small (approximately 180 ms longer than when unaffected by tDCS), the results do provide clues that brain activity associated with deceptive responding, particularly for memorized or to-be-learned information, varies as a function of the deceptive response type (i.e., deceptive foil endorsement or target denial). This "temporary lesion/enhancement" finding of deceptive memory response differences is reinforced by similar conclusions from the fMRI studies of Abe et al. (2008) and Browndyke et al. (2008) and has applicability to neuropsychological practice where most SVTs rely on the detection of deceptively false recognition memory responses. In addition, contrary to the Karim et al. (2010) approach of tDCS-mediated cortical inhibition, Priori and colleagues were interested to see what the effect of excitability would have on deceptive behavior. The two tDCS study results, however, are complimentary to the notion that PFC engagement in general is integral to deceptive behavior and suggest that the magnitude of aPFC and DLPFC activity during deception is inversely associated with deceptive success and associated behavioral and physiological indicators of deception.

The few studies that have employed rTMS to investigate deception have found similarly interesting, but often contradictory, results to the Karim et al. (2010) and Priori et al. (2008) tDCS studies. Unlike tDCS, which may generally have inhibitory (i.e., cathodal tDCS) or excitatory (i.e., anodal tDCS) action on the cortex, rTMS is more focally disruptive and has greater temporal resolution to tDCS. For instance, a single rTMS pulse to the occipital cortex 80–100 ms after visual stimulus presentation has the capacity to completely mask an individual's perception of the stimulus, essentially producing temporary and reversible cortical blindness. Using this more refined and stronger "virtual lesion" technique (which incidentally is not without risk of seizure), Luber, Fisher, Appelbaum, Ploesser, and Lisanby (2009) discovered that single rTMS pulse in the posterior midline/precuneus region 240 ms after the presentation of GKT (Lykken, 1959) stimuli resulted in significantly slower response times during deception relative to truthful responding. But, similar rTMS pulse presentations in the right and left DLPFC had no effect on lie or truth response times. The authors attributed the surprising lack of rTMS response in the DLPFC to the relative task ease of their variation on the GKT. Although not a wholly satisfying explanation for the DLPFC noneffect, the results suggesting that temporary disruption of the parietal cortex may affect deceptive success highlights the possible contribution of self-referential thinking in deception decisions and/or posterior working memory processes critical to the speed of deceptive responses. The optimal 240 ms stimulus onset asynchrony (SOA) delay for rTMS application by Luber et al. suggests that disruption of posterior working memory regions is a more likely explanation of their deception response slowing results.

Karton and Bachmann (2011), in the only other study to date that has used rTMS to manipulate deceptive behavior, found that the application of 5–10 min of 1 Hz stimulation to the left or right DLPFC had a measurable effect on deceptive response tendency relative to control stimulation in the posterior cortex. Dissociation between left and right DLPFC stimulation was noted, such that rTMS inhibition of the left DLPFC resulted in a significant increase in deceptive responses, whereas deception decreased after right DLPFC inhibition. The working memory demands of the Karton and Bachmann study were minimal (i.e., lie or truth responses to simple red or blue colored circle stimuli), and participants were unprompted and free to choose when to engage in deception or truthfulness. The simple application of rTMS to either the left or right DLPFC essentially exerted a general tendency toward one behavioral choice or the other. The laterality effects found by Karton and Bachmann suggest that a right DLPFC unfettered by dominant left control (i.e., left DLPFC rTMS inhibition) may be critical to deceptive tendency, whereas inhibition of the aPFC, as demonstrated via tDCS by Karim et al. (2010), may be important to deceptive success.

Lie Detection Using Advanced Techniques

At present, the right to privacy ceases with a judicial warrant. Courts can order your car or house searched and exposure of your sensitive computer files and documents. Privacy limitations even extend to one's own body. Blood tests, DNA samples, and drug screens are all commonplace in criminal processing and judicial proceedings. By extension of the logic behind these legal bodily searches, there are no current legal limitations on a court's ability to also order an individual to submit to a brain scan in the near future.

The Cephos Corporation (Pepperell, MA; http://www.cephoscorp.com), a privately held firm specifically licensed to perform brain-based lie detection and holder of current and pending patents, makes the following claim regarding the use of fMRI for the purpose of lie detection, " . . . it provides a means of detecting deception which cannot be circumvented by trained, skillful, or remorseless liars" (Kozel, 2011). This claim may eventually prove to be so, but evidence on differentiating lies from truth outside of controlled experimental paradigms is wholly lacking, and the resilience of fMRI lie detection to countermeasures is presently counterfactual to the claims earlier (Ganis, Rosenfeld, Meixner, Kievit, & Schendan, 2011). For instance, subtle movements of the head could significantly interfere with fMRI data acquisition or examined individuals could intentionally "jitter" their response types and times to create statistical uncertainty, obscuring any differences between lie and truth responses. In addition, scientific evidence supporting the detection of deceptive behavior or malingering in nonnormal controls is exceedingly sparse (Wu et al., 2010). The respected cognitive neuroscientist Michael Gazzaniga cogently argues that these and other considerations render brain scanning technology "not ready for prime time" for the purpose of deception detection and other criminal/legal applications (Carey, 2011).

Despite glaring limitations and warnings, the search for a better fMRI lie detection mouse trap" continues. Recent evidence suggests that the application of advanced data signal processing methods to fMRI data may hold promise in reasonably accurate lie versus truth discrimination (Davatzikos et al., 2005; Jin et al., 2009). However, the high dimensionality of traditional fMRI data makes it generally unsuitable for direct use in standard dimension reduction and feature selection signal processing algorithms. Jin et al. (2009) reported that standard entry of traditional 3 mm^3 isotropic voxels from deception fMRI paradigm data into partial least squares (PLS) or random frequency (RF) data reduction methods results in impractical glacial processing times and generally poor truth versus lie classification (< 60% accuracy). Their preliminary examination of support vector machine (SVM) data reduction for deception classification purposes was similarly poor, with an accuracy of 55.2%. This, then, led the researchers to apply various feature detection methods and determine the optimal number of feature sets shared by all (i.e., ensemble feature detection) that then provided the best SVM discrimination results.

Although values are not explicitly stated in the Jin et al. (2009) article, a graph of their combined feature selection and data reduction technique output suggests that deception detection accuracy was approximately 83%, with a sensitivity of 85%, specificity of 81%, and positive predictive value (PPV) of 83%. Their results clearly suggest that the combination of feature selection and data reduction techniques is superior to either alone. When the features in their fMRI data that yielded these optimal discrimination values were mapped back to a representative brain atlas space, the regions with the largest concentration of contributing voxels to the truth versus lie discrimination were in the bilateral supplementary motor area (SMA; BA 6 & 8), left opercular region (BA 48), and right putamen. The finding of SMA activity being discriminative of deception relative to truth conditions also shows up consistently in more traditional approaches to fMRI data analysis (Bles & Haynes, 2008; Browndyke et al., 2008; Kozel, Revell, et al., 2004).

On the contrary, Davatzikos et al. (2005) was more successful in generating SVM-based classification accuracy of deception versus truth conditions by focusing only on activation patterns in their data that were difficult by other means to distinguish between truth and lie conditions. A data-training approach to establish the fMRI pattern most discriminative of truth versus lie resulted in a 99.3% separation and a classification accuracy equal to 87.9% (90% sensitivity, 85.8% specificity). But, these impressive results are based on group aggregates of discriminative patterns. When Davatzikos et al. applied the SVM classification methods to individual subject responses via leave-one-subject-out cross validation, the average classification performance remained the same (i.e., 88.6% with 90.9% sensitivity and 86.4% specificity).

As demonstrated, these advanced signal processing methods certainly hold promise and have classification accuracy near the upper range of that stated for traditional polygraph methods (i.e., 65%–95%; Stern, 2004). However, a few glaring practical limitations exist that call into question the feasibility of a fMRI deception detection "mouse trap", the most notable of which is the reliance of these signal processing methods on training data and their specificity to the fMRI task paradigm that contributed to the data. It is one thing to be highly accurate in discriminating between truth and lie conditions in a contrived laboratory scenario but quite another to argue that the discriminating fMRI data pattern is valid for the myriad of possible criminal/real-world scenarios. Davatzikos et al. (2005) admitted as much by stating in their article, "The main conclusion from this study is not that a universal classifier can be built that detects truthful from nontruthful responses, but rather that sophisticated classification methods can be trained . . . to identify certain patterns of brain activity" (p. 667). With this, we can see that the practical application of a fMRI lie detector (using pattern classification methods) is limited largely by a general lack of normative brain pattern data for all the possible scenarios where deception may be a factor. The ecological validity for these advanced methods in practical lie detection for criminal or medicolegal use is charitably unknown, if not nonexistent, regardless of any optimistic claims to the contrary. As a result, fMRI "lie detection" in its current form is not likely to survive a rigorous *Daubert* challenge for scientific admissibility (Klein, 1994; Mossman, 2003).

CONCLUSION

It is clear from the weight of evidence that deception and malingering behavior requires additional engagement of prefrontal brain regions relative to those required for truthful or adequate task effort. Apart from executive control regions shared as a function of increased working memory load, task switching, and inhibitory control demanded by deceptive responding, activity in the VLPFC and temporoparietal junction appear to be distinct to deceptive behavioral responses. Hemispheric differences between the right and left prefrontal cortex (PFC) regions appear to play a part in deception success and intent with the relative importance of the right PFC being implicated in the rTMS and tDCS "virtual lesion," as well as traditional loss-of-function studies. From the available evidence, the detection of deceptive intent is dependent on limbic and orbitofrontal engagement. However, the relative contributions of these areas to deceptive behavior and its detection are still a mystery waiting for further investigation. It is also clear that the functional neuroanatomical underpinnings of deceptive behavior and malingering share many common regions, most notably those involved in the increased executive demands associated with deception. Although, activity unique to SVT performance and inadequate cognitive effort is even more open to debate.

To date, there have only been a handful of studies to even address the functional substrates specific to the malingering of cognitive deficits (Allen et al., 2007; Browndyke et al., 2008; Larsen et al., 2010; Lee et al., 2005; Mak & Lee, 2006), and only one study has examined SVT performance in sample patients who are impaired (Wu et al., 2010). The cognitive neuroscience of malingering is still in its infancy. There are fundamental questions yet to be addressed (e.g., "How does malingering behavior manifest itself in patients with documented brain damage?") and practical considerations to be vaulted (e.g., fMRI task construction/presentation limitations, ecologically valid approximations of actual test-taking behavior) before we gain a more comprehensive understanding of the neuroanatomical underpinnings of malingering behavior.

Advanced neuroimaging and current stimulation technologies have provided the ability to not only delve into the fundamental processes governing deception and malingering, but also the ability to manipulate deceptive behavior and elucidate previous intangibles, such as morality. The application of advanced brain scanning technology in the legal and criminal justice fields will, as Michael Gazzaniga warns, "begin to influence how the public views justice and responsibility" (Carey, 2011). For instance, how will the resolution of individuals' inner thoughts to external examination intersect with their Fifth Amendment right to avoid self-incrimination or Fourth Amendment protection from unreasonable search and seizure? It is incumbent on those choosing these avenues of investigation to heed the promethean warnings of Shelley (1818) and consider any potential adverse societal consequences of latent "deception intent" detection and deception control technologies—as implied by the results of recent fMRI "lie detection" algorithms and tDCS/rTMS loss-of-function deception studies.

To maintain a balance among the drive for knowledge, legal/business interests, and potential social consequences, investigations into the cognitive neuroscience of deceptive behavior and malingering should include the input of legal scholars and bioethicists at the investigator and institutional review board levels. In this brave new world of latent intent detection and potential cognitive control, the "cognitive liberty" of individuals must be considered (Wolpe, Foster, & Langleben, 2005). Once the proverbial lid of the box has been opened (which arguably has happened), we are only left with the hope that positive societal consequences will buffet against the demons of humankind's lesser nature.

ACKNOWLEDGMENTS

The author would like to acknowledge Katherine Rief, BS (The Advisory Board Co., Washington, DC) for her contributions to the deception and false memory activation likelihood estimation (ALE) meta-analyses discussed in this chapter; the methods and results of which are detailed in the chapter Appendix. No conflicts of interest are claimed by either the chapter author or acknowledged contributors.

REFERENCES

Abe, N. (2009). The neurobiology of deception: Evidence from neuroimaging and loss-of-function studies. *Current Opinion in Neurology*, 22(6), 594–600.

Abe, N. (2011). How the brain shapes deception: An integrated review of the literature. *The Neuroscientist*, 17(5), 560–574.

Abe, N., Fujii, T., Hirayama, K., Takeda, A., Hosokai, Y., Ishioka, T., . . . Mori, E. (2009). Do parkinsonian patients have trouble telling lies? The neurobiological basis of deceptive behaviour. *Brain*, 132(Pt. 5), 1386–1395.

Abe, N., Okuda, J., Suzuki, M., Sasaki, H., Matsuda, T., Mori, E., . . . Fujii, T. (2008). Neural correlates of true memory, false memory, and deception. *Cerebral Cortex*, 18(12), 2811–2819.

Abe, N., Suzuki, M., Mori, E., Itoh, M., & Fujii, T. (2007). Deceiving others: Distinct neural responses of the prefrontal cortex and amygdala in simple fabrication and deception with social interactions. *Journal of Cognitive Neuroscience*, 19(2), 287–295.

Abe, N., Suzuki, M., Tsukiura, T., Mori, E., Yamaguchi, K., Itoh, M., & Fujii, T. (2006). Dissociable roles of prefrontal and anterior cingulate cortices in deception. *Cerebral Cortex*, 16(2), 192–199.

Abel, S., Dressel, K., Kümmerer, D., Saur, D., Mader, I., Weiller, C., & Huber, W. (2009). Correct and erroneous picture naming responses in healthy subjects. *Neuroscience Letters*, 463(3), 167–171.

Allen, M. D., Bigler, E. D., Larsen, J., Goodrich-Hunsaker, N. J., & Hopkins, R. O. (2007). Functional neuroimaging evidence for high cognitive effort on the Word Memory Test in the absence of external incentives. *Brain Injury*, 21(13–14), 1425–1428.

Anderson, S. W., Bechara, A., Damasio, H., Tranel, D., & Damasio, A. R. (1999). Impairment of social and moral behavior related to early damage in human prefrontal cortex. *Nature: Neuroscience*, 2(11), 1032–1037.

Ardolf, B. R., Denney, R. L., & Houston, C. M. (2007). Base rates of negative response bias and malingered neurocognitive dysfunction among criminal defendants referred for neuropsychological evaluation. *The Clinical Neuropsychologist*, 21(6), 899–916.

Benjamini, Y., & Hochberg, Y. (1995). Controlling the false discovery rate: A practical and powerful approach to multiple testing. *Journal of the Royal Statistical Society*, 57(1), 289–300.

Bhatt, S., Mbwana, J., Adeyemo, A., Sawyer, A., Hailu, A., & Vanmeter, J. (2009). Lying about facial recognition: An fMRI study. *Brain and Cognition*, 69(2), 382–390.

Bles, M., & Haynes, J. D. (2008). Detecting concealed information using brain-imaging technology. *Neurocase*, 14(1), 82–92.

Boaz, T. L., Perry, N. W., Raney, G., Fischler, I. S., & Shuman, D. (1991). Detection of guilty knowledge with event-related potentials. *Journal of Applied Psychology, 76*(6), 788–795.

Browndyke, J. N., Paskavitz, J., Sweet, L. H., Cohen, R. A., Tucker, K. A., Welsh-Bohmer, K. A., . . . Schmechel, D. E. (2008). Neuroanatomical correlates of malingered memory impairment: Event-related fMRI of deception on a recognition memory task. *Brain Injury, 22*(6), 481–489.

Byrne, R. W., & Corp, N. (2004). Neocortex size predicts deception rate in primates. *Proceedings of the Royal Society: Biological Sciences, 271*(1549), 1693–1699.

Carey, B. (2011, November 1). Decoding the brain's cacophony. *The New York Times.* Retrieved from http://www.nytimes.com/2011/11/01/science/telling-the-story-of-the-brains-cacophony-of-competing-voices.html

Chikazoe, J., Konishi, S., Asari, T., Jimura, K., & Miyashita, Y. (2007). Activation of right inferior frontal gyrus during response inhibition across response modalities. *Journal of Cognitive Neuroscience, 19*(1), 69–80.

Christ, S. E., Van Essen, D. C., Watson, J. M., Brubaker, L. E., & McDermott, K. B. (2009). The contributions of prefrontal cortex and executive control to deception: Evidence from activation likelihood estimate meta-analyses. *Cerebral Cortex, 19*(7), 1557–1566.

Cohen, J. D., Perlstein, W. M., Braver, T. S., Nystrom, L. E., Noll, D. C., Jonides, J., & Smith, E. E. (1997). Temporal dynamics of brain activation during a working memory task. *Nature, 386*(6625), 604–608.

Damasio, A. R. (1996). The somatic marker hypothesis and the possible functions of the prefrontal cortex. *Philosophical Transactions of the Royal Society of London: Biological Sciences, 351*(1346), 1413–1420.

Davatzikos, C., Ruparel, K., Fan, Y., Shen, D. G., Acharyya, M., Loughead, J. W., . . . Langleben, D. D. (2005). Classifying spatial patterns of brain activity with machine learning methods: Application to lie detection. *Neuroimage, 28*(3), 663–668.

Dennis, N. A., Kim, H., & Cabeza, R. (2008). Age-related differences in brain activity during true and false memory retrieval. *Journal of Cognitive Neuroscience, 20*(8), 1390–1402.

Eickhoff, S. B., Laird, A. R., Grefkes, C., Wang, L. E., Zilles, K., & Fox, P. T. (2009). Coordinate-based activation likelihood estimation meta-analysis of neuroimaging data: A random-effects approach based on empirical estimates of spatial uncertainty. *Human Brain Mapping, 30*(9), 2907–2926.

Etcoff, N. L., Ekman, P., Magee, J. J., & Frank, M. G. (2000). Lie detection and language comprehension. *Nature, 405*(6783), 139.

Farwell, L. A., & Donchin, E. (1986). The "brain detector." P300 in the detection of deception? *Psychophysiology, 24,* 434.

Farwell, L. A., & Donchin, E. (1991). The truth will out: Interrogative polygraphy ("lie detection") with event-related brain potentials. *Psychophysiology, 28*(5), 531–547.

Ganis, G., Kosslyn, S. M., Stose, S., Thompson, W. L., & Yurgelun-Todd, D. A. (2003). Neural correlates of different types of deception: An fMRI investigation. *Cerebral Cortex, 13*(8), 830–836.

Ganis, G., Rosenfeld, J. P., Meixner, J., Kievit, R. A., & Schendan, H. E. (2011). Lying in the scanner: Covert countermeasures disrupt deception detection by functional magnetic resonance imaging. *Neuroimage, 55*(1), 312–319.

Genovese, C. R., Lazar, N. A., & Nichols, T. (2002). Thresholding of statistical maps in functional neuroimaging using the false discovery rate. *Neuroimage, 15*(4), 870–878.

Goldstein, E. R. (1923). Reaction times and the consciousness of deception. *American Journal of Psychology, 34,* 562–581.

Green, P. (2003). *Green's word memory test for Windows: User's manual.* Edmonton, Canada: Green's.

Grèzes, J., Berthoz, S., & Passingham, R. E. (2006). Amygdala activation when one is the target of deceit: Did he lie to you or to someone else? *Neuroimage, 30*(2), 601–608.

Grèzes, J., Frith, C., & Passingham, R. E. (2004). Brain mechanisms for inferring deceit in the actions of others. *Journal of Neuroscience, 24*(24), 5500–5505.

Harada, T., Itakura, S., Xu, F., Lee, K., Nakashita, S., Saito, D. N., & Sadato, N. (2009). Neural correlates of the judgment of lying: A functional magnetic resonance imaging study. *Neuroscience Research, 63*(1), 24–34.

Heun, R., Jessen, F., Klose, U., Erb, M., Granath, D. O., & Grodd, W. (2004). Response-related fMRI of veridical and false recognition of words. *European Psychiatry, 19*(1), 42–52.

Ito, A., Abe, N., Fujii, T., Ueno, A., Koseki, Y., Hashimoto, R., . . . Mori, E. (2011). The role of the dorsolateral prefrontal cortex in deception when remembering neutral and emotional events. *Neuroscience Research, 69*(2), 121–128.

Jin, B., Strasburger, A., Laken, S. J., Kozel, F. A., Johnson, K. A., George, M. S., & Lu, X. (2009). Feature selection for fMRI-based deception detection. *BMC Bioinformatics, 10*(Suppl. 9), S15.

Johnson, R. Jr., Henkell, H., Simon, E., & Zhu, J. (2008). The self in conflict: The role of executive processes during truthful and deceptive responses about attitudes. *Neuroimage, 39*(1), 469–482.

Karim, A. A., Schneider, M., Lotze, M., Veit, R., Sauseng, P., Braun, C., & Birbaumer, N. (2010). The truth about lying: Inhibition of the anterior prefrontal cortex improves deceptive behavior. *Cerebral Cortex, 20*(1), 205–213.

Karton, I., & Bachmann, T. (2011). Effect of prefrontal transcranial magnetic stimulation on spontaneous truth-telling. *Behavioral Brain Research*, 225(1), 209–214.

Kim, H., & Cabeza, R. (2007). Trusting our memories: Dissociating the neural correlates of confidence in veridical versus illusory memories. *Journal of Neuroscience*, 27(45), 12190–12197.

Klein, R. D. (1994). Daubert v Merrell Dow: Scientific evidence in the courtroom. *Journal of the American Medical Association*, 271(20), 1578.

Kozel, F. A. (2011). *U.S. Patent No. 7,899,524*. Southlake, TX: U.S. Patent and Trademark Office.

Kozel, F. A., Johnson, K. A., Mu, Q., Grenesko, E. L., Laken, S. J., & George, M. S. (2005). Detecting deception using functional magnetic resonance imaging. *Biological Psychiatry*, 58(8), 605–613.

Kozel, F. A., Padgett, T. M., & George, M. S. (2004). A replication study of the neural correlates of deception. *Behavioral Neuroscience*, 118(4), 852–856.

Kozel, F. A., Revell, L. J., Lorberbaum, J. P., Shastri, A., Elhai, J. D., Horner, M. D., . . . George, M. S. (2004). A pilot study of functional magnetic resonance imaging brain correlates of deception in healthy young men. *Journal of Neuropsychiatry and Clinical Neuroscience*, 16(3), 295–305.

Laird, A. R., Fox, P. M., Price, C. J., Glahn, D. C., Uecker, A. M., Lancaster, J. L., . . . Fox, P. T. (2005). ALE meta-analysis: Controlling the false discovery rate and performing statistical contrasts. *Human Brain Mapping*, 25(1), 155–164.

Lancaster, J. L., Tordesillas-Gutiérrez, D., Martinez, M., Salinas, F., Evans, A., Zilles, K., . . . Fox, P. T. (2007). Bias between MNI and Talairach coordinates analyzed using the ICBM-152 brain template. *Human Brain Mapping*, 28(11), 1194–1205.

Langleben, D. D., Loughead, J. W., Bilker, W. B., Ruparel, K., Childress, A. R., Busch, S. I., & Gur, R. C. (2005). Telling truth from lie in individual subjects with fast event-related fMRI. *Human Brain Mapping*, 26(4), 262–272.

Langleben, D. D., Schroeder, L., Maldjian, J. A., Gur, R. C., McDonald, S., Ragland, J. D., . . . Childress, A. R. (2002). Brain activity during simulated deception: An event-related functional magnetic resonance study. *Neuroimage*, 15(3), 727–732.

Larsen, J. D., Allen, M. D., Bigler, E. D., Goodrich-Hunsaker, N. J., & Hopkins, R. O. (2010). Different patterns of cerebral activation in genuine and malingered cognitive effort during performance on the Word Memory Test. *Brain Injury*, 24(2), 89–99.

Lee, T. M., Au, R. K., Liu, H. L., Ting, K. H., Huang, C. M., & Chan, C. C. (2009). Are errors differentiable from deceptive responses when feigning memory impairment? An fMRI study. *Brain and Cognition*, 69(2), 406–412.

Lee, T. M., Liu, H. L., Chan, C. C., Ng, Y. B., Fox, P. T., & Gao, J. H. (2005). Neural correlates of feigned memory impairment. *Neuroimage*, 28(2), 305–313.

Lee, T. M., Liu, H. L., Tan, L. H., Chan, C. C., Mahankali, S., Feng, C. M., . . . Gao, J. H. (2002). Lie detection by functional magnetic resonance imaging. *Human Brain Mapping*, 15(3), 157–164.

Lissek, S., Peters, S., Fuchs, N., Witthaus, H., Nicolas, V., Tegenthoff, M., . . . Brüne, M. (2008). Cooperation and deception recruit different subsets of the theory-of-mind network. *Public Library of Science ONE*, 3(4), e2023.

Luber, B., Fisher, C., Appelbaum, P. S., Ploesser, M., & Lisanby, S. H. (2009). Non-invasive brain stimulation in the detection of deception: Scientific challenges and ethical consequences. *Behavioral Sciences and the Law*, 27(2), 191–208.

Lykken, D. T. (1959). The GSR in the detection of guilt. *Journal of Applied Psychology*, 43(6), 385–388.

Lykken, D. T. (1974). Psychology and the lie detector industry. *American Psychologist*, 29(10), 725–739.

Mak, E. G., & Lee, T. M. (2006). Detection of feigned memory impairments using a Chinese word task. *Psychological Reports*, 98(3), 779–788.

Marchewka, A., Brechmann, A., Nowicka, A., Jednoróg, K., Scheich, H., & Grabowska, A. (2008). False recognition of emotional stimuli is lateralised in the brain: An fMRI study. *Neurobiology of Learning and Memory*, 90(1), 280–284.

Mertens, R., & Allen, J. J. (2008). The role of psychophysiology in forensic assessments: Deception detection, ERPs, and virtual reality mock crime scenarios. *Psychophysiology*, 45(2), 286–298.

Mittenberg, W., Patton, C., Canyock, E. M., & Condit, D. C. (2002). Base rates of malingering and symptom exaggeration. *Journal of Clinical and Experimental Neuropsychology*, 24(8), 1094–1102.

Mohamed, F. B., Faro, S. H., Gordon, N. J., Platek, S. M., Ahmad, H., & Williams, J. M. (2006). Brain mapping of deception and truth telling about an ecologically valid situation: Functional MR imaging and polygraph investigation—initial experience. *Radiology*, 238(2), 679–688.

Mossman, D. (2003). Daubert, cognitive malingering, and test accuracy. *Law and Human Behavior*, 27(3), 229–249.

Nuñez, J. M., Casey, B. J., Egner, T., Hare, T., & Hirsch, J. (2005). Intentional false responding shares neural substrates with response conflict and cognitive control. *Neuroimage*, 25(1), 267–277.

Phan, K. L., Magalhaes, A., Ziemlewicz, T. J., Fitzgerald, D. A., Green, C., & Smith, W. (2005). Neural correlates of telling lies: A functional magnetic resonance imaging study at 4 Tesla. *Academic Radiology*, 12(2), 164–172.

Priori, A, Mameli, F, Cogiamanian, F, Marceglia, S, Tiriticco, M, Mrakic-Sposta, S, Ferrucci, R, Zago, S, Polezzi, D, Sartori, G. (2008). Lie-specific involvement of dorsolateral prefrontal cortex in deception. *Cereb Cortex* 18(2):451–455.

Rosenfeld, J. P., Nasman, V. T., Whalen, R., Cantwell, B., & Mazzeri, L. (1987). Late vertex positivity in event-related potentials as a guilty knowledge indicator: A new method of life detection. *International Journal of Neuroscience*, 34(1–2), 125–129.

Rosenfeld, J. P., Reinhart, A. M., Bhatt, M., Ellwanger, J., Gora, K., Sekera, M., Sweet, J. (1998). P300 correlates of simulated malingered amnesia in a matching-to-sample task: Topographic analyses of deception versus truthtelling responses. *International Journal of Psychophysiology*, 28(3), 233–247.

Rosenfeld, J. P., Soskins, M., Bosh, G., & Ryan, A. (2004). Simple, effective countermeasures to P300-based tests of detection of concealed information. *Psychophysiology*, 41(2), 205–219.

Schatz, P., & Browndyke, J. (2002). Applications of computer-based neuropsychological assessment. *Journal of Head Trauma Rehabilitation*, 17(5), 395–410.

Shelley, M. (1818). *Frankenstein or, the modern Prometheus*. London, UK: Lackington, Hughes, Harding, Mavor, & Jones.

Spence, S. A., Farrow, T. F., Herford, A. E., Wilkinson, I. D., Zheng, Y., & Woodruff, P. W. (2001). Behavioural and functional anatomical correlates of deception in humans. *Neuroreport*, 12(13), 2849–2853.

Spence, S. A., Hunter, M. D., Farrow, T. F., Green, R. D., Leung, D. H., Hughes, C. J., & Ganesan, V. (2004). A cognitive neurobiological account of deception: Evidence from functional neuroimaging. *Philosphical Transactions of the Royal Society of London: Biological Sciences*, 359(1451), 1755–1762.

Spence, S. A., Kaylor-Hughes, C., Farrow, T. F., & Wilkinson, I. D. (2008). Speaking of secrets and lies: The contribution of ventrolateral prefrontal cortex to vocal deception. *Neuroimage*, 40(3), 1411–1418.

Stern, P. C. (2004). The polygraph and lie detection. In P.C. Stern (Ed.), *Report of the National Research Council Committee to review the scientific evidence on the polygraph* (pp. 340–357). Washington, DC: The National Academies Press.

Stuss, D. T., Gallup, G. G. Jr., & Alexander, M. P. (2001). The frontal lobes are necessary for "theory of mind." *Brain*, 124(Pt. 2), 279–286.

Talairach, J., & Tournoux, P. (1988). *Co-planar stereotaxic atlas of the human brain: 3-dimensional proportional system: an approach to cerebral imaging*. New York, NY: Thieme Medical.

Tian, F., Sharma, V., Kozel, F. A., & Liu, H. (2009). Functional near-infrared spectroscopy to investigate hemodynamic responses to deception in the prefrontal cortex. *Brain Research*, 1303, 120–130.

Tombaugh, T. (1996). *Test of memory malingering manual*. New York, NY: MultiHealth Systems.

Turkeltaub, P. E., Eden, G. F., Jones, K. M., & Zeffiro, T. A. (2002). Meta-analysis of the functional neuroanatomy of single-word reading: Method and validation. *Neuroimage*, 16(3 Pt. 1), 765–780.

Turner, M. S., Cipolotti, L., Yousry, T. A., & Shallice, T. (2008). Confabulation: Damage to a specific inferior medial prefrontal system. *Cortex*, 44(6), 637–648.

Vendemia, J. M., Buzan, R. F., & Simon-Dack, S. L. (2005). Reaction time of motor responses in two-stimulus paradigms involving deception and congruity with varying levels of difficulty. *Behavioral Neurology*, 16(1), 25–36.

Von Zerssen, G. C., Mecklinger, A., Opitz, B., & von Cramon, D. Y. (2001). Conscious recollection and illusory recognition: An event-related fMRI study. *European Journal of Neuroscience*, 13(11), 2148–2156.

Wertheimer, M., King, D. B., Peckler, M. A., Raney, S., & Schaef, R. W. (1992). Carl Jung and Max Wertheimer on a priority issue. *Journal of the History of the Behavioral Sciences*, 28(1), 45–56.

Willison, J., & Tombaugh, T. N. (2006). Detecting simulation of attention deficits using reaction time tests. *Archives of Clinical Neuropsychology*, 21(1), 41–52.

Winner, E., Brownell, H., Happé, F., Blum, A., & Pincus, D. (1998). Distinguishing lies from jokes: Theory of mind deficits and discourse interpretation in right hemisphere brain-damaged patients. *Brain and Language*, 62(1), 89–106.

Wolpe, P. R., Foster, K. R., Langleben, D. D. (2005). Emerging neurotechnologies for lie-detection: Promises and perils. *American Journal of Bioethics*, 5(2), 39–49.

Wu, T., Allen, M., Goodrich-Hunsaker, N., Hopkins, R., & Bigler, E. D. (2010). Functional neuroimaging of symptom validity testing in traumatic brain injury. *Psychology, Injury and Law*, 3, 50–62.

Yang, Y., Raine, A., Lencz, T., Bihrle, S., Lacasse, L., & Colletti, P. (2005). Prefrontal white matter in pathological liars. *British Journal of Psychiatry*, 187, 320–325.

Yang, Y., Raine, A., Narr, K. L., Lencz, T., LaCasse, L., Colletti, P., Toga, A. W. (2007). Localisation of increased prefrontal white matter in pathological liars. *British Journal of Psychiatry*, 190, 174–175.

Zannino, G. D., Barban, F., Caltagirone, C., & Carlesimo, G. A. (2008). Do confabulators really try to remember when they confabulate? A case report. *Cognitive Neuropsychology*, 25(6), 831–852.

APPENDIX 14.1

ACTIVATION LIKELIHOOD ESTIMATION ANALYSES METHODS

A thorough search of the research literature on false memory and deception was conducted using the U.S. National Library of Medicine PubMed database. The search was limited to functional neuroimaging articles published between 1990 and 2010 that met the following search parameters for false memory or deception/malingering articles: False memory articles = [(((("1990/01/01"[Publication Date]: "2010/01/01"[Publication Date])) AND (false memory)) AND (brain[Title/Abstract])) AND (((fMRI[Title/Abstract]) OR PET[Title/Abstract]) OR imaging[Title/Abstract])]. Deception/malingering articles = [(((("1990/01/01"[Publication Date]: "2010/01/01"[Publication Date])) AND (brain[Title/Abstract])) AND (((fMRI[Title/Abstract]) OR PET[Title/Abstract]) OR imaging[Title/Abstract])) AND ((((deception[Title/Abstract]) OR lie[Title/Abstract]) OR malinger[Title/Abstract]) OR malingering[Title/Abstract])]. These searches yielded 45 unique articles for false memory and 108 unique articles for deception/malingering.

The resulting false memory articles were narrowed further to 10 investigations that used functional neuroimaging to examine brain processes involved in unintentional false recognition. Additional three studies were excluded because of lack of analyzable stereotactic spatial coordinates, which resulted in a final total of seven false memory studies from which 53 individual foci were retained for meta-analysis (see Table 14.1).

Because the PubMed database search does not discriminate the context and connotation of search terms, the term "lie" was often included in deception/malingering results such as "the disease *lies* on a continuum," as opposed to the deceptive connotation of the word. Sixty-two studies were excluded from the original 108 deception study search results for this reason. The remaining 46 deception studies were then interrogated for the primary cognitive aspect of the task paradigms used to assess deception. Only task paradigms that included a

TABLE 14.1 Research Studies Included in Deception and False Memory Activation Likelihood Estimation Meta-analyses

Study Type	Research Article	Participant *n*	Contrast Type	Number of Foci
Deception Studies	(Abe, et al., 2006)	14	Main effect of deception	4
	(Abe, et al., 2007)	16	Main effect of deception	7
	(Abe, et al., 2008)	20	Main effect of deception	20
	(Bhatt, et al., 2009)	18	Lie > Truth (unfamiliar faces)	9
			Lie > Truth (familiar faces)	4
	(Browndyke, et al., 2008)	7	Malingered misses > normal hits	7
			Malingered false alarms > Normal correct rejections	7
	(Kozel, Padgett, et al., 2004)	10	Lie > Truth	11
	(Kozel, Revell, et al., 2004)	10	Lie > Truth	10
	(Kozel, et al., 2005)	31	Lie > Truth	17
	(Lee, et al., 2009)	10	Malingered > Truthful response	8
				Total = 104
False Memory Studies	(Abe, et al., 2008)	20	False > true recognition	10
	(Abel, et al., 2009)	34	False > true recognition	3
	(Dennio, Kim, & Cabeza, 2008)	33	Main effect of false retrieval	8
	(Heun, et al., 2004)	15	Main effect of false recognition	6
	(Kim & Cabeza, 2007)	16	High confidence false recognition	7
	(Marchewka, et al., 2008)	23	False > True recognition	9
	(von Zerssen, Mecklinger, Opitz, & von Cramon, 2001)	12	False > Correct retrieval	10
				Total=53

memory component in the measurement of lying and/or deception were included in the analysis so they could be more consistently compared to the false memory analysis. Functional imaging contrasts reported in the paired down list of deception studies reflected the main effect of deception relative to a truth condition. Again, to be included, all studies must have reported spatial coordinates in standard stereotactic atlas space. On the basis of these two analysis entry requirements, 37 additional deception studies were excluded leaving 9 final studies with 102 individual foci for meta-analysis (see Table 14.1).

Once all of the resulting studies were aggregated, spatial coordinates (x, y, z) from the relevant functional imaging contrasts were standardized to a common stereotactic atlas space to allow for direct cross comparison. Study coordinates reported in Talairach atlas space (Talairach & Tournoux, 1988) were converted to Montreal Neurological Institute (MNI) space using a Lancaster transform (Lancaster et al., 2007). The number of subjects included in each contributing study contrast was also recorded as parameter to aid in the weighing of individual study significance in the meta-analyses.

Activation likelihood estimate (ALE) analyses (Eickhoff et al., 2009; Laird et al., 2005) were conducted separately for false memory and deception/malingering studies (see Table 14.1) by modeling reported individual study MNI foci as a three-dimensional Gaussian function smoothed with a 12 mm full width half maximum (FWHM) kernel (Turkeltaub, Eden, Jones, & Zeffiro, 2002) to allow enough spatial overlap among foci for statistical comparison. Statistical significance was evaluated using the standard ALE permutation procedure with a minimum of 5,000 permutations per solution. ALE analyses were corrected for multiple comparisons using a false discovery rate procedure (FDR; Benjamini & Hochberg, 1995; Genovese, Lazar, & Nichols, 2002) and thresholded for cluster size to conservatively control for Type I error. To exceed established analysis thresholds, ALE analysis clusters were required to be statistically significant at FDR $q < .01$ with a minimum volume of 100 mm^3. Two output maps were produced, reflecting the separate false memory and deception ALE meta-analyses.

ACTIVATION LIKELIHOOD ESTIMATION ANALYSES RESULTS

Peak MNI coordinates, Brodmann areas, and cluster sizes for significant ALE regional commonalities are summarized in Table 14.2 illustrating the two separate ALE analyses. The ALE value noted in Table 14.2 is the maximum ALE value for a particular statistically significant common cluster. This maximum value was found at the local extrema coordinate reported for each significant ALE cluster (i.e., spatial location of the most statistically significant voxel within a cluster). All ALE values are significant based on an FDR of $q < .01; k \geq 100$mm^3. The significant common clusters from each ALE analysis are overlaid on a single brain template in Figure 14.1.

The ALE analysis aggregating studies that focused on false memory found six clusters that were statistically significant. These clusters were centered in the medial frontal gyrus (Cluster 1), the left and right claustrum (Clusters 2 & 6), the inferior frontal gyrus (Cluster 3), the anterior cingulate (Cluster 4), and the middle frontal gyrus (Cluster 5). Although seven other clusters were reported in the analysis output, these clusters were each driven by a single study and did not reflect commonality across studies. These single study clusters were excluded in subsequent analysis and the ALE results figures.

Numerous clusters of significance were apparent when the ALE model was run with contrasts depicting activations during deception. These clusters were centered in the inferior frontal gyrus (Clusters 1 & 3), the red nucleus (Cluster 2), the precuneus (Clusters 4 & 11), the middle frontal gyrus (Clusters 5 & 9), the cingulate gyrus (Cluster 7), the superior frontal gyrus (Cluster 8), the superior temporal gyrus (Clusters 10 & 12), and the parahippocampal gyrus/amygdala area (Cluster 13). The large number of common active clusters associated with deception not only emphasizes the complexity of the process of lying but also the general robustness of activity in these common regions across the various deception task paradigms.

TABLE 14.2 Significant Regions of Brain Activity Associated With Deception and False Memory Studies

Common Brain Activity by Study Type		Cluster Number	Location (Brodmann Area)	Local Extrema			Cluster Volume (mm³)	ALE value (×10⁻³)
				x	y	z		
Deception studies	Right hemisphere	1	Inferior frontal gyrus (BA 44)	56	16	12	4,664	3.09
		2	Midbrain, red nucleus	4	−20	−8	632	1.24
		3	Inferior frontal gyrus (BA 46)	44	40	−6	568	1.56
		4	Precuneus (BA 7)	8	−60	68	568	1.91
		5	Middle frontal gyrus (BA 9)	40	42	30	456	1.35
		6	Medial frontal gyrus (BA 10)	12	56	−4	368	1.23
		7	Cingulate gyrus (BA 31)	6	−28	34	296	1.21
		8	Superior frontal gyrus (BA 6)	24	16	60	280	1.06
		9	Middle frontal gyrus (BA 47)	−44	36	−6	1,624	2.27
		10	Sup. temporal gyrus (BA 39)	−50	−56	34	928	1.46
		11	Precuneus (BA 7)	−14	−46	58	640	1.97
		12	Superior temporal gyrus (BA 22)	−44	−26	4	440	1.34
		13	Parahippocampal gyrus, amygdala	−26	0	−26	328	1.16
False Memory Studies	Right Hemisphere	1	Medial frontal gyrus (BA 6)	4	18	44	872	1.53
		2	Claustrum, gray matter	28	24	−10	816	1.65
		3	Inferior frontal gyrus (BA 9)	40	14	28	520	1.28
	Left hemisphere	4	Anterior Cingulate (BA 32)	0	50	4	920	1.77
		5	Middle frontal gyrus (BA 8)	−36	30	42	816	1.38
		6	Claustrum, Gray Matter	−28	24	−4	768	1.30

Note: ALE meta-analyses critical statistical threshold for interstudy regions of common activation established at FDR $q < 0.01$ and k (extent) $\geq 100mm^3$. ALE − activation likelihood estimation; BA − Brodmann area.

Cognitive Performance Validity Assessment in Mild Traumatic Brain Injury, Physical Pain, and Posttraumatic Stress

15

Kevin J. Bianchini, Kelly L. Curtis, & Kevin W. Greve

It is becoming increasingly necessary for neuropsychologists, especially those working in a civil forensic context, to address complaints of pain and reactive psychological conditions in the course of their evaluations of persons claiming brain dysfunction because of head trauma. Chronic pain (CP) after traumatic brain injury (TBI), for example, occurs in 75% of patients with mild traumatic brain injury (MTBI) and 32% of patients with moderate-to-severe TBI (Nampiaparampil, 2008). Cognitive complaints are common even after MTBI (Larrabee, 2005). However, because cognitive symptoms are not specific to neurological injury, they are also often a feature of conditions not associated with brain damage or dysfunction, such as CP or posttraumatic stress disorder (PTSD; Brewin, Kleiner, Vasterling, & Field, 2007; Eccleston, 1994, 1995; Krietler & Niv, 2007; Nicholson, 2000; Oien, Nelson, Lamberty, & Arbisi, 2011). In addition to the genuine cognitive, psychological, and somatic consequences and correlates of an injury, illness, or traumatic stress, these problems are potentially compensable; therefore, malingering is a potential issue (Mittenberg, Patton, Canyock, & Condit, 2002).

Malingering is an act of will, and its specific manifestation(s) depends on the idiosyncrasies of individual cases, including claimants' beliefs regarding the effects of their injury and efforts to avoid detection (Greve & Bianchini, 2004). Thus, in both feigned and genuine cases, a mixed symptom presentation would not be unexpected. A mixed symptom presentation is incentivized in the American civil justice system in which compensation is largely related to the magnitude of *disability* attributed to an injury. Compensation may be attached to three factors: (a) cost of past and future medical care, (b) wage loss from total inability to work or from a reduced level of employment, and (c) loss of ability to care for self or others (e.g., need for physical assistance). As a result, the addition of ancillary symptoms and related disability that further compromise claimants' functional status can increase the potential value of claims.

For example, if an individual with a low back injury is released to light or sedentary duty, then the presence of cognitive symptoms that prevent him or her from effectively working as a security guard would change the claim from one of partial wage loss to one of total wage loss. Likewise, a patient with head injury whose cognitive symptoms have largely resolved but who has unremitting posttraumatic headaches may claim the need for indefinite pain management, the potential costs of which may further increase the value of the claim. In cases of genuine injury or illness causally linked to the injury in question, adding that value to the claim is reasonable and justified. However, this also means that intentionally exaggerated or feigned disability can artificially increase the potential compensation for a claim and that a multidimensional (cognitive, psychological, and/or somatic) presentation may be more valuable still.

Approximately one third of persons evaluated by neuropsychologists in a compensable or incentivized context are malingering (Ardolf, Denney, & Houston, 2007; Bianchini, Curtis, & Greve, 2006; Chafetz, 2008; Greve et al., 2006; Greve, Ord, Bianchini, & Curtis, 2009; Larrabee, 2005; Mittenberg et al., 2002). Given the high rate of malingering in compensated contexts (cf., Mittenberg et al., 2002), performance and symptom validity must be assessed comprehensively (American Academy of Clinical Neuropsychology, 2007; Bush et al., 2005) and throughout the course of the neuropsychological evaluation (Boone, 2009). There is a consensus in neuropsychology that validity and malingering can be reliably detected (Heilbronner, Sweet, Morgan, Larrabee, & Millis, 2009), and failure to assess validity must be justified (Bush et al., 2005; Heilbronner et al., 2009).

The purpose of this chapter is to summarize the symptom validity test[1] (SVT) literature in MTBI/concussion, CP, and PTSD. Over the last two decades, numerous SVTs have been developed and empirically validated, mostly with TBI populations. In the past decade, their validation has been expanded to other populations, most notably CP (Greve & Bianchini, 2009) and also PTSD (e.g., Freeman, Powell, & Kimbrell, 2008; Hall & Hall, 2006; Morel, 2008; Rogers, Payne, Correa, Gillard, & Ross, 2009). A comprehensive review of this topic is beyond the scope of a single chapter. In addition to summarizing the extensive literature on these broad topics, the focus of this chapter will be narrowed to cognitive SVTs for the following reasons.

First, by far the most comprehensive and methodologically sound work has been on cognitive SVTs, whereas the research on techniques to detect malingered psychological and physical presentations lags somewhat behind. Second, genuine cognitive complaints are common in both CP and PTSD, and malingered complaints in those domains would not be seen as unreasonable. Thus, clinicians should examine cognition and cognitive symptom validity in these patient populations. Third, the extensive data on the diagnostic accuracy of cognitive SVTs developed in persons with known brain pathology can be generalized to cases in which there is no brain injury claim (Bianchini, Etherton, & Greve, 2004). Fourth, the research methodologies that have been applied so effectively to cognitive SVT development can easily be adapted to the validation of measures of psychological and physical symptom exaggeration.

Finally, Slick, Sherman, and Iverson (1999) provided a now well-studied system for diagnosing malingered neurocognitive dysfunction (MND) which is relevant for a malingered cognitive presentation regardless of the alleged etiology of the cognitive dysfunction. This system has been modified such that it can be more directly applied to CP and even PTSD (Bianchini, Greve, & Glynn, 2005; Larrabee, Greiffenstein, Greve, & Bianchini, 2007).

COGNITIVE PERFORMANCE VALIDITY TESTING: A GENERAL OVERVIEW

Measures of cognitive performance validity are intended to determine if an individual has underperformed on tests of perceptual or cognitive ability and may take

---

[1] In this chapter, the term "symptom validity test" is used to refer to any test, score, or other formal indicator used to assess the validity of performance on cognitive tests or the accuracy of self-report on questionnaires or in structured interviews.

two general forms: stand-alone SVTs, and embedded indicators derived from clinical measures of cognitive ability. Stand-alone SVTs are independent tests specifically designed to detect attempts to misrepresent the status of a cognitive or perceptual function. Among the earliest stand-alone SVTs were those devised by André Rey, namely the Dot Counting Test and the 15-Item Test (for discussion, see Lezak, Howieson, & Loring, 2004). The Rey 15-Item Test is one of the most frequently given SVTs (Slick, Tan, Strauss, & Hultsch, 2004) despite its limited diagnostic value (Reznek, 2005), although its use is likely in decline with the development of more sophisticated measures. These and similar SVTs have been subjected to extensive modern research to determine and improve the diagnostic accuracy (for recent review, see Boone & Lu, 2007, and Nitch & Glassmire, 2007).

A second variety of stand-alone SVTs, the forced-choice SVT, is of more recent vintage but has come to have a central place in the batteries of most psychologists engaged in the assessment of persons with incentive to appear disabled. Initially described for use among patients presenting suspicious perceptual deficits (Brady & Lind, 1961; Grosz & Zimmerman, 1965; Pankratz, Fausti, & Peed, 1975), Pankratz (1983) is credited with naming this procedure "symptom validity testing" and with adapting it to questions of exaggerated memory complaints (Heubrock & Petermann, 1998). Numerous stand-alone forced-choice SVTs using various stimuli and methodological variations have been published (Bianchini, Mathias, & Greve, 2001), although only a handful are commonly used in clinical practice (Slick et al., 2004). Among the more popular and well-studied tests are the Test of Memory Malingering (TOMM; Tombaugh, 1996), Word Memory Test (WMT; Green, Allen, & Astner, 1996; Green, 2005), and Portland Digit Recognition Test (PDRT; Binder, 1990, 1993).

The value of stand-alone SVTs in the detection of malingering is evident; they are probably among the most accurate and well-studied SVTs. However, stand-alone SVTs have some disadvantages. First, they are sensitive primarily to feigned memory impairment so they provide limited coverage of other relevant behavioral domains. Therefore, if malingerers choose to exaggerate cognitive problems other than memory problems, they may go undetected by these measures. Moreover, these SVTs may be vulnerable to active efforts to avoid detection (e.g., coaching). Because they are readily identifiable by their format and because there is considerable information available about them on the Internet (Bauer & McCaffrey, 2006), some well-prepared malingerers may go undetected. Finally, stand-alone SVTs require additional testing time, and they do not speak as directly to the validity of performance on specific clinical measures.

Embedded or internal SVTs, in contrast, are derived from standard clinical tests and procedures that are used as a routine part of the psychological test battery rather than being an independent test. They may consist of a single specially developed test score (e.g., reliable digit span [RDS]; Greiffenstein, Baker, & Gola, 1994), multiple scores combined in various ways (e.g., vocabulary minus digit span from the Wechsler Adult Intelligence Scale-Revised [WAIS-R], Mittenberg, Theroux-Fichera, Zielinski, & Heilbronner, 1995; linear shrinkage model for the California Verbal Learning Test [CVLT], Millis & Volinsky, 2001), or simply a standard clinical score that has demonstrated validity in differentiating malingering from nonmalingering cases (e.g., Working Memory Index [WMI] from the Wechsler Adult Intelligence Scale-Third Edition [WAIS-III], Etherton, Bianchini, Ciota, Heinly, & Greve, 2006).

Embedded SVTs have drawn considerable research and clinical interest because (a) they enhance the sensitivity of the entire malingering battery without requiring extra administration time; (b) they can provide direct information about the validity of performance on specific tests (Mathias, Greve, Bianchini, Houston, & Crouch, 2002; Meyers & Diep, 2000; Meyers & Volbrecht, 2003); (c) they may be less susceptible to coaching than SVTs (Ashendorf, O'Bryant, & McCaffrey, 2003; Mathias et al., 2002); and (d) they can be used to evaluate performance validity in the absence of specialized techniques. The development of malingering detection data for standard clinical measures has become a popular enterprise in the last 10 years, as the content of Boone (2007) and Larrabee (2007) texts demonstrate. Validity data for almost every commonly administered neuropsychological test is available. This is illustrated in the Morgan and Sweet (2009) casebook on malingering that contains five appendices (Sweet, 2009) of bibliographies of specific validity indicators.

Combining both stand-alone SVTs and embedded indicators allows the comprehensive evaluation of performance validity throughout the evaluation (Boone, 2009), while providing direct information on the validity of performance on specific clinical tests. With embedded indicators, there is no additional time or cost obstacle to a thorough assessment of validity even in the most constrained evaluations. The role of these various tests and indicators is the *detection* of invalid test performance that may contribute to inaccurate and/or unreliable clinical decisions (e.g., regarding diagnostic impressions, treatment recommendations, and prognostications). Findings from these indicators, when positive, may also contribute to the formal diagnosis of malingering.

COGNITIVE PERFORMANCE VALIDITY TESTING IN SELECTED POPULATIONS

Mild Traumatic Brain Injury

TBIs are one of the leading causes of mortality and morbidity in the world and can have a serious impact on an individual's behavioral, psychological, and cognitive functioning. In the United States alone, approximately 1.5 million people sustain a TBI each year. Roughly 250,000–290,000 people are hospitalized because of TBI, approximately 50,000 die, and 125,000 are still considered disabled after 1 year (Dikmen et al., 2009; Scherer & Madison, 2005). Of those persons who present to the hospital sustaining a TBI, between 50% (Scherer & Madison, 2005) and 90% (Larrabee, 2005; Rose, 2005) have TBIs that are mild in nature. Based on incidence data from 1995, the Centers for Disease Control and Prevention estimated that the total lifetime cost (direct and indirect costs) for all TBI is around $60 billion, $16.7 billion (29%) of which is allocated to the treatment of MTBI (also known as concussion) alone (Thurman, 2001). Given these statistics, it is important to study outcome in these populations, particularly MTBI.

To effectively assess a person's condition and establish an appropriate treatment plan, a clinician must be able to accurately classify the level of brain injury that a person has sustained. According to current classification systems, head injury severity is not defined in terms of symptoms, test results, or functional outcome but rather by the neurological or physiological signs present at the time of the injury (Alexander, 1995; Arciniegas, Anderson, Topkoff, & McAllister, 2005; Binder, 1997; Ruff, 2005). These acute injury characteristics include (a) duration of coma (if any), (b) alterations of consciousness (feeling dazed, disorientation, etc.), (c) length of posttraumatic amnesia, (d) objective findings on standard neuroimaging techniques, and (e) whether focal neurological signs are present (Arciniegas et al., 2005; Bernstein, 1999; Dikmen, Machamer, Winn, & Temkin, 1995).

There is a general consensus that moderate or severe TBIs are easier to classify, mainly because the injury characteristics are more easily identifiable, and objective neuropathological findings are usually present in these cases (McCrea, 2008). On the other hand, with MTBI, the lack of gross objective findings (Miller, 2001; Satz et al., 1999), quick symptom resolution, and delays in seeking immediate medical attention (if at all; McCrea, 2008) make it hard to establish whether an individual has even sustained an injury (Ruff, Iverson, Barth, Bush, & Broshek, 2009). This complexity is particularly challenging for the clinician because MTBI is the most common cause of referral to neuropsychologists conducting forensic assessments in personal injury litigation (Ruff & Richardson, 1999).

In 1993, the Mild Traumatic Brain Injury Committee of the Head Injury Interdisciplinary Special Interest Group of the American Congress of Rehabilitation Medicine (ACRM) developed criteria of what MTBI encompasses that have been widely used in subsequent empirical research on MTBI (Ruff et al., 2009). In particular, the ARCM criteria for MTBI require at least one of the following: (a) any period of loss of consciousness; (b) any loss of memory for events immediately before or after the accident; (c) any alteration in mental state at the time of the accident; or (d) focal neurological deficits that may or may not be transient. In addition, the severity of the injury cannot exceed the following: (a) loss of consciousness of approximately 30 min or less; (b) after 30 min, an initial Glasgow Coma Scale of 13–15; and (c) posttraumatic amnesia not more than 24 hr.

In 2009, Ruff and colleagues published a comparison of the two classification systems and provided recommendations for clinicians regarding how to assess the diagnostic criteria that these systems outline. It is important to note that, regardless of the classification system used, each stresses the importance of using a "multidimensional definition that incorporates information on the biomechanics, acute injury characteristics, and clinical course to assist clinicians in making the most accurate diagnosis of mild TBI" (McCrea et al., 2009, p. 1369). In all cases, there must be at least some alteration of consciousness to diagnose a brain injury.

Once it has been determined that an individual sustained an MTBI, clinicians have ample sources of information describing the natural course of recovery. The neuropsychological literature has consistently found complete resolution of symptoms within 3 months in cases of single uncomplicated MTBI (Belanger, Curtiss, Demery, Lebowitz, & Vanderploeg, 2005; Binder, Rohling, & Larrabee, 1997; Carroll et al., 2004; Dikmen et al., 2009; Dikmen et al., 1995; Frenchman, Fox, & Maybery, 2005; Schretlen & Shapiro, 2003). However, despite this large body of evidence indicating rapid recovery, a small minority of patients who sustained MTBIs experience persisting subjective symptoms and alleged disability (Alexander, 1995; Ingebrigsten, Waterloo, Marup-Jensen, Attner, & Romner, 1998; Karzmark, Hall, & Englander, 1995; Macleod, 2010; Ryan & Warden, 2003; Smith-Seemiller, Fow, Kant, & Franzen, 2003; Wood, 2004). Identifying the cause(s) of these persisting problems is an important purpose of the neuropsychological evaluation.

In the absence of objective brain pathology, symptoms persisting for more than a year are often associated with premorbid psychological factors, emotional problems, pain, and/or stress (Belanger et al., 2005; Carroll et al., 2004). It is also important to recognize the potential for malingering in cases in which there is a potential for financial compensation. It is well established that financial incentive is related to outcome in brain injury in general, and the effect of money is strongest at the mild end of the TBI severity continuum (Binder, 1986; Binder & Rohling, 1996; Paniak et al., 2002; Price & Stevens, 1997; Reynolds, Paniak, Toller-Lobe, & Nagy, 2003; Youngjohn et al., 1995). Carroll et al. (2004) found that the most consistent predictor of poor outcome was the presence of litigation. Bianchini et al. (2006) showed that the rates of invalid performance and diagnosable malingering increased as the amount of potential compensation increased. The base rate of malingering among persons with a history of MTBI is between 30% and 40%, whereas it is only about 10% in patients with a history of moderate-to-severe TBI (Bianchini et al., 2006; Larrabee, 2005; Mittenberg et al, 2002). Thus, the failure to assess validity and malingering, particularly in MTBI cases, is likely to result in grossly inaccurate conclusions regarding the cognitive and disability status of some claimants.

Until recently, the development and validation of symptom validity indicators focused almost exclusively on TBI, with particular emphasis on symptom validity assessment with MTBI cases. Providing a thorough review of all of the symptom validity indicators (both stand-alone and embedded) that have been studied throughout the history of the development of SVT methods is beyond the scope of this chapter; however, the readers are referred to various excellent reference works (e.g., Boone, 2007; Larrabee, 2007; Morgan & Sweet, 2009). Research on cognitive performance validity assessment in TBI cases continues, particularly with cross validation of existing indicators and the development of new indicators (e.g., RDS; Ylioja, Baird, & Podell, 2009). In fact, the volume of research on some indicators has been sufficiently large as to justify meta-analysis (e.g., WAIS, digit span subtest; Jasinski, Berry, Shandera, & Clark, 2011).

Tables 15.1 and 15.2 provide a summary of the research that has been conducted on validity testing in MTBI cases since 2008 for stand-alone SVTs and embedded performance validity indicators, respectively. These tables are designed to facilitate the use of these measures by clinicians. Along with sample characteristics and validity indicators examined, cutoffs (as determined by the highest likelihood ratios) and associated sensitivity and false positive error rates are included. All of the research summarized in these tables has employed criterion-groups designs.

There are several simulator or criterion-groups studies examining the performance of existing or new stand-alone or embedded validity indicators published since 2008 that are not included in the tables because their samples are comprised of mixed clinical patients, patients with mixed-severity TBI, or patients without TBI (e.g., psychiatric, learning disabled), rather than focusing on MTBI only (e.g., Barker, Horner, & Bachman, 2010; Booksh, Pella, Singh, & Gouvier, 2010; Bortnik et al., 2010; Chafetz, 2011; Davis, Wall, Ramos, Whitney, & Barisa, 2010; Gunn, Batchelor, & Jones, 2010; Harrison, Edwards, Armstrong, & Parker 2010; Kim, Boone, Victor, Marion, et al., 2010; Kim, Boone, Victor, Lu, et al., 2010; Krishnan & Donders, 2011;

TABLE 15.1 Criterion Groups Study Examining Specificity and Sensitivity in Stand-Alone Symptom Validity Tests in Mild Traumatic Brain Injury

Authors	n	Sample	Validity Indicator	Cutoff	FP	Sens %
Greve, Ord et al., 2008	43 27	TBI not MND TBI MND	Portland Digit Recognition Test	≤ 21 easy ≤ 18 hard ≤ 44 total	2 2 2	28 33 38
			Test of Memory Malingering	≤ 48 (T2) ≤ 44 (Ret)	2 2	50 35
			Word Memory Test	≤ 77.5 (IR) ≤ 77.5 (DR) ≤ 70.0 (C1)	2 2 2	50 47 45

Note. C1 = consistency score 1; DR = delayed recognition; FP = false positive error rate; IR = immediate recognition; MND = malingered neurocognitive dysfunction; *n* = sample size; Ret = retention; sens = sensivity; TBI = traumatic brain injury; T2 = Trial 2.

TABLE 15.2 Criterion Groups Studies Examining Specificity and Sensitivity of Embedded Indicators in Mild Traumatic Brain Injury

Authors	n	Sample	Validity Indicator	Cutoff	FP	Sens %
Curtis et al., 2009	26	MTBI not MND	WAIS-III verbal IQ	≤ 70	4	26
	31	MTBI MND	WAIS-III performance IQ	≤ 75	4	39
			WAIS-III full scale IQ	≤ 70	0	26
			WAIS-III Verbal Comprehension Index	≤ 70	8	29
			WAIS-III Perceptual Organization Index	≤ 75	0	33
			WAIS-III Working Memory Index	≤ 70	4	26
			WAIS-III Processing Speed Index	≤ 70	8	36
Curtis et al., 2010	24	MTBI not MND	Seashore Rhythm Test-correct	≤ 20	4	37
	27	MTBI MND	Speech Sounds Perception Test-errors	≥ 13	4	59
Greve, Lotz et al. 2008	44	MTBI not MND	WAIS-III eVIQ minus VIQ	≥ 25	2	34
	38	MTBI MND	WAIS-III ePIQ minus PIQ	≥ 25	5	29
			WAIS-III eFSIQ minus FSIQ	≥ 25	7	34
Greve, Curtis et al., 2009	62	TBI not MND	California Verbal Learning Test-II recognition hits	≤ 8	2	29
	35	TBI MND	California Verbal Learning Test-II linear shrinkage	≥ 3	2	31
Greve, Heinly et al., 2009	55	MTBI not MND	Wisconsin Card Sorting Test-failure to maintain set	≥ 4	0	18
	38	MTBI MND	Wisconsin Card Sorting Test-Suhr & Boyer's formula	≥ 4.5	2	24
			Wisconsin Card Sorting Test-King et al.'s formula	≥ 1.5	2	16
Kirkwood et al., 2011	224	Pediatric MTBI (credible)	WAIS-III digit span scaled score	≤ 4	1	38
	37	Pediatric MTBI (noncredible)	WAIS-III reliable digit span	≤ 5	0	27
			WAIS-III digit span forward (raw)	≤ 5	1	24
			WAIS-III Digit Span Backward (raw)	≤ 4	3	24
Ord et al., 2010	31	MTBI not MND	Connors' Continuous Performance Test-II omissions (raw)	> 30	6	33
	27	MTBI MND	Connors' Continuous Performance Test-II hit reaction time S.E.	> 16	3	41
Wolfe et al., 2010	124	Moderate-to-severe TBI	California Verbal Learning Test-II logistic regression formula	≥ 0.6293	10	49
	29	MTBI MND				
Ylioja et al., 2009	29	PPCS–valid	Wechsler Memory Scale-III reliable spatial span	≤ 6	14	55
	33	PPCS–invalid				

Note. e = estimated; FP = false positive error rate; IQ = intelligence quotient; MND = malingered neurocognitive dysfunction; MTBI = mild traumatic brain injury; n = sample size; PPCS = persistent postconcussion syndrome; SE = standard error; sens = sensitivity; TBI = traumatic brain injury; WAIS-III = Wechsler Adult Intelligence Scale-Third Edition.

Lindstrom, Coleman, Thomassin, Southall, & Lindstrom, 2011; Lindstrom, Lindstrom, Coleman, Nelson, & Gregg, 2009; Martins & Martins, 2010; Miller et al., 2011; Pivovarova, Rosenfeld, Dole, Green, & Zapf, 2009; Powell, Locke, Smigielski, & McCrea, 2011; Schroeder & Marhsall, 2010; Schutte, Millis, Axelrod, & VanDyke, 2011; Singhal, Green, Ashaye, Shankar, & Gill, 2009; Solomon et al., 2010; Suhr, Sullivan, & Rodriguez, 2011; Whiteside, Wald, & Busse, 2011). These types of studies offer valuable information about performance validity; many are summarized in Bianchini, Curtis, and Greve (in press).

Examination of Tables 15.1 and 15.2 shows that most of the research recently conducted has examined the use of embedded indicators to detect malingered from nonmalingered performance. With the exception of one study (Kirkwood, Hargrave, & Kirk, 2011), the research conducted in this time frame used the Slick et al., (1999) classification system for MND. One study examined the efficacy of a new embedded indicator (Ylioja et al., 2009), whereas the remaining studies served as cross validations for already established indicators and tests such as the PDRT, TOMM, and WMT (Greve, Ord, Curtis, Bianchini, & Brennan, 2008), and various indicators from the WAIS-III/IV (Curtis, Greve, & Bianchini, 2009; Greve, Lotz, & Bianchini, 2008; Kirkwood et al., 2011), CVLT-II (Greve, Curtis, Bianchini, & Ord, 2009; Wolfe, Millis, Hanks, Fichtenberg, Larrabee, & Sweet, 2010), Continuous Performance Test-II (CPT-II; Ord, Boettcher, Greve, & Bianchini, 2010), Seashore Rhythm and Speech Sounds Perception Tests (Curtis, Greve, Brasseux, & Bianchini, 2010), and Wisconsin Card Sorting Test (WCST; Greve, Heinly, Bianchini, & Love, 2009). Without exception, all of the indicators achieved specificity of at least 90%, more often 95% or higher. Sensitivity ranged from 16% (WCST, King et al.'s formula) to almost 60% (Speech Sounds Perception Test—errors; reliable spatial span).

Chronic Pain

CP occurs when pain persists beyond the normal recovery time that it takes for tissue to heal from an injury, which is typically around 3 months (Pappagallo & Werner, 2008), although some researchers suggest 6 months is when pain transitions from acute to chronic (Hart, Martelli, & Zasler, 2000; Tunks, Crook, & Weir, 2008). CP is a major cause of morbidity and significantly impacts society in both direct and indirect ways. According to the Joint Commission on the Accreditation of Healthcare Organizations, approximately 33% of Americans will experience CP at some point in time in their lives, and more than half of all Americans report experiencing current or CP within the last year (Porter-Moffitt et al., 2006). The median prevalence of benign CP is 15% (ranging from 2% to 40%, depending on the specific study), with the most frequent pain sites being lower back, neck, and shoulder (Verhaak, Kerssens, Dekker, Sorbi, & Bensing, 1998).

Between $90 billion (Turk, 2002) and $125 billion (Hendler, 1997 as cited in Meyers & Diep, 2000; Nicholson & Martelli, 2004) is expended annually on health care in the United States to diagnose and treat CP. Other costs that cannot be directly measured are also accrued. CP accounts for a significant amount of lost work productivity, time off of work, and income replacement in the United States and accounts for approximately 25% of all workers' compensation claims filed and 33% of total medical compensation costs (Guo et al., 1995; Guo, Tanaka, Halperin, & Cameron, 1999). It also has a significant impact on an individual's everyday functioning and can severely limit one's social interactions and ability to accomplish nonwork related tasks (Gatchel, Bernstein, Stowell, & Pransky, 2008).

It is currently well accepted that the pathophysiology of chronic pain is not entirely or clearly understood (Waddell, McCulloch, Kummel, & Venner, 1980), and physical or diagnostic characteristics of injuries associated with pain do not fully explain symptomatic or functional outcomes (Boden, Davis, Dina, Patronas, & Wiesel, 1990). This lack of clear association between tissue damage and CP perception has led to the investigation of psychological factors in search of an explanation for some of this unexplained variance. Research has confirmed that identifiable psychosocial factors are related to outcome (see Linton, 2000, for a review). Moreover, the financial incentive associated with workers' compensation claims and personal injury litigation is also significantly associated with outcome (Harris, Mulford, Solomon, van Gelder, & Young, 2005; Rainville, Sobel, Hartigan, & Wright, 1997; Rohling, Binder, & Langhinrichsen-Rolling, 1995).

Patients with CP may complain of or manifest cognitive symptoms such as impaired memory or concentration. There are no known meta-analyses summarizing the extent of cognitive problems in CP populations; however, various commentaries and reviews provide an overview of the most frequently reported cognitive problems in CP (see Hart et al., 2000; Hart, Wade, & Martelli, 2003; Krietler & Niv, 2007; Nicholson, 2000; Nicholson, Martelli, & Zasler, 2001). In general, CP, independent from TBI, appears to have an adverse effect on cognitive functioning. This effect appears to be most salient on aspects of attention, concentration, speed of processing, and executive control, particularly on tasks that are complex and demanding (Eccleston, 1994, 1995; Krietler & Niv, 2007; Nicholson, 2000). The overlap between cognitive effects of CP and TBI is evident.

Some cognitive symptoms likely accompany the experience of pain, arising as a consequence of pain-related depression, distraction caused by the presence of pain, or as a side effect of sedating medications such as narcotic analgesics (Eccleston, 1994, 1995; Ravnkilde et al., 2002). However, cognitive complaints by litigating patients with pain without head injury sometimes exceed those reported by nonlitigating patients with head injury (Iverson & McCracken, 1997; Iverson, King, Scott, & Adams, 2001). Early research on this topic has shown documentation of malingered cognitive impairment in patients whose primary complaints are of pain (Bianchini et al., 2004; Greve, Bianchini, & Ameduri, 2003; Larrabee, 2003).

The prevalence of malingering in patients with CP has been a subject of debate. Estimates have ranged from as low as 1.25% to 10% (Fishbain, Cutler, Rosomoff, & Rosomoff, 1999) to as high as 40% (Kay & Morris-Jones, 1998; Leavitt & Sweet, 1986; Mittenberg et al., 2002). The Fishbain et al. (1999) estimates were based on a flawed analysis of the existing data (see Greve, Ord, et al., 2009, for a discussion). On the other hand, methodological issues raise concerns about the precision of the higher estimates. Greve, Ord, et al. (2009) used two different methods of determining the base rate of malingering in a psychologically-referred sample of patients with CP overall and in subgroups with different contextual variables (e.g., attorney- vs. doctor-referred). Definitive evidence of malingering was found in 10% of cases and the overall prevalence ranged from 20% to 45%, depending on the method of diagnosis and model assumptions. The rate of cognitive malingering was just as high. Thus, malingering alone is a significant issue in the cognitive assessment of the patient with CP, and methods for the detection of invalid cognitive test performance are necessary.

The application of SVT methods to the psychological assessment of CP has lagged behind TBI. As a result, there are fewer indicators that have been directly validated in patients with CP. Early studies found that some SVTs are insensitive to pain (Conder, Allen, & Cox, 1992; Green, Iverson, & Allen, 1999) and that underperformance is under volitional control in some patients with pain (Gervais et al., 2001). Other research that includes TBI and pain samples has demonstrated that diagnostic statistics derived from patients with documented brain pathology (i.e., TBI) are generalizable to patients with pain (Greve, Ord, et al., 2008; Greve, Curtis, et al., 2009). Moreover, the false positive error rate is lower at a given cutoff in CP than in TBI.

Over the past 5 years, the number of studies assessing the diagnostic accuracy of various SVTs and embedded indicators in CP patients has expanded significantly.

TABLE 15.3 Simulator and Criterion-Groups Studies Examining Specificity and Sensitivity of Stand-Alone Symptom Validity Tests in Chronic Pain

Authors	n	Sample	Validity Indicator	Cutoff	FP	Sens %
			Simulator Studies			
Etherton, Bianchini, Greve, Ciota et al., 2005	20	Undergrad volunteers – control	Test of Memory Malingering	≤ 45 (T2)	0	85
	20	Cold-pressor induced pain		≤ 45 (Ret)	0	75
	20	Sim pain-related memory deficit				
			Criterion Groups			
Greve, Ord et al., 2008	42	Non-MPRD clinical pain	Portland Digit Recognition Test	≤ 21 easy	2	63
	58	MPRD clinical pain		≤ 18 hard	2	56
				≤ 39 total	2	56
			Test of Memory Malingering	≤ 45 (T2)	2	48
				≤ 40 (Ret)	2	44
			Word Memory Test	≤ 62.5 (IR)	2	48
				≤ 62.5 (DR)	2	52
				≤ 57.5 (C1)	2	26
Greve, Bianchini, Etherton et al., 2009	76	Non-MPRD clinical pain	Portland Digit Recognition Test	≤ 25 easy	3	45 / 51[a]
	109	MPRD clinical pain		≤ 20 hard	7	45 / 46[a]
	29	Undergrad volunteers pain sim		≤ 30 total	8	59 / 62[a]
Greve, Etherton et al., 2009	118	Non-MPRD clinical pain	Test of Memory Malingering	≤ 48 (T2)	0	45
	216	MPRD clinical pain		≤ 48 (Ret)	1	48

Note. C1 = consistency score 1; DR = delayed recognition; FP = false positive error rate; IR = immediate recognition; MPRD = malingered pain-related disability; n = sample size; Ret = retention; sens = sensitivity; sim = simulator; T2 = Trial 2; undergrad = undergraduate.
[a]Represents sensitivity data for the simulator group.

Tables 15.3 and 15.4 provide information regarding the sensitivity and specificity of several stand-alone and embedded indicators in CP samples. The information presented in these tables provides clinicians data specifically applicable to patients with CP as well as providing comparisons regarding classification accuracy between CP and MTBI populations.

Our laboratory has conducted several simulator and criterion-groups studies examining the ability of existing indicators to distinguish between malingering and nonmalingering patients with CP. Regarding stand-alone indicators, one study used simulators with the TOMM (Etherton, Bianchini, Ciota, & Greve, 2005) and three employed criterion-groups validation to examine the efficacy of the PDRT, TOMM, and WMT (Greve, Bianchini, Etherton, Ord, & Curtis, 2009; Greve, Etherton, Ord, Bianchini, & Curtis, 2009; Greve, Ord, Curtis, Bianchini, & Brennan, 2008). All showed false positive error rates less than 5%, and sensitivity ranged from 26% (WMT consistency; Greve, Ord, et al., 2008) to 85% (TOMM Trial 2; Etherton, Bianchini, Ciota, et al., 2005).

The embedded indicators that have been examined in CP come from the WAIS-III and CVLT-II. Three simulator studies examined RDS, the WMI score, and Process-

TABLE 15.4 Simulator and Criterion-Groups Studies Examining Specificity and Sensitivity of Embedded Validity Indicators in Chronic Pain

Authors	n	Sample	Validity Indicator	Cutoff	FP	Sens %
			Simulator Studies			
Etherton, Bianchini, Ciota et al., 2005	20	Undergrad volunteers – controls	Reliable digit span	≤ 7	0	65
	20	Undergrad volunteers – cold pressor pain				
	20	Undergrad volunteers – sim pain				
Etherton, Bianchini, Ciota et al., 2006 (Study 1)	20	Undergrad volunteers – controls	Working Memory Index	≤ 80	0	65
	20	Undergrad volunteers – cold pressor pain				
	20	Undergrad volunteers – sim pain				
Etherton, Bianchini, Heinly et al., 2006 (Study 1)	20	Undergrad volunteers – controls	Processing Speed Index	≤ 80	0 / 5[a]	95
	20	Undergrad volunteers – cold pressor pain				
	20	Undergrad volunteers – proc distraction				
	20	Undergrad volunteers – sim pain				
			Criterion Groups			
Etherton, Bianchini, Greve, & Heinly, 2005	53	Nonmalingering clinical pain	Reliable digit span	≤ 6	0	37
	35	Definite MND clinical pain		≤ 7	8	60
Etherton, Bianchini, Ciota et al., 2006 (Study 2)	49	Nonmalingering patients with clinical pain	Working Memory Index	≤ 70	4	47
	32	Definite MND patients with clinical pain				
Etherton, Bianchini, Heinly et al., 2006 (Study 2)	48	Nonmalingering patients with clinical pain patients	Processing Speed Index	≤ 75	8	69
	32	Definite MND patients with clinical pain				
Greve, Curtis et al., 2009	38	Non-MPRD clinical pain	California Verbal Learning Test-II recognition hits	≤ 7	3	24
	41	MPRD clinical pain	California Verbal Learning Test-II linear shrinkage	≥ 3	3	37
Greve et al., 2010	176	Non-MPRD clinical pain	Reliable digit span	≤ 6	1	24
	185	MPRD clinical pain		≤ 7	15	49

Note. FP = false positive error rate; MPRD = malingered pain related disability; *n* = sample size; proc = procedural distraction group; Ret = retention; sens = sensitivity; sim = simulator; T2 = Trial 2; undergrad = undergraduate.
[a]FP rate = 0% in the control and procedural distraction groups; 5% in the cold pain group;

ing Speed Index (PSI; Etherton, Bianchini, Ciota, et al., 2006; Etherton, Bianchini, Greve, & Heinly, 2005; Etherton, Bianchini, Heinly, & Greve, 2006). Two of the studies earlier also employed criterion-groups validation as a second part to their studies in studying WMI and PSI (Etherton, Bianchini, Heinly, et al., 2006; Etherton, Bianchini, Ciota, et al., 2006). Two additional criterion-groups studies examined RDS (Etherton, Bianchini, Ciota, et al., 2005; Greve, Bianchini, Etherton, Meyers, Curtis, & Ord, 2010). The remaining criterion-groups study examined the use of the CVLT-II in detecting malingering from nonmalingering in CP (Greve, Curtis, et al., 2009). Examination of Table 14.4 shows that the performance of the indicators in CP is similar to their performance in MTBI.

Post-Traumatic Stress Disorder

PTSD requires exposure to "an event or events that involved actual or threatened death or serious injury, or a threat to the physical integrity of self and others" (American Psychiatric Association [APA], 2000, p. 467) and the presence of a constellation of symptoms including (a) persistent reexperiencing of the event, (b) avoidance of reminders of the event, and (c) increased autonomic arousal. The diagnosis of PTSD relies entirely on subjective report, making it especially vulnerable to exaggeration and malingering (Guriel & Fremouw, 2003). What constitutes a "traumatic event" is subjective, and how a person interprets and reacts to such event is variable (Hall & Hall, 2006; Resnick, 1997).

Exposure to a traumatic event is relatively common, with roughly 50% (40%–60%) of community adults having experienced some type of trauma at some point in their lives (Kessler, Sonnega, Bromet, Hughes, & Nelson, 1995, as cited in Taylor, Frueh, & Asmundson, 2007). However, it is estimated that less than 10% of exposed persons actually develop PTSD (APA, 2000; Arbisi & Nelson, 2011; Kessler et al., 2005; Taylor et al., 2007), although these estimates vary as a function of the type of trauma experienced as well as the population being studied (Guriel & Fremouw, 2003).

Malingering is estimated to occur in approximately 20%–30% of PTSD personal injury claimants (Lees-Haley, 1997) and about 20%–25% of compensation-seeking combat veterans (Frueh, Hamner, Cahill, Gold, & Hamlin, 2000, as cited in Taylor et al., 2007). These rates are similar to the 30% base rates of malingering that are reported in both MTBI and CP populations. Malingering is a particular concern in the Veterans Affairs (VA) health care system because PTSD is one of the most highly compensated disabilities (Oboler, 2000). Approximately 95% of veterans diagnosed with PTSD apply for financial compensation, usually in the form of psychiatric disability (Frueh et al., 2000, as cited in Taylor et al., 2007; Rosen & Taylor, 2007).

Although PTSD is primarily considered a psychiatric disorder rather than a neurological disorder (Demakis, Gervais, & Rohling, 2008), cognitive deficits in PTSD have been reported. Meta-analyses examining the impact of PTSD on cognitive functioning have indicated a small-to-moderate effect on overall cognitive functioning (d = 0.215 [Brewin, et al., 2007]; d = 0.30 [Oien, et al., 2011]). In particular, problems with attention, learning and memory, and executive function have been documented (Oien et al., 2011; Solomon & Mikulincer, 2006; Taylor et al., 2007).

Given the prevalence of malingering in PTSD populations, as well as the presence of multidimensional symptom presentations (i.e., psychiatric and cognitive), validity issues are important moderators for clinicians to study so they can distinguish individuals with PTSD from those who are malingering PTSD when financial incentive for disability or impairment is present (Demakis et al., 2008). In fact, malingering is such a salient concern that the *Diagnostic and Statistical Manual of Mental Disorders* (4th ed., text rev.; *DSM-IV-TR*) explicitly cautions clinicians to rule out malingering before diagnosing PTSD (APA, 2000). The routine failure to do so likely compromises most general PTSD research and threatens the clinical and forensic diagnosis of PTSD (Morel & Shepherd, 2008; Rosen, 2006; Rosen & Taylor, 2007).

Over the past decade, there has been a steadily increasing body of research on the methods that can be employed to detect PTSD malingering. Thus, so far, the empirical investigation has almost exclusively relied on identifying malingered performance with questionnaire-based methods (Morel, 1998). Some of the self-report measures that have been consistently examined in this area include the Minnesota Multiphasic Personality Inventory-2 (MMPI-2; Butcher, Dahlstrom, Graham, Tellegen, & Kaemmer, 1989), Trauma Symptom Inventory (TSI; Briere, 1995), and Personality Assessment Inventory (PAI; Morey, 1991), as well as the Structured Interview of Reported Symptoms (SIRS; Rogers, 1992). It is unfortunate that the confidence in the accuracy of these methods is limited for several reasons: (a) little of the existing research has been cross validated; (b) clinically appropriate comparison groups have either not been used or are underused; and/or (c) studies using criterion-groups research has not been conducted (Guriel & Fremouw, 2003).

Relatively few studies exist that examine cognitive exaggeration in PTSD using well-known and empirically validated symptom validity measures. Rosen and Powel (2003) provided a case report of an individual diagnosed with PTSD who failed the PDRT at below-chance levels (PDRT total = 22 / 72, p = 0.001). Demakis et al. (2008) examined the rates of cognitive and psychological exaggeration in claimants with symptoms of PTSD who were evaluated in a medicolegal context. Altogether, 29% of the patients failed at least one cognitive symptom validity measure (WMT, Computerized Assessment of Response Dias [CARB], TOMM; Millis & Volinsky [2001] CVLT algorithm) at published cutoffs. Further analyses showed a negative relationship between failure rates and neuropsychological performance. That is, individuals who failed two or more cognitive SVTs scored worse on measures of neuropsychological functioning than individuals failing one cognitive SVT.

Greiffenstein and Baker (2008) conducted a study looking at physical symptoms and cognitive validity in a sample of 799 individuals dually diagnosed with PTSD and persistent postconcussion syndrome (PPCS). Cognitive exaggeration was measured using Trial 2 and the retention trial of the TOMM as well as RDS. Cutoffs associated with the 90% and 99% specificity rates (i.e., 10% and 1% false positive error rates, respectively) were used to determine the percentage of individuals in each group who exhibited invalid performance. As observed in the Demakis et al. (2008) study, results from this study showed a "dose-response" relationship between rates of failure and diagnostic category, with the highest failure rates being observed for the group dually diagnosed with PTSD and PPCS.

The findings of the Demakis et al. (2008) and Greiffenstein and Baker (2008) studies address the necessity of assessing cognitive validity in PTSD populations. However, neither study included participants who were formally diagnosed with PTSD, but rather they endorsed PTSD symptomatology. Moreover, neither study provided data (e.g., diagnostic statistics) that are helpful in detecting malingered PTSD.

There has only been one SVT that has been developed to measure performance validity specifically for PTSD. In 1995, Morel developed a forced-choice SVT, the Morel Emotional Numbing Test (MENT), which detects simulated impairment of facial affect recognition in individuals with alleged PTSD (Morel, 1995, 1998). It is a stand-alone test of symptom validity that assesses the (in)ability to recognize facial expressions and is highly resistant to most neurological illnesses (Morel & Marshman, 2008). In general, results from studies have shown that military veteran disability claimants, some of whom were diagnosed with PTSD, obtain significantly more errors than clinical comparison groups (Morel, 1998). A meta-analysis of results from studies using the MENT has shown that the test exhibits high sensitivity (0.73) and specificity (0.97; Morel & Shepherd, 2008). However, independent validation of this test has not yet been conducted and is needed.

The Diagnosis of Malingering

The research described in the previous sections focused on the ability of tests and scores to accurately identify invalid cognitive test performance and to determine at what point those scores are consistent with an intentional effort to appear disabled. Using those data to conclude that an individual is, in fact, malingering (i.e., diagnosis as opposed to simple detection) requires a second level of inference (Heilbronner et al., 2009). Malingering is neither a diagnosis in *DSM* nor does *DSM* outline any true criteria for determining if an individual is malingering. Instead, *DSM-IV* simply lists conditions which, if present, mean that malingering should be suspected. Terms are not operationally defined, and no standards are described. However, detailed and comprehensive systems for the diagnosis of malingering have been published.

Compiling and integrating various research criteria used in studies of neuropsychological malingering, Slick et al., (1999) developed a set of explicit criteria for the diagnosis of MND. By requiring multiple positive indications of malingering (from cognitive testing and self-report), this system further reduces the risk of false positive errors. The Bianchini et al. (2005) criteria for malingered pain-related disability (MPRD) are similar to those of Slick et al. (1999) but differ by giving equal weight to signs of cognitive, psychological, and physical malingering. The study of malingering in TBI cases and more recently MPRD has been facilitated by these formal diagnostic systems. The forensic assessment and diagnosis of malingering has benefitted as well from these diagnostic systems and from the research based on them. There are no formal criteria for the diagnosis of malingered PTSD. However, the conceptual framework underpinning modern malingering diagnosis is relevant to PTSD.

Past attempts to define malingering have often placed the clinician in the position of inferring intention from a single event or finding (e.g., *DSM*). Instead, the Slick et al. (1999) criteria for MND and the Bianchini et al. (2005) criteria for MPRD consider multiple, highly improbable events as indicative of intent. This is a more comprehensive approach that relies heavily on objective, quantitative indicators of exaggeration as opposed to a qualitative assessment of specific or single behavior. Larrabee, Greiffenstein, Greve, and Bianchini (2007) have articulated the conceptual basis of this more modern approach:

> It is not necessary to rely on single events that unequivocally demonstrate intent because the MND and MPRD criteria are based on behaviors and symptom reports that are atypical for and not representative of expected clinical findings in genuine, unequivocal neurological, psychiatric, or developmental disorders. (p. 338)

The application of the Slick et al. (1999) system is limited because it specifically focuses on cognition, and evidence of *cognitive* malingering is necessary for a diagnosis of MND. In contrast, although the Bianchini et al. (2005) system was developed with CP in mind, their framework can reasonably be applied to any potentially compensable condition, including PTSD. This application of the MPRD system is appropriate because the focus is on malingering of disability and not simply on a single medical or psychological condition or behavioral domain in which disability might manifest (i.e., cognition).

Because the focus of the MPRD criteria is on the exaggeration of *disability* and not etiology or condition, reliable evidence of exaggerated disability, regardless of the behavioral domain, is what is needed for a diagnosis. What may be lacking in some potentially compensable conditions is data on specific indicators in that population to demonstrate at what level a finding becomes "atypical for and not representative of expected clinical findings'' for the condition in question. The routine inclusion of various nonmalingering clinical samples in the study of performance and self-report validity will help address this issue. An explicit system for the diagnosis of malingered PTSD does not exist in the literature; however, the MPRD system adapts very well to the problem of PTSD because it explicitly includes parameters for the exaggeration of psychological symptoms and the exaggeration of mental impairment through SVT performances.

SUMMARY AND DISCUSSION

MTBI, pain conditions/syndromes, and PTSD are clinical conditions with which patients commonly present for evaluation by neuropsychologists. Patients with these conditions report varied symptoms that are sometimes linked to disability in the context of civil litigation. Such claims of disability are directly related to damages in litigation. The disability claim may be based on symptoms from multiple behavioral domains including cognitive, emotional, and physical symptoms (Bianchini et al, 2005).

Cognitive impairment is documented in brain trauma, chronic pain, and PTSD. The presence of cognitive impairment can add value to a compensation claim, particularly in conditions in which the injury is not primarily cognitive (e.g., CP, psychiatric injury) because it may result in a relatively higher level of disability. Because cognitive disability can add value to a compensation claim, there is incentive to exaggerate or fabricate cognitive impairment. Thus, cognitive SVTs are important for the evaluation of these three conditions despite the diversity of primarily physical, cognitive, and emotional sources for symptoms and disability.

This chapter provides clinicians and researchers with an accessible reference on the use of cognitive SVT measures in the three target populations. In this chapter, we have presented the empirical literature for the use of various cognitive SVTs in patients with pain and posttraumatic stress. The recent literature on SVTs in the MTBI has been described here. Good earlier summaries of the research on the use of these measures in patients with MTBI are available and are cited in this chapter.

We offer the following recommendations for the use of SVT:

1. Carefully review the relevant research and make judgments regarding performance validity based on the generalizability of the particular research samples to the examinee who is the subject of inquiry. Data and interpretive recommendations in test manuals may be modified by new research. It is the clinicians' responsibility to stay current with the literature on the SVTs they use for validity assessment.
2. Base decisions about performance validity on the specificity of observed scores in the context of the nature of the clinical/forensic/research question and circumstances of the assessment. Clinicians should be aware of those situations in which SVT failure may be more likely even at relatively conservative cutoffs.
3. Be aware that, in general, a single positive SVT finding may be sufficient to raise concern about the validity of a specific test result but may not be sufficient for a diagnosis of malingering. It is also possible that a single positive finding (excluding a significantly below-chance score on a forced-choice SVT) is an anomaly and does not indicate that evaluation results are compromised.

4. Use a multimethod (performance, self-report), multidomain (cognitive, psychological, physical) validity assessment approach to ensure a comprehensive assessment of validity regardless of the alleged condition or clinical presentation. The accuracy of conclusions rests almost entirely on the validity of test data. Failure to detect invalid test results may lead to misdiagnosis and worse (e.g., unnecessary medical treatments).

5. All data from an evaluation should be analyzed within a formal diagnostic system such as those of Slick et al. (1999) or Bianchini et al. (2005). These systems protect against false positive diagnostic errors by requiring multiple relatively independent positive findings at relatively strict cutoffs to diagnose malingering.

CONCLUSIONS

There is a large body of empirical literature that provides the basis for examining symptom validity and malingering in MTBI samples. Continued research on embedded measures will help protect the ability of psychologists to detect invalid cognitive performance, particularly given efforts (e.g., coaching) to reduce the effectiveness of freestanding SVTs. There is a growing literature on the use of cognitive SVTs in patients with pain, but more research is needed particularly in the area of physical capacity assessment. Cognitive SVTs validated with moderate and severe TBI groups can be applied to patients with pain.

There is a small body of research on the use of symptom validity measures with patients claiming PTSD. As with pain populations, data on cognitive SVTs from persons with significant brain pathology can be helpful in PTSD cases. Work in this area may further benefit from the use of specific malingering diagnostic criteria such as those proposed by Bianchini et al. (2005) for use in CP. Overall, research on, and clinical application of, symptom validity assessment methods is well developed in patients with TBI, but continued work is needed in patients with pain and PTSD. The framework for further development in these conditions is present and awaits only the researchers and data.

REFERENCES

Alexander, M. P. (1995). Mild traumatic brain injury: Pathophysiology, natural history, and clinical management. *American Academy of Neurology*, 45(7), 1253–1260.

American Academy of Clinical Neuropsychology. (2007). American Academy of Clinical Neuropsychology (AACN) practice guidelines for neuropsychological assessment and consultation. *The Clinical Neuropsychologist*, 21(2), 209–231.

American Psychiatric Association. (2000). *Diagnostic and statistical manual of mental disorders* (4th ed., text rev.). Washington, DC: Author.

Arbisi, P. A., & Nelson, N. (2011, June). *The neuropsychology of posttraumatic stress disorder*. A workshop presented at the 9th Annual Conference of the American Academy of Clinical Neuropsychology, Washington, DC.

Arciniegas, D. B., Anderson, C. A., Topkoff, J., & McAllister, T. W. (2005). Mild traumatic brain injury: A neuropsychiatric approach to diagnosis, evaluation, and treatment. *Neuropsychiatric Disease and Treatment*, 1(4), 311–327.

Ardolf, B. R., Denney, R. L., & Houston, C. M. (2007). Base rates of negative response bias and malingered neurocognitive dysfunction among criminal defendants referred for neuropsychological evaluation. *The Clinical Neuropsychologist*, 21(6), 899–916.

Ashendorf, L., O'Bryant, S. E., & McCaffrey, R. J. (2003). Specificity of malingering detection strategies in older adults using the CVLT and WCST. *The Clinical Neuropsychologist*, 17(2), 255–262.

Barker, M. D., Horner, M. D., & Bachman, D. L. (2010). Embedded indices of effort in the repeatable battery for the assessment of neuropsychological status (RBANS) in a geriatric sample. *The Clinical Neuropsychologist*, 24(6), 1064–1077.

Bauer, L., & McCaffrey, R. J. (2006). Coverage of the Test of Memory Malingering, Victoria Symptom Validity Test, and Word Memory Test on the Internet: Is test security threatened? *Archives of Clinical Neuropsychology*, 21(1), 121–126.

Belanger, H. G., Curtiss, G., Demery, J. A., Lebowitz, B. K., & Vanderploeg, R. D. (2005). Factors moderating neuropsychological outcomes following mild traumatic brain injury: A meta-analysis. *Journal of the International Neuropsychological Society*, 11(3), 215–227.

Bernstein, D. M. (1999). Subject review: Recovery from mild head injury. *Brain Injury*, 13(3), 151–172.

Bianchini, K. J., Curtis, K. L., & Greve, K. W. (in press). Detection of malingering in mild traumatic brain injury, chronic pain, and posttraumatic stress disorder. In S. Bush & D. Carone (eds.), *MTBI, symptom validity assessment, and malingering*.

Bianchini, K. J., Curtis, K. L., & Greve, K. W. (2006). Compensation and malingering in traumatic brain injury: A dose-response relationship? *The Clinical Neuropsychologist*, 20(4), 831–847.

Bianchini, K. J., Etherton, J. L., & Greve, K. W. (2004). Diagnosing cognitive malingering in patients with work-related pain: Four cases. *Journal of Forensic Neuropsychology*, 4, 65–85.

Bianchini, K. J., Greve, K. W., & Glynn, G. (2005). On the diagnosis of malingered pain-related disability: Lessons from cognitive malingering research. *The Spine Journal*, 5(4), 404–417.

Bianchini, K. J., Mathias, C. W., & Greve, K. W. (2001). Symptom validity testing: A critical review. *The Clinical Neuropsychologist*, 15(1), 19–45.

Binder, L. M. Persisting symptoms after mild head injury: a review of the postconcussive syndrome. *J Clin Exp Neuropsychol*. 1986 Aug;8(4): 323–46.

Binder, L. M. (1990). Malingering following minor head trauma. *The Clinical Neuropsychologist*, 4, 25–36.

Binder, L. M. (1993). *Portland Digit Recognition Test manual* (2nd ed.). Portland, OR: Author.

Binder, L. M. (1997). A review of mild head trauma. Part II: Clinical implications. *Journal of Clinical and Experimental Neuropsychology*, 19(3), 432–457.

Binder, L. M., & Rohling, M. L. (1996). Money matters: A meta-analytic review of financial incentives on recovery after closed-head injury. *American Journal of Psychiatry*, 153(1), 7–10.

Binder, L. M., Rohling, M. L., & Larrabee, G. J. (1997). A review of mild head trauma. Part I: Meta-analytic review of neuropsychological studies. *Journal of Clinical and Experimental Neuropsychology*, 19(3), 421–431.

Boden, S. D., Davis, D. O., Dina, T. S., Patronas, N. J., & Wiesel, S. W. (1990). Abnormal magnetic-resonance scans of the lumbar spine in asymptomatic subjects. A prospective investigation. *Journal of Bone and Joint Surgery*, 72(3), 403–408.

Booksh, R. L., Pella, R. D., Singh, A. N., & Gouvier, W. D. (2010). Ability of college students to simulate ADHD on objective measures of attention. *Journal of Attention Disorders*, 13(4), 325–338.

Boone, K. B. (2007). *Assessment of feigned cognitive impairment: A neuropsychological perspective*. New York, NY: Guilford Press.

Boone, K. B. (2009). The need for continuous and comprehensive sampling of effort/response bias during neuropsychological examinations. *The Clinical Neuropsychologist*, 23(4), 729–741.

Boone, K. B., & Lu, P. H. (2007). Non-forced-choice effort measures. In G. J. Larrabee (Ed.), *Assessment of malingered neuropsychological deficits* (pp. 27–43). New York, NY: Oxford University Press.

Bortnik, K. E., Boone, K. B., Marion, S. D., Amano, S., Ziegler, E., Cottingham, M. E., . . . Zeller, M. A. (2010). Examination of various WMS-III Logical Memory scores in the assessment of response bias. *The Clinical Neuropsychologist*, 24(2), 344–357.

Brady, J. P., & Lind, D. L. (1961). Experimental analysis of hysterical blindness. *Archives of General Psychiatry*, 4, 331–339.

Brewin, C. R., Kleiner, J. S., Vasterling, J. J., & Field, A. P. (2007). Memory for emotionally neutral information in posttraumatic stress disorder: A meta-analytic investigation. *Journal of Abnormal Psychology*, 116(3), 448–463.

Briere, J. (1995). *Trauma symptom inventory professional manual*. Odessa, FL: Psychological Assessment Resources.

Bush, S. S., Ruff, R. M., Tröster, A. I., Barth, J. T., Koffler, S. P., Pliskin, N. H., . . . Silver, C. H. (2005). Symptom validity assessment: Practice issues and medical necessity NAN policy & planning committee. *Archives of Clinical Neuropsychology*, 20(4), 419–426.

Butcher, J. N., Dahlstrom, W. G., Graham, J. R., Tellegen, A., & Kaemmer, B. (1989). *Minnesota Multiphasic Personality Inventory-2 (MMPI-2): Manual for administration and scoring*. Minneapolis, MN: University of Minnesota Press.

Carroll, L. J., Cassidy, J. D., Peloso, P. M., Borg, J., von Holst, H., Holm, L., . . . Pépin, M. (2004). Prognosis for mild traumatic brain injury: Results of the WHO Collaborating Centre Task Force on Mild Traumatic Brain Injury. *Journal of Rehabilitation Medicine*, (43), 84–105.

Chafetz, M. D. (2008). Malingering on the social security disability consultative exam: Predictors and base rates. *The Clinical Neuropsychologist*, 22(3), 529–546.

Chafetz, M. (2011). Reducing the probability of false positives in malingering detection of social security disability claimants. *The Clinical Neuropsychologist, 25*(7), 1–14.

Conder, R., Allen, L., & Cox, D. (1992). *Manual for the computerized assessment of response bias.* Durham, NC: CogniSyst.

Curtis, K. L., Greve, K. W., & Bianchini, K. J. (2009). The Wechsler Adult Intelligence Scale-III and malingering in traumatic brain injury: Classification accuracy in known groups. *Assessment, 16*(4), 401–414.

Curtis, K. L., Greve, K. W., Brasseux, R., & Bianchini, K. J. (2010). Criterion groups validation of the Seashore Rhythm Test and Speech Sounds Perception Test for the detection of malingering in traumatic brain injury. *The Clinical Neuropsychologist, 24*(5), 882–897.

Davis, J. J., Wall, J. R., Ramos, C. K., Whitney, K. A., & Barisa, M. T. (2010). Using grip strength force curves to detect simulation: A preliminary investigation. *Archives of Clinical Neuropsychology, 25*(3), 204–211.

Demakis, G. J., Gervais, R. O., & Rohling, M. L. (2008). The effect of failure on cognitive and psychological symptom validity tests in litigants with symptoms of post-traumatic stress disorder. *The Clinical Neuropsychologist, 22*(5), 879–895.

Dikmen, S. S., Corrigan, J., Levin, H. S., Machamer, J., Stiers, W., & Weisskopf, M. G. (2009). Cognitive outcome following traumatic brain injury. *Journal of Head Trauma Rehabilitation, 24*(6), 1–9.

Dikmen, S. S., Machamer, J. E., Winn, H. R., & Temkin, N. R. (1995). Neuropsychological outcome at 1-year post head injury. *Neuropsychology, 9*, 80–90.

Eccleston, C. (1994). Chronic pain and attention: A cognitive approach. *British Journal of Clinical Psychology, 33*(Pt. 4), 535–547.

Eccleston, C. (1995). Chronic pain and distraction: An experimental investigation into the role of sustained and shifting attention in the processing of chronic persistent pain. *Behavioral Research and Therapy, 33*(4), 391–405.

Etherton, J. L., Bianchini, K. J., Ciota, M. A., & Greve, K. W. (2005). Reliable digit span is unaffected by laboratory-induced pain: Implications for clinical use. *Assessment, 12*, 101–106.

Etherton, J. L., Bianchini, K. J, Ciota, M. A., Heinly, M. T., & Greve, K. W. (2006). Pain, malingering and the WAIS-III Working Memory Index. *The Spine Journal, 6*, 61–71.

Etherton, J. L., Bianchini, K. J., Greve, K. W., & Ciota, M. A. (2005). Test of Memory Malingering performance is unaffected by laboratory-induced pain: Implications for clinical use. *Archives of Clinical Neuropsychology, 20*(3), 375–384.

Etherton, J. L., Bianchini, K. J., Greve, K. W., & Heinly, M. T. (2005). Sensitivity and specificity of reliable digit span in malingered pain-related disability. *Assessment, 12*, 130–136.

Etherton, J. L., Bianchini, K. J., Heinly, M. T., & Greve, K. W. (2006). Pain, malingering, and performance on the WAIS-III Processing Speed Index. *Journal of Clinical and Experimental Neuropsychology, 28*, 1218–1237.

Fishbain, D. A., Cutler, R., Rosomoff, H. L., & Rosomoff, R. S. (1999). Chronic pain disability exaggeration/malingering and submaximal effort research. *Clinical Journal of Pain, 15*(4), 244–274.

Freeman, T., Powell, M., & Kimbrell, T. (2008). Measuring symptom exaggeration in veterans with chronic posttraumatic stress disorder. *Psychiatry Research, 158*(3), 374–380.

Frenchman, K. A., Fox, A. M., & Maybery, M. T. (2005). Neuropsychological studies of mild traumatic brain injury: A meta-analytic review of research since 1995. *Journal of Clinical and Experimental Neuropsychology, 27*(3), 33–351.

Frueh, B. C., Hamner, M. B., Cahill, S. P., Gold, P. B., & Hamlin, K. L., (2000). Apparent symptom overreporting in combat veterans evaluated for PTSD. *Clinical Psychology Review, 20*(7), 853–885.

Gatchel, R. J., Bernstein, D., Stowell, A. W., & Pransky, G. (2008). Psychosocial differences between high-risk acute vs. chronic low back pain patients. *Pain Practice, 8*(2), 91–97.

Gervais, R. O., Russell, A. S., Green, P., Allen, L. M. 3rd, Ferrari, R., Pieschl, S. D. (2001). Effort testing in patients with fibromyalgia and disability incentives. *J Rheumatol.* Aug 28(8), 1892–9.

Goebel, J. A., Sataloff, R. T., Hanson, J. M., Nashner, L. M., Hirshout, D. S. & Sokolow, C. C. (1997). Posturographic evidence of nonorganic sway patterns in normal subjects, patients, and suspected malingerers. *Otolaryngology Head and Neck Surgery, 117*(4), 292–302.

Green, P. (2005). *Green's Word Memory Test for Windows. User's manual and program.* Edmonton, Alberta, Canada: Green's.

Green, P., Allen, L. M., & Astner, K. (1996). *The Word Memory Test: A user's guide to the oral and computer-administered forms, US Version 1.1.* Durham, NC: CogniSyst.

Green, P., Iverson, G. L. & Allen, L. (1999). Detecting malingering in head injury litigation with the Word Memory Test. *Brain Inj.* Oct 13(10) 813–9.

Greiffenstein, M. F., & Baker, W. J. (2008). Validity testing in dually diagnosed post-traumatic stress disorder and mild closed head injury. *The Clinical Neuropsychologist, 22*(3), 565–582.

Greiffenstein, M. F., Baker, W. J., & Gola, T. (1994). Validation of malingered amnesia measures with a large clinical sample. *Psychological Assessment*, 6, 218–224.

Greve, K. W., & Bianchini, K. J. (2004). Setting empirical cut-offs on psychometric indicators of negative response bias: A methodological commentary with recommendations. *Archives of Clinical Neuropsychology*, 19(4), 533–541.

Greve, K. W., & Bianchini, K. J. (2009). Schmerz und Beschwerdenvalidierrung [Symptom validity testing in pain]. In T. Merten & D. Dettenborn (Eds.), *Diagnostik der Beschwerdenvalidität* (pp. 193–229). Berlin, Germany: Deutsch Psychologen Verlag GmbH.

Greve, K. W., Bianchini, K. J., & Ameduri, C. J. (2003). Use of a forced-choice test of tactile discrimination in the evaluation of functional sensory loss: A report of 3 cases. *Archives of Physical Medicine and Rehabilitation*, 84(8), 1233–1236.

Greve, K. W., Bianchini, K. J., Black, F. W., Heinly, M. T., Love, J. M., Swift, D. A., & Ciota, M. (2006). The prevalence of cognitive malingering in persons reporting exposure to occupational and environmental substances. *NeuroToxicology*, 27(6), 940–950.

Greve, K. W., Bianchini, K. J., Etherton, J. L., Meyers, J. E., Curtis, K. L., & Ord, J. S. (2010). The reliable digit span test in chronic pain: Classification accuracy in detecting malingered pain-related disability. *The Clinical Neuropsychologist*, 24(1), 137–152.

Greve, K. W., Bianchini, K. J., Etherton, J. L., Ord, J. S., & Curtis, K. L. (2009). Detecting malingered pain-related disability: Classification accuracy of the Portland Digit Recognition Test. *The Clinical Neuropsychologist*, 23(5), 850–869.

Greve, K. W., Binder, L. M., & Bianchini, K. J. (2009). Rates of below-chance performance in forced-choice symptom validity tests. *The Clinical Neuropsychologist*, 23(3), 534–544.

Greve, K. W., Curtis, K. L., Bianchini, K. J., & Ord, J. (2009). Are the original and second edition of the California Verbal Learning Test equally accurate in detecting malingering? *Assessment*, 16, 237–248.

Greve, K. W., Etherton, J. L., Ord, J., Bianchini, K. J., & Curtis, K. L. (2009). Detecting malingered pain-related disability: Classification accuracy of the test of memory malingering. *The Clinical Neuropsychologist*, 23, 1250–1271.

Greve, K. W., Heinly, M. T., Bianchini, K. J., & Love, J. M. (2009). Malingering detection with the Wisconsin Card Sorting Test in mild traumatic brain injury. *The Clinical Neuropsychology*, 23(2), 343–362.

Greve, K. W., Lotz, K. L., & Bianchini, K. J. (2008). Observed versus estimated IQ as an index of malingering in traumatic brain injury: Classification accuracy in known groups. *Applied Neuropsychology*, 15(3), 161–169.

Greve, K. W., Ord, J. S., Bianchini, K. J., & Curtis, K. L. (2009). The prevalence of malingering in chronic pain patients referred for psychological evaluation in a medico-legal context. *Archives of Physical Medicine & Rehabilitation*, 90, 1117–1126.

Greve, K. W., Ord, J., Curtis, K. L., Bianchini, K. J., & Brennan, A. (2008). Detecting malingering in traumatic brain injury and chronic pain: A comparison of three forced-choice symptom validity tests. *The Clinical Neuropsychologist*, 22, 896–918.

Grosz, H. J., & Zimmerman, J. (1965). Experimental analysis of hysterical blindness: A follow-up report and new experimental data. *Archives of General Psychiatry*, 13, 255–260.

Gunn, D., Batchelor, J., & Jones, M. (2010). Detection of simulated memory impairment in 6- to 11-year-old children. *Child Neuropsychology*, 16(2), 105–118.

Guo, H. R., Tanaka, S., Cameron, L. L., Seligman, P. J., Behrens, V. J., Ger, J., . . . Putz-Anderson, V. (1995). Back pain among workers in the United States: National estimates and workers at high risk. *American Journal of Industrial Medicine*, 28(5), 591–602.

Guo, H. R., Tanaka, S., Halperin, W. E., & Cameron, L. L. (1999). Back pain prevalence in US industry and estimates of lost workdays. *American Journal of Public Health*, 89(7), 1029–1035.

Guriel, J., & Fremouw, W. (2003). Assessing malingered posttraumatic stress disorder: A critical review. *Clinical Psychology Review*, 23(7), 881–904.

Hall, R. C., & Hall, R. C. (2006). Malingering of PTSD: Forensic and diagnostic considerations, characteristics of malingerers and clinical presentations. *General Hospital Psychiatry*, 28(6), 525–535.

Harris, I., Mulford, J., Solomon, M., van Gelder, J. M., & Young, J. (2005). Association between compensation status and outcome after surgery: A meta-analysis. *Journal of the American Medical Association*, 293(13), 1644–1652.

Harrison, A. G., Edwards, M. J., Armstrong, I., & Parker, K. C. (2010). An investigation of methods to detect feigned reading disabilities. *Archives of Clinical Neuropsychology*, 25(2), 89–93.

Hart, R. P., Martelli, M. F., & Zasler, N. D. (2000). Chronic pain and neuropsychological functioning. *Neuropsychology Review*, 10(3), 131–149.

Hart, R. P., Wade, J. B., & Martelli, M. F. (2003). Cognitive impairment in patients with chronic pain: The significance of stress. *Current Pain and Headache Reports*, 7(2), 116–126.

Heilbronner, R. L., Sweet, J. J., Morgan, J. E., Larrabee, G. J., & Millis, S. R. (2009). American Academy of Clinical Neuropsychology Consensus Conference Statement on the neuropsychological assessment of effort, response bias, and malingering. *The Clinical Neuropsychologist*, 23(7), 1093–1129.

Hendler, N. (1997). Diagnosis: Reduced disability costs. *Risk Management*, 44(10), 14–18.

Heubrock, D., & Petermann, F. (1998). Neuropsychological assessment of suspected malingering: Research results, evaluation techniques, and further directions of research and application. *European Journal of Psychological Assessment*, 14(3), 211–225.

Hirsch, G., Beach, G., Cooke, C., Menard, M., & Locke, S. (1991). Relationship between performance on lumbar dynamometry and Wadell score in a population with low-back pain. *Spine*, 16(9), 1039–1043.

Ingebrigsten, T., Waterloo, K., Marup-Jensen, S., Attner, E., & Romner, B. (1998). Quantification of post-concussion symptoms 3 months after minor head injury in 100 consecutive patients. *Journal of Neurology*, 245(9), 609–612.

Iverson, G. L. (2005). Outcome from mild traumatic brain injury. *Current Opinions in Psychiatry*, 18(3), 301–317.

Iverson, G. L. (2007). Indentifying exaggeration and malingering. *Pain Practice*, 7(2), 94–102.

Iverson, G. L., King, R. J., Scott, J. G., & Adams, R. L. (2001). Cognitive complaints in litigating patients with head injuries or chronic pain. *Journal of Forensic Neuropsychology*, 2, 19–30.

Iverson, G. L., & McCracken, L. M. (1997). "Postconcussive" symptoms in persons with chronic pain. *Brain Injury*, 11(11), 783–790.

Jasinski, L. J., Berry, D. T., Shandera, A. L., & Clark, J. A. (2011). Use of the Wechsler Adult Intelligence Scale digit span subtest in malingering detection: A meta-analytic review. *Journal of Clinical and Experimental Neuropsychology*, 33(3), 300–314.

Karzmark, P., Hall, K., & Englander, J. (1995). Late-onset post-concussion symptoms after mild brain injury: The role of premorbid, injury-related, environmental, and personality factors. *Brain Injury*, 9(1), 21–26.

Kay, N. R., & Morris-Jones, H. (1998). Pain clinic management of medico-legal litigants. *Injury*, 29(4), 305–308.

Kessler, R. C., Berglund, P., Demler, O., Jin, R., Merikangas, K. R., & Walters, E. E. (2005). Lifetime prevalence and age-of-onset distributions of DSM-IV disorders in the National Comorbidity Survey Replication. *Archives of General Psychiatry*, 62(6), 593–602.

Kessler, R. C., Sonnega, A., Bromet, E., Hughes, M., & Nelson, C. B. (1995). Posttraumatic stress disorder in the National Comorbidity Survey. *Archives of General Psychiatry*, 52(12), 1048–1060.

Kim, M. S., Boone, K. B., Victor, T., Marion, S. D., Amano, S., Cottingham, M. E., . . . Zeller, M. E.. (2010). The Warrington Recognition Memory Test for words as a measure of response bias: Total score and response time cutoffs developed on "real world" credible and noncredible subjects. *Archives of Clinical Neuropsychology*, 25(1), 60–70.

Kim, N., Boone, K. B., Victor, T., Lu, P. Keatings, C., & Mitchell, C. (2010). Sensitivity and specificity of a digit symbol recognition trial in the identification of response bias. *Archives of Clinical Neuropsychology*, 25(5), 420–428.

Kirkwood, M. W., Hargrave, D. D., & Kirk, J. W. (2011). The value of the WISC-IV digit span subtest in detecting noncredible performance during pediatric neuropsychological examinations. *Archives of Clinical Neuropsychology*, 26(5), 377–384.

Krempl, G. A., & Dobie, R. A. (1998). Evaluation of posturography in the detection of malingering subjects. *American Journal of Otolaryngology*, 19(5), 619–627.

Krietler, S., & Niv, D. (2007). Cognitive impairment in chronic pain. *Pain Clinical Uupdates: International Association for the Study of Pain*, 15(4), 1–4.

Krishnan, M., & Donders, J. (2011). Embedded assessment of validity using the continuous visual memory test in patients with traumatic brain injury. *Archives of Clinical Neuropsychology*, 26(3), 176–183.

Lange, R. T., Iverson, G. L., Brooks, B. L., & Rennison, V. L. (2010). Influence of poor effort on self-reported symptoms and neurocognitive test performance following mild traumatic brain injury. *The Journal of Clinical and Experimental Neuropsychology*, 32(9), 961–972.

Larrabee, G. J. (2003). Exaggerated pain report in litigants with malingered neurocognitive dysfunction. *The Clinical Neuropsychologist*, 17(3), 395–401.

Larrabee, G. J. (2005). Assessment of malingering. In G. J. Larrabee (Ed.), *Forensic neuropsychology: A scientific approach* (pp. 115–158). New York, NY: Oxford University Press.

Larrabee, G. J. (2007). *Assessment of malingered neuropsychological deficits*. New York, NY: Oxford University Press.

Larrabee, G. J., Greiffenstein, M. F., Greve, K. W., & Bianchini, K. J. (2007). Refining diagnostic criteria for malingering. In G. J. Larrabee (Ed.), *Assessment of Malingered Neuropsychological Deficits* (pp. 334–371). New York, NY: Oxford University Press.

Leavitt, F., & Sweet, J. J. (1986). Characteristics and frequency of malingering among patients with low back pain. *Pain*, 25(3), 357–364.

Lees-Haley, P. R. (1997). MMPI-2 base rates for 492 personal injury plaintiffs: Implications and challenges for forensic assessment. *Journal of Clinical Psychology*, 53(7), 745–755.

Lezak, M. D., Howieson, D. B., & Loring, D. W. (2004). *Neuropsychological assessment* (4th ed.). New York, NY: Oxford University Press.

Lindstrom, W., Coleman, C., Thomassin, K., Southall, C. M., & Lindstrom, J. H. (2011). Simulated dyslexia in postsecondary students: Description and detection using embedded validity indicators. *The Clinical Neuropsychologist*, 25(2), 302–322.

Lindstrom, W. A. Jr., Lindstrom, J. H., Coleman, C., Nelson, J., & Gregg, N. (2009). The diagnostic accuracy of symptom validity tests with postsecondary students with learning disabilities: A preliminary investigation. *Archives of Clinical Neuropsychology*, 24(7), 659–669.

Linton, S. J. (2000). A review of the psychological risk factors in back and neck pain. *Spine*, 25(9), 1148–1156.

Lynch, W. J. (2004). Determination of effort level, exaggeration, and malingering in neurocognitive assessment. *Journal of Head Trauma Rehabilitation*, 19(3), 277–283.

MacLeod, A. D. S. (2010). Post concussion syndrome: The attraction of the psychological by the organic. *Medical Hypotheses*, 74(6), 1033–1035.

Martins, M., & Martins, I. P. (2010). Memory malingering: Evaluating WMT criteria. *Applied Neuropsychology*, 17(3), 177–182.

Mathias, C. W., Greve, K. W., Bianchini, K. B., Houston, R. J., & Crouch, J. A. (2002). Detecting malingered neurocognitive dysfunction using the reliable digit span in traumatic brain injury. *Assessment*, 9(3), 301–308.

McCrea, M. (2008). *Mild traumatic brain injury and post-concussion syndrome: The new evidence base for diagnosis and treatment.* New York, NY: Oxford University Press.

McCrea, M., Iverson, G. L., McAllister, T. W., Hammeke, T. A., Powell, M. R., Barr, W. B., & Kelly, J. P. (2009). An integrated review of recovery after mild traumatic brain injury (MTBI): Implications for clinical management. *The Clinical Neuropsychologist*, 23(8), 1368–1390.

Meyers, J. E., & Diep, A. (2000). Assessment of malingering in chronic pain patients using neuropsychological tests. *Applied Neuropsychology*, 7(3), 133–139.

Meyers, J. E., & Volbrecht, M. E. (2003). A validation of multiple malingering detection methods in a large clinical sample. *Archives of Clinical Neuropsychology*, 18(3), 261–276.

Mild Traumatic Brain Injury Committee of the Head Injury Interdisciplinary Special Interest Group of the American Congress of Rehabilitation Medicine. (1993). Definition of mild traumatic brain injury. *Journal of Head Trauma Rehabilitation*, 8(3), 86–87.

Miller, J. B., Millis, S. R., Rapport, L. J., Bashem, J. R., Hanks, R. A., & Axelrod, B. N. (2011). Detection of insufficient effort using the advanced clinical solutions for the Wechsler Memory Scale, fourth edition. *The Clinical Neuropsychologist*, 25(1), 160–172.

Miller, L. (2001). Not just malingering: Syndrome diagnosis in traumatic brain injury litigation. *Neurorehabilitation*, 16(2), 109–122.

Millis, S. R., & Volinsky, C. T. (2001). Assessment of response bias in mild head injury: Beyond malingering tests. *Journal of Clinical and Experimental Neuropsychology*, 23(6), 809–828.

Mittenberg, W., Patton, C., Canyock, E. M., & Condit, D. C. (2002). Base rates of malingering and symptom exaggeration. *Journal of Clinical and Experimental Neuropsychology*, 24(8), 1094–1102.

Mittenberg, W., Theroux, S., Aguila-Puentes, G., Bianchini, K., Greve, K., & Rayls, K. (2001). Identification of malingered head injury on the Wechsler Adult Intelligence Scale-3rd edition. *The Clinical Neuropsychologist*, 15(4), 440–445.

Mittenberg, W., Theroux-Fichera, S., Zielinski, R. E., & Heilbronner, R. L. (1995). Identification of malingered head injury on the Wechsler Adult Intelligence Scale-Revised. *Professional Psychology: Research and Practice*, 26(5), 491–498.

Morel, K. R. (1995). Use of the binomial theorem in detecting factitious posttraumatic stress disorder. *Anxiety Disorders Practice Journal*, 2(1), 55–62.

Morel, K. R. (1998). Development and preliminary validation of a forced-choice test of response bias for posttraumatic stress disorder. *Journal of Personality Assessment*, 70(2), 299–314.

Morel, K. R. (2008). Comparison of the Morel Emotional Numbing Test for posttraumatic stress disorder to the Word Memory Test in neuropsychological evaluations. *The Clinical Neuropsychologist*, 22(2), 350–362.

Morel, K. R. & Marshman, K. C. (2008). Critiquing symptom validity tests for posttraumatic stress disorder: A modification of Hartman's criteria. *Journal of Anxiety Disorders*, 22(8), 1542–1550.

Morel, K. R., & Shepherd, B. E. (2008). Developing a symptom validity test for posttraumatic stress disorder: Application of the binomial distribution. *Journal of Anxiety Disorders*, 22(8), 1297–1302.

Morey, L. C. (1991). *Personality assessment inventory: Professional manual.* Tampa, FL: Psychological Assessment Resources.

Morgan, J., & Sweet, J. (Eds.) (2009). *Neuropsychology of malingering casebook.* New York, NY: Taylor & Francis.

Nampiaparampil, D. E. (2008). Prevalence of chronic pain after traumatic brain injury: A systematic review. *Journal of the American Medical Association*, 300(6), 711–719.

Nicholson, K. (2000). Pain, cognition and traumatic brain injury. *Neurorehabilitation*, 14(2), 95–103.

Nicholson, K., & Martelli, M. F. (2004). The problem of pain. *Journal of Head Trauma Rehabilitation*, 19(1), 2–9.

Nicholson, K., Martelli, M. F., & Zasler, N. D. (2001). Does pain confound interpretation of neuropsychological test results? *NeuroRehabilitation*, 16(4), 225–230.

Nitch, S. R., & Glassmire, D. M. (2007). Non-forced-choice measures to detect noncredible cognitive performance. In K. B. Boone (Ed.), *Assessment of feigned cognitive impairment: A neuropsychological perspective* (pp. 78–102). New York, NY: Guilford Press.

Oboler, S. (2000). Disability evaluations under the Department of Veterans Affairs. In R. D. Rodinelli & R. T. Katz (Eds.), *Impairment rating and disability evaluation* (pp. 187–217). Philadelphia, PA: W. B. Saunders.

Oien, M. L., Nelson, N. W., Lamberty, G. J., & Arbisi, P. A. (2011). Neuropsychological function in posttraumatic stress disorder: A meta-analytic review. *The Clinical Neuropsychologist*, 25, 555.

Ord, J. S., Boettcher, A. C., Greve, K. W., & Bianchini, K. J. (2010). Detection of malingering in mild traumatic brain injury with the Conners' Continuous Performance Test-II. *Journal of Clinical and Experimental Neuropsychology*, 32(4), 380–387.

Paniak, C., Reynolds, S., Toller-Lobe, G., Melnyk, A., Nagy, J., & Schmidt, D. (2002). A longitudinal study of the relationship between financial compensation and symptoms after treated mild traumatic brain injury. *Journal of Clinical and Experimental Neuropsychology*, 24(2), 187–193.

Pankratz, L. (1983). A new technique for the assessment and modification of feigned memory deficit. *Perceptual and Motor Skills*, 57(2), 367–372.

Pankratz, L., Fausti, S. A., & Peed, S. (1975). A forced-choice technique to evaluate deafness in the hysterical or malingering patient. *Journal of Consulting and Clinical Psychology*, 43(3), 421–422.

Pappagallo, M., & Werner, M. (2008). *Chronic pain: A primer for physicians*. Chicago, IL: Remedica.

Pivovarova, E., Rosenfeld, B., Dole, T., Green, D., & Zapf, P. (2009). Are measures of cognitive effort and motivation useful in differentiating feigned from genuine psychiatric symptoms? *International Journal of Forensic Mental Health*, 8, 271–278.

Porter-Moffitt, S., Gatchel, R. J., Robinson, R. C., Deschner, M., Posamentier, M., Polatin, P., & Lou, L. (2006). Biopsychosocial profiles of different pain diagnostic groups. *Journal of Pain*, 7(5), 308–318.

Powell, M. R., Locke, D. E., Smigielski, J. S., & McCrea, M. (2011). Estimating the diagnostic value of the trail making test for suboptimal effort in acquired brain injury rehabilitation patients. *The Clinical Neuropsychologist*, 25(1), 108–118.

Price, J. R. & Stevens, K. B. Psycholegal implications of malingered head trauma. *Appl Neuropsychol.* 1997;(1): 75–83.

Rainville, J., Sobel, J. B., Hartigan, C., & Wright, A. (1997). The effect of compensation involvement on the reporting of pain and disability by patients referred for rehabilitation of chronic low back pain. *Spine*, 22(17), 2016–2024.

Ravnkilde, B., Videbech, P., Clemmensen, K., Egander, A., Rasumssen, N. A., & Rosenberg, R. (2002). Cognitive deficits in major depression. *Scandinavian Journal of Psychology*, 43(3), 239–251.

Resnick, P. (1997). Malingering of posttraumatic disorders. In R. Rogers (Ed.), *Clinical assessment of malingering and deception* (2nd ed., pp.130–152). New York, NY: Guilford Press.

Reynolds, S., Paniak, C., Toller-Lobe, G., & Nagy, J. (2003). A longitudinal study of compensation-seeking and return to work in a treated mild traumatic brain injury sample. *Journal of Head Trauma Rehabilitation*, 18(2), 139–147.

Reznek, L. (2005). The Rey 15-item memory test for malingering: A meta-analysis. *Brain Injury*, 19(7), 539–543.

Rogers, R. (1992). *Structured interview of reported symptoms*. Odessa, FL: Psychological Assessment Resources.

Rogers, R. (1997). Researching dissimulation. In R. Rogers (Ed.), *Clinical assessment of malingering and deception* (2nd ed., pp. 398–426). New York, NY: Guilford Press.

Rogers, R., Payne, J. W., Correa, A. A., Gillard, N. D., & Ross, C. A. (2009). A study of the SIRS with severely traumatized patients. *Journal of Personality Assessment*, 91(5), 429–438.

Rohling, M. L., Allen, L. M., & Green, P. (2002). Who is exaggerating cognitive impairment and who is not? *CNS Spectrums*, 7(5), 387–395.

Rohling, M. L., Binder, L. M., & Langhinrichsen-Rolling, J. (1995). Money matters: A meta-analytic review of the association between financial compensation and the experience and treatment of chronic pain. *Health Psychol.* Nov 14(6), 537–47.

Rose, J. M. (2005). Continuum of care model for managing mild traumatic brain injury in a workers' compensation context: A description of the model and its development. *Brain Injury*, 19(1), 39–53.

Rosen, G. M. (2006). DSM's cautionary guideline to rule out malingering can protect the PTSD data base. *Journal of Anxiety Disorders*, 20(4), 530–535.

Rosen, G. M. & Powell, J. E. (2003). Use of a symptom validity test in the forensic assessment of Posttraumatic Stress Disorder. *Anxiety Disorders*, 17, 361–367

Rosen, G. M., & Taylor, S. (2007). Pseudo-PTSD. *Journal of Anxiety Disorders*, 21(2), 201–210.

Ruff, R. (2005). Two decades of advances in understanding of mild traumatic brain injury. *Journal of Head Trauma Rehabilitation*, 20(1), 5–18.

Ruff, R. M., & Richardson, A. M. (1999). Mild traumatic brain injury. In J. J. Sweet (Ed.), *Forensic Neuropsychology: Fundamentals and Practice* (pp. 315–338). New York: Psychology Press.

Ruff, R. M., Iverson, G. L., Barth, J. T., Bush, S. S., & Broschek, D. K. (2009). Recommendations for diagnosing a mild traumatic brain injury: A National Academy of Neuropsychology education paper. *Archives of Clinical Neuropsychology*, 24(1), 3–10.

Ryan, L. M., & Warden, D. L. (2003). Post concussion syndrome. *International Review of Psychiatry*, 15(4), 310–316.

Sackett, D. L., & Haynes, R. B. (2002). The architecture of diagnostic research. *British Medical Journal*, 324(7336), 539–541.

Satz, P. S., Alfano, M. S., Light, R. F., Morgenstern, H. F., Zaucha, K. F., Asarnow, R. F., & Newton, S. (1999). Persistent post-concussive syndrome: A proposed methodology and literature review to determine the effects, if any, of mild head and other bodily injury. *Journal of Clinical and Experimental Neuropsychology*, 21(5), 620–628.

Scherer, M., & Madison, C. F. (2005). Moderate and severe traumatic brain injury. In G. J. Larrabee (Ed.). *Forensic neuropsychology: A scientific approach* (pp. 237–270). New York, NY: Oxford University Press.

Schretlen, D. J., & Shapiro, A. M. (2003). A quantitative review of the effects of traumatic brain injury on cognitive functioning. *International Review of Psychiatry*, 15(4), 341–349.

Schroeder, R. W., & Marshall, P. S. (2010). Validation of the sentence repetition test as a measure of suspect effort. *The Clinical Neuropsychologist*, 24(2), 326–343.

Schutte, C., Millis, S., Axelrod, B., & VanDyke, S. (2011). Derivation of a composite measure of embedded symptom validity indices. *The Clinical Neuropsychologist*, 25(3), 454–462.

Singhal, A., Green, P., Ashaye, K., Shankar, K. & Gill, D. (2009). High specificity of the medical symptom validity test in patients with very severe memory impairment. *Archives of Clinical Neuropsychology*, 24(8), 721–728.

Slick, D. J., Sherman, E. M., & Iverson, G. L. (1999). Diagnostic criteria for malingering neurocognitive dysfunction: Proposed standards for clinical practice and research. *The Clinical Neuropsychologist*, 13(4), 545–561.

Slick, D. J., Tan, J. E., Strauss, E. H., & Hultsch, D. F. (2004). Detecting malingering: A survey of experts' practices. *Archives of Clinical Neuropsychology*, 19(4), 465–473.

Smith-Seemiller, L., Fow, N. R., Kant, R., & Franzen, M. D. (2003). Presence of post-concussion syndrome in patients with chronic pain vs mild traumatic brain injury. *Brain Injury*, 17(3), 199–206.

Solomon, R. E., Boone, K. B., Miora, D., Skidmore, S., Cottingham, M., Victor, T., . . . Zeller, M. (2010). Use of the WAIS-III picture completion subtest as an embedded measure of response bias. *The Clinical Neuropsychologist*, 24(7), 1243–1256.

Solomon, Z., & Mikulincer, M. (2006). Trajectories of PTSD: A 20-year longitudinal study. *American Journal of Psychiatry*, 163(4), 659–666.

Stevens, A., Friedel, E., Mehren, G., & Merten, T. (2008). Malingering and uncooperativeness in psychiatric and psychological assessment: Prevalence and effects in a German sample of claimants. *Psychiatry Research*, 157(1–3), 191–200.

Suhr, J. A., Sullivan, B. K., & Rodriguez, J. L. (2011). The relationship of noncredible performance to continuous performance test scores in adults referred for attention-deficit/hyperactivity disorder evaluation. *Archives of Clinical Neuropsychology*, 26(1), 1–7.

Sweet, J. (2009). Forensic bibliography: effort/malingering and other common forensic topics encountered by clinical neuropsychologists (pp. 566-630). In J. Morgan & J. Sweet (eds.), *Neuropsychology of Malingering Casebook*. New York: Taylor & Francis.

Taylor, S., Frueh, B. C., & Asmundson, G. J. (2007). Detection and management of malingering in people presenting for treatment of posttraumatic stress disorder. Methods, obstacles, and recommendations. *Journal of Anxiety Disorders*, 21(1), 22–41.

Thurman, D. J. (2001). The epidemiology and economics of head trauma. In L. Miller & R. Hayes (Eds.), *Head trauma: Basic, preclinical, and clinical directions*. New York: John Wiley and Sons.

Tombaugh, T. (1996). *Test of Memory Malingering manual*. New York, NY: MultiHealth Systems.

Trueblood, W., & Schmidt, M. (1993). Malingering and other validity considerations in the neuropsychological evaluation of mild head injury. *Journal of Clinical and Experimental Neuropsychology*, 15(4), 578–590.

Tunks, E. R., Crook, J., & Weir, R. (2008). Epidemiology of chronic pain with psychological comorbidity: Prevalence, risk, course, and prognosis. *Canadian Journal of Psychiatry*, 53(4), 224–234.

Turk, D. C. (2002). A diathesis-stress model of chronic pain and disability following traumatic injury. *Pain Research Management*, 7(1), 9–19.

Verhaak, P. F., Kerssens, J. J., Dekker, J., Sorbi, M. J., & Bensing, J. M. (1998). Prevalence of chronic benign pain disorder among adults: A review of the literature. *Pain*, 77(3), 231–239.

Waddell, G., McCulloch, J. A., Kummel, E., & Venner, R. M. (1980). Nonorganic physical signs in low-back pain. *Spine*, (Phila PA 1976). 1980 Mar-Apr; 5(2), 117–125.

Whiteside, D., Wald, D., & Busse, M. (2011). Classification accuracy of multiple visual spatial measures in the detection of suspect effort. *The Clinical Neuropsychologist*, 25(2), 287–301.

Wolfe, P. L., Millis, S. R., Hanks, R., Fichtenberg, N., Larrabee, G. J., & Sweet, J. J. Effort indicators within the California Verbal Learning Test-II (CVLT-II). *Clin Neuropsychol.* 2010 Jan 24(1), 153–68.

Wood, R. L. (2004). Understanding the 'miserable minority': A diathesis-stress paradigm for post-concussional disorder. *Brain Injury*, 18(11), 1135–1153.

Ylioja, S. G., Baird, A. D., & Podell, K. (2009). Developing a spatial analogue of the reliable digit span. *Archives of Clinical Neuropsychology*, 24(8), 729–739.

Youngjohn, J. R. Confirmed attorney coaching prior to neuropsychological evaluation. *Assessment* 1995; 2:279–83.

Arbisi, P. A. (2011, June). *The neuropsychology of posttraumatic stress disorder*. A workshop presented at the 9th Annual Conference of the American Academy of Clinical Neuropsychology, Washington, DC.

Symptom Validity Assessment of Mild Traumatic Brain Injury Cases in Disability and Civil Litigation Contexts

16

Michael D. Chafetz

The modern era of disability legislation was heralded by the Americans with Disabilities Act (ADA, 1990), which was based on the Education for the Handicapped Act (1975; Colker, 2005). As Colker (2005) noted, the public climate regarding disabilities had its hostile side: Senator Thomas Eagleton (D-Mo.) had to be replaced as the vice presidential running mate in 1972 by presidential candidate George McGovern after rather negative public reaction when he disclosed that he had received treatment for mental illness. In 1988, when presidential candidate Michael Dukakis refused to disclose medical records amid rumors about treatment for mental illness, President Reagan responded to a question about this refusal by saying, "Look, I'm not going to pick on an invalid." However, at about the same time in August 1988, Vice President Bush urged Congress to enact the ADA. Bills were introduced in the Senate and House of Representatives. The Senate Bill passed on a 76-8 vote in September 1989, and the House Bill passed on a 403-20 vote: in May 1990. The House bill was the product of more than 20 hearings and four committee reports. President George H. W. Bush, whose son Neil has dyslexia, had commanded Attorney General Richard Thornburgh to work with Congress on developing this disability legislation. Thornburgh and his wife had already become advocates for individuals with disabilities after their son, Peter, suffered a traumatic brain injury (TBI) in a 1960 motor vehicle accident (Colker, 2005).

Although disability programs are well intended, there has always been concern about cheating. For example, Stevens (1986) wrote about rabbis discovering in the second century BC that some people were feigning disabilities to take advantage of relief programs. In modern times, during the immediate backlash to the ADA, several writers spoke of the windfalls that people with questionable impairments (and their lawyers) would obtain in their pursuit of disability claims (Colker, 2005). Associated Press writer, Stephen Ohlemacher (2010), in interviewing Dan Allsup, communications director of an Illinois company that represents disability applicants, pointed out concern about fraud, with Allsup opining that Social Security's stringent definition of disability is part of a process that helps eliminate malingerers. As described in more detail later in this chapter, this very stringent definition of disability actually incentivizes claimants toward intentional exaggeration of their problems (Chafetz, 2010).

Case vignettes are significantly masked and should not be identifiable.

Disability contracts are ultimately about limitations on the abilities to work, although the abilities to engage in play and leisure activities, perform family roles, and engage in meaningful social interactions often come into the analysis. Depending on the institution with which the claimant has a contract (e.g., Social Security Administration [SSA], Veterans Administration [VA], private disability carrier), different analyses are emphasized. For example, the Department of Defense (DoD) is largely interested in physical conditions that make members unfit to continue military duties, and compensation is intended to provide an offset to the interruption of a military career. By contrast, disability in the VA is based on a service-connected impairment whether or not it impedes a military career, and the compensation is based on expected future losses in civilian earnings (Buddin & Kappur, 2005).

In civil litigation, the concern regarding disability status is ultimately about liability and damages (Greiffenstein, 2008). How disabled a claimant/plaintiff has become will factor into the damages claim amount, but the suit will also be concerned with liability—whether the actual injury claim arose from the actions of the defendant. Thus, in civil litigation, it becomes critical to determine whether there indeed was a TBI resulting from the fall, motor vehicle accident, fight, explosion, and so forth. The parties to the lawsuit will argue over this on the damages, along with how severe and long lasting was the injury and the limitations it produced.

By its very nature, mild traumatic brain injury (MTBI), particularly without secondary complications (e.g., subarachnoid bleed, subdural hematoma), usually follows with good recovery in a relatively short period (Iverson & Lange, 2011; McCrea, 2008) and is not typically disabling over time (Iverson & Lange, 2011). By the time a long-term disability or a civil litigation claimant reaches the office of the neuropsychologist, numerous factors other than MTBI will need to be considered regarding his or her contribution to symptom maintenance. These factors may include (but are not limited to) motivation regarding work (Chafetz, Prentkowski, & Rao, 2011) or money (Bianchini, Curtis, & Greve, 2006), psychosocial factors and personality functioning (Bianchini, 2010), diagnosis threat and confusion over the nature of a MTBI (Suhr & Gunstad, 2002a), and even the politics regarding the treatment of veterans and military personnel coming home from a combat theater, with the expressed goal of the VA to be overinclusive in the screenings of TBI (Iverson, Langlois, McCrea, & Kelly, 2009).

This chapter describes the process, role expectations, and activities of the neuropsychologist who is engaged in answering referral questions in disability and other civil medicolegal contexts when MTBI is part of the claim. The ethics and role boundaries of the consultation are described along with the nature of the referral questions. Symptom validity issues provide an important component to the neuropsychologist's understanding of the claimant's presentation. Motivational aspects of the claimant's presentation are considered critical factors in the analysis of a claim.

ETHICS AND ROLE BOUNDARIES

Training for clinical work in psychology and neuropsychology typically involves learning the importance of developing a treatment alliance. In most clinical contexts, the patient and the psychologist work together to obtain the proper diagnosis, establish treatment goals, and effect positive change, often with an analysis of attachment styles that may affect the alliance (Diener & Monroe, 2011). Within this relationship, the psychologist is truly biased in favor of the patient's welfare and is invested in helping the patient become more effective and feel better. Unless the psychologist also receives forensic training, there is little preparation for the psychologist's role in an independent psychological or neuropsychological examination (traditionally called IME, from independent medical examination).

One of the main boundary issues in an IME is the absence of a typical doctor–patient relationship, which is the primary reason for the use of the term "independent." The bias of being the claimant's treatment provider is removed from the independent consultation. Greenberg and Shuman (1997) and Strasburger, Gutheil, and Brodsky (1997) have written eloquently of how the roles of treatment provider and forensic examiner are "irreconcilable." Bush (2005) has provided clear delineation of the roles of the neuropsychologist in the independent examination and suggested a third role—that of clinical examiner—who may testify to any aspect of the examination. In the typical disability or litigation context, the referring party (e.g., the Disability Determinations Services [DDS], VA, IME company, insurance company, or defense counsel) is the client. The examinee must be informed of this relationship and the absence of a typical doctor–patient relationship. This author uses an IME consent form in which he offers respect for the dignity and person of the examinee, but if the examinee needs treatment or advice, it must be obtained from the examinee's own doctors. This consent form is forthcoming concerning expectations of the evaluation, states that no recordings will be permitted, and advises claimants to do his or her best and respond accurately because any finding to the contrary may have a negative impact on the claim. In fact, as reported by Chafetz (2010), the local DDS for SSA required a similar warning: "Failure to do your best on these tests may result in an unfavorable decision on the claim."

Examiners must be competent in the forensic arena (Heilbrun, DeMatteo, Marczyk, & Goldstein, 2008), which cannot be automatically assumed by competence in the clinical arena (Greenberg & Shuman, 2007). The clinical forensic boundary issues are important because of several factors: responding to the actual client in the case (insurance company vs. patient); answering the right questions (what is a useful treatment plan for the patient vs. whether the examinee has been availed of a useful treatment plan); and examining issues regarding examinee motivation (seeking help for a clinical problem vs. seeking compensation for a disabling problem). Consider how the blurring of boundaries by a treatment provider who agrees to opine as an expert in civil litigation can be exploited by an attorney in a deposition or trial: "Well, doctor, you say you are an expert in the field, but when you said the patient had memory problems did you not even consider that the patient's subjective sense of memory problems could actually be measured by testing?" What is perfectly acceptable in a clinical arena may be wholly inadequate in a forensic arena.

Moreover, the examiner in a disability claim might get more restricted responses from the claimant if the neutral objective stance of the disability examiner (Greenberg & Shuman, 1997) is interpreted as coldness by the claimant, who may well have expectations about the adversarial nature of the claim. This issue of examiner interpersonal style can theoretically also be true for litigation, particularly when it becomes necessary for the claimant to be examined by "the other side." As the evaluator is paid by the third party, the claimant may believe that the evaluator is not truly independent. However, as Greiffenstein (2009) noted, it is a myth that examiner bias "causes" poor effort because there is no evidence that bias or even the position of the defense examiner (rather than the plaintiff examiner) causes distortion. In this author's experience, examiners' respect for the claimant goes a long way toward developing a working rapport with the claimant, thus facilitating a more open exchange. There are several touchstones of empathy for the examiner such as overcoming obstacles (e.g., internship applications and interviews), being confronted with a critical examination, or feeling disrespected by an adjustor at an insurance company. The claimant's anxiety about an independent examination can easily be understood by the examiner who is always respectful and considerate and yet still is objective and evaluative.

TYPES OF DISABILITY CASES

This section will present an analysis of military compensation and Social Security disability cases with particular discussion of claimants who are low functioning and of motivational analysis.

Military Compensation

According to Buddin and Kapur (2005), the Code of Federal Regulations focuses the percentage rankings of VA disability compensation on the earnings loss of veterans who are disabled. In particular, the ranking is based on the average impairment in earning capacity. There are no allowances for pain and suffering (as in civil litigation) unless these factors in some way affect civilian earnings. The primary consideration involves what the individual could have earned without the disability compared to with the disability, and it is ranked according to levels. In contrast, disability in the Social Security system is based on total inability to work (Social Security Advisory Board, 2003). As Chafetz (2010) described, this extreme definition of disability has been viewed as contrary to work motivation because compensation is conditional on a claimant demonstrating a total inability to work, when only the individuals who are most impaired cannot work even part-time and/or in very low-functioning positions (e.g., store greeter, ticket taker). Thus, in Social Security disability claims, claimants might be hesitant to engage in work-related activities that would undermine their claim for benefits. This disincentive is not as likely to carry forward into the VA disability claim because the cutoff is not so critical, although claimants might see exaggeration as a route toward a higher percentage ranking.

Moreover, although disability compensation in civilian life is tied to the employee's earnings before the injury, this is not so in VA compensation. As Buddin and Kapur (2005) stated, a private and a major who both lose a foot are both entitled to the same benefit, whereas experience and earning potential would in the civilian disability arena result in much higher compensation for the higher paid individual (i.e., the major).

TBI has become recognized as the signature injury of the wars in Afghanistan (Operation Endurance Freedom [OEF]) and Iraq (Operation Iraqi Freedom [OIF]; Howe, 2009). Classification of TBI is considered as mild (MTBI) if there is no finding on structural imaging[1], loss of consciousness (LOC) is not more than 30 min, posttraumatic amnesia (PTA) does not occur for more than 1 day, the Glasgow Coma Scale (GCS) rating total ranges from 13 to 15, and there is some alteration of mental status that may last just a moment or for up to 24 hr (Howe, 2009; Iverson & Lange, 2011; McCrea, 2008). Both the LOC and the alteration of mental state characteristics require further refinement because orthostatic hypotension and the vasovagal (syncopal) response (occurring from sudden pain or anxiety-producing events) can both cause similar mental alterations for brief periods (France, France, & Patterson, 2006; Ropper & Samuels, 2009), and thus would not necessarily indicate that a brain injury

---

[1] A positive finding on neuroimaging has been classified by some clinicians/researchers as a complication of MTBI, but in the military, it is considered as evidence of moderate TBI.

has taken place. Moreover, characteristics often associated with depression (e.g., subjective concentration and memory complaints, and irritability) often are diagnosed as "postconcussion syndrome" even in the absence of the individual meeting criteria for a concussion (Iverson, 2006).

Approximately 11.2%–22.8% of veterans referred for postdeployment screening after returning from OEF or OIF screen positive for MTBI (Iverson et al., 2009). As Iverson et al. (2009) indicated, these estimates may be high because it was the expressed intent of the VA to be overinclusive in the screenings. Howe (2009) analyzed mechanisms by which blasts can produce brain injury, along with more conventional forms of brain injury in the combat theater (e.g., motor vehicle accidents), but all the classification systems indicate that the initial characteristics of the neurological response, rather than the type of force, define the levels of the brain injury, if one has indeed occurred. After 3 months, the neuropsychological results of patients who have sustained uncomplicated MTBI and have no significant comorbid medical/psychiatric problems or litigation are indistinguishable from those of persons who have not sustained such injuries (Iverson & Lange, 2011; Rohling et al., 2011).

Combat can involve such intense experiences that some soldiers return from the combat theater with confusion and emotional disarray. In addition to having been exposed to blasts or having sustained more conventional forms of TBI, some combat veterans return with hypervigilance, guilt, and the suite of posttraumatic stress disorder (PTSD) symptoms of avoidance, reexperiencing, and physiological reactivity (American Psychiatric Association, 2000). In studies systematically reviewed by Carlson, Kehle, and Meis (2009), approximately 32%–66% of military TBI subjects were also found to have PTSD, whereas 14%–56% of nonmilitary TBI subjects also had PTSD. Care must be taken in the analysis of these cases, particularly with late-developing symptoms involving compensable claims; as Greiffenstein and Baker (2008) have shown, a high proportion of late postconcussion syndrome cases fail symptom validity measures, and the rates are higher when cases involve both late postconcussion *and* posttraumatic stress claims. This study went further to question whether the threat perceptions necessary to trigger PTSD could be encoded during the amnestic state of the TBI if the dual claim is resulting from the same event, but combat experiences are so complex, it is likely that multiple events could be defining PTSD trauma even if only one event caused the TBI. Of course, the analysis would be based on individual experience, but as Greiffenstein and Baker (2008) pointed out, late-appearing dual diagnosis is thoroughly intertwined with secondary gain.

Moreover, symptom specificity is a problem in the differential diagnosis process. Vasterling et al. (2006) showed that deployment compared to nondeployment was associated with negative emotions and decreased neuropsychological test scores. Depression, more than head injury, accounts for elevated levels of concussion symptoms (Iverson, 2006; Suhr & Gunstad, 2002b). PTSD itself can lead to neuropsychological problems (Samuelson et al., 2006), but in compensation contexts, PTSD symptomology can be exaggerated or simulated (Merten, Thies, Schneider, & Stevens, 2009; Rubenzer, 2009). The following military postdeployment case vignette provides an example of delineating issues of PTSD and MTBI in the context of a disability evaluation, considering that differential diagnosis is important in assessing symptom validity (i.e., attributing symptoms to the proper diagnosis).

Case Vignette Delineating Post-Traumatic Stress Disorder and Mild Traumatic Brain Injury Issues in War Veteran

A 28-year-old marine seen for an IME in 2010 had been deployed as a gunner on a Humvee while participating in security for convoys. He was very close with the members of his unit. In fact, after another incident in which his team leader was killed, he still wore the name of this leader on his watch in the leader's honor. He had vengeance in his mind from the death of his team leader, but when he killed a man, he started putting himself in that man's place, wondering if that man was just defending his family and way of life. He was also scared and did not know what would have happened if he had not shot the man. The MTBI was caused when a rocket-propelled grenade (RPG) blasted in close quarters in an alley between his vehicle and another. In this RPG incident, he recalls the blast noise and his body hitting inside the turret. He did not bleed out of his ears or nose. His superior officer told him he had been unconscious when he fell. He got up a few moments later, feeling dazed and having ringing in his ears. He recalls getting up and going to the aide station and being told he had a slight concussion, and he recalls going back to base and having dinner. This marine met criteria for MTBI at the time. He was treated while on active duty for orthopedic problems, PTSD, and symptoms attributed to MTBI, but at the time of the IME 5 years later, he was still reporting short-term memory loss. The current neuropsychological examination (IME) showed no deficits, and in fact, he had strong memory abilities. On mental speed tasks, he was hypervigilant for errors, which was considered a finding related to PTSD watchfulness that had generalized. He fit criteria for PTSD and major depressive disorder, and it was thought that chronic pain was a factor in his poor adjustment and continuing irritability. Although this veteran had no failures on symptom validity testing, the accuracy of his symptom report was carefully determined by delineating PTSD and depression symptoms from issues associated with his MTBI.

War veterans may have reasons for a late-developing dysphoria that are not the direct result of combat. For example, relationships may change dramatically once the medical board disability process begins. One highly decorated veteran of four tours in OIF and OEF told this examiner how bad life was for him at the moment because he no longer enjoyed respect for his accomplishments and skills now that he was away from his unit and dealing only with people who looked at him as escaping his responsibilities through his disability claim.

Additional postdeployment complications have been portrayed in the award-winning 2008 war film directed by Kathryn Bigelow, *Hurt Locker*. Many combat veterans seeking disability have attested to the relevance of this film to this author. This film followed the stories of a U.S. Army Explosive Ordinance Disposal (EOD) team working in the Iraq War. The character of Sergeant First Class William James thrived on the clarity of mission and purpose and the adrenaline rush of his specialty. When he returned from theater, his life at home could not come close to the thrill and clarity of his missions and the camaraderie of his team. The following vignette provides an illustration of the *Hurt Locker* phenomenon in a military veteran who had suffered a MTBI and whose providers all thought he had PTSD.

Case Vignette of *Hurt Locker* Phenomenon

A 32-year-old truck driver had served in Iraq as a gunner and saw several men wounded. One member of his team bled out from a leg wound and died. A suicide bomber killed civilians on a bus, and the driver had to participate in the postblast analysis. Children had died in this explosion, and he was horrified. When he came home from his tour, he was angry at politicians with the war in general, and he began abusing alcohol. His marriage dissolved. Within a couple of years, he returned to Iraq to work as a truck driver for a private security contractor. He made several runs off of the base, but on the 12th run, his truck ran over two land mines. The vehicle was fully armored, and he did not experience blast pressures. However, he was jolted severely, injuring his back, and his helmeted (Kevlar) head hit the cab and his jaw separated. He had brief alteration of consciousness (a few seconds), but he recalled the blasts. He did have clear memories afterward. He was seen for a private disability IME about 1.5 years later. There was no measurable cognitive disorder. He had dysphoria, hypervigilance, and strange dreams, but he did not endorse a significant level of PTSD symptomology on testing. He did not avoid war movies and in fact enjoyed watching *Saving Private Ryan*. He liked playing video combat games to calm himself. He was distressed that his medical conditions would not allow him to return to combat theater. In fact, he developed a neighborhood watch program in which at night he walked the "perimeter" of his house and neighborhood. He talked about the danger of looters, but the risks appeared much lower than security issues he faced in Iraq. He appeared to be reenacting missions of security and protection from danger. His problems were not related to MTBI but were not particular to PTSD either. He was dysphoric largely from missing the thrill of the combat theater and not being permitted to return because of medical problems that included diabetes and pancreatitis.

Social Security Disability Compensation and the Low-Functioning Claimant

The SSA has two systems designed to help disabled individuals with monetary benefits: (a) Social Security Disability Insurance (SSDI), which is for workers (and their dependents) who have paid into the Social Security trust fund; and (b) Supplemental Security Income (SSI), which is for individuals who are disabled (and their dependents) with limited income and assets (Morton, 2010). According to SSA, a person is disabled if "unable to engage in any substantial gainful activity" because of a medically determinable physical or mental impairment. The disability must have lasted or be expected to last for a continuous period of at least 12 months or be expected to result in death (http://www.socialsecurity.gov/dibplan/dqualify4.htm; see also Chafetz, 2010; Morton, 2010).

Although some writers (see Ohlemacher, 2010) have suggested that this extreme definition of disability helps to eliminate fraud, in reality, it is just the opposite, with an incentive created in which claimants must demonstrate (sometimes in dramatic fashion) that they are so impaired as to have absolutely *no* ability to work (Chafetz, 2010). If they can work part-time, then their abilities do not fit the SSA definition of disability and denial of benefits is more likely. In a base-rate paper, Chafetz (2008) revealed high rates of symptom validity problems typically more than 40% in SSI/ SSDI claimants.

In numerous policy statements and clarifications, SSA has made it clear that the use of symptom validity testing, which is considered critical in assessing the validity of the findings (Heilbronner, Sweet, Morgan, Larrabee, & Millis, 2009), is not to be used in any programmatic way for disability evaluations. It is beyond the scope of this chapter to go into extensive detail about SSA's reasoning, but Chafetz (2010) refuted SSA's points using data from the burgeoning scientific literature on symptom validity and has not received any notice of argument to the contrary by any SSA psychologist. For example, SSA has been concerned that malingering cannot be "proven" with tests, but it was pointed out that rigorous studies of symptom validity test (SVT) classification accuracy are available, along with methods that significantly reduce the likelihood of false positive identification of a valid-performing claimant as malingering (Chafetz, 2010, 2011).

There is a rightful discussion about the use of symptom validity testing for claimants with intellectual disability (Salekin & Doane, 2009; Victor & Boone, 2007), which is especially important in arenas such as Social Security disability in which there is a high proportion of claimants who are low functioning (Chafetz, 2008, 2010; Chafetz, Abrahams, & Kohlmaier, 2007).

Chafetz et al. (2007) developed an 11-item scale (now termed the Symptom Validity Scale [SVS][2] for individuals who are low functioning) in which embedded measures from the history, the author's mental/cognitive status examination, and the Wechsler intelligence scales (adults or children) were validated individually, and as a whole scale, showed use in assessing effort of claimants with low levels of intellectual functioning. Claimants who are low functioning and are providing invalid response do so, at least to some extent, in a way that is different than claimants who are higher functioning. For example, a variable developed by Mittenberg, Theroux-Fichera, Zielinski, and Heilbronner (1995; see also Iverson & Tulsky, 2003) in which Wechsler Adult Intelligence Scale-Third Edition (WAIS-III) vocabulary minus digit span (V-DS) ≥ 3 scaled score points, which is a validity indicator in the identification of malingered brain injury in claimants who are higher functioning, had to be eliminated in the SVS for individuals who are low functioning. In these claimants who are low functioning, the vocabulary-scaled score was infrequently high, and there was little correlation in this difference score with other measures of symptom validity.

This author has sought to assure SSA that neuropsychologists are doing everything in their power *not* to mislabel honest claimants as malingering when a claimant who is low functioning might fail a validity indicator. In one study, multiple failures of symptom validity indicators were seen to yield a very small rate of false positive identifications ($< 1\%$; Chafetz, 2011). There was good convergence in these findings empirically (in the database) and by calculations using the chaining of likelihood ratios (as in Larrabee, 2008). In essence, if a claimant fails a single validity indicator, there is some likelihood (e.g., 8% false positive level) that the failure is caused by other factors (e.g., low intellectual functioning, internal distress), but if a claimant fails three indicators, there is little likelihood ($< 1\%$) that this claimant has been misidentified. Moreover, this author believes that the use of a profile analysis across easy and difficult subtests (Howe & Loring, 2009; Singhal, Green, Ashaye, Shankar, & Gill, 2009) to show severe impairment (as in dementia) holds some promise in being able to eliminate claimants who are severely impaired from being mislabeled as malingerers, although more classification accuracy studies will need to be done on claimants, particularly those at risk for malingering. Profile analysis procedures have been developed for the Word Memory Test, Medical Symptom Validity Test (MSVT), and the nonverbal MSVT (Green, 2003/2005, 2004, 2008).

As Chafetz et al. (2007) demonstrated, claimants for Social Security disability benefits have meaningful correlations between effort and IQ. Therefore, the evidence necessary for a disability decision becomes clouded when it is hard to delineate poor effort from truly impaired intellectual functioning. Salekin and Doane (2009) pointed out that most normative studies of SVTs in which cutoffs were established have not been performed with individuals who are low-functioning, and it is simplistic to think that the usual cutoffs would apply in those who are intellectually disabled (ID). Both Victor and Boone (2007) and Salekin and Doane (2009) cited studies showing higher false positive rates of SVT failure by individuals who are ID. In one oft-cited study of residential individuals who are ID, Hurley and Deal (2006) showed

---

[2] The SVS was originally termed the Disability Determinations Malingering Rating Scale, but the term was broadened to include claimants who are low functioning in all types of examinations and to remove the automatic connotation of malingering when noncredible behavior was observed and documented.

that 41% of individuals with mental retardation (MR) failed the usual cutoff on the Test of Memory Malingering (TOMM). In this study, there was no significant correlation between TOMM performance and IQ, which indicated that effort had little or no effect on IQ scores.

Although Salekin and Doane (2009) correctly pointed out that the clinician's job is to delineate bona fide strengths and weaknesses from those that are simulated, these authors tend to lump together various levels of MR into one category of intellectual disability. Recognition memory is largely retained in mild MR (Green, 2004) and in early dementia (Merten, Bossink, & Schmand, 2007). Investigators (Green, 2004; Richman et al., 2006) have shown that children with mild MR (mean verbal IQ of 65) obtained a mean of 95% correct on the MSVT immediate recognition (IR) and delayed recognition (DR) effort subtests. However, a higher proportion of non–compensation-seeking subjects with more severe levels of MR (Victor & Boone, 2007) or more advanced dementia (Merten et al., 2007; Teichner & Wagner, 2004) fail recognition-based symptom validity testing.

In another frequently-cited study, Simon (2007) showed that a large proportion of adjudicated (incarcerated) individuals who are low functioning with no incentive to feign impairment passed the usual cutoff on the TOMM, obtaining a mean Trial 2 score of 48.7 and a mean retention trial of 49.4. None of these MR subjects fell below the cutoff on the retention trial. Many of these subjects had other Axis I disorders. Marshall and Happe's (2007) findings showed that adults with mild MR have high ($\geq$ 89%) passing rates for the forced-choice portion of the California Verbal Learning Test-II (CVLT-II; Delis, Kramer, Kaplan, & Ober, 2000), the V-DS difference score, and the Rarely Missed Index from the Wechsler Memory Scale-III (WMS-III; Psychological Corporation, 1997), although specificity figures were low for the Rey 15-Item Test and the Dot Counting Test.

The differences between the Hurley and Deal (2006) study, which found a high percentage of failures on a SVT, and the others, might have to do with the sample characteristics. For example, in the Simon (2007) study, the individuals were already adjudicated and thus had no need to dissimulate. Although the subjects in the Hurley and Deal (2006) study were in a residential home and not applying for compensation, the proportion of subjects who were receiving Social Security Disability Insurance was unknown. What is known from the Chafetz et al. (2011) study (see subsequent discussion) is that the failure rate for low functioning disability claimants was quite high, and that the only SVT failures (6.7%) in the state rehabilitation group (also low functioning) were those referred by the local disability determinations office, and presumably, they were attempting to protect their disability payments. Thus, the motivation and understanding of the purpose of testing of SVT failing subjects in the Hurley and Deal (2006) may not have been entirely clear.

Concerning motivation, a key factor in the performance on any cognitive or effort test, Chafetz et al. (2011) compared the rates of SVT failure in three referral groups equated for low intellectual functioning (mean IQ < 75) but differing in motivation: (a) DDS: claimants seeking compensation for a total inability to work; (b) Louisiana Rehabilitation Service (LRS): claimants seeking to work to obtain compensation; and (c) Department of Children and Family Services (DCFS): parents seeking to have their children returned from state custody. The rates of dual SVT failure were as follows: DDS (45.5%); LRS (6.7%); and DCFS (0.0%). The DCFS parents were striving to impress, doing everything in their power to have the state return their children to them, and none of them failed SVTs. In the LRS group in which claimants were purportedly seeking to work, the dual failure rate was quite small, but further analysis revealed an interesting point: all of the failures in the LRS group were from individuals who had been sent to LRS from the local DDS, as (2006) the agencies cooperate in attempting to find work for individuals who are disabled but who have residual strengths. Although most LRS claimants passed symptom validity testing, it could well be that these particular individuals who failed were simply cooperating with the DDS mandate, but in fact, still operating under the DDS motivation for compensation. As discussed by Chafetz (2010), the high failure rate in the DDS group can in part be attributed to the SSA requirement of *total* inability to work, and thus claimants were likely trying to prove their intellectual disabilities as best as they could. Thus, this study showed that motivation (to work or to have their children returned) was critically important in SVT failure by these claimants who are low functioning, but low IQ per se was not a factor as it was equated in the three groups.[3]

What if the claimant with low IQ who also intentionally performed poorly on the neuropsychological evaluation in a desperate attempt to gain disability income? This point was considered by Chafetz et al. (2007) when regression equations were developed between IQ and the total score on the SVS for individuals who are low functioning. The relationship between the SVS total score and IQ was established in four groups: adult TOMM study, adult MSVT study, child TOMM study, and child MSVT study. The regression weight in both adult studies was approximately 1 and in both child studies was 1.6. Thus, for each SVS total point in a failed adult protocol, the full scale IQ (FSIQ) score moves down by 1 point. For each SVS total point in a failed child protocol, the IQ score moves down by 1.6 points. In the Chafetz et al. (2007) study, the fact that both the TOMM and MSVT studies produced the same weights with adults and with children was considered a replication of the weights findings for both adults and children, indicating reliability of this method in both adults and children.

In a study of malingering by proxy, Chafetz and Prentkowski (2011) showed the use of these regression weights. The parent of a 9-year-old boy was seeking SSDI on his behalf. On the Wechsler Intelligence Scale for Children-Third Edition (WISC-III), the boy obtained a FSIQ of 40 with scaled scores of 1 on all of the subtests, which is regarded as noncredible given that neuropsychological strengths and weaknesses typically are present in mental retardation (Mahone & Slomine, 2008). His TOMM Trial 1 and 2 scores were 14/50 and 9/50, respectively, which were both significantly below chance ($p < .01$) based on the binomial calculation. On the SVS, his total score of 23 was in the definite malingering range (Chafetz et al, 2007). If these 23 points are then multiplied by the regression weight (for children) of 1.62 ($23 \times 1.62 = 37.26$ points), it is considered that the IQ dropped 37 points because of effort problems alone. Adding these 37 points to his IQ of 40 gives an estimated IQ of 77, now in the borderline to low average range given the usual 95% confidence interval. If this method were to be used in practice, the local DDS would have information that the child appears not to be so impaired to warrant disability benefits (Morton, 2010).

For the present chapter, the data from Chafetz et al. (2007) and Chafetz (2008) were reanalyzed to seek the regression weights for the MSVT and the TOMM with respect to IQ in adults. The equation for the MSVT DR variable (entered as 100% − DR) is as follows: 68.9−0.25 DR = IQ ($r = -.78$; $F[1, 42] = 63.4$, $p < .001$). The equation for the TOMM Trial 2 variable (entered as 50− T2) is as follows: 68.1−0.43 T2 = IQ

---

[3] In fact, the DDS group originally had somewhat lower IQ than the other two groups, but this difference was caused by effort, based on SVT failure. When only the claimants who passed SVTs were considered, there was no significant difference in IQ between the three groups: DDS, LRS, and DCFS.

($r = -.68$; $F[1, 125] = 106.3$, $p < .001$). By using these weights, along with the SVT score, the examiner can now estimate for the DDS what the IQ might have been if the MSVT DR score had been 100% (full effort) or the TOMM Trial 2 score had been 50 (full effort). If the MSVT is used, IQ goes down by 0.25 points for every 1% or 1.25 points for each item missed (5%) on DR. If the TOMM is used, IQ goes down by 0.43 for every item missed (2%) on Trial 2. If the TOMM were on a 100-point scale and rescaled so that each unit missed corresponded to 5% (as on the MSVT), the IQ would drop by 1.075 points for each 5% drop, a slightly flatter rate. The reader who is working in the DDS arena may use this regression tool to estimate for the DDS what the IQ might have been if the claimant had not failed the MSVT or the TOMM.

PRIVATE DISABILITY AND CIVIL LITIGATION CASES

This section considers factors involved in private disability and civil litigation cases.

Private Disability

Private disability cases are also about an inability to work, but the particular contract with the carrier will determine whether the inability to work is a short- or long-term disability issue, whether it is for the claimant's particular work occupation or for any employment to which he or she might be suited, and whether it is about a total inability to work versus having limitations that restrict the claimant to doing only part-time work (Green, 2009). The neuropsychologist in these cases may be dealing directly with the disability carrier as the client (see "Ethics and Role Boundaries" section of this chapter) or might be engaged with an IME company whose job is to facilitate the referral from the private carrier or attorney group to the neuropsychologist and arrange the examination with the claimant. These IME companies are often quite professional (sometimes run by psychologists) and have developed clean boundaries and a professional set of referral questions that go directly to the crux of the problems. The IME neuropsychologist must be clear that the decision of disability is only within the scope of the disability carrier, according to the terms of the disability contract (Green, 2009). The neuropsychologist's role is to determine whether there are cognitive or emotional limitations that restrict the claimant's performance of work duties. The particular referral questions help guide the neuropsychologist into examining preexisting factors and uncovering how much these factors contribute to the claimant's current limitations. The questions also guide the neuropsychologist into deciding whether factors subsequent to the injury (e.g., divorce, death in the family) are contributing to the limitations currently experienced.

Bianchini (2010) described motivation and/or emotional factors that can prolong disability presentations. These factors include attorney involvement (Bernacki & Tao, 2008), administrative delays (Sinnott, 2009), and childhood psychological trauma (Harkonmäki et al., 2007), any of which can affect the claimant's motivation and/or emotional state. The following information covers other motivational and/or behavioral factors involved in these disability cases.

A frequent question concerning motivation involves whether there are "secondary gain" factors that may be applicable in deciding about the claimant's behavior and whether the claimant is truly limited from participating in work activities. Sigmund Freud (1959) described two types of gain: primary and secondary. In Freud's use of the term, a primary gain involved a decrease in anxiety through a psychological mechanism that resulted in the production of a symptom of the illness. There may be psychological conflict that is relieved by the symptom production, leading to what we now call conversion or other somatoform problems. Freud described secondary gain as an advantage (interpersonal or social) attained by the patient as a consequence of the illness. In modern terms, malingering is often associated with secondary gain factors because it involves significant compensation or avoidance of duty or punishment. The following case illustrates the importance of distinguishing between primary and secondary gain factors in the analysis of a disability claimant.

Case Vignette About Primary Versus Secondary Gain

A 59-year-old insurance case manager with a master's degree in social work and running his own consulting business lost his wife to heart disease in 2003. He was treated with medication for the loss, but during the ensuing years, he had numerous other stressors, including the incarceration of close assistants for drug dealing, an Internal Revenue Service audit, and dealing with the aftermath of a tornado that damaged his neighborhood. He maintained a high level of functioning and was highly responsible, always taking care of his clients and always being prepared for his work in court. In 2005, he remarried happily. He had considerable savings and investment income, and his wife made a nice living as a corporate executive. In 2007, he tripped and fell face down. Although he had frequently dealt with head injury cases with neuropsychologists, he declined to go to a hospital, choosing instead to lie down. He developed bruising over large areas of his face and was miserable for several days, taking some time off to recuperate. Within weeks of this incident, the aforementioned tornado damaged his neighborhood, causing him to shut down his business for a couple of weeks while he relocated to temporary quarters and dealt with the insurance claims. During this time, he had frequent headaches and began refusing further business. He also experienced memory problems. He eventually obtained a magnetic resonance imaging (MRI) of the brain, which showed an anomaly interpreted as a "prior ischemic event" in the white matter of the right frontal lobe. Given his previous experience with head injury cases, he self-diagnosed this problem as a contrecoup injury to his brain, although he did not obtain a neuropsychological evaluation. He started to believe he was no longer capable of his former high level of performance, and he started to decrease his case management business even further. He then stopped working and claimed disability benefits through his private policy, and the case came to this examiner after several denials in 2010. A subsequent MRI of the brain was normal, but he believed he could not perform at his previously high level of accomplishment, and he feared failing in court. He failed the MSVT with scores of 85%, 80%, 75%, 100%, and 55%. He also could reliably recite only four digits forward (although getting a total reliable digit span score of 8), and he had a poor delayed recognition score on the Repeatable Battery for the Assessment of Neuropsychological Status (RBANS; with an effort index [EI] score of 2), but he did well on many cognitive ability tests except those that were obviously about attention and memory. An EI of 2 on the RBANS has been shown to have adequate specificity (Armistead-Jehle & Hansen, 2011), but it is noteworthy that all 2 points came from poor recognition memory. These findings were initially conceived by this examiner as being about alleviating his anxiety and fear of failing in his high level work (primary gain) rather than about achieving compensation (secondary gain), particularly as he enjoyed good investment income. However, a significant factor was that his disability policy required him to prove *total* inability to work so he could not even return part-time to get up to speed. His awareness of his disability contract terms, coupled with his desire to maintain his low-stress life, suggested that secondary gain factors were more likely operating in this case.

At frequent times, claimants will have a motivational conflict, particularly the approach-avoidance conflict (Elliot, 2008) in which they are moving toward a positive goal that simultaneously has negative attributes (e.g., returning to a hated high-paying job). The conflicted claimant vacillates, approaching the positive goal, but then when the goal is getting near at hand, the claimant will back away as the negative attributes of that goal become more apparent. The tension is relieved when the claimant gets far from the goal, but then approach begins all over again because the claimant realizes just how desirable the goal may be. Sometimes there is a double approach-avoidance conflict operating within the same system. For example, a worker who is injured may long to return to his or her job but fear failure should he or she return. At the same time, the worker who is injured may enjoy spending more time at home but find household duties to be very stressful. Thus, this worker is drawn both to his or her prior job and to his or her home, but there are aspects of both that he or she is driven to avoid. This vacillation can confound treatment, delaying a disability case beyond any psychological problems that may be apparent.

Case Vignette on Double Approach-Avoidance Conflict

A 31-year-old security specialist working for a private company in Iraq was seen for a neuropsychological IME 3 years after a slip and fall in which he hurt his head and neck. He was deployed at a high-level security work and special missions. At one point, he came off active duty, received special training, and began working in units guarding high-level personnel. He thrived on the clarity of mission and purpose and loved his job. He indicated having an adrenalin rush for the danger and the mission. His slip and fall occurred on a wet floor with no retrograde amnesia and uncertain anterograde amnesia. MRI of the brain was negative. After returning to duty within a few weeks, he later suffered a bite from a poisonous snake. He returned home for medical care and never rotated back to Iraq. He was seen about 2.5 years after the snake bite. He failed the Word Memory Test and the MSVT and showed inconsistent behaviors, walking with difficulty with a cane coming in but not using the cane going out to the car where his brother was waiting. Neuropsychological examination revealed no deficits. He was happy at home, involved with his wife and young son, but admitted that being a househusband as his sole occupation would "drive me batty." On the other side, he clearly missed the camaraderie, mission, authority, and clarity of his work, but he had become deconditioned and felt that he would embarrass himself if he were to return (not to mention failing the physical). A double approach-avoidance conflict was considered with vacillation back and forth (in his mind) between returning to work and staying home with his family. The approach-avoidance conflict at home had become stronger as he continued enjoying activities with his young son. The approach-avoidance conflict at work involved a strong desire to return with an equally strong desire to preserve his memories of competence and so not to embarrass himself by failing the physical. It is interesting to consider that failing SVTs would suggest that the avoidance component was stronger than the approach component.

It is common that when a patient goes to an emergency room (ER) after sustaining a concussion, even if medically cleared to return home, the patient is given a warning sheet detailing the signs and symptoms that are important to consider if one has had a "traumatic brain injury." Of course, many patients routinely use the Internet to look up symptoms and outcomes, and it is certainly not hard to find advice on what to do if your brain has been injured. The concept of "diagnosis threat" (Suhr & Gunstad, 2002a) was put forth as a way of describing the self-fulfilling prophecy in the reduced neuropsychological performance of people who believe they "have" a TBI. Under the influence of diagnosis threat, people are acting in accordance with their beliefs but are otherwise ignorant of the long-term outcomes and healing involved following MTBI. As Iverson et al. (2009) has indicated, the VA has been intentionally overinclusive about TBI in postdeployment screenings. Considerable information is being disseminated about TBI to veterans, and in many medical board examinations long after the recovery period, this author has seen veterans with strong beliefs in their brain pathology.

Civil Litigation

Although private disability cases may ultimately involve an adversarial situation with the claimant retaining an attorney as the claim continues on through appeals, the civil litigation case is clearly adversarial. A plaintiff has been or feels wronged or hurt and sues the defendant for damages. In cases involving TBI, the plaintiff may have sought evaluation with a neuropsychologist directly, via another health care professional, or the plaintiff's attorney may have referred to a neuropsychologist. The defendant is also entitled to have the plaintiff undergo an IME, although ethically (and practically) the examination done by the neuropsychologist retained by the plaintiff's attorney may be sufficient. A good account of the basics of forensic neuropsychology can be found in Greiffenstein (2008).

Because the plaintiff is seeking monetary damages, the motivation of the plaintiff is frequently perceived as being about seeking compensation. However, complex human motivations about a sense of justice, righting the wrong, punishing the perpetrator, or taking down the Goliath (e.g., a large company) frequently become part of the plaintiff's presentation. The adversarial system is a huge enterprise, and plaintiffs frequently have to cope with having their backgrounds investigated and being under surveillance, and the urge to speak out and possibly exaggerate may become more prominent as the wheels of justice grind slowly. On the other hand, if a wealthy defendant has attacked a plaintiff, a prison sentence after a criminal trial may not be enough to convince the plaintiff that justice has been served, and a civil suit might be launched for monetary damages. Is this about seeking compensation or about seeing that real punishment and restitution is done? It is only by thorough examination of symptom validity in the individual case that neuropsychologists can get a better handle on these questions.

An important point in the science of the development of symptom validity testing can be said to be the publication of the Slick, Sherman, and Iverson (1999) article on malingered neurocognitive dysfunction, which set forth clear guidelines subsequently used for the development of known groups studies (Heilbronner et al., 2009). The known groups format permitted psychologists to construct rigorous classification-accuracy studies, which produced known error rates for SVTs that could stand up to challenge in court. The development of these studies is one major reason that the use of psychologists and neuropsychologists in court has risen exponentially over the 1978–2008 period, whereas the use of psychiatrists and neuropsychiatrists in court has risen generally with the increase in court cases (Kaufmann, 2009).

Malingering involves the intentional production or exaggeration of symptoms for the purpose of gain (e.g., money, medications) or to avoid duty or imprisonment (Slick et al., 1999). The following case provides an example of malingering encountered in a neuropsychological IME performed at the request of defense counsel in a civil litigation case.

Independent Medical Examination Vignette

A 38-year-old electrician was body slammed by his supervisor during an altercation at work 2 years prior to the IME. The primary injury was to his shoulder. A neuropsychologist consulted by the plaintiff indicated that the plaintiff had cognitive decline because of a head injury, and there was a claim for damages because of TBI that yielded cognitive problems. However, there was no evidence of TBI. There was no retrograde or anterograde amnestic loss and no loss of consciousness. The plaintiff appeared aware of the implications of the lawsuit. When the examiner asked him about details of the event, he quickly said that witnesses had told him the supervisor left the room after the altercation, but then he later confirmed that he himself saw the supervisor leave the room, indicating no anterograde loss. He failed the nonverbal MSVT and obtained a raw score of 32 on the SVS (previously known as the Fake Bad Scale or FBS) of the MMPI-2 (103T). A score this high has no known false positives (Larrabee, 2007). He also obtained a poor recognition score on a verbal memory test embedded within the examination. There were numerous other inconsistencies in self-report and testing, which fit Slick et al.'s (1999) A, B, and C criteria, and a diagnosis of malingering was given.

One of the more interesting aspects of the human condition occurs when malingering is produced at the direction of another (e.g., parent, spouse), a condition referred to as malingering by proxy (Slick et al., 1999). Chafetz and Prentkowski (2011) presented the case of a 9-year-old child whose parent was seeking Social Security Disability benefits on his behalf. The child's scores on symptom validity testing were significantly below chance, indicating awareness and intent to produce invalid responding. The following is a civil litigation case from the archives of this author that shows a similar process in the legal arena.

Adult Malingering by Proxy Vignette

In 2002, the husband of a 49-year-old woman called this author's office for an appointment. She had been involved in a motor vehicle accident the year before in which she was at a stop sign and turned left, and the next thing she knew, she was in her car with significant pain in her left knee. The husband indicated that there was no lawsuit and that they had not retained an attorney. This statement was in fact not true, and the examiner only learned this fact 4 years later when he was asked to provide a deposition in this matter. An attorney had been retained at the time of the original evaluation. The lawsuit had been filed in the name of the patient and her husband. In later papers, the husband's name appeared first. According to her statements in the interview, she recalled everything up to starting to make the turn and thus had no retrograde loss. She estimated having lost consciousness for about 20–30 min, but there was no objective evidence for this LOC. She got out of the vehicle. The police arrested her, thinking she was drunk, but the charges were dropped. The husband picked her up and wanted to take her to ER, but she started screaming to take her home. They went to ER the next day, and she was found to have a knee injury and scalp laceration. Later, computed tomography (CT) and MRI scans of the brain and electroencephalogram (EEG) were normal. At the neuropsychological evaluation a year later, she reported headaches, trouble getting started, stuttering (never having stuttered before), and problems with attention and short-term memory. During the neuropsychological examination, she failed the TOMM (with scores of 45, 46, and 44 for the three sections of the test) but passed all other symptom validity measures. However, there were numerous inconsistencies present that satisfied Slick et al.'s (1999) B and C criteria for malingered neurocognitive dysfunction. The results of the cognitive ability tests were mostly in the low average to average range. At the time, the Barona regression equation (Barona, Reynolds, & Chastain, 1984) was used to estimate premorbid functioning, which was in the high average range. In a notable manner, at the deposition, the deposing attorney for the plaintiff (perhaps in a gambit) suggested that the facts (notably education) given to the examiner were incorrect and asked the examiner to recalculate the Barona estimate, which was now in the middle of the average range; the suggestion was that this couple had been intentionally misleading. The examiner learned that they had been involved in other lawsuits on her behalf. By the time of the deposition, she was reported to be anxious and miserable and even worse off. After the deposition, the husband wrote to the examiner to introduce into the patient's file a more comprehensive account of her achievements and how badly she had declined. He fired lawyers and hired new ones. Two years later, the examiner was contacted by a new attorney in the case, who rapidly settled after the examiner reported his findings to the new attorney.

CONCLUSION

This chapter examined the world of disability and civil litigation concerning cases of MTBI with coverage of possible malingering. Although MTBI usually resolves completely in a relatively short period, yielding no lasting neuropsychological deficits by the time of a disability evaluation, numerous factors come into play in the assessment of these cases including the need to consider differential diagnostic issues when considering symptom attribution. The factors are better understood by examining the motivation of the claimant, which is facilitated through the use of symptom validity testing. Findings of valid performance can also be of value. The special case of the claimant who is low functioning was addressed, and the ethics and role boundaries of the neuropsychologist in these cases were explored.

REFERENCES

American Psychiatric Association. (2000). *Diagnostic and statistical manual of mental disorders* (4th ed., text rev.). Washington, DC: Author.

Americans with Disabilities Act, 42 U.S.C § 12101 (1990). Retrieved from http://www.ada.gov/pubs/adastatute08.htm

Armistead-Jehle, P., & Hansen, C. L. (2011). Comparison of the repeatable battery for the assessment of neuropsychological status effort index and stand-alone symptom validity tests in a military sample. *Archives of Clinical Neuropsychologist*, 26(7), 592–601.

Barona, A., Reynolds, C., & Chastain, R. (1984). A demographically based index of premorbid intelligence for the WAIS-R. *Journal of Consulting and Clinical Psychology*, 52(5), 885–887.

Belanger, H. G., Kretzmer, T., Yoash-Gantz, R., Pickett, T., & Tupler, L. A. (2009). Cognitive sequelae of blast-related versus other mechanisms of brain trauma. *Journal of the International Neuropsychological Society*, 15(1), 1–8.

Bernacki, E. J., & Tao, X. G. (2008). The relationship between attorney involvement, claim duration, and workers' compensation costs. *Journal of Occupation and Environmental Medicine*, 50(9), 1013–1018.

Bianchini, K. J. (2010). The financial incentive effect: It's not just malingering. *The Clinical Neuropsychologist*, 24(4), 556.

Bianchini, K. J., Curtis, K. L., & Greve, K. W. (2006). Compensation and malingering in traumatic brain injury: A dose-response relationship? *The Clinical Neuropsychologist*, 20(4), 831–847.

Buddin, R., & Kapur, K. (2005). *An analysis of military disability compensation*. Santa Monica, CA: Research ANd Development Corporation.

Bush, S. S. (Ed.). (2005). Ethical challenges in forensic neuropsychology. In *A casebook of ethical challenges in neuropsychology* (pp. 10–70). New York, NY: Psychology Press.

Carlson, K., Kehle, S., & Meis, L. (2009). *The assessment and treatment of individuals with history of traumatic brain injury and post-traumatic stress disorder: A systematic review of the evidence*. Washington, DC: Department of Veteran Affairs.

Chafetz, M. D. (2008). Malingering on the social security disability consultative exam: Predictors and base rates. *The Clinical Neuropsychologist*, 22(3), 529–546.

Chafetz, M. D. (2010). Symptom validity issues in the psychological consultative examination for social security disability. *The Clinical Neuropsychologist*, 24(6), 1045–1063.

Chafetz, M. D. (2011). Reducing the probability of false positives in malingering detection of social security disability claimants. *The Clinical Neuropsychologist*, 25(7), 1239–1252.

Chafetz, M. D., Abrahams, J. P., & Kohlmaier, J. (2007). Malingering on the social security disability consultative examination: A new rating scale. *Archives of Clinical Neuropsychology*, 22(1), 1–14.

Chafetz, M. D., & Prentkowski, E. (2011). A case of malingering by proxy in a social security disability psychological consultative examination. *Applied Neuropsychology*, 18(2), 143–149.

Chafetz, M. D., Prentkowski, E., & Rao, A. (2011). To work or not to work: Motivation (not low IQ) determines SVT findings. *Archives of Clinical Neuropsychology*, 26(4), 306–313.

Colker, R. (2005). *The disability pendulum: The first decade of the Americans with disabilities act*. New York, NY: New York University Press.

Delis, D. C., Kramer, J. H., Kaplan, E., & Ober, B. A. (2000). *California verbal learning test* (2nd ed.). San Antonio, TX: Psychological Corporation.

Diener, M. J., & Monroe, J. M. (2011). The relationship between adult attachment style and therapeutic alliance in individual psychotherapy: A meta-analytic review. *Psychotherapy*, 48(3), 237–248.

Education of All Handicapped Children Act of 1975, Pub. L. 94–142 § 1400. Retrieved from http://www.scn.org/~bk269/94-142.html

Elliot, A. J. (Ed.). (2008). *Approach and avoidance motivation. In Handbook of approach and avoidance motivation* (pp. 3–16). New York, NY: Psychology Press.

France, C. R., France, J. L., & Patterson, S. M. (2006). Blood pressure and cerebral oxygenation responses to skeletal muscle tension: A comparison of two physical maneuvers to prevent vasovagal reactions. *Clinical Physiology and Functional Imaging* 26(1), 21–25.

Freud, S. (1959). *Freud's psychoanalytic procedure, standard edition*. London, UK: Hogarth Press.

Green, P. (2003/2005). *Manual for the word memory test*. Edmonton, Canada: Green's Publishing.

Green, P. (2004). *Manual for the medical symptom validity test*. Edmonton, Canada: Green's Publishing.

Green, P. (2008). *Manual for the nonverbal medical symptom validity test*. Edmonton, Canada: Green's Publishing.

Green, J. (2009). Disability insurance case management: External consultant. In J. E. Morgan & J.J. Sweet (Eds.), *Neuropsychology of malingering casebook* (pp. 457–465). New York, NY: Psychology Press.

Greenberg, S. A., & Shuman, D. W. (1997). Irreconcilable conflict between therapeutic and forensic roles. *Professional Psychology: Research and Practice*, 28, 50–57.

Greenberg, S. A., & Shuman, D. W. (2007). When worlds collide: Therapeutic and forensic roles. *Professional Psychology: Research and Practice*, 38(2), 129–132.

Greiffenstein, M. F. (2008). Basics of forensic neuropsychology. In J. E. Morgan & J. H. Ricker (Eds.), *Textbook of clinical neuropsychology* (pp. 905–941). New York, NY: Taylor & Francis.

Greiffenstein, M. F. (2009). Clinical myths of forensic neuropsychology. *The Clinical Neuropsychologist*, 23(2), 286–296.

Greiffenstein, M. F., & Baker, W. J. (2008). Validity testing in dually diagnosed post-traumatic stress disorder and mild closed head injury. *The Clinical Neuropsychologist*, 22(3), 565–582.

Harkonmäki, K., Korkeila, K., Vahtera, J., Kivimäki, M., Suominen, S., Sillanmäki, L., & Koskenvuo, M. (2007). Childhood adversities as a predictor of disability retirement. *Journal of Epidemiology and Community Health*, 61(6), 479–484.

Heilbronner, R. L., Sweet, J. J., Morgan, J. E., Larrabee, G. J., & Millis, S. R. (2009). American Academy of Clinical Neuropsychology Consensus Conference Statement on the neuropsychological assessment of effort, response bias, and malingering. *The Clinical Neuropsychologist*, 23(7), 1093–1129.

Heilbrun, K., DeMatteo, D., Marczyk, G., & Samuelson, K.W.>Goldstein, A. M. (2008). Standards of practice and care in forensic mental health assessment: Legal, professional, and principles-based considerations. *Psychology, Public Policy, and Law*, 14(1), 1–26.

Howe, L. L. (2009). Giving context to post-deployment post-concussive-like symptoms: Blast-related potential mild traumatic brain injury and comorbidities. *The Clinical Neuropsychologist*, 23(8), 1315–1337.

Howe, L. L., & Loring, D. W. (2009). Classification accuracy and predictive ability of the medical symptom validity test's dementia profile and general memory impairment profile. *The Clinical Neuropsychologist*, 23(2), 329–342.

Hurley, K. E., & Deal, W. P. (2006). Assessment instruments measuring malingering used with individuals who have mental retardation: Potential problems and issues. *Mental Retardation*, 44, 112–119.

Iverson, G. L. (2006). Misdiagnosis of the persistent postconcussion syndrome in patients with depression. *Archives of Clinical Neuropsychology*, 21(4), 303–310.

Iverson, G. L., & Lange, R. T. (2011). Mild traumatic brain injury. In M. R. Schoenberg & J. G. Scott (Eds.), *The little black book of neuropsychology: A syndrome-based approach* (pp. 697–720), New York, NY: Springer Publishing.

Iverson, G. L., Langlois, J .A., McCrea, M. A., & Kelly, J. P. (2009). Challenges associated with post-deployment screening for mild traumatic brain injury in military personnel. *The Clinical Neuropsychologist*, 23(8), 1299–1314.

Iverson, G. L., & Tulsky, D. S. (2003). Detecting malingering on the WAIS-III. Unusual digit span performance patterns in the normal population and in clinical groups. *Archives of Clinical Neuropsychology*, 18(1), 1–9.

Kaufmann, P.M. (2009). Protecting raw data and psychological tests from wrongful disclosure: A primer on the law and other persuasive strategies. *The Clinical Neuropsychologist*, 23(7), 1130–1159.

Larrabee, G. J. (Ed.). (2007). Evaluation of exaggerated health and injury symptomatology. In *Assessment of malingered neuropsychological deficits* (pp. 264–286). New York, NY: Oxford University Press.

Larrabee, G. J. (2008). Aggregation across multiple indicators improves the detection of malingering: Relationship to likelihood ratios. *The Clinical Neuropsychologist*, 22(4), 666–679.

Mahone, E. M., & Slomine, B. S. (2008). Neurodevelopmental disorders. In J. E. Morgan & J. H. Ricker (Eds), *Textbook of clinical neuropsychology* (pp. 105–127). New York, NY: Taylor & Francis.

Marshall, P., & Happe, M. (2007). The performance of individuals with mental retardation on cognitive tests assessing effort and motivation. *The Clinical Neuropsychologist*, 21(5), 826–840.

McCrea, M. (2008). *Mild traumatic brain injury and post-concussion syndrome: The new evidence base for diagnosis and treatment.* New York, NY: Oxford University Press.

Merten, T., Bossink, L., & Schmand, B. (2007). On the limits of effort testing: Symptom validity tests and the severity of neurocognitive symptoms in nonlitigant patients. *Journal of Clinical and Experimental Neuropsychology*, 29(3), 308–318.

Merten, T., Thies, E., Schneider, K., & Stevens, A. (2009). Symptom validity testing in claimants with alleged posttraumatic stress disorder: Comparing the morel emotional numbing test, the structured inventory of malingered symptomatology, and the word memory test. *Psychological Injury and Law*, 2, 284–293.

Mittenberg, W. Theroux-Fichera ,S., Zielinski, R.E., & Heilbronner, R.L. (1995). Identification of malingered head injury on the Wechsler Adult Intelligence Scale-Revised. *Professional Psychology: Research and Practice*, 26, 491–498.

Morton, D. A., III. (2010). *Nolo's guide to social security disability* (5th ed.). Berkeley, CA: Nolo.

Ohlemacher, S. (2010). *Social security disability system bogged down with requests.* Retrieved from http://www.oneidadispatch.com/articles/2010/05/09/news/doc4be763e825022593194203.txt?viewmode=fullstory

Psychological Corporation. (1997). *WAIS-III/WMS-III technical manual.* San Antonio, TX: Harcourt Brace.

Richman, J., Green, P., Gervais, R., Flaro, L Merten, T. Brockhaus, R., & Ranks, D. (2006). Objective tests of symptom exaggeration in independent medical examinations. *Journal of Occupational and Environmental Medicine*, 48(3), 303–311.

Rohling, M. L., Binder, L. M., Demakis, G. J., Larrabee, G. J., Ploetz, D. M., & Langhinrichsen-Rohling, J. (2011). A meta-analysis of neuropsychological outcome after mild traumatic brain injury: Re-analyses and reconsiderations of Binder et al. (1997), Frencham et al. (2005), and Pertab et al. (2009). *The Clinical Neuropsychologist*, 25(4), 608–623.

Ropper, A., & Samuels, M. (2009). *Adams and Victor's principles of neurology* (9th ed.). New York, NY: McGraw-Hill.

Rubenzer, S. (2009). Posttraumatic stress disorder: Assessing response style and malingering. *Psychological Injury and Law*, 2(2), 114–142.

Salekin, K. L., & Doane, B. M. (2009). Malingered intellectual disability: The value of available measures and methods. *Applied Neuropsychology*, 16(2), 105–113.

Samuelson, K.W., Neylan, T.C., Metzler, T.J., Lenoci, M., Rothlind, J., Henn-Haase, C., . . . Marmar, C. R. (2006). Neuropsychological functioning in posttraumatic stress disorder and alcohol abuse. *Neuropsychology*, 20(6), 716–726.

Simon, M. J. (2007). Performance of mentally retarded forensic patients on the Test of Memory Malingering. *Journal of Clinical Psychology*, 63(4), 339–344.

Singhal, A., Green, P., Ashaye, K., Shankar, K., & Gill, D. (2009). High specificity of the medical symptom validity test in patients with very severe memory impairment. *Archives of Clinical Neuropsychology*, 24(8), 721–728.

Sinnott, P. (2009). Administrative delays and chronic disability in patients with acute occupational low back injury. *Journal of Occupational and Environmental Medicine*, 51(6), 690–699.

Slick, D. J., Sherman, E. M., & Iverson, G. L. (1999). Diagnostic criteria for malingered neurocognitive dysfunction: Proposed standards for clinical practice and research. *The Clinical Neuropsychologist*, 13(4), 545–561.

Social Security Advisory Board (2003). The Social Security Definition of Disability. Washington, DC: Social Security Advisory Board.

Stevens, J. (1986). Is it organic or is it functional. Is it hysterical or malingering? *The Psychiatric Clinics of North America*, 9(2), 241–254.

Strasburger, L. H., Gutheil, T. G., & Brodsky, A. (1997). On wearing two hats: Role conflict in serving as both psychotherapist and expert witness. *The American Journal of Psychiatry*, 154(4), 448–456.

Suhr, J. A., & Gunstad, J. (2002a). "Diagnosis threat": The effect of negative expectations on cognitive performance in head injury. *Journal of Clinical and Experimental Neuropsychology*, 24(4), 448–457.

Suhr, J. A., & Gunstad, J. (2002b). Postconcussive symptom report: The relative influence of head injury and depression. *Journal of Clinical and Experimental Neuropsychology*, 24(8), 981–993.

Teichner, G., & Wagner, M. T. (2004). The test of memory malingering (TOMM): Normative data from cognitively intact, cognitively impaired, aoond elderly patients with dementia. *Archives of Clinical Neuropsychology*, 19(3), 455–464.

Vasterling, J. J., Proctor, S. P., Amoroso, P., Kane, R., Heeren, T., & White, R. F. (2006). Neuropsychological outcomes of army personnel following deployment to the Iraq war. *The Journal of the American Medical Association*, 296(5), 519–529.

Victor, T. L., & Boone, K. B. (2007). Identification of feigned mental retardation. In K. B. Boone (Ed.), *Assessment of feigned cognitive impairment: A neuropsychological perspective* (pp. 310–345). New York, NY: Guilford Press.

Symptom Validity Assessment and Sports Concussion 17

Stephen N. Macciocchi & Steven Broglio

To place symptom validity testing in sports concussion in proper perspective, a brief historical review of sports concussion assessment is necessary. Sports concussion was a generally unstudied clinical problem in the United States until interest in mild traumatic brain injury (MTBI) began to draw the attention of researchers in the mid-1980s. MTBI has been a controversial diagnosis since early animal studies identified a pathophysiological correlate of brief loss of consciousness, and uncontrolled clinical studies found MTBI to be associated with persisting cognitive impairment (Barth, Macciocchi, Giordani, Rimel, Jane, & Boll, 1983; Ommaya & Generalli, 1974). Subsequent research recognized several co-occurring disorders in persons with MTBI that had the potential to bias outcome studies (Levin et al., 1987). Researchers quickly learned that studying MTBI in the emergency room (Alves, Macciocchi, & Barth, 1993) and medical settings (Davidoff, Morris, Roth, & Bleiberg, 1985), presented methodological challenges. As a result, after some deliberation, researchers turned to settings where MTBI could be studied in persons without numerous co-occurring disorders and where methodological challenges were less prominent. After some analysis of biomechanics- and methodology-friendly environments, sports concussion was born as an empirical model for MTBI (Barth et al., 1989).

Once sports were identified as an opportunistic environment to study MTBI, a large prospective study of sports concussion was initiated with funding from the Pew Foundation in 1983. Over several years, more than 2,000 football players were enrolled and administered baseline testing followed by postconcussion assessments consisting of cognitive tests and symptom checklists (Macciocchi, Barth, Alves, Rimel, & Jane, 1996). At the time, formal symptom validity testing was not used routinely in clinical settings, let alone in research settings, although many such tests were being developed at the time. Moreover, part of the motivation for seeking out sports settings was the presumption that athletes were different from persons frequenting emergency rooms following a MTBI. Athletes were presumed to be healthy, motivated, generally without significant cognitive problems, and willing to comply with the demands of research participation.

At that time, sports concussion was not viewed as a clinical problem, and resistance to viewing sports concussion as a health concern was widespread. Athletes, athletic trainers, and especially coaches, many of whom were former football players, viewed concussion as a trivial injury that was part of the game. There was no societal mandate for treating sports concussion as a health care problem, and athletes were rarely, if ever, assessed on a clinical basis. Part of the reason investigators selected sports settings for research in the first place was the belief that athletes would always exert optimal effort during testing, which would limit measurement bias because of suboptimal effort, a problem that was commonly encountered in clinical populations. As a result, investigators never considered the value of symptom validity testing in an environment where athletes were, by definition, highly motivated to perform well and return to play following what was then perceived to be a minor injury in the larger scheme of things.

Once sports concussion became identified as a valid research model of MTBI, many clinicians and researchers began to study the problem in earnest (Collins et al., 1999; Guskiewicz et al., 2003; McCrea, Kelly, Randolph, Cisler, & Berger, 2002; Pellman, Lovell, Viano, Casson, & Tucker, 2004). As research on sports concussion became more prevalent, the scope of the problem became more apparent. Many new investigators gravitated to sports concussion research, and much more funding was made available so these investigators could address some of the pressing empirical issues in sports concussion. Although sports concussion research began to flourish, clinical considerations also gained momentum as evidenced by the development of sports concussion management guidelines (Guskiewicz et al., 2004; Kelly & Rosenberg, 1997; McCrory et al., 2009).

As clinical and research endeavors in sports concussion increased, sports concussion was slowly pushed into the public's awareness. Enterprising neuropsychologists were developing concussion-specific batteries, sideline assessment techniques, and symptom checklists designed to assist in concussion management. Shortly thereafter, computerized assessment measures were developed and became more popular and widely used (Erlanger et al., 2003; Iverson, Lovell, & Collins, 2003). Today, computerized assessment is commonplace in high school, college, and professional sports. Computerized assessment has several advantages when applied to the large numbers of athletes that are being assessed in current athletic environments, but one limitation is the lack of embedded symptom validity indicators that have been externally validated.

Symptom validity assessment in mainstream clinical neuropsychology has advanced rapidly from simple behavioral observations that were the standard practice in the 1980s, to the development of many freestanding and embedded symptom validity (effort) measures that exist today. Research on symptom validity assessment has increased exponentially, and the list of symptom validity tests and methods for assessing symptom validity is extensive (Heilbronner, Sweet, Morgan, Larrabee, & Millis, 2009). Readers will find extensive discussion of these approaches in various clinical populations in other chapters. Because symptom validity issues in sports populations have generally been believed to be nonexistent or have been ignored, there is very limited research on symptom validity assessment in athletes. In the discussion that follows, we review situations that typically raise validity concerns, and we describe measures that may be of value in assessing the validity of clinical data in sports populations. We focus on three basic domains: self-reported symptoms, postural stability, and cognition.

SYMPTOM ASSESSMENT

Symptom minimization and symptom magnification can both affect the clinician's judgment regarding an athlete's injury and readiness to return to play. Therefore, both minimization and magnification of symptoms must be considered by the clinician.

Symptom Minimization

It is unfortunate that neuropsychologists do not always have multiple measurement models at their disposal. As a result, the most difficult assessment of validity involves the determination of whether symptom reports are accurate. When baseline testing became commonplace, athletes quickly realized that comparisons to baseline were critical to return to play, which created an environment ripe for manipulation. Athletic teammates constantly talk with one another and share information about examinations, potential problems, and ways to optimize what they believe to be in their best interest. Generally speaking, such discussions involve ways to get back to play as soon as possible.

For instance, if an athlete is referred for more comprehensive evaluation because of persisting impairment on computerized measures and balance testing, without any self-reported symptoms, the focus of validity assessment must be on minimization or denial of symptoms. This scenario is relatively common and is challenging for clinicians because they are less skilled at detecting symptom denial than symptom magnification. When there is persisting impairment on cognitive and/or balance tests and athletes also deny symptoms, underreporting must be considered. Formal freestanding symptom validity tests of cognitive effort will be of no value when underreporting occurs. The optimal way to address this situation is to closely examine the athletes' history of concussion, initial symptom reports, and resolution of symptoms over time. In some cases, atypical symptom presentation and resolution will be present.

As an example, athletes who sustain a severe concussion with posttraumatic confusion, balance and/or dizziness problems, and headache immediately following the injury and then report complete resolution of symptoms within 24 hr merit closer scrutiny. In addition, athletes who have very high symptom scores at 24-hr postinjury and then have complete resolution of symptoms at 48 or 72 hr require closer examination. Clinicians have access to well-documented patterns of symptom recovery, and these patterns can serve as a guideline for symptom resolution. However, for the most part, clinicians are in the unenviable role of determining when symptom reports are invalid based on very little, other than knowledge of brain–behavior relationships.

In some cases, help comes in the form of supplementary testing. For instance, in the case of an athlete who initially had balance and/or dizziness problems immediately postinjury and then denied these symptoms at 24 hr, postural stability testing may prove helpful. In some cases, athletes deny balance problems on self-report measures, but when subjected to a balance test, they become "dizzy" and have to stop the test or perform well below normative and baseline data (Broglio, Sosnoff, & Ferrara, 2009). Although the objective and potentially confrontational nature of these findings may not deter all athletes from minimizing symptoms, in most cases, the athletes will reassess their situation and be more open to discussing the validity of their postinjury symptom reports.

Symptom Magnification

Prior to the advent of baseline testing, athletes were only administered symptom checklists postinjury, and determining impairment was based on traditional normative comparisons. The precision of normative comparisons is always difficult to assess, especially with symptom reports, but because most athletes were attempting to return to participation, clinicians assumed athletes would generally underreport symptoms. Following the media blitz about concussions and the possible long-term impact of multiple concussions, athletic participants are beginning to present with abnormal reactions to concussive injuries, which include abnormal symptom reports.

The most common presentation is an athlete who has sustained a concussion and views the concussion as a legitimate way to avoid further participation. In such cases, clinicians often see a disproportionate number and severity of symptoms as well as protracted symptoms. For instance, athletes will have symptoms that persist for several months following a questionable concussion. In some cases, these athletes' symptoms become more frequent and severe over time, and new symptoms may arise. In most cases, these athletes are ambivalent about return to play. Systematic assessment of symptom frequency and severity can provide valuable information on recovery or lack thereof. Computerized instruments such as the ImPACT (Iverson et al., 2003) have embedded symptom scales, but other measures of postconcussive symptoms have been validated for use in concussion management (Piland, Ferrara, Macciocchi, Broglio, & Gould, 2010).

In most cases, athletes who have atypical and perplexing symptom recovery also have co-occurring psychological problems such as depression and anxiety, and when looking at their personality organization, there is a great departure from what is normally observed in most dedicated athletes. Most successful athletes have narcissistic and compulsive personality traits. Depressive, dependent, avoidant, and/or schizoid personality traits are rare and may be informative in the context of other clinical findings.

Knowledge of brain–behavior relationships is critical when assessing symptom validity, but in the case of symptom magnification (compared to minimization), clinicians are on somewhat more firm empirical ground, in part because symptom magnification is often accompanied by suboptimal effort on cognitive tests. Such dissimulation can be detected with stand-alone and/or embedded effort indicators as well as validity scales from measures such as the Minnesota Multiphasic Personality Inventory-2-Restructured Form (Ben-Porath & Tellegen, 2008). Nevertheless, clinical judgment is critical because clinical experience suggests that athletes who magnify symptoms have complex reasons for not wanting to return to play. Because the culture of sports regarding concussion has only recently changed, clinicians have not yet systematically studied symptom magnification in athletes. Based on clinical observation and some emerging patterns of test findings, there appear to be a subgroup of athletes who want to avoid continued participation. Having persisting symptoms from a concussion is one way to legitimately cease participation with the backing of the medical staff.

Some features to look for in these cases are deviations from normal injury and recovery symptoms patterns, excessive concern about the impact of single or multiple concussions, an atypical personality organization for highly successful athletes, poor performance on freestanding effort tests, academic achievement that surpasses athletic prowess, and somatic preoccupation. Diagnosing the problem is rarely difficult because of multiple sources of information, but providing the athlete with feedback and discussing the implications of the assessment can be complicated. Chapter 6 provides a feedback model that may be helpful to clinicians working in this area.

Because our society values sports so highly, many young participants in athletics are not really athletes at all but simply persons who have been thrust into athletics for various reasons. The difference between being an athlete and participating in athletics is important. In most cases, athletes rarely evidence symptom magnification. Persons who value academic or occupational goals more highly than athletics and want to stop participating in sports that have a risk of concussion usually do so without duress and seem relieved when given the opportunity to move on to other pursuits.

POSTURAL STABILITY ASSESSMENT

Postural stability (PS) has proven to be an important component of sports concussion assessment (Broglio, Macciocchi, & Ferrara, 2007). Using PS as a measurement strategy allows for assessment of different symptom domains than those assessed on cognitive measures. It is unfortunate that PS assessment requires expensive technology and expertise that neuropsychologists typically do not acquire in the normal course of training. Nonetheless, if PS equipment is available, the validity of various physical symptoms can be addressed. To understand how PS can be used in validity assessments, a brief review of PS measurement models are presented.

PS is the ability to maintain a center of gravity (COG) within the limits of stability (LOS). LOS can be thought of as an imaginary cone with the narrow end at the feet and broadening as it rises. When standing still under normal circumstances, there is a sway in the anterior/posterior and medial/lateral directions within the LOS that is controlled by minute muscle contractions at the ankle and hip. Sway varies between people and circumstances, but the average individual can sway approximately 12.5° angle in the anterior/posterior direction and 16° angle laterally. If the magnitude of sway is sufficient to move the COG beyond the edge of the cone (perturbation), then a stepping strategy must be employed to avoid falling.

Contracting the appropriate musculature in the appropriate sequence requires the integration of three afferent signals received by the brain from the body. The first signal is the ability of the body to "feel" the location of the body and its extremities in relation to the surface on which it is standing (somatosensory). The feet and ankles provide the central nervous system (CNS) with the necessary information to maintain postural equilibrium. The second signal (visual) is received via the eyes and uses fixed objects as a reference to body motion to maintain PS. As stance requirements become more complex, cues from the visual system are integrated with the somatosensory information that helps maintain upright and stable posture. The third signal is from the vestibular system located within the inner ear and functions to supply information on the body's gravitational, linear, and angular accelerations of the head in relation to inertial space (Guskiewicz, 1999). Under normal circumstances, the vestibular system plays a small role in maintaining postural stability because it does not provide reference of the body to an external object, but if inappropriate or conflicting information is supplied to the somatosensory (moving or compliant support surface) and visual (moving visual field) systems, the vestibular system will resolve the conflict between the two to maintain the body within the LOS (El-Kashlan, Shepard, Asher, Smith-Wheelock, & Telian, 1998; Nashner, Black, & Wall, 1982; Nashner & Peters, 1990).

In combination, signals from the three systems are simultaneously transmitted and integrated to the brain, and an efferent signal is returned to the musculature via a feedback mechanism (Swanik, Lephart, Giannantonio, & Fu, 1997). Some investigators have suggested that PS is maintained through both feedback and feed-forward mechanisms. The concept of feed-forward mechanism suggests that balance centers send preprogramed signals to the periphery based on prior experiences in a given set of conditions. These signals may be modified based on position of the body in relation to the environment and of individual segments in relation to each other that are provided by the feedback pathway (Swanik et al., 1997). This combined system appears to be the most scientifically plausible. If balance was strictly a feedback process, a large delay would occur from the time stimuli were induced, the afferent signal was transmitted and interpreted, and an efferent impulse was finally sent and the appropriate muscles reacted accordingly. In the feed-forward model, afferent and efferent signals are continually being sent to maintain postural equilibrium.

Concussion and Postural Stability

A number of domains may be affected by concussion, including cognition and postural control (Broglio & Puetz, 2008). At the time of injury, there appears to be a functional change in one or more of the three balance systems previously described, and/or the brain is less able to integrate afferent signals, which ultimately leads to equilibrium problems or dizziness. The degree and duration of instability following concussion varies based on injury severity but can be quantified using force plate technology. One system that has proven especially beneficial to clinicians for concussion management is the NeuroCom Sensory Organization Test (SOT). The SOT implements six different testing conditions that manipulate or remove the visual, vestibular, or somatosensory inputs alone or in combination (see Figure 17.1).

During each trial, the subject stands on a force platform that tracks center of pressure (COP) motion. Based on the testing condition and the individual's sway,

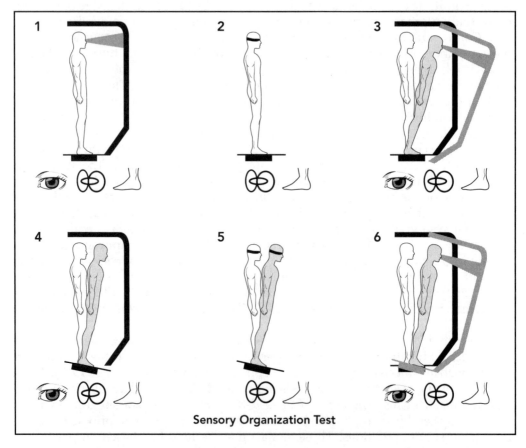

Sensory Organization Test

FIGURE 17.1 The six conditions of the NeuroCom Sensory Organization Test. Each condition manipulates or removes the visual, vestibular, and/or somatosensory system. Figure used courtesy of NeuroCom International, Inc.

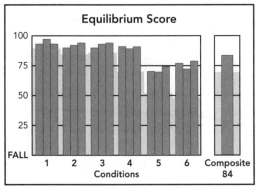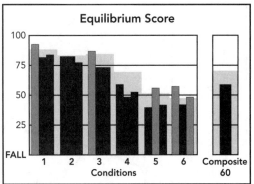

FIGURE 17.2 Sensory Organization Test performance of a healthy young adult (college athlete) prior to concussion (left) and following concussion (right).

the floor and/or walls may move in conjunction with the COP. For example, in Condition 6, for every degree forward the participant leans, the floor and walls move the same amount. The combination of the six conditions has proven particularly useful by allowing clinicians to identify abnormalities in an individual's ability to use and integrate visual, vestibular, and somatosensory inputs while balancing (Nashner, 1997). The SOT has been adopted for a number of clinical uses, including discriminating between those with and without pathologies related to aging (Hirabayashi & Iwasaki, 1995; Peterka & Black, 1990), disease (Arokoski, Leinonen, Arokoski, Aalto, & Valtonen, 2006; Hirsch, Toole, Maitland, & Rider, 2003; Nallegowda et al., 2004), and concussion (Guskiewicz, Ross, & Marshall, 2001; Peterson, Ferrara, Mrazik, Piland, & Elliot, 2003).

Clinical interpretation of SOT performance includes scores for composite balance and ratio scores that estimate the contribution of each of the sensory inputs (Nashner, 1997). Higher balance scores (those approaching 100) indicate less sway, whereas lower scores indicate the individual has approached or exceeded the LOS. Under normal, noninjured conditions, young healthy adults produce a composite balance score between 75 and 95. Figure 17.2 demonstrates the performance of a college athlete with no known injuries and with deficits in postural control as noted on the SOT by declines in the composite balance score. A closer look at the postural control mechanism indicates suppressed visual and vestibular ratios, which are believed to influence the overall ability to maintain balance. These changes are not thought to be related to damage in the systems themselves but rather impairment in how the information is being integrated and therefore is used to generate efferent motor responses (Guskiewicz, Riemann, Perrin, & Nashner, 1997; Guskiewicz et al., 2001). In the acute postconcussion stage, the changes to postural control can be rather large, and the SOT therefore demonstrates a 62% sensitivity when the individual is evaluated within 24 hr of injury (Broglio et al., 2007).

Interpreting Change on the Sensory Organization Test

Some clinical models of concussion management call for serial testing of the individual who is injured following injury, with testing typically occurring on days 1, 3, 5, and 10 postinjury. In this paradigm, healthy young adults demonstrated a 10% improvement in the composite balance score between Day 1 and 5 with no performance change between Day 5 and 10 (Peterson et al., 2003). Wrisely et al. (2007) reported a consistent improvement in the composite balance score of young adults

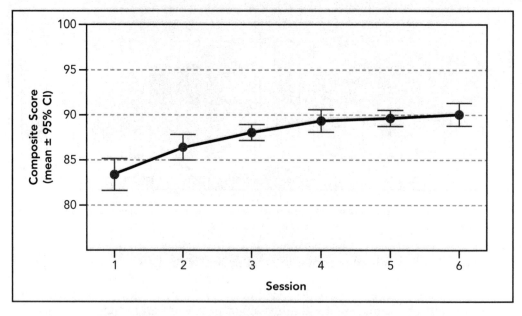

FIGURE 17.3 Change in composite scores over time. CI = confidence interval. Adapted from "Learning Effects of Repetitive Administrations of the Sensory Organization Test in Healthy Young Adults," by D. M. Wrisley, M. J. Stephens, S. Mosley, A. Wojnowski, J. Duffy, and R. Burkard, 2007, *Archives of Physical Medicine and Rehabilitation*, 88(8), pp. 1049–1054. Copyright 2007 by Elsevier.

when the test was administered every second or third day over a 2-week interval. By the fourth administration, however, performance leveled off with no additional improvements (see Figure 17.3). In addition, the scores remained the same when administered 30 days later (Session 6), indicating the maintenance of the learned postural task.

The known learning effects demonstrated on the SOT not only make the clinical interpretation of data difficult but also suggest that practice effects should be observed, which helps with assessing self-reported balance problems. Although there are no broadly accepted guidelines available for the interpretation of changes scores on the SOT, one investigation applied Reliable Change Index (RCI) to a group of young adults who are concussed and nonconcussed (see Table 17.1) and found that

TABLE 17.1 Reliable Change Scores for the NeuroCom Sensory Organization Test

Change Scores	RCI Value	Composite Balance	Somatosensory Ratio	Visual Ratio	Vestibular Ratio
95% CI	1.96	9.75	10.08	11.93	25.69
90% CI	1.65	8.48	8.46	9.99	22.41
85% CI	1.44	7.65	7.41	8.73	20.27
80% CI	1.28	7.01	6.60	7.75	18.63
75% CI	1.15	6.48	5.92	6.95	17.27
70% CI	1.04	6.02	5.34	6.24	16.08

Note. CI = confidence interval; RCI = Reliable Change Index. Adapted from "Reliable Change of the Sensory Organization Test," by S. P. Broglio, M. S. Ferrara, K. Sopiarz, and M. S. Kelly, 2008, *Clinical Journal of Sport Medicine*, 18(2), pp. 148–154. Copyright 2008 by Wolters Kluwer Health.

the 75% confidence interval provided the highest sensitivity and specificity to injury (Broglio, Ferrara, Sopiarz, & Kelly, 2008). For example, relative to a preinjury assessment, a postinjury composite balance score decline that is 6.48 or more is believed to reflect a concussion. Following the acute stage of injury, performance on the SOT appears to be restored to preinjury levels by 3-day postinjury in young adults (Guskiewicz et al., 1997; Guskiewicz et al., 2001). This restoration represents a return of total COP motion (postural sway) to preinjury levels. More complex analysis of COP motion (i.e., approximate entropy [ApEn] analysis), however, has shown ongoing changes to postural control at the same time point.

Symptom Validity and the Sensory Organization Test

Malingering on preconcussion and postconcussion testing is reported anecdotally by clinicians but rarely quantified. Athletes may choose to perform poorly on a baseline examination so that postmorbid deficits will be masked, allowing for a more rapid return to play. On the contrary, an athlete may elect to feign poor performance on a postinjury test to avoid return to play for a myriad of reasons, including lack of desire to play or conflict with coaching staff. There have been several attempts to identify malingering on neuropsychological tests and to ensure a high level of effort during testing, but little has been done relative to postural control testing, although several clinical considerations merit attention.

It is more important that following a baseline assessment, all data including postural control should be reviewed with validity concerns in mind. When looking at postural data, one factor that raises concerns about test validity is the presence of a consistent sinusoidal COP pattern throughout the duration of the trial (Allum & Shepard, 1999). In these instances, the athlete is performing in a manner that seems to reflect impairment but is actually consistent with an irregular sway pattern. Some investigators have tried to quantify poor performance using a stepwise linear discriminate function analysis with the SOT data and were able to correctly identify poor performance produced via nonphysiological causes at 95.5% of the time (Cevette, Puetz, Marion, Wertz, & Muenter, 1995). It may also be possible to apply ApEn estimations, which mathematically evaluate the regularity of sway patterns to these data as a screening tool. Those with lower ApEn scores would be suspected of faking poor performance because there would be a consistent and predictable pattern of motion relative to the irregular pattern seen with normal performance. In other words, atypical patterns of postural stability have been identified, and these measures can be used if test data appear unreliable to clinicians.

Following concussive injuries, clinicians should be aware of other nonquantifiable characteristics of an individual intentionally generating an impaired performance. For example, an athlete who reports dizziness and/or balance difficulties but has a comparable performance on the SOT relative to the baseline evaluation would be a suspect. In this instance, the clinician should question an overreporting of symptoms or determine whether the baseline assessment was suboptimal. In addition, the ability of the athlete to easily walk into the clinic and onto the SOT support surface, but perform poorly on the SOT, particularly Condition 1, should raise suspicion. Athletes who perform more poorly on the easiest conditions (Conditions 1, 2, and 3) relative to the more difficult conditions (Conditions 5 and 6) are highly suspect for suboptimal effort. Finally, athletes who demonstrate the same degree of sway on all trials, even though the later conditions will inherently generate more motion, are also suspect of performing suboptimally (Allum & Shepard, 1999; Cevette et al., 1995).

COGNITIVE ASSESSMENT

Freestanding Effort Tests and Multiple Baselines

Prior to the advent of baseline testing, suboptimal effort was rarely considered relevant in sports concussion assessment and management. Now that baseline examinations are commonly employed, athletes have an opportunity to perform suboptimally on baseline testing with the expectation that impaired baseline testing would obscure the effects of a concussion when tested postinjury. The number of athletes who have used this strategy and will attempt to use it in the future is not known, but prominent National Football League (NFL) athletes such as Peyton Manning have openly talked about performing suboptimally to reduce the likelihood of finding impairment postinjury (Sean Leahy, USA Today: April 27, 2011). In addition, research has shown that athletes' effort can be suboptimal when being examined at baseline, even when using effort tests with low sensitivity (Hunt, Ferrara, Miller, & Macciocchi, 2007).

Assessing performance validity is critical during the baseline examination. The baseline testing model is essentially a quasi-experimental pretest–posttest design that has several threats to internal and external validity—the most prominent of which are history and instrumentation (Campbell & Stanley, 1963). Athletes have several preoccurring and co-occurring disorders that can affect test performance. Learning disorders, intellectual limitations, substance use, and prior brain injury can all impair performance on neuropsychological measures at baseline. Clinicians must make a determination of whether the baseline examination is valid, given the athlete's history and performance on cognitive measures.

There are methods for addressing validity issues at baseline. First, although computerized assessment platforms typically have embedded validity measures, freestanding effort tests can always be administered at baseline. There are many instruments available, but brief tests with high sensitivity and specificity such as the Medical Symptom Validity Test (Green, 2004) are highly recommended. This instrument has several subtests (immediate recall, delayed recall, paired associate learning, and free recall) that can be integrated into the baseline examination with relative ease. Because symptom report and health history are routinely collected, the delays encountered during effort testing can be filled with self-report measures or an interview. Baseline is the time to make sure the athlete is giving optimal effort, and putting time into enhancing the validity of baseline measures is critical to interpreting postconcussive data at a later date.

Another method for optimizing validity is employing a multiple baseline design recommended by Hinton-Bayre, even though the original intention of the design was to limit practice effects and not to optimize effort (Hinton-Bayre, Geffen, Geffen, McFarland, & Frijs, 1999). Multiple baseline designs were originally recommended because of the practice effects observed on many neuropsychological instruments used in sports concussion research. Hinton-Bayre observed that practice effects were generally limited after a second assessment at baseline. When using multiple baseline assessments, problems with irregular and erratic performance may be evident. If so, steps can be taken to resolve discrepancies. Although Hinton-Bayre recommends multiple assessments in close proximity at baseline, many athletes have baseline testing when entering an athletic program and are concussed 2–3 years later after considerable maturation has occurred. Maturation is a threat in pretest–posttest designs, and if the baseline examination is not current, the result may be an underestimate of functioning at the time of injury. In other words, the baseline is biased toward not finding a change in cognitive skills postinjury (Type II error). As such, it seems prudent to have multiple baselines during a young athlete's career to assure maturation bias does not occur.

Embedded Validity Indicators

Computer assessment has, with few exceptions, replaced more traditional neuropsychological assessment in sports settings. Computer platforms are more logistically feasible when doing baseline assessment for large groups and in theory are more user-friendly for clinicians in the sports environment. Computer assessment is not without problems, however, and several issues regarding psychometrics remain to be resolved despite the proliferation of these instruments (Broglio, Ferrara, Macciocchi, Baumgartner, & Elliott, 2007; Randolph, McCrea, & Barr, 2005).

There are several computer platforms that are commonly used in sports concussion assessment, including ImPACT and HeadMinder Concussion Resolution Index (CRI). Each computer platform has validity indexes, but existing research on the sensitivity and specificity of these validity measures is somewhat limited. Readers should consult manuals for specific instruments to determine what validity indicators seem most appropriate given the context of the examinations being used. As an example, ImPACT recommends several validity indicators, including X and O total incorrect > 30, word memory < 69%, design memory < 50%, three letters < 10, and impulse composite score > 30 (D. Tauchen: Impacttest.com). There is limited data on whether these indicators adequately capture athletes who exert suboptimal effort. As a result, pairing computerized programs with freestanding effort tests can be very helpful in detecting problematic task engagement.

Although computer assessment has essentially taken the place of traditional neuropsychological assessment in most situations, at times, a more extensive and traditional examination is clinically warranted. In most cases, a traditional examination would only be administered if the athlete has (a) protracted symptomatology- and/or (b) an atypical pattern of performance on computerized measures- and/or (c) an unusual pattern or severity of self-reported symptoms. There are differences of opinion on what neuropsychological measures should be used when conducting the examination, but the most prudent methodology would include using tests that have used in sports concussion research over the past two decades. It is more important that concussion has a well-defined pathophysiology that makes the use of many neuropsychological tests focused on intellectual, academic, sensorimotor, and visuoperceptual skills inappropriate because of sensitivity problems. In general, attention, processing speed, and learning and memory would be expected to be the primary neurocognitive skills impacted by a concussion.

CONCLUSION

Athletic populations create challenges for clinicians who must evaluate symptom validity. The most common scenarios involve assessing the validity of baseline data and assessing the validity of atypical recovery following concussion. Clinicians have several measures available to help with determinations regarding symptom validity, including cognitive tests with embedded symptom validity indicators, freestanding effort tests, postural stability testing, and structured symptom reports. Because research on symptom validity and effort in athletic populations is very limited, clinicians must use all empirical data available and, most importantly, exercise prudent clinical judgment. Although symptom validity assessment in sports populations is in its infancy, there is no reason to expect that suboptimal effort would have any less effect on test findings than is apparent in other clinical populations.

REFERENCES

Allum, J. H., & Shepard, N. T. (1999). An overview of the clinical use of dynamic posturography in the differential diagnosis of balance disorders. *Journal of Vestibular Research*, 9(4), 223–252.

Alves, W., Macciocchi, S. N., & Barth, J. T. (1993). Post concussive symptoms after uncomplicated mild head injury. *Journal of Head Trauma Rehabilitation*, 8, 48–59.

Arokoski, J. P., Leinonen, V., Arokoski, M. H., Aalto, H., & Valtonen, H. (2006). Postural control in male patients with hip osteoarthritis. *Gait & Posture*, 23(1), 45–50.

Barth, J. T., Alves, W., Ryan, T., Macciocchi, S. N., Rimel, R., Jane, J., & Nelson, W. (1989). Mild head injury in sports: Neuropsychological sequelae and recovery of function. In H. Levin, H. Eisenberg, & A. Benton (Eds.), *Mild head injury* (pp. 257–275). New York, NY: Oxford University Press.

Barth, J. T., Macciocchi, S. N., Giordani, B., Rimel, R., Jane, J., & Boll, T. (1983). Neuropsychological sequelae of minor head injury. *Neurosurgery*, 13(5), 529–533.

Ben-Porath, Y. S., & Tellegen, A. (2008). *Minnesota multiphasic personality inventory-2 restructured form.* Minneapolis, MN: University of Minnesota Press.

Broglio, S. P., Ferrara, M. S., Macciocchi, S. N., Baumgartner, T. A., & Elliott, R. (2007). Test-retest reliability of computerized concussion assessment programs. *Journal of Athletic Training*, 42(4), 509–514.

Broglio, S. P., Ferrara, M. S., Sopiarz, K., & Kelly, M. S. (2008). Reliable change of the sensory organization test. *Clinical Journal of Sport Medicine*, 18(2), 148–154.

Broglio, S. P., Macciocchi, S. N., & Ferrara, M. S. (2007). Sensitivity of the concussion assessment battery. *Neurosurgery*, 60(6), 1050–1057.

Broglio, S. P., & Puetz, T. W. (2008). The effect of sport concussion on neurocognitive function, self-report symptoms, and postural control: A meta-analysis. *Sports Medicine*, 38(1), 53–67.

Broglio, S. P., Sosnoff, J. J., & Ferrara, M. S. (2009). The relationship of athlete-reported concussion symptoms and objective measures of neurocognitive function and postural control. *Clinical Journal of Sport Medicine*, 19(5), 377–382.

Campbell, D. T., & Stanley, J. C. (1963). *Experimental and quasi-experimental designs for research.* Chicago, IL: Rand McNally.

Cevette, M. J., Puetz, B., Marion, M. S., Wertz, M. L., & Muenter, M. D. (1995). A physiologic performance on dynamic posturography. *Otolaryngology—Head and Neck Surgery*, 112(6), 676–688.

Collins, M. W., Grindel, S. H., Lovell, M. R., Dede, D. E., Moser, D. J., Phalin, B. R., . . . McKeag, D. B. (1999). Relationship between concussion and neuropsychological performance in college football players. *The Journal of the American Medical Association*, 282(10), 964–970.

Davidoff, G., Morris, J., Roth, E., & Bleiberg, J. (1985). Cognitive dysfunction and mild closed head injury in traumatic spinal cord injury. *Archives of Physical Medicine and Rehabilitation*, 66(8), 489–491.

El-Kashlan, H. K., Shepard, N. T., Asher, A. M., Smith-Wheelock, M., & Telian, S. A. (1998). Evaluation of clinical measures of equilibrium. *The Laryngoscope*, 108(3), 311–319.

Erlanger, D., Feldman, D., Kutner, K., Kaushik, T., Kroger, H., Festa, J., . . . Broshek, D. (2003). Development and validation of a web-based neuropsychological test protocol for sports-related return-to-play decision-making. *Archives of Clinical Neuropsychology*, 18(3), 293–316.

Green, P. (2004). *Green's medical symptom validity test (MSVT) for Microsoft Windows: User's manual.* Edmonton, Canada: Green's Publishing.

Guskiewicz, K. M. (1999). Regaining balance and postural equilibrium. In W. E. Prentice (Ed.), *Rehabilitation techniques in sports medicine* (3rd ed., pp. 107–133). Boston, MA: WCB/McGraw-Hill.

Guskiewicz, K. M., Bruce, S. L., Cantu, R. C., Ferrara, M. S., Kelly, J. P., McCrea, M., . . . Valovich McLeod, T. C. (2004). National Athletic Trainers' Association position statement: Management of sport-related concussion. *Journal of Athletic Training*, 39(3), 280–297.

Guskiewicz, K. M., McCrea, M., Marshall, S. W., Cantu, R. C., Randolph, C., Barr, W., . . . Kelly, J. P. (2003). Cumulative effects associated with recurrent concussion in collegiate football players: The NCAA concussion study. *The Journal of the American Medical Association*, 290(19), 2549–2555.

Guskiewicz, K. M., Riemann, B. L., Perrin, D. H., & Nashner, L. M. (1997). Alternative approaches to the assessment of mild head injury in athletes. *Medicine and Science in Sports and Exercise*, 29(Suppl. 7), S213–S221.

Guskiewicz, K. M., Ross, S. E., & Marshall, S. W. (2001). Postural stability and neuropsychological deficits after concussion in collegiate athletes. *Journal of Athletic Training*, 36(3), 263–273.

Heilbronner, R. L., Sweet, J. J., Morgan, J. E Larrabee, G. J., & Millis, S. R. (2009). American Academy of Clinical Neuropsychology Consensus Conference Statement on the neuropsychological assessment of effort, response bias, and malingering. *The Clinical Neuropsychologist*, 23(7), 1093–1129.

Hinton-Bayre, A. D., Geffen, G. M., Geffen, L. B., McFarland, K. A., & Frijs, P. (1999). Concussion in contact sports: Reliable change indices of impairment and recovery. *Journal of Clinical and Experimental Neuropsychology*, 21(1), 70–86.

Hirabayashi, S., & Iwasaki, Y. (1995). Developmental perspective of sensory organization on postural control. *Brain & Development*, 17(2), 111–113.

Hirsch, M. A., Toole, T., Maitland, C. G., & Rider, R. A. (2003). The effects of balance training and high-intensity resistance training on persons with idiopathic Parkinson's disease. *Archives of Physical Medicine and Rehabilitation*, 84(8), 1109–1117.

Hunt, T., Ferrara, M., Miller, L. S., & Macciocchi, S. N. (2007). The effect of effort on baseline neuropsychological test scores in high school football athletes. *Archives of Clinical Neuropsychology*, 22(5), 615–621.

Iverson, G. L., Lovell, M. W., & Collins, M. R. (2003). Interpreting change on the ImPACT following sports concussion. *The Clincial Neuropsychologist*, 17(4), 460–467.

Kelly, J. P., & Rosenberg, J. H. (1997). Diagnosis and management of concussion in sports. *Neurology*, 48(3), 575–580.

Levin, H. S., Mattis, S., Ruff, R. M., Eisenberg, H. M., Marshall, L. F., Tabaddor, K., . . . Frankowski, R. F. (1987). Neurobehavioral outcome following minor head injury: A three-center study. *Journal of Neurosurgery*, 66(2), 234–243.

Macciocchi, S. N., Barth, J. T., Alves, W., Rimel, R. W., & Jane, J. A. (1996). Neuropsychological functioning and recovery after mild head injury in collegiate athletes. *Neurosurgery*, 39(3), 510–514.

McCrea, M., Kelly, J. P., Randolph, C., Cisler, R., & Berger, L. (2002). Immediate neurocognitive effects of concussion. *Neurosurgery*, 50(5), 1032–1042.

McCrory, P., Meeuwisse, W., Johnston, K., Dvorak, J., Aubry, M., Molloy, M., & Cantu, R. (2009). Consensus statement on concussion in sport, 3rd International Conference on Concussion in Sport held in Zurich, November 2008. *Clinical Journal of Sport Medicine*, 19(3), 185–200.

Nallegowda, M., Singh, U., Handa, G., Khanna, M., Wadhwa, S., Yadav, S. L., . . . Behari, M. (2004). Role of sensory input and muscle strength in maintenance of balance, gait, and posture in Parkinson's disease: A pilot study. *American Journal of Physical Medicine & Rehabilitation*, 83(12), 898–908.

Nashner, L. M. (1997). Computerized dynamic posturography. In G. P. Jacobson, C. W. Newman, & J. M. Kartush (Eds.), *Handbook of balance function testing* (pp. 280–305). St Louis, MO: Mosby Year Book.

Nashner, L. M., Black, F. O., & Wall, C., III. (1982). Adaptation to altered support and visual conditions during stance: Patients with vestibular deficits. *The Journal of Neuroscience*, 2(5), 536–544.

Nashner, L. M., & Peters, J. F. (1990). Dynamic posturography in the diagnosis and management of dizziness and balance disorders. *Neurological Clinics*, 8(2), 331–349.

Ommaya, A. K., & Gennarelli, T. A. (1974). Cerebral concussion and traumatic unconsciousness: Correlation of experimental and clinical observations of blunt head injuries. *Brain*, 97(4), 633–654.

Pellman, E. J., Lovell, M. R., Viano, D. C., Casson, I. R., & Tucker, A. M. (2004). Concussion in professional football: Neuropsychological testing—Part 6. *Neurosurgery*, 55(6), 1290–1305.

Peterka, R. J., & Black, F. O. (1990). Age-related changes in human posture control: Sensory organization tests. *Journal of Vestibular Research*, 1(1), 73–85.

Peterson, C. L., Ferrara, M. S., Mrazik, M., Piland, S. G., & Elliot, R. (2003). Evaluation of neuropsychological domain scores and postural stability following cerebral concussion in sports. *Clinical Journal of Sport Medicine*, 13(4), 230–237.

Piland, S. G., Ferrara, M. S., Macciocchi, S. N., Broglio, S. P., & Gould, T (2010). Investigation of baseline self-report concussion symptom scores. *Journal of Athletic Training*, 45(3), 273–278.

Randolph, C., McCrea, M., & Barr, W. B. (2005). Is neuropsychological testing useful in the management of sport-related concussion? *Journal of Athletic Training*, 40(2), 139–152.

Swanik, C. B., Lephart, S. M., Giannantonio, F. P., & Fu, F. H. (1997). Reestablishing proprioception and neuromuscular control in the ACL-injured athlete. *Journal of Sport Rehabilitation*, 6, 182–206.

Wrisley, D. M., Stephens, M. J., Mosley, S., Wojnowski, A., Duffy, J., & Burkard, R. (2007). Learning effects of repetitive administrations of the sensory organization test in healthy young adults. *Archives of Physical Medicine and Rehabilitation*, 88(8), 1049–1054.

Symptom Validity Assessment of Military and Veteran Populations Following Mild Traumatic Brain Injury   18

Shane S. Bush & Christopher J. Graver

Uncomplicated mild traumatic brain injury (MTBI), commonly referred to as *concussion*, disrupts normal cerebral functioning through a series of acute metabolic changes (Giza & Hovda, 2001, 2004; Iverson, 2005; Iverson, Lange, Gaetz, & Zasler, 2007). During the acute to subacute period following injury, cognitive and behavioral changes are typically experienced and observed. Most persons who sustain MTBIs recover quickly and completely (i.e., less than 3 months; Belanger & Vanderploeg, 2005; Binder, Rohling, & Larrabee, 1997; Frencham, Fox, & Maybery, 2005; Iverson, 2005; Schretlen & Shapiro, 2003). However, a very small percentage (about 5%) of persons report various nonspecific cognitive, physical, and emotional symptoms many months or years following an event that included an MTBI (Iverson, 2005; McCrea, 2008). Although such nonspecific symptoms may be misattributed by patients or by well-meaning but misinformed health care professionals to the neurological effects of the remote MTBI, the symptoms in most cases more accurately reflect emotional difficulties, physical pain, adverse effects of medications, or other factors including intentional exaggeration or fabrication of symptoms (Iverson, 2005; Luis, Vanderploeg, & Curtiss, 2003; Meares et al., 2011). An important role for neuropsychologists is to clarify the nature, extent, and validity of such symptoms so that appropriate education, treatment, and/or disability determinations can be provided.

PREVALENCE OF TRAUMATIC BRAIN INJURY IN MILITARY AND VETERAN POPULATIONS

Approximately 28,000 traumatic brain injuries (TBIs) are sustained yearly by U.S. military service members, most of which are mild (Marion, Curley, Schwab, & Hicks, 2011). According to a paper published by the RAND Corporation (2008), there were 320,000 TBIs suffered by Operation Iraqi Freedom/Operation Enduring Freedom (OIF/OEF) veterans prior to the paper's publication in 2008. As many as 360,000 TBIs have been reported elsewhere as having been sustained during OIF and OEF (Zoroya, 2009). These figures have been widely cited in the media, and TBI has been repeatedly labeled as "the signature wound of the war"; however, the tally is an inaccurate extrapolation from unpublished survey data and screening tools of nonspecific symptoms. To be more accurate, medical chart reviews from 2000 to 2010 have documented 202,281 TBIs sustained by military personnel in all settings, not just OIF/OEF veterans (Department of Defense [DoD], 2011). Of those, 155,623 were MTBIs; 36,125 were moderate-to-severe TBI; 3,451 were penetrating TBI; and 7,082 were unable to be classified by severity. These statistics are consistent with other published studies showing that approximately 85% of all TBIs are mild in nature (Bazarian, McClung, Shah, Cheng, Flesher, & Kraus, 2005). The exact numbers of combat-related TBIs is unknown, but Zoroya noted only 4,471 OIF/OEF TBIs officially listed by the Pentagon as of 2007. Even if this number is an underestimate, it is still well below the figures provided by the media.

Funding for brain injury treatment and research was approximately $1 billion in 2007–2008 (Zoroya, 2009). In addition, the Veterans Administration (VA) instituted mandatory screening and evaluation of every veteran deployed to OIF/OEF presenting for care (U.S. Department of Veterans Affairs, 2007). Furthermore, resources from neuropsychology, neurology, psychiatry, and psychology that were already in place to manage TBI sequelae are essentially being duplicated in TBI clinics. According to a report to the Congress, the operating budget and procurement funding of the Defense and Veterans Brain Injury Center (DVBIC) in Washington, DC was approximately $36 million for 2009 (Rice, 2009). A recent report from the DoD also reported, "TBI clinics in military facilities are increasing the number of staff and case managers . . . as well as the Defense Centers of Excellence (DCoE) Outreach Center," which is a 24/7 call center for TBI resources and information (Burgess, 2010). At present, TBI is not among the top 10 most prevalent service-connected disabilities for veterans receiving compensation (Department of Veterans Affairs, Veterans Benefits Administration, 2010).

TRAUMATIC BRAIN INJURY–RELATED BENEFITS AND INCENTIVE FOR DISSIMULATION

Most TBIs are classified as mild, which are categorically different from moderate-to-severe TBIs and enjoy full resolution of symptoms on objective testing by 90 days without the need for specialized intervention (McCrea, 2008; Rohling et al., 2011). But subjective symptoms reports may persist beyond this recovery window for multiple reasons. Dikmen, Machamer, Fann, and Temkin (2010) found that symptom reporting following TBI was significantly related to age, gender, preinjury alcohol abuse, preinjury psychiatric history, and severity of TBI. Because individuals with MTBI tend to recover rapidly without specialized treatment, this leaves only 4,138 persons with moderate-to-severe TBIs in need of specialized, long-term treatment across the entire military in 2010 (DoD, 2011). Nevertheless, the magnanimous attention to TBI by the government in recent years has paved the way for extraordinary financial benefits for soldiers and veterans with claimed residual symptoms of concussion, as well as providing a method for avoiding duties, deployment, and continued service without having to repay enlistment bonuses, which can be as much as $40,000. In addition, Traumatic Service Members' Group Life Insurance (TSGLI) will pay $25,000–$100,000 for traumatic injury(s) from a single event (TSGLI, 2011). Furthermore, a 100% disability rating by the military or VA results in a total estimated lifetime monetary benefit of approximately $1.6 million with additional amounts authorized for spouses and/or dependents, as well as many other nonmonetary benefits, and it lays the foundation for Social Security disability benefits (Whittaker, 2010).

Bianchini, Curtis, and Greve (2006) found a dose-response relationship between financial compensation and malingering. With compensation of this magnitude, the concern for malingered neurocognitive dysfunction as a result of concussion is prominent. Moreover, involvement in Rule 706 inquiries ("sanity boards") has demonstrated that claims of concussion sequelae have been presented as a means to excuse inappropriate and irresponsible behaviors as well as diminish or limit culpability in criminal circumstances (e.g., driving under the influence [DUI], domestic violence). Thus, because of the numerous and significant potential benefits associated with a TBI diagnosis, there is abundant incentive for military personnel and veterans to exaggerate or fabricate symptoms in the context of concussion. At the same time, the VA system maintains an assumption of disability, which facilitates the pursuit of disability benefits by allowing service members to apply for benefits even before they have been found unfit for duty by military health care professionals.

Although Braverman (1978) suggested that there would be public hostility toward malingering individuals because their undeserved financial gain comes at the cost of services to deserving individuals, such hostility is not necessarily apparent in today's society based on specific direction from the VA to give veterans the "benefit of the doubt" regarding their symptoms and illnesses. Whereas the reasonable doubt rule (Pension, Bonuses, and Veterans' Relief, 2009) states that benefit should be given in cases where evidence is equivocal, in practice, many health care providers in the VA system interpret this instruction to take patients' statements as fact without collateral verification or objective evaluation. This implicit interpretation was formalized in 2010 when the VA no longer required independent verification of the stressor, easing veterans' ability to obtain service connection for their claimed illness (Associated Press, 2010). This philosophy is so extreme that clinicians who apply critical thinking and assess the credibility and validity of symptoms have been excused from employment with the VA for the express reason that using instruments to detect exaggerated or feigned symptoms is not giving the benefit of the doubt (Poyner, 2010).

The military and veterans disability systems are structured in such a way as to offer incentive for maintaining illness, as well as encouraging more serious symptom presentation (Burkett & Whitely, 1998). In addition, the military has created special groups called Warrior Transition Battalions (WTBs) where soldiers who are chronically ill and/or anticipating medical separation are located. Such soldiers are relieved of normal duties, and their only responsibilities are to attend medical appointments and check in regularly with a case manager. Anecdotally, there are soldiers with claims of enduring cognitive sequelae of concussion several years postinjury that have reported spending their days in the WTB engaged in a range of activities from playing computer games to running various business ventures on the side while they continue to collect active duty pay. Soldiers also admitted during neuropsychological evaluations to sharing information about illnesses, symptoms, benefits, and examinations, as well as advice about specific examiners to request or avoid during their medical boards. They have been overheard discussing the Test of Memory Malingering (TOMM; Tombaugh, 1996) in particular and appear to have been coached on it, rendering the TOMM a questionable instrument for continued use in military and veteran populations. In all likelihood, the WTB environment creates an iatrogenic peer group dynamic that makes continued illness and dissimulation more likely to occur, similar to findings of negative group therapy outcomes of high-risk adolescents (Dishion, Poulin, & Burraston, 2001).

Clinical experience has revealed that despite the consequences for malingering outlined in the "Uniform Code of Military Justice" (UCMJ), prosecution under the UCMJ is not, to our knowledge, generally pursued even when objective testing indicates intentional feigning of symptoms (e.g., significantly below chance performance on forced-choice tests), and additional evidence (e.g., publicly available videos) demonstrates cognitive and physical functioning at a level sufficient for independence with daily activities. In the context of exceptional financial benefits, an inclusive benefit-of-the-doubt philosophy and a lack of consistency enforcing consequences for exaggerated/fabricated symptoms, it is perhaps no wonder that poor effort and symptom exaggeration are common in military and veteran populations, necessitating a thorough and objective examination of symptom validity in any evaluation, regardless of rank or situation.

Although some clinical services provided to veterans have no potential for secondary gain and are purely clinical in nature, evaluating active duty personnel and veterans who may receive new or increased benefits based on neuropsychological findings carries many similarities to forensic evaluations in personal injury cases. For example, information in clinical reports may be used in determinations about benefits, including financial compensation. Establishing clinical diagnoses and pursuing treatment often provide the foundation for disability claims and VA service connection. Various publications, including *How to Receive Disability for PTSD* (Latham, 1992) and *Posttraumatic Stress Disorder: How to Apply for 100 Percent Total Disability Rating* (Hill, 1993), outline how to obtain VA benefits, including using clinical services to lay the foundation for such pursuits. In particular, Hill stated, "You will need to be involved in treatment to get 100 percent disability for PTSD, but you will not have to remain in treatment once you receive your award" (p. 11). As Burkett and Whitley (1998) stated, "With such powerful monetary incentives in place, it's naïve to think that all, or even most, of those (Vietnam) veterans who claim they suffer from PTSD . . . ever served in Vietnam" (p. 239), let alone were truly traumatized by the experience. Thus, as in civilian medicolegal evaluation and treatment contexts, neuropsychologists must be aware that financial pursuits may affect the clinical presentations of some patients. Clinicians are best able to help their patients when the patients present in a valid manner, determined in part with psychometric measures.

In contrast to postservice veterans, active duty soldiers in the medical evaluation board (MEB) process have access to attorney advisors from the office of the judge advocate general who can review their findings and assist with appeals. Neuropsychologists in such forensic contexts have roles as neutral examiners rather than treatment providers. In the clinic of the second author (CG), service members undergoing medical board evaluations are notified of this neutral examiner, nontreatment relationship, and they are explicitly informed that results or recommendations from the evaluation will not be provided to them, but rather a decision about medical retention standards will be provided to the medical board to incorporate into their narrative summary.

PREVALENCE OF DISSIMULATION IN MILITARY AND VETERAN POPULATIONS

There are several studies and resources supporting a significant rate of exaggeration and/or malingering in veterans populations, with associated costs in the billions of dollars (Department of Veterans Affairs Office of Inspector General, 2005; Freeman, Powell, & Kimbrell, 2008; Frueh et al., 2003; Frueh, Hamner, Cahill, Gold, & Hamlin, 2000). For example, a study by the Department of Veterans Affairs Office of Inspector General (2005) found that approximately 25% of veterans with posttraumatic stress disorder (PTSD) had insufficient evidence of a traumatic stressor at a cost of almost $20 billion for questionable claims. The review showed that raters relied on " . . . the veteran's unsubstantiated testimony or secondary source information such as buddy statements or information taken from Internet websites to determine the veteran's combat status and/or the occurrence of claimed stressors" (Department of Veterans Affairs Office of Inspector General, 2005, pp. 47–48). In addition, veterans were attending treatment regularly until a service connection was obtained, after which approximately 40% of them came to appointments one-fifth as often, and some stopped seeking care entirely. Furthermore, a cross check of federal tax databases in 2004 found 8,846 veterans deemed "unemployable" by the VA who were earning incomes, some in excess of $50,000 annually (Associated Press, 2010). Burkett and Whitely (1998) documented cases of individuals who were service-connected for PTSD but never saw military combat, some of whom never served in the military. Sheila Rauch, Director of the Veterans Affairs Returning Veterans' Mental Health Program in Ann Arbor, Michigan acknowledged that veterans may embellish symptoms to obtain service-connected benefits for PTSD and recommended that clinicians assess symptom validity in such evaluations (Rauch, 2010). Despite these recommendations, Poyner (2010) encountered only one standardized assessment of symptom magnification by VA examiners in more than 100 cases reviewed.

Contexts in which the potential for financial gain exist, including disability payments or benefits, are considered forensic. Neuropsychological services provided in such contexts may be clinical (i.e., promoting treatment or care) or forensic (i.e., assisting a trier of fact or administrative decision maker with decisions about impairment and causality). For military personnel or veterans who have a stated purpose of pursuing service-connected benefits or who may be pursuing an increased percentage of service connection, neuropsychological services should be considered forensic in nature. There is a wide range of reported base rates of malingered neurocognitive dysfunction in nonmilitary and military forensic disability contexts. Larrabee (2003) summarized 11 studies and found the overall base rate of malingering in nonmilitary forensic contexts to be approximately 40%. This percentage is consistent with other estimated base rates of malingering following concussions that approach 40% in compensation-seeking individuals, as opposed to the estimated 9% base rate of malingering following moderate-to-severe TBI (Mittenberg, Patton, Canyock, & Condit, 2002). In a criminal forensic setting, concussion was the most frequently malingered illness, occurring in approximately 45% of all cases (Ardolf, Denney, & Houston, 2007).

More specific to military personnel, one study reported that 25% of active duty service members with claims of blast trauma in OIF/OEF were excluded because of suspicions of poor effort or malingering, but that study was not specifically designed to detect poor effort, and it used a relatively insensitive symptom validity measure (e.g., California Verbal Learning Test, 2nd edition [CVLT-II] forced choice), so 25% is likely an underestimate (Belanger, Kretzmer, Yoash-Gantz, Pickett, & Tupler, 2009). A small study of OIF/OEF active duty soldiers with claims of concussion found that approximately 17% performed below established cutoffs for suboptimal effort on multiple symptom validity tests (SVTs) including the Medical Symptom Validity Test (MSVT) and TOMM (Whitney, Shepard, Williams, Davis, & Adams, 2009). None of the 17% had a genuine memory impairment profile on the MSVT.

Armistead-Jehle and Hansen (2011) found an 8%–30% failure rate on symptom validity measures among active duty personnel reporting a history of MTBI/concussion and/or various mental health conditions, including PTSD and depression. These authors noted that differences among sample subgroups likely accounted for the differences in failure rates, with midlevel career officers having the lowest rate of SVT failure. There are unpublished data on several hundred service members indicating that 54%–57% of military concussion cases fall below cutoffs (indicating noncredible performance) on the MSVT, nonverbal Medical Symptom Validity Test (NV-MSVT), or Word Memory Test (WMT; Graver & Shurak, in press). In a study of veterans with reported histories of concussions, evidence of poor effort on SVTs was discovered in approximately 58% of the sample (Armistead-Jehle, 2010).

STANDARD OF PRACTICE

Clinicians must determine whether each examinee's presentation and test results are valid. However, clinicians are not particularly good at making such determinations based on clinical judgment and behavioral observations alone (Dawes, Faust, & Meehl, 1989; Ekman & O'Sullivan, 1991; Faust, 1995; Faust, Hart, Guilmette, & Arkes, 1988; Hickling, Blanchard, Mundy, & Galovski, 2002; Morel, 2010; Reid, 2000; Richman et al., 2006; see also Chapter 2 of this volume by Guilmette). Nonetheless, neuropsychological evaluations are encountered in practice with minimal-to-no SVTs to objectively assess effort. Typically in such cases, clinicians provide subjective assurances of good effort and valid results in their reports without formally assessing symptom validity, a process that is inconsistent with current standards in the field of neuropsychology (Bush et al., 2005; Heilbronner, Sweet, Morgan, Larrabee, & Millis, 2009). Except for patients with cognitive impairment severe enough to require 24-hr supervision or assistance, the use of empirically based measures (stand-alone SVTs, embedded indicators) to determine symptom validity is the standard of practice (Bush et al., 2005; Heilbronner et al., 2009). Multiple texts capture this essential aspect of neuropsychological practice and present summaries of much of the extensive scientific literature published on symptom validity assessment (e.g., Boone, 2007; Carone & Bush, in press; Larrabee, 2007; Sweet & Morgan, 2009).

Assessment Procedures and Measures

The assessment of symptom validity typically involves multiple procedures and measures. All aspects of the neuropsychological evaluation have the potential to inform the examiner about the validity of the examinee's presentation and symptoms, and a convergence of information provides increased confidence in the accuracy of symptom validity determinations. Such procedures include the review of records, behavioral observations, interviews of the examinee and others, and use of standardized tests. An emphasis is placed on assessing consistencies and inconsistencies within and between these sources of information, as well as assessing levels of performance and patterns of performance on neuropsychological measures and SVTs, scales, and indicators (Slick, Sherman, & Iverson 1999). Selection of standardized measures should be based in large part on their psychometric properties for a given population. Selection and use of symptom validity measures and procedures should be determined by the clinician based on an understanding of relevant scientific and professional literature, in the context of a given examinee, and should not be limited or prohibited by facility administration policies, insurance carriers, or other nonscientific requirements.

At least one psychologist (Poyner, 2010) was told that the psychodiagnostic services that she provided to veterans were no longer needed because her use of symptom validity measures implied an assumption of malingering and failed to give veterans the benefit of the doubt regarding the presence of a compensable disorder. She stated,

> Based on my clinical experience, a "benefit of the doubt" mindset demonstrates that an underlying political climate influences what are otherwise supposed to be objective and professional assessments of psychiatric disability claims. It is problematic that the VA sends veterans to highly trained, objectively focused psychologists, but apparently prefers psychologists base their "findings" on less than scientific bases—bases that seem

grounded in misplaced benevolence and/or political expediency, rather than empirical data . . . This kind of tacit (or in my case not-so-tacit) expectation poses serious ethical concerns for professionals such as myself, and undermines the integrity of the VA system and its disability adjudication processes. Altogether, these concerns also suggest that limited VA resources are routinely wasted or misallocated, and are therefore diverted from serving the needs of those who should truly be service connected for mental illnesses, courageous men and women who have given so much to our country and deserve the services and benefits the VA system was designed to provide. (p. 131)

Informing clinicians that they cannot use procedures that are part of the current standard of practice or appropriately interpret and report SVT results places them in untenable ethical and professional positions and prohibits them from making the accurate diagnoses and determinations for which they are responsible.

The Office of the Assistant Secretary of Defense (2008) published a memorandum providing clinical guidance on symptom management in MTBI cases. The memorandum describes assessment procedures, including neuropsychological assessment, but does not mention symptom validity issues or assessment. In addition, the memorandum provides several assessment measures in an appendix, but none of the measures has a symptom validity scale, index, or other psychometrically-based indicator of the veracity of the examinee's self-report. More recently, however, a Pentagon telecommunication, specified as All Army Activities (ALARACT) 214/2011, MTBI Campaign, Annex C, stated that neuropsychological evaluations must include a measure of effort.

Review of Records

A thorough review of the medical records is a valuable part of the neuropsychological evaluation. Clinicians working in military and VA settings typically have access to multiple electronic databases through the military and VA; there is a shared VA/DoD database providing access to records in each system. Although neuropsychologists who work outside of these systems and do not have such access to electronic records may obtain veterans' records through a *Freedom of Information Act* (1996) request, such procedures are not practical for most clinical or forensic purposes. Clinicians may pursue, or have patients pursue, records from the VA or a military medical facility by submitting written requests with appropriate releases; however, immediate access, comparable to that available to VA or DoD employees, is typically unavailable. Clinicians are encouraged to have patients attempt to obtain these records at the time of scheduling so that hard copies can be brought to the appointment. Military medical facilities tend to be expedient with these requests, and some facilities will provide these records within a few minutes if the patient appears in person to the patient administration section.

Sometimes notes or other records are missing, incomplete, or otherwise unavailable, but if theater-of-operation notes are available, they will document downrange medical visits with complaints and treatments through the Armed Forces Health Longitudinal Technology Application (AHLTA), an electronic medical record, or through the Medical Protection System (MEDPROS), which tracks all immunizations, medical readiness, and deployability data for army soldiers. In addition, hard copies of handwritten theater notes are sometimes available through the medical board if requested. Thus, failure to have documentation of the injury may not necessarily rule out its occurrence but should incite caution when self-reported injuries are the only available source of information. When medically evacuated from OIF/OEF combat theaters, military personnel almost always receive a TBI screening at Landstuhl Region Medical Center (LRMC), which is documented in the medical record. Nevertheless, one of the most common shortcomings in evaluations opining residual deficits of concussion is a failure to review these records for a more complete and thorough history. It is common to see concussions diagnosed months or years after deployment based on patients' self-report when a review of the medical chart shows that concussion screenings downrange or at LRMC were negative.

It is essential that all relevant information be clearly documented in the neuro-psychological report. Verification of the injury is the first step. In many DoD and VA cases, concussions frequently have occurred several years before the disability evaluation. Relevant dates of injury should be clearly documented in the evaluation, given their importance for understanding the recovery course and expected residual symptoms. If the patient's injuries are not documented medically, DoD clinicians can still take advantage of candid access to the patient's command personnel for verification of experiences and injuries. Examples of military personnel claiming TBI without verification of combat trauma by their commands are common. Although it may be possible for military personnel to sustain symptoms of a mild concussion and not inform medical personnel or others who would bring the injury to the attention of the command, such injuries would have to be very mild and would resolve quickly and completely, or they would surely be noticed.

In addition, clinicians need to consider, in case conceptualization, the discrepancy present when patients with negative concussion screens, normal neuropsychological results, or no cognitive complaints at mandatory postdeployment exams, later report cognitive and neurologic symptoms because of concussion. It is helpful to ask patients at some point why they did not report symptoms at the postemployment exams to see if there is any reasonable explanation. Clinicians can use the entirety of the medical record to assess for inconsistencies that are a key component of the criteria set forth by Slick et al. (1999) for determining malingered neurocognitive dysfunction. This process requires time and diligence, but it can assist in the documentation of escalating symptoms over time, establishing the temporal proximity of symptom onset to the claimed injury, and lead to better diagnostic clarification and treatment suggestions.

Another issue worth noting in the record review is whether the patients ever sought treatment for the claimed symptoms and, if so, complied with the treatment. A commonly cited reason for noncompliance with medical treatment is forgetfulness to attend appointments or implement treatments secondary to the concussion, which, depending on the acuity of the injury, may be highly implausible and more indicative of motivation factors. Cognitive symptoms secondary to concussion may also be used to avoid punishment because of a failure to report to a formation or duty station, complete assigned tasks, keep uniform or quarters up to military standards, and various other infractions. These infractions, as well as any potential legal issues, should be documented because they raise suspicion of exaggeration/malingering in the context of a condition that typically resolves relatively rapidly and is not expected to result in chronic amnesia for antisocial behaviors. Other aspects of the evaluation that raise concern for exaggerated/malingered symptoms include discontent with the military, complaints of inadequate care (despite copious medical visits), seeking evaluations from non-DoD providers without authorization and using those results to bolster the disability case, and congressional complaints that directly relate to compensable conditions.

Clinical Interview

The interview of patients can help clarify and expand on information obtained from the records. At least a moderate level of knowledge regarding military environments and equipment is useful for detecting implausible reports of injuries. For instance, soldiers might make incredible reports of being thrown dozens of feet through the air by grenades (as typically seen in Hollywood movies) with resulting TBI but no other physical injuries. A basic understanding of the principle of a grenade as fragmentation ordinance, not a large concussive blast, helps the clinicians to realize the potential embellishment or prevarication, especially if the soldiers report being within the lethal radius without visible physical injury.

Clinicians should also realize that improvised explosive devices (IEDs) are often standard ordinance such as mortars or land mines that are deployed or detonated in unconventional ways. As such, a lethal blast radius can be estimated in many cases. Vehicle born IEDs (VBIEDs) tend to be more forceful, and the blast radius is more difficult to gauge because of their variability in size and explosive material. Nevertheless, blast force strong enough to cause disruption of brain functioning would likely disrupt other bodily systems resulting in symptoms such as dyspnea, tinnitus, or vertigo (for a basic review of these injuries, see University Hospitals Emergency Medical Services [EMS] Training & Disaster Preparedness Institute, 2011). Knowledge of whether the soldiers were mounted (in a vehicle) or dismounted (on foot) as well as the type of vehicle (M1 Abrams tank vs. high mobility multipurpose wheeled vehicle [Humvee]) helps to gauge the relative risk of injury versus what is being reported. Similar to what might be encountered in tort cases, the claimed mechanism of injury may be unlikely to yield sufficient force to cause a concussion, but service members may rely on the relative naïveté of civilian clinicians for embellishment of military situations.

In addition, for unsophisticated simulators, reports of the relationship between loss of consciousness, posttraumatic amnesia, retrograde amnesia, and altered mental status may be inconsistent with the typical concussive sequelae (Paniak, MacDonald, Toller-Lobe, Durand, & Nagy, 1998). Therefore, all aspects of the claimed concussion mechanism should be elicited. The evaluation should also elicit any problems noted with functioning downrange or the need for medical evacuation. Clinicians may not fully appreciate the rigorous physical and cognitive demands of the austere deployed environment, but the strenuous routine and close quarters with squad members relying on each other will likely unmask any residual concussion symptoms. The incongruities between concussed soldiers who continue to function in combat but then claim an inability to function in the less demanding environment of in-country garrison is worthwhile to document and should raise concern for the veracity of the claimed level of disability.

Clinicians should note when reported levels of dysfunction are discrepant with examinees' complaints. For example, an examinee who reports significant cognitive deficits as a result of an MTBI but has completed higher education or has worked at an intellectually demanding job since the injury occurred is demonstrating a discrepancy between reported problems and objective functioning. Examinees may also call attention to a decline in abilities from premorbid levels, claiming all problems started or worsened significantly during military service or deployment to establish the military connection necessary for benefits eligibility. However, as several researchers have revealed, examinees commonly overestimate their premorbid functioning, even when they have no incentive to exaggerate symptoms; therefore, examinee estimates of their premorbid functioning cannot be accepted in isolation as an accurate or reliable marker of preinjury abilities (Ferguson, Mittenberg, Barone, & Schneider, 1999; Gunstad & Suhr, 2001; Mittenberg, DiGiulio, Perrin, & Bass, 1992). Premorbid functioning should be assessed to the extent possible through records, transcripts, collateral reports, and objective testing.

A final consideration includes the context in which the complaints arose, such as during a postdeployment exam versus a MEB; this context helps establish external incentive. There is a certain disability level that needs to be reached to qualify for lifetime monthly disability payments as well as free medical care and priority access to care. Intimate knowledge of the disability ratings process by the patient should make the clinician wary, especially when accompanied by an appeal of findings or an expressed desire to reach a certain disability rating. This suspicion is heightened when other claims for financial compensation are taking place such as VA service connection, Social Security Disability Insurance (SSDI), and TSGLI. Although interviews of collateral sources of information (e.g., spouses, friends) are also important to consider, the clinician should be aware that the informant may be under pressure to report the patient's symptoms in an exaggerated manner. For example, some soldiers and veterans make claims of being totally dependent on a spouse for the purpose of being found incompetent to manage affairs. The result can be a hefty annual salary to the spouse as a "caregiver" that is likely more than the spouse would earn in a traditional occupation.

Behavioral Observations

Examinees may be observed in the exam room or in other settings such as hallways, cafeterias, and parking lots. Observations of examinees outside of the exam room, which may be planned or occur by chance, can be particularly informative. The observations made in military and veteran contexts are similar to those made in civilian contexts. An emphasis is placed on determining consistencies or inconsistencies between reported functioning and observed functioning as well as on atypical and overly impaired presentations. Examples of overly impaired presentations may include the use of assistive devices (e.g., sunglasses, canes, wheelchairs) or service dogs when there is (a) no concomitant documented disability, (b) no recommendation for their use, or (c) persistent implementation despite medical recommendations against their use. A very slow, labored, or dramatic approach to the examination should raise concern. Individuals wishing to call attention to exaggerated or fabricated deficits may comment that they feel "stupid" or "retarded" because they perform worse than children with intellectual disabilities on SVTs, although such comments may also reflect underlying psychiatric conditions.

Test Measures

The psychological, neuropsychological, and symptom validity tests used with military and veteran populations are essentially the same as those used with civilian populations and are reviewed in detail in Chapters 8 through 13 of this volume. As required by professional ethics (American Psychological Association, 2002; Standard 9.01, Bases for Assessments), "Psychologists base the opinions contained in their recommendations, reports, and diagnostic or evaluative statements, including forensic testimony, on information and techniques sufficient to substantiate their findings . . . " and "provide opinions of the psychological characteristics of individuals only after they have conducted an examination of the individuals adequate to support their statements or conclusions." Thus, for examinees who report or have clear documentation of having sustained an MTBI, clinicians select the measures that they deem indicated for a given evaluation.

ACCURACY IN DIAGNOSIS AND DOCUMENTATION

Descriptions of symptom validity results in neuropsychological evaluation must avoid ambiguity. When the available information does not permit the clinician to be certain regarding examinee effort and honesty or the presence of malingering, the use of probabilistic language (e.g., Slick et al., 1999) is preferred to convey the likelihood of a condition being present, rather than vacillating between potential illnesses that are rarely equally likely. The use of base rates and knowledge of the illness should be used in decision making (Elstein, 1999). For example, if symptom validity testing is failed and the results are deemed invalid, clinicians should address the likelihood of residual cognitive symptoms secondary to concussion given what is known about typical recovery as well as other information from the history, interview, and collateral sources. Ambiguous conclusions are ineffectual for commanders who rely on such information for fitness-for-duty determinations. In addition, ambiguous descriptions or explanations of results (e.g., "Although the patient scored below cutoffs on two symptom validity tests, the scores were not below chance, and the patient appeared to try his best, with an element of anxiety affecting his performance; therefore, the results are considered valid.") leave disability evaluators in a quandary that may lead to application of the benefit-of-the-doubt doctrine (38 U.S.C. § 5107) described previously. In addition, without clarity in diagnosis, the risk of iatrogenic illness and inappropriate treatment is increased.

It is common to encounter clinical notes that attribute all symptoms to a concussion. For example, one neurologist's medical note attributed the patient's restless leg syndrome to a concussion. This example of misattribution highlights the importance of considering alternative etiologies and clearly explaining any ruled out diagnoses lest other conditions remain uninvestigated and disability ratings are made on incomplete information. Although exaggeration of symptoms is necessary for a diagnosis of malingering, it is not sufficient. There are other reasons for symptom exaggeration, and although it may still be intentional, when primary gain is present (e.g., "cry for help"), factitious disorder is a more appropriate diagnosis. Other possibilities for invalid test scores can include a lack of motivation secondary to severe psychiatric illness, disinterest or disengagement, distraction because of severe pain, overmedication, or even burnout when multiple neuropsychological evaluations occur over a short period, as might happen in the medical board process.

There are treatment providers in the disability system who act as advocates for patients and may unintentionally endorse a biased view as part of their health care provision. It is unfortunate that there are also providers who go beyond advocating for the patients' best interest and enable malingered symptoms. One of the ways this occurs is by providing a skewed interpretation of ambiguous language in reports. Clinicians can mitigate this tendency with a careful choice of diction. For example, some providers interpret "inconclusive findings" as being a problem with the neuropsychological tests, rather than a problem with the effort and motivation of the patient. This inaccurate interpretation of the wording in reports may be avoided by using more specific terms such as "exaggeration" or "poor effort" when appropriate. In addition, specifying that the results underestimate the patients' true cognitive abilities more accurately conveys the nature of the problem with the test data than "invalid" or "unknown." Comparing obtained SVT scores to those of groups of individuals known to have much more significant impairment (e.g., older adults with dementia who require 24-hr care or children with mental retardation) can help illustrate the findings in a manner that all reasonable clinicians will understand and accept.

The use of established diagnostic criteria is central to a responsible and ethical neuropsychological evaluation. The criteria set forth by Slick et al. (1999) provide a more comprehensive diagnostic system than the *Diagnostic and Statistical Manual of Mental Disorders* (4th ed., text rev.; *DSM-IV-TR*; American Psychiatric Association,

2000) for the diagnosis of malingered neurocognitive dysfunction. Use of the terms *possible*, *probable*, and *definite* malingered neurocognitive dysfunction communicates the clinicians' confidence in the diagnosis to an appropriate degree. Use of the term "malingered neurocognitive dysfunction" also specifies the condition that is being malingered because patients can have other genuine medical or psychiatric problems that clinicians would want to take care not to imply were malingered as well, without additional supportive evidence. Likewise, because neuropsychological evaluations sometimes reveal malingered psychiatric disorders, determinations of exaggerated and fabricated psychiatric symptoms should also be described in clear terms in neuropsychological reports.

The diagnosis provided by the clinicians should be based on established diagnostic criteria, emphasizing objective evidence without undue influence of emotional, political, or social factors. In appropriate clinical environments, the clinician's chain of command, including supervisors and administrators (a) understands the standard of practice regarding symptom validity assessment; (b) supports the use of objective psychometric measures of effort and honesty; and (c) encourages clinicians to report their findings as accurately as possible. Clinical environments that do not offer these necessary qualities are requiring clinicians to practice in a manner that is inconsistent with ethical and professional standards of practice.

Providing a clinical diagnosis instead of a determination of malingering when criteria for malingering are met is unethical (Ethical Standard 5.01, Avoidance of False or Deceptive Statements) and fails to serve the best interests of the examinee, the clinician, and society. There are numerous reported examples of veterans who fraudulently received psychiatric disability benefits and, when caught, faced criminal charges in civilian courts that resulted in large fines and incarceration (Morel, 2010; Department of Veterans Affairs Office of Inspector General, 2007). Such individuals, the government agencies involved, and tax payers would have been much better served if the clinicians had detected and clearly reported the invalid presentation at the outset.

In the case of medical boards in the military, the findings are eventually forwarded to the physical evaluation board, which includes nonmedical providers. Thus, neuropsychologists can be most effective by writing reports with a broad audience in mind, avoiding professional jargon or vague and confusing terms, and potentially explaining or providing education on neuropsychological points that may not be readily apparent to an untrained individual.

PROVIDING EDUCATION AND FEEDBACK REGARDING INVALID RESULTS

Neuropsychologists can provide a valuable service by educating psychology colleagues, other health care providers, and administrators about the importance of symptom validity assessment in the evaluation of military personnel and veterans who clearly have, or may have, a history of MTBI. Although experience suggests that some otherwise well-meaning professionals can be quite resistant to learning about the prevailing practices and scientific literature regarding symptom validity assessment, opening such a dialogue and striving to maintain the dialogue can be advantageous to all parties. The sharing of such information can occur during staff meetings, case conferences or grand rounds presentations, journal clubs, and other educational contexts. It may be particularly valuable to introduce trainees to the MTBI and symptom validity assessment literature so that their appreciation of the issues is established when they become licensed practitioners.

Bringing in neuropsychology colleagues who may be considered authorities on the topic to present an overview to the staff at a given institution offers an outside perspective that may be better received than the same information provided by someone within the institution; the authors of the National Academy of Neuropsychology and American Academy of Clinical Neuropsychology position papers (Bush et al., 2005; Heilbronner, Sweet, Morgan, Larrabee, Millis, and Conference Participants, 2009) or the recently published texts on the topic (Boone, 2007; Carone & Bush, in press; Larrabee, 2007; Morgan & Sweet, 2009) are examples of those who may be considered authorities.

Examinees are informed at the outset of neuropsychological evaluations during the consent process that they should try their best on the tests and respond honestly throughout the evaluation. Although there is some variability among clinicians about how much information on this topic to convey to examinees at the outset, it is typical for neuropsychologists to inform examinees that their effort and honesty will be assessed. Some clinicians inform examinees that specific tests or other measures of effort and honesty will be used during the evaluation and that disingenuous presentations will likely be detected. However, some clinicians avoid this practice under the assumption that it may produce more sophisticated malingerers. Regardless of which approach is used, there is a widespread agreement that it is unacceptable for clinicians to state which symptom validity measures will be used or give patients information that would allow them to identify a specific symptom validity measure. Likewise, such specific information is not shared with examinees following evaluations.

When neuropsychological evaluations are performed for clinical (vs. forensic) purposes, examinees are typically offered a feedback session to discuss the results of the evaluation and recommendations. Feedback sessions commonly include discussion of symptom validity. When examinees have presented in a valid manner and the test results are considered valid for interpretations, a brief statement to that effect may be offered prior to discussion of the results of the neurocognitive ability measures and psychological tests.

When examinee dissimulation and invalid SVT results are present, such information is typically conveyed to the examinee, if the evaluation was performed in a context in which feedback is expected. Examinee responses to such information vary considerably, from the acknowledgment that an attempt was made to mislead the examiner (rare) and that the examinee was not fully engaged in the evaluation (more common), to adamant denials (common), and threats of formal complaint or physical violence against the neuropsychologist (uncommon but depends on the setting). Neuropsychologists conveying such information understand the implications of the information that they are providing and typically want to facilitate understanding and appropriate resolution of the case. Carone, Iverson, and Bush (2010) presented a model that may be of value to both clinicians and examinees when discussing determinations of dissimulation and malingering. The model "emphasizes the need for professionalism and respect for the patient as well as the need for objective data-driven decisions" (p. 774), which allows neuropsychologists to "broach a complex subject matter in a scientifically and professionally accurate, but sensitive, manner" (p. 775). Chapter 6 provides an updated review of this feedback model by Carone et al.

Even if exaggeration of cognitive symptoms is detected, there may be other genuine conditions worthy of attention. Using this approach can help maintain rapport and facilitate communication about recommendations that may still be clinically relevant and advantageous to the patient. Some examples include normalizing subjective complaints that are common in the general population; education about concussion recovery to mitigate any iatrogenic illness; referrals to learn better coping skills, given that symptom exaggeration may be secondary to immature or exhausted coping mechanisms; treatment for ongoing psychological illness and insomnia, which are very common in service members with ongoing complaints; and investigations of other medical conditions that may be credible and would provide an alternative explanation for current complaints.

CONCLUSIONS

Neuropsychologists who provide services to military personnel and veterans routinely evaluate those who report persisting symptoms following MTBIs. An essential part of neuropsychological evaluations is establishing that examinees presented in a valid manner, provided adequate effort on neurocognitive tests, and responded honestly to interview questions and self-report psychological tests and scales. Neuropsychologists want to find that military personnel and veterans presented in a valid manner and get no joy or satisfaction from determining that a service member or veteran fabricated or exaggerated symptoms. However, history has established that some military personnel and veterans misrepresent their true symptoms and functioning for primary or secondary gain. In some evaluation contexts, the percentage of examinees who dissimulate constitutes a sizeable minority of examinees. Therefore, to best serve examinees, government institutions, and the public, neuropsychologists who evaluate military personnel or veterans who present with persisting neurocognitive symptoms following an MTBI must be vigilant about symptom validity issues and use quantitative measures of symptom validity in their evaluations.

Assessment of symptom validity requires a multimethod approach that typically includes review of records, behavioral observations, clinical interview, and objective testing. Psychometric assessment of effort and honesty is the standard of practice in neuropsychology. Use of multiple objective measures and indicators of effort is expected of neuropsychologists who evaluate military personnel or veterans, with the rigor of such assessment corresponding to the base rates of dissimulation with various patient populations. For example, fewer measures of symptom validity may be needed when there is no potential for secondary gain, whereas more extensive assessment of symptom validity is needed when the potential exists for new or increased disability compensation or other benefits or avoidance of military duty. Neuropsychologists are responsible for determining the optimal methods and procedures for assessing symptom validity with each examinee. Attempts by others to restrict the clinician's judgment place the clinician in a position that is generally inconsistent with professional ethics.

Neuropsychologists have much to offer military personnel and veterans who have sustained MTBIs including (a) establishing whether a TBI was sustained; (b) determining neurocognitive strengths and weaknesses; (c) establishing the presence of factors that are not directly related to neurological trauma that may be contributing to persisting symptoms such as emotional distress, physical pain, medications, and external incentive; (d) providing education to patients, their families, and other health care providers; (e) offering recommendations for treatments such as psychotherapy, psychiatric care, and pain management; and (f) providing cognitive rehabilitation services to help patients compensate for objectively verified cognitive deficits, regardless of the etiology. Providing such services to military personnel and veterans can be a very rewarding endeavor for clinical neuropsychologists.

REFERENCES

American Psychiatric Association. (2000). *Diagnostic and statistical manual of mental disorders* (4th ed., text rev.). Washington, DC: Author.

American Psychological Association. (2002). Ethical principles of psychologists and code of conduct. *American Psychologist*, 57(12), 1060–1073.

Ardolf, B. R., Denney, R. L., & Houston, C. M. (2007). Base rates of negative response bias and malingered neurocognitive dysfunction among criminal defendants referred for neuropsychological evaluation. *The Clinical Neuropsychologist*, 21(6), 899–916.

Armistead-Jehle, P. (2010). Symptom validity test performance in U.S. veterans referred for evaluation of mild TBI. *Applied Neuropsychology*, 17(1), 52–59.

Armistead-Jehle, P., & Hansen, C. L. (2011). Comparison of the Repeatable Battery for the Assessment of Neuropsychological Status Effort Index and Stand-Alone Symptom Validity Tests in a Military Sample. *Archives of Clinical Neuropsychology*, 26(7), 592–601.

Associated Press. (2010). *VA's PTSD rules an invitation for false claims.* Retrieved from http://www.oregonlive.com/news/index.ssf/2010/05/vas_ptsd_rules_an_invitation_f.html

Bazarian, J. J., McClung, J., Shah, M. N., Cheng, Y. T., Flesher, W., & Kraus, J. (2005). Mild traumatic brain injury in the United States, 1998–2000. *Brain Injury*, 19(2), 85–91.

Belanger, H. G., Kretzmer, T., Yoash-Gantz, R., Pickett, T., & Tupler, L. A. (2009). Cognitive sequelae of blast-related versus other mechanisms of brain trauma. *Journal of the International Neuropsychological Society*, 15(1), 1–8.

Belanger, H. G., & Vanderploeg, R. D. (2005). The neuropsychological impact of sports-related concussion: A meta-analysis. *Journal of the International Neuropsychological Society*, 11(4), 345–357.

Bianchini, K. J., Curtis, K. L., & Greve, K. W. (2006). Compensation and malingering in traumatic brain injury: A dose-response relationship? *The Clinical Neuropsychologist*, 20(4), 831–847.

Binder, L. M., Rohling, M. L., & Larrabee, G. J. (1997). A review of mild head trauma. Part I: Meta-analytic review of neuropsychological studies. *Journal of Clinical and Experimental Neuropsychology*, 19(3), 421–431.

Boone, K. B. (2007). *Assessment of feigned cognitive impairment: A neuropsychological perspective.* New York, NY: Guilford Press.

Braverman, M. (1978). Post-injury malingering is seldom a calculated ploy. *Occupational Health & Safety*, 47(2), 36–40.

Burgess, M. A. (2010). *New developments lead to early TBI detection.* Retrieved from U.S. Department of Defense, American Forces Press Services website: http://www.defense.gov/news/newsarticle.aspx?id=58587

Burkett, B., & Whitely, G. (1998). *Stolen valor: How the Vietnam generation was robbed of its heroes and history.* Dallas, TX: Verity Press.

Bush, S. S., Ruff, R. M., Tröster, A. I., Barth, J. T., Koffler, S. P., Pliskin, N. H., . . . Silver, C. H. (2005). Symptom validity assessment: Practice issues and medical necessity NAN policy & planning committee. *Archives of Clinical Neuropsychology*, 20(4), 419–426.

Carone, D. A., & Bush, S. S. (Eds). (in press). Mild traumatic brain injury: Symptom validity assessment and malingering. New York, NY: Springer Publishing.

Carone, D. A., Iverson, G. L., & Bush, S. S. (2010). A model to approaching and providing feedback to patients regarding invalid test performance in clinical neuropsychological evaluations. *The Clinical Neuropsychologist*, 24, 759–778.

Dawes, R. M., Faust, D., & Meehl, P. E. (1989). Clinical versus actuarial judgment. *Science*, 243(4899), 1668–1674.

Department of Defense. (2011). *Worldwide numbers for traumatic brain injury* (non-combat and combat injuries). Retrieved from http://www.dvbic.org/TBI-Numbers.aspx

Department of Veterans Affairs Office of Inspector General. (2005). *Review of state variances in VA disability compensation payments* (#05-00765-137). Retrieved from http://www.va.gov/oig/52/reports/2005/VAOIG-05-00765-137.pdf

Department of Veterans Affairs Office of Inspector General. (2007). *Semiannual report to Congress: October 1, 2006–March 31, 2007, Volume 57.* Retrieved from http://www.va.gov/oig/publications/semiann/reports.asp

Department of Veterans Affairs, Veterans Benefits Administration. (2010). *Annual benefits report, fiscal year 2010.* Retrieved from http://www.vba.va.gov/REPORTS/abr/2010_abr.pdf

Dikmen, S. A., Machamer, J., Fann, J. R., & Temkin, N. R. (2010). Rates of symptom reporting following traumatic brain injury. *Journal of the International Neuropsychological Society*, 16(3), 401–411.

Dishion, T. J., Poulin, F., & Burraston, B. (2001). Peer group dynamics associated with iatrogenic effect in group interventions with high-risk young adolescents. *New Directions for Child and Adolescent Development*, (91), 79–92.

Ekman, P., & O'Sullivan, M. (1991). Who can catch a liar? *American Psychologist, 46*(9), 913–920.

Elstein, A. S. (1999). Heuristics and biases: Selected errors in clinical reasoning. *Academic Medicine, 74*(7), 791–794.

Faust, D. (1995). The detection of deception. *Neurologic Clinics, 13*(2), 255–265.

Faust, D., Hart, K., Guilmette, T. J., & Arkes, H. R. (1988). Neuropsychologists' capacity to detect adolescent malingerers. *Professional Psychology: Research and Practice, 19*, 508–515.

Ferguson, R. J., Mittenberg, W., Barone, D. F., & Schneider, B. (1999). Postconcussion syndrome following sports-related head injury: Expectation as etiology. *Neuropsychology, 13*(4), 582–589.

Freedom of Information Act, 5 U.S.C. § 552, Pub. L. No. 104-231, 110 Stat. 3048. (1996). FOIA Update, Vol. XVII, No. 4. Retrieved from http://www.justice.gov/oip/foia_updates/Vol_XVII_4/page2.htm

Freeman, T., Powell, M., & Kimbrell, T. A. (2008). Measuring symptom exaggeration in veterans with chronic posttraumatic stress disorder. *Psychiatric Research, 158*(3), 374–380.

Frencham, K. A., Fox, A. M., & Maybery, M. T. (2005). Neuropsychological studies of mild traumatic brain injury: A meta-analytic review of research since 1995. *Journal of Clinical and Experimental Neuropsychology, 27*(3), 334–351.

Frueh, B. C., Elhai, J. E., Gold, P. B., Monnier, J., Magruder, K. M., Keane, T. M., & Arana, G. W. (2003). Disability compensation seeking among veterans evaluated for posttraumatic stress disorder. *Psychiatric Services, 54*(1), 84–91.

Frueh, B. C., Hamner, M. B., Cahill, S. P., Gold, P. B., & Hamlin, K. L. (2000). Apparent symptom overreporting in combat veterans evaluated for PTSD. *Clinical Psychology Review, 20*(7), 853–885.

Giza, C. C., & Hovda, D. A. (2001). The neurometabolic cascade of concussion. *Journal of Athletic Training, 36*(3), 228–235.

Giza, C. C., & Hovda, D. A. (2004). The pathophysiology of traumatic brain injury. In M. R. Lovell, R. J. Echemendia, J. T. Barth, & M. W. Collins (Eds.), *Traumatic brain injury in sports* (pp. 45–70). Lisse, The Netherlands: Swets & Zeitlinger.

Graver, C. J., & Shurak, N. R. (in press). Base rates of suboptimal effort in military personnel claiming cognitive deficits following concussion.

Gunstad, J., & Suhr, J. A. (2001). "Expectation as etiology" versus "the good old days": Postconcussion syndrome symptom reporting in athletes, headache sufferers, and depressed individuals. *Journal of the International Neuropsychological Society, 7*(3), 323–333.

Heilbronner, R. L., Sweet, J. J., Morgan, J. E., Larrabee, G. J., & Millis, S. (2009). American Academy of Clinical Neuropsychology consensus conference statement on the neuropsychological assessment of effort, response bias, and malingering. *The Clinical Neuropsychologist, 23*(7), 1093–1129.

Hickling, E., Blanchard, E., Mundy, E., & Galovski, T. (2002). Detection of malingered MVA-related posttraumatic stress disorder: An investigation of the ability to detect professional actors by experienced clinicians, psychological tests, and psychophysiological assessment. *Journal of Forensic Psychology Practice, 2*, 33–53.

Hill, R. (1993). *Posttraumatic stress disorder: How to apply for 100 percent total disability rating*. Lee's Summit, MO: Vietnam Doorgunners Association.

Iverson, G. L. (2005). Outcome from mild traumatic brain injury. *Current Opinion in Psychiatry, 18*(3), 301–317.

Iverson, G. L., Lange, R. T., Gaetz, M., & Zasler, N. D. (2007). Mild TBI. In N. D. Zasler, H. T. Katz, & R. D. Zafonte (Eds.), *Brain injury medicine: Principles and practice* (pp. 333–371). New York, NY: Demos Medical Publishing.

Latham, D. (1992). *How to receive disability for PTSD*. Aurora, IN: Latham Publishing.

Larrabee, G. J. (2003). Detection of malingering using atypical performance patterns on standard neuropsychological tests. *The Clinical Neuropsychologist, 17*(3), 410–425.

Larrabee, G. J. (2007). *Assessment of malingered neuropsychological deficits*. New York, NY: Oxford University Press.

Luis, C. A., Vanderploeg, R. D., & Curtiss, G. (2003). Predictors of postconcussion symptom complex in community dwelling male veterans. *Journal of the International Neuropsychological Society, 9*(7), 1001–1015.

Marion, D. W., Curley, K. C., Schwab, K., & Hicks, R. R. (2011). Proceedings of the military mTBI diagnostics workshop. *Journal of Neurotrauma, 28*(4), 517–516.

McCrea, M. (2008). *Mild traumatic brain injury and postconcussion syndrome: The new evidence base for diagnosis and treatment*. New York, NY: Oxford University Press.

Meares, S., Shores, E. A., Taylor, A. J., Batchelor, J., Bryant, R. A., Baguley, I. J., . . . Marosszeky, J. E. (2011). The prospective course of postconcussion syndrome: The role of mild traumatic brain injury. *Neuropsychology, 25*(4), 454–465.

Mittenberg, W., DiGiulio, D. V., Perrin, S., & Bass, A. E. (1992). Symptoms following mild head injury: Expectation as aetiology. *Journal of Neurology, Neurosurgery, and Psychiatry, 55*(3), 200–204.

Mittenberg, W., Patton, C., Canyock, E. M., & Condit, D. C. (2002). Base rates of malingering and symptom exaggeration. *Journal of Clinical and Experimental Neuropsychology*, 24(8), 1094–1102.

Morel, K. R. (2010). *Differential diagnosis of malingering versus posttraumatic stress disorder: Scientific rationale and objective psychometric methods.* New York, NY: Nova Science Publishers, Inc.

Office of the Assistant Secretary of Defense. (2008). *Memorandum: Symptom management in mild traumatic brain injury.* Retrieved from http://evans.amedd.army.mil/srp/pdf/final%20HA%20mTBI%20-CONUS%20recs.pdf

Paniak, C., MacDonald, J., Toller-Lobe, G., Durand, A., & Nagy, J. (1998). A preliminary normative profile of mild traumatic brain injury diagnostic criteria. *Journal of Clinical and Experimental Neuropsychology*, 20(6), 852–855.

Pensions, Bonuses, and Veterans' Relief, 38 C.F.R. § 3.102 (2009).

Poyner, G. (2010). Psychological evaluations of veterans claiming PTSD disability with the Department of Veterans Affairs: A clinician's viewpoint. *Psychological Injury and Law*, 3(2), 130–132.

RAND Corporation. (2008). *Invisible wounds: Mental health and cognitive care needs of America's returning veterans.* Retrieved from http://www.rand.org/pubs/research_briefs/RB9336/index1.html

Rauch, S. A. (2010). Posttraumatic stress disorder. *Audio-Digest Psychiatry*, 39(3). Retrieved from http://www.cme-ce-summaries.com/psychiatry/ps3903.html

Reid, W. H. (2000). Malingering. *Law and Psychiatry*, 6(4), 226–228.

Rice, C. M. (2009). *Report to Congress on expenditures for activities on traumatic brain injury and posttraumatic stress disorder for 2009.* Retrieved from http://www.tricare.mil/tma/congressionalinformation/downloads/201063/Annual%20Report%20-%20Section%201634(b).pdf

Richman, J., Green, P., Gervais, R., Flaro, L., Merten, T., Brockhaus, R., & Ranks, D. (2006). Objective tests of symptom exaggeration in independent medical examinations. *Journal of Occupational and Environmental Medicine*, 48(3), 303–311.

Rohling, M. L., Binder, L. M., Demakis, G. J., Larrabee, G. J., Ploetz, D. M. & Langhinrichsen-Rohling, J., (2011). A meta-analysis of neuropsychological outcome after mild traumatic brain injury: re-analyses and reconsiderations of Binder et al. (1997), Frencham et al. (2005), and Pertab et al. (2009).

Schretlen, D. J., & Shapiro, A. M. (2003). *A quantitative review of the effects of traumatic brain injury on cognitive functioning.* International Review of Psychiatry, 15(4), 341–349.

Slick, D. J. Sherman, E. M. S. & Iverson, G. L. (1999). Diagnostic criteria for malingered neurocognitive dysfunction: Proposed standards for clinical practice and research. *The Clinical Neuropsychologist*, 13, 545–561.

Sweet, J. J., & Morgan, J. E. (Eds.). (2009). *The neuropsychology of malingering casebook.* New York, NY: Taylor & Francis.

Tombaugh, T. N. (1996). *TOMM: Test of memory malingering.* North Tonawanda, NY: Multi-Health Systems.

Traumatic Service Members' Group Life Insurance. (2012). *Procedural guide: Traumatic injury protection under service members' group life insurance (TSGLI).* Retrieved from http://www.insurance.va.gov/sglisite/tsgli/tsgliguide/tsgliproceduresguide.pdf

University Hospitals EMS Training & Disaster Preparedness Institute. (2011). *Blast injuries.* Retrieved from http://www.emsconedonline.com/pdfs/EMT-%20BLAST%20INJURIES-Trauma.pdf

U.S. Department of Veterans Affairs. (2007). Screening and evaluation of possible traumatic brain injury in operation enduring freedom (OEF) and operation Iraqi freedom (OIF) veterans. *VHA directive 2010–012:* Retrieved from http://www.va.gov/vhapublications/ViewPublication.asp?pub_ID=2176

Whitney, K. A. Shepard, P. H., Williams, A. L., Davis, J. J., & Adams, K. M. (2009). The Medical Symptom Validity Test in evaluation of Operation Iraqi Freedom/Operation Enduring Freedom soldiers: A preliminary study. *Archives of Clinical Neuropsychology*, 24(2), 145–152.

Whittaker, P. (2010, April). Medical boards and mental health. *Paper presented at the Madigan Healthcare System Disability Evaluation System Seminar, Tacoma, WA.*

Zoroya, G. (2007). Scientists: Brain injuries from war worse than thought. *USA Today.* Retrieved from http://www.usatoday.com/news/world/iraq/2007-09-23-traumatic-brain-injuries_N.htm

Zoroya, G. (2009). Officials: Troops hurt by brain-injury focus. *USA Today.* Retrieved from http://www.usatoday.com/news/washington/2009-04-15-researchers-brain-injury_N.htm

DISCLAIMER

The opinions or assertions contained herein are the private views of the authors and are not to be construed as official or reflecting the views of the Department of the Army, Department of Defense, or Veterans Administration.

Symptom Validity Assessment With Special Populations

Jacobus Donders & Michael W. Kirkwood

This chapter reviews the current state of the art of using symptom validity tests (SVTs) with pediatric mild traumatic brain injury (MTBI) and other special populations. The first half of this chapter describes the use of various SVTs with pediatric populations. The second half reviews application of these procedures with adult populations that have specific neurological and/or psychiatric conditions. Suggestions for future research are made throughout the chapter.

ASSESSMENT OF EFFORT IN PEDIATRIC POPULATIONS

In adult populations, research on methodologies to identify response bias has grown exponentially in the last two decades. Relying on objective tools to evaluate noncredible effort and response bias in children is no less important because subjective judgment alone is unlikely to be consistently accurate (Faust, Hart, & Guilmette, 1988; Faust, Hart, Guilmette, & Arkes, 1988). Although developmental competencies need to be considered when evaluating any pediatric population, research has now established that school-age children can readily pass several SVTs using cutoffs established with adults.

Children below age 5 or 6 years with a wide range of learning and neurologic problems can pass the Test of Memory Malingering (TOMM; Constantinou & McCaffrey, 2003; Donders, 2005; Kirk et al., 2011; MacAllister, Nakhutina, Bender, Karantzoulis, & Carlson, 2009). The Word Memory Test (WMT) and Computerized Assessment of Response Bias (CARB) require some facility with reading and numbers so they are inappropriate for early–elementary-aged children. However, on the primary effort indices, children who are older than 10 years typically score above adult cutoffs on the CARB (Courtney, Dinkins, Allen, & Kuroski, 2003). On the WMT, no age effect has been found in children with at least a third-grade reading level (Green & Flaro, 2003). The Medical Symptom Validity Test (MSVT) is similar to the WMT but is shorter and easier and has been successfully used with children as young as second or third grade (Blaskewitz, Merten, & Kathmann, 2008; Carone, 2008; Kirkwood & Kirk, 2010).

How often children display noncredible effort during neuropsychological evaluations has been investigated in several case series. Donders (2005) examined the performance of 100 general pediatric patients on the TOMM and found two boys with a history of noncompliant behavior who put forth insufficient effort. In another study using a mixed outpatient sample, Kirk et al. (2011) found that 4 of 101 children failed the TOMM, with 3 of the 4 also failing another SVT. MacAllister et al. (2009) reported that 2 of 60 pediatric patients with epilepsy performed poorly on the TOMM because of effort-related problems. In a study by Carone (2008) that included 38 children with moderate-to-severe traumatic brain injury (TBI) and other types of serious neurological dysfunction, 2 children were judged to have failed the MSVT because of noncredible effort. A much higher rate of suboptimal effort was found by Chafetz, Abrahams, and Kohlmaier (2007) during U.S. Social Security disability determination evaluations. In their compensation-seeking sample, the TOMM was administered to 96 children and the MSVT to 27 children with failure rates of 28% and 37%, respectively.

Scant attention has been focused on whether invalid effort occurs in pediatric MTBI populations specifically. The only identified work in the area is several publications by Kirkwood and colleagues using data from a consecutive clinical case series from an outpatient concussion program. Patients in the series were considered eligible if they were aged 8–17 years at the time of evaluation. All patients sustained blunt head trauma within the previous 12 months and were referred because of concerns or questions about the effects of underlying brain injury. Children who had intracranial pathology on neuroimaging were included if their Glasgow Coma Scale (GCS) score was never less than 13. Exclusionary criteria were forensic referral, neurosurgical intervention, injury resulting from abuse, and non-TBI such as hypoxia, stroke, or infectious illness.

The first publication using this MTBI case series was focused on the base rate of noncredible effort (Kirkwood & Kirk, 2010). Of the 193 eligible participants, 33 (17%) failed at least one of the three primary effort indices of the MSVT. The group who failed the MSVT was no different than those who passed in terms of injury severity or premorbid developmental learning, attention, or reading problems. After accounting for possible false positives and false negatives on the MSVT, 17% of the sample was judged to have exerted suboptimal effort.

Kirkwood, Yeates, Randolph, and Kirk (2011) recently examined whether performance on the MSVT has implications for ability-based test performance, in an updated version of the case series presented in Kirkwood and Kirk (2010). The updated analysis was based on 276 children. Again, no background or injury-related variable differentiated those who passed from those who failed the MSVT. Performance on the MSVT was correlated significantly with performance on all ability-based tests and explained more than one third (38%) of the variance on a summary index representing performance across the entire range of ability tests. Participants failing the MSVT also performed significantly worse on nearly all neuropsychological tests. Effect sizes were large across most standardized tests, comparable to those seen in similar studies of adults, including samples with financial incentive to perform poorly (Constantinou, Bauer, Ashendorf, Fisher, & McCaffrey, 2005; Lange, Iverson, Brooks, & Rennison, 2010). Even performance on very simple tasks such as the time it took to recite the alphabet, days of the week, or months of the year differed significantly between groups, with participants failing the MSVT taking roughly twice as long as those passing. Group differences were actually least apparent on tests of vocabulary and single-word reading, two skills that might have been predicted to be most related to performance on the verbally based MSVT, if the MSVT primarily measured ability rather than effort.

The practical implications of these data are clear. Following MTBI, a sizable minority of children and adolescents appears to put forth suboptimal effort during neuropsychological examinations, even when external incentives may not be readily apparent. Not unlike studies with adults after MTBI, the SVT performance in pediatric patients also appears to have a substantial impact on ability-based test scores. The findings have potential implications for research as well. The relatively large number of children who have displayed noncredible effort after MTBI raises questions about data collected from previous studies. To date, no identified pediatric MTBI outcome study has incorporated an objective means to evaluate performance validity or symptom exaggeration. As such, previous pediatric studies that have reported persistent postconcussive cognitive deficits or documented cases of "postconcussion syndrome" need to be interpreted cautiously.

The question of why children exert noncredible effort during a neuropsychological evaluation is complex, although it is clear that noncredible effort cannot be equated simply with "malingering." The underlying motivations are apt to include both conscious and unconscious processes and attempts to profit externally and to fulfill internal psychological needs. To illustrate the varied motivations that can be seen in children, Kirkwood, Kirk, Blaha, and Wilson (2010) presented six clinical cases in which invalid performance was apparent. The reasons for the noncredible effort included social motivations, school avoidance, sports avoidance, family factors, and psychogenesis. Simple noncompliance is also apt to explain some cases of noncredible effort in children (Carone, 2008; Donders, 2005). In compensation-seeking contexts, motivations are especially challenging to discern, with some children likely feigning in an attempt to seek indirect approval or attention from family members and others acting more directly to achieve an external incentive, either on their own accord or after explicit coaching. Of note, although children are undoubtedly capable of feigning in pursuit of financial gain after TBI (Lu & Boone, 2002; McCaffrey & Lynch, 2009), compensation-seeking behavior did not drive most of noncredible effort cases in the previously described MTBI case series, in contrast to what is commonly encountered with adults after MTBI. In the most recent analysis (Kirkwood et al., 2011), for example, no participants reported seeking disability compensation, and only 6% of the children who failed the MSVT reported attorney involvement or planned litigation, versus 8% who passed the MSVT.

Regardless of whether a practitioner fully appreciates why a school-age child fails a SVT, such performance should raise questions about the reliability and validity of all collected data. Of course, performance on any SVT depends, in part, on the particular demands of the task and can vary for a multitude of reasons including true impairment and temporary fluctuations in arousal, attention, emotional state, and effort. Determining whether a child is responding in a consistently biased fashion or providing invalid effort in general not only requires careful examination of SVT performance but also a solid understanding of the natural history of the presenting condition; a scrutiny of the child's developmental, medical, educational, and environmental background; and a thorough consideration of the consistency and plausibility of the behavioral, self-report, and test data. How to handle noncredible effort once identified in a clinical evaluation has been largely unexplored in the pediatric literature. Donders (2011) did, however, describe a gentle but confrontational approach that was successful in improving the effort of an oppositional teen. Carone, Iverson, and Bush (2010) also recently proposed a comprehensive model for providing feedback to adults who display invalid performance, which undoubtedly also has a good deal of relevance in considering appropriate ways to discuss noncredible effort with children and their caregivers.

SYMPTOM VALIDITY ASSESSMENT OF OLDER ADULTS WITH COGNITIVE DECLINE

With demographic shifts toward greater longevity and a growing proportion of the population who have passed the traditional retirement age, referrals for evaluation of possible mild cognitive impairment (MCI) or dementia are becoming increasingly frequent in the practice of neuropsychologists who see adult patients. This is one example of a group of conditions where a false positive error (i.e., mistaking genuine impairment for invalid performance) can arguably be considered to be more serious than a false negative one when using SVTs, given the fact that the former could potentially lead to conclusions that might deprive patients from various potentially beneficial therapeutic interventions. For example, if a patient with true dementia of the Alzheimer type were denied a trial of an acetylcholinesterase inhibitor on the basis of an erroneously presumed invalid effort, there might be an increased risk for more rapid progression of the disease. On the contrary, it has also been demonstrated that insufficient effort is a significant predictor of poor success of treatment for chronic neurological conditions (Van Hout, Wekking, Berg, & Deelman, 2008).

It cannot be just assumed that anybody with a diagnosed serious neurological condition, including MCI or dementia, will put forth good effort during neuro-psychological evaluations, so accurate assessment of symptom validity remains important. Although early investigations found concerning rates of false positives when traditional SVT cutoffs were applied, more recent studies of SVTs in persons with MCI or dementia have shown promising results, as long as some special considerations are kept in mind. When the conventional cutoffs are used, many stand-alone and embedded SVTs have poor specificity for persons with dementia. This has been found with tasks as diverse as the TOMM (Teichner & Wagner, 2004), the Victoria Symptom Validity Test (VSVT; Loring, Larrabee, Lee, & Meador, 2007), and the Wechsler Memory Scale-Revised (WMS-R) discriminant function (Hilsabeck et al., 2003). Dean, Victor, Boone, Philpott, and Hess (2009) found that in a large group of patients with various forms of dementia and no incentive to feign cognitive impairment, most effort indices were associated with specificities only in the 30%–70% range when conventional criteria were used. The exception was the vocabulary minus digit span indicator, which maintained specificity $\geq$ 90% across all dementia severity groups. Dean and colleagues suggested possible adjustments of the cutoffs for the other SVT indices to achieve acceptable (i.e., $\geq$ 90%) specificity, but those cutoffs have not yet been cross validated.

Specific criteria for the determination of the possibility of a "genuine memory impairment" or "dementia" profile have been developed for some other commonly used SVTs including the WMT, MSVT, and nonverbal Medical Symptom Validity Test (NV-MSVT; Howe, Anderson, Kaufman, Sachs, & Loring, 2007; Singhal, Green, Ashaye, Shankar, & Gill, 2009). This pattern analysis involves a more detailed actuarial profile analysis that considers the relative performance on all of the test's indices (i.e., not only those in which the conventional cutoffs were based). Some investigators, who were apparently not aware of this option, have recommended against the use of these specific tests in cases of dementia (e.g., Rudman, Oyebode, Jones, & Bentham, 2011). However, Martins and Martins (2010) demonstrated that this recommendation is not appropriate. They found that with only the traditional cutoffs for the WMT immediate recall, delayed recall, and consistency indices, almost two thirds of their patients with MCI who had no secondary gain issues were misclassified as providing poor effort. However, they also demonstrated that specificity could be improved to about 95% when the actuarial criteria for the genuine memory impairment profile were used. Similar results, with specificity > 90%, were reported by Howe and Loring (2009) regarding the dementia profile criteria for the MSVT in a sample of patients referred to a memory disorders clinic which had no medicolegal or financial incentive to underperform and by Green, Montijo, and Brockhaus (2011) with the WMT and MSVT in a sample of patients with MCI (97% specificity). Henry,

Merten, Wolf, and Harth (2010) also found high specificity (> 98%) when actuarial dementia profile analysis was applied to the results from the NV-MSVT in a mixed older adult neurological sample, of which about one third had dementia. In contrast, Axelrod and Schutte (2010) did not find support for the efficacy of the dementia profile for the MSVT, but they applied this algorithm to a very heterogeneous clinical sample, most of whom most likely did not have MCI or dementia.

At present, the consensus in the literature appears to be that the originally published cutoffs for many SVTs may not be applicable in cases of MCI or dementia, but with either adjusted cutoffs or actuarial profile analysis, specificity can be likely improved to acceptable (≥ 90%) levels. It is important, however, that adjusted cutoffs for the TOMM, Warrington Recognition Memory Test, and other instruments that have recently been suggested (Dean et al., 2009) be cross validated with independent samples. In addition, the algorithm for the dementia profile for tests such as the WMT, MSVT, and NV-MSVT should not be applied in cases where there is no independent evidence (e.g., frontotemporal atrophy on brain magnetic resonance imaging [MRI] or collateral information from an independent source with no secondary gain contingencies) to suggest the likelihood of a clinical diagnosis of MCI or dementia. A goal for future research is the exploration of increasing sensitivity of various SVTs to poor effort in cases of MCI and dementia while maintaining acceptable specificity. In addition, no published studies have yet reported on the effect of MTBI on the neuropsychological test performance of persons with premorbid MCI or dementia; this kind of information is also sorely needed.

SYMPTOM VALIDITY TEST PERFORMANCE BY PATIENTS WITH OTHER NEUROLOGICAL IMPAIRMENT

The assessment of effort or symptom validity in patients with other kinds of independently verified neurological impairment also needs to be addressed. This is another example where the potential price of false positive errors would be high because it might deny that such patients needed rehabilitation services or disability benefits. Yet, suboptimal effort has been reported to occur in about one fifth of patients who are clinically referred seeking outpatient treatment for sequelae of acquired brain injury (Locke, Smigielski, Powell, & Stevens, 2008). The findings in the literature have been somewhat mixed but generally encouraging regarding the use of the most common SVTs for patients with various forms of neurological impairment.

Slick and colleagues (2003) reported on a small retrospective case series of nonlitigating patients with profound memory impairment because of conditions ranging from Korsakoff syndrome to aneurysm of the anterior communicating artery. All of these six patients obtained perfect or near perfect scores on the VSVT. Goodrich-Hunsaker and Hopkins (2009) also reported that three patients with profound amnesia as the result of bilateral hippocampal atrophy, as documented on MRI, scored above the conventional cutoff scores on the WMT. Using a larger (n = 32) sample of persons with long-standing mental retardation, Brockhaus and Merten (2004) reported an excellent specificity of almost 97% when using the same criteria. Encouraging results, with specificities ≥ 89%, were reported by Marshall and Happe (2007) for the California Verbal Learning Test-Second Edition (CVLT-II) forced-choice score, the Wechsler Adult Intelligence Scale-Third Edition (WAIS-III) vocabulary minus digit span difference, and the Wechsler Memory Scale-Third Edition (WMS-III) rarely missed items index in a large (n = 100) sample of adults with a history of developmental delay and full scale IQ scores in the 51–74 range. Using a slightly higher functioning sample but with overall ability level below average (< 80),

Chafetz, Prentkowski, and Rao (2011) demonstrated that motivational context had a major impact on failure rates on the MSVT, with a > 50% rate in those seeking disability as compared to a 0% rate in those seeking to retain or regain custody of their children. In contrast, Merten, Bossink, and Schmand (2007) found that most of their nonlitigating patients with conditions ranging from cerebrovascular disease to encephalitis failed several SVT indexes. They suggested that the conventional cutoffs for the TOMM could be applied with confidence for persons with a Mini-Mental State Examination (MMSE) score ≥ 24, but that caution was needed with the WMT in this population. The actuarial profile analysis for the possibility of a genuine memory impairment or dementia profile was not investigated in that study.

Other studies have explored the results of SVTs with various neurological conditions where cognitive impairment is common, although not universal. Woods and colleagues (2003) reported high specificity (98%) of the Hiscock Digit Memory Test (HDMT) in a sample of noncompensation-seeking persons with HIV-associated neurocognitive disorder. Drane and colleagues (2006) reported that almost 92% of their patients with epileptic seizures (defined as *definite ictal EEG [electroencephalography] abnormalities*) passed the conventional cutoffs on the WMT, whereas only about half of their patients with psychogenic nonepiletic seizures (who had episodes of unresponsiveness or behavioral abnormality in the absence of epileptiform EEG changes) did. They concluded that this suggested a motivational component to the presentation of the patients in the latter group.

Several studies have examined performance on SVTs in persons with severe TBI. Macciocchi, Seel, Alderson, and Godsall (2006) reported excellent specificity (99%) of the VSVT in a 9-month series of consecutive admissions to an acute inpatient rehabilitation program of persons with TBI who had a median GCS score of 7. Batt, Shores, and Chekaluk (2008) reported that, for patients with more than a week of posttraumatic amnesia or coma after severe TBI, the TOMM had reasonable specificity of 84%, but the WMT misclassified 44% of the same individuals. It is unfortunate that these authors did not apply the actuarial criteria for the genuine memory impairment or dementia profile. Donders and Boonstra (2007) reported excellent specificity (95%) of the conventional WMT cutoff scores for persons with severe TBI (i.e., coma ≥ 24 hr) who did not have a complicating prior psychiatric history. In addition, Donders and Strong (2011) demonstrated that length of coma and pass or fail of the standard WMT cutoffs made independent contributions to overall learning on the CVLT-II, suggesting that the effects of injury severity and validity of effort can clearly be dissociated.

In general, the balance of the studies in the literature suggest that the most common SVTs, including TOMM, VSVT, and WMT, can be used without a high risk for false positives in a wide range of neurological conditions. Less common SVTs, such as the Rey Dot Counting Test, have had more mixed results across studies (Boone et al., 2002; Marshall & Happe, 2007). Of course, no SVT should be used in isolation, and there is very little research on the effect of MTBI on individuals with preexisting neurological problems such as multiple sclerosis or epilepsy. This is regrettable because persons with chronic neurological problems can potentially have some degree of diminishment of either brain or cognitive reserve capacity (Stern, 2007). It does not appear that a remote prior history of MTBI is likely to affect cognitive performance of persons who sustain a new MTBI (Dawson, Batchelor, Meares, Chapman, & Marosszeky, 2007), but this relationship has not yet been fully explored in persons with a history of moderate-to-severe TBI. Bornstein and colleagues (1993) did not find an effect of a history of MTBI on the neuropsychological test performance of persons with HIV, but this is one of the very few studies in this area, which is in need of additional research of the specific impact on SVT performance. In addition, more research is needed on the effect of prescription medications on SVT performance in persons with bona fide neurological conditions because there is some research emerging that suggests benzodiazepines, in particular, may have some effect in this regard (Loring et al., 2011).

ASSESSMENT OF EFFORT IN PATIENTS WITH PSYCHIATRIC CONDITIONS

There are a number of psychiatric conditions where key features of the clinical syndrome could hypothetically affect motivation for participation in neuropsychological assessment. For example, either severe apathy or depression could theoretically affect test effort even though it is clear that the two are distinctly different constructs, particularly in populations who also have dementia or other neurological conditions (Butterfield, Cimino, Oelke, Hauser, & Sanchez-Ramos, 2010; Levy et al., 1998; Starkstein, Ingram, Garau, & Mizrahi, 2005). Likewise, negative symptoms of schizophrenia, such as avolition, could potentially explain poor motivation during testing, but it is important to realize that this may reflect distinct underlying striato-cortical pathology and not necessarily willful underperformance (Barch & Dowd, 2010; Meisenzahl, Schmitt, Scheuerecker, & Möller, 2007; Simon et al., 2010). However, accurate measurement of effort during assessment would still be important because apathy at baseline is known to be a significant risk factor for future functional decline in community-dwelling older adults (Clarke, Ko, Lyketsos, Rebok, & Eaton, 2010) as well as for conversion from MCI to dementia (Chilovi et al., 2009). Likewise, avolition has been related to poorer functional outcomes in schizophrenia (Foussias & Remington, 2010).

When persons pass SVTs, there is little evidence for an effect of depression on cognitive test performance (Rohling, Green, Allen, & Iverson, 2002). However, this begs the question of how valid SVTs are in psychiatric populations. Regarding depression, the studies on the applicability of SVTs are encouraging. Ashendorf, Constantinou, and McCaffrey (2004) demonstrated that level of depression did not affect performance on the TOMM in a large sample of community-dwelling older adults. Even more convincingly, Rees, Tombaugh, and Boulay (2001) found that none of 26 consecutive inpatients from an affective disorders unit scored below the conventional cutoff point for the second or retention trials of the TOMM. Likewise, Gierok, Dickson, and Cole (2005) found that only 1 out of 20 psychiatric inpatients with various diagnoses but without secondary gain incentives failed these TOMM criteria. Yanez, Fremouw, Tennant, Strunk, and Coker (2006) did find slightly lower but still acceptable specificity (85%–90%) in 20 patients with very high levels of depression. Furthermore, O'Bryant, Finlay, and O'Jile (2007) demonstrated that performance on the TOMM did not correlate significantly with standardized measures of anxiety and depression in a larger mixed clinical sample. Thus, the TOMM in particular has been validated for use with patients with depression. There has been relatively less research with other SVTs in samples with clinical depression. In addition, none of the above studies formally assessed apathy. These are goals for future research. Such studies should be feasible now that there are specific diagnostic criteria for the concept of apathy (Mulin et al., 2011), and several reliable and valid instruments for its assessment are available (Clarke et al., 2011).

In the area of psychotic disorders, the findings have been more mixed. Egeland and colleagues (2003) described that patients with schizophrenia had "close to normal" scores on the VSVT, but they did not provide actual data on classification accuracy for that test. Duncan (2005) reported a specificity of 92% using the conventional cutoffs for the TOMM in a sample of psychiatric inpatients with various psychotic disorders. Moreover, he demonstrated that the presence of impairment of concentration, as defined by performance on a continuous performance test, did not significantly increase the risk of false positives with those cutoffs. In contrast, Gorissen, Sanz, and Schmand (2005) found that 72% of patients with schizophrenia spectrum disorders failed the WMT when the conventional cutoffs for that test were used. They attributed this to lack of mental effort as a manifestation of the negative symptoms of schizophrenia including apathy and avolition. However, they did not investigate to what degree the results would have been different if the criteria for the genuine memory impairment or dementia profile had been applied. In fact, no study has yet been published regarding such actuarial profile analysis of the WMT, MSVT, or NV-MSVT in patients with psychotic disorders. This is another goal for future research.

The current consensus in the literature appears to be that conventional cutoffs for most SVTs can be applied with reasonable confidence for patients with mood disorders who do not have psychotic symptoms. The situation is less clear regarding psychotic disorders, and SVTs should be applied with more caution in that population until future research clarifies the use of adjusted cutoffs or actuarial profile analysis. Such research should also address the impact of MTBI on the SVT and other test performance in patients with schizophrenia or other psychotic disorders. In addition, in light of a growing literature of significant SVT failure rates in self-referred nonlitigating individuals who seek academic accommodations for conditions ranging from learning disability to attention deficit hyperactivity disorder (Suhr, Hammers, Dobbins-Buckland, Zimak, & Hughes, 2008; Sullivan, May, & Galbally, 2007), more research is needed on the role of MTBI in such populations.

Some research has been done in the area of SVT performance of persons who incurred uncomplicated MTBI after relatively more benign prior psychiatric histories, such as outpatient psychotherapy for anxiety disorder or several years of receiving a low dose of selective serotonin reuptake inhibitor for dysthymic disorder. Such prior history has been shown to be associated with an almost fourfold increased relative risk for failure of validity criteria on the TOMM or the CVLT-II forced-choice index in persons with MTBI, even in the absence of financial compensation seeking (Moore & Donders, 2004). Similar results have been reported for the WMT using the conventional cutoffs (Donders & Boonstra, 2007). In both studies, which spanned the full range of TBI severity, ≤ 5% of the cases who were classified by the SVT as having invalid effort had (a) coma ≥ 24 hr and (b) no history of premorbid psychiatric problems. It should be noted that none of these studies found any statistically significant correlation between measures of injury severity (e.g., length of coma) and level of performance on the SVT used, suggesting that it was very unlikely that the findings could be attributed to organic effects of novel-acquired brain dysfunction. Furthermore, it is also unlikely that the findings can be explained by other factors that can be comorbid with MTBI such as pain (Etherton, Bianchini, Greve, & Ciota, 2005). Some individuals with uncomplicated MTBI with longstanding prior emotional or psychosocial adjustment difficulties may just be making reattribution errors associated with underestimation of their premorbid problems and selective augmentation of cognitive and somatic symptoms. It is important to note that this does not occur exclusively in a context of financial compensation seeking. Like Drane and colleagues (2006) have suggested regarding their patients with psychogenic nonepileptic seizures, SVT failure in persons with uncomplicated MTBI superimposed on a premorbid outpatient psychiatric history cannot be automatically equated with intentional exaggeration or fabrication of deficits. However, it means that the findings are attributable to something other than neurologic dysfunction.

CONCLUSIONS

Several SVTs can be applied with confidence in pediatric populations (e.g., pediatric MTBI) and with adults with a wide range of neurological disorders or depressive spectrum disorders. When applied with older adults with dementia, cutoffs may need to be adjusted downward (e.g., for TOMM), and/or actuarial profile analysis is advisable (e.g., for WMT or MSVT). For patients with psychotic disorders, these instruments need to be used with caution. It is important to appreciate that failure of SVTs in any of these populations does not necessarily equate with malingering. Failed SVTs inform the examiner about the likely invalidity of findings, but the reason for that invalidity needs to be determined on a case-by-case basis. A priority for future research is the clarification of SVT performance and its correlates in patients who sustain MTBI that is superimposed on a preexisting neurologic or psychiatric history.

REFERENCES

Ashendorf, L., Constantinou, M., & McCaffrey, R. J. (2004). The effect of depression and anxiety on the TOMM in community-dwelling older adults. *Archives of Clinical Neuropsychology*, 19(1), 125–130.

Axelrod, B. N., & Schutte, C. (2010). Analysis of the dementia profile on the Medical Symptom Validity Test. *The Clinical Neuropsychologist*, 24(5), 873–881.

Barch, D. M., & Dowd, E. C. (2010). Goal representations and motivational drive in schizophrenia: The role of prefrontal-striatal interactions. *Schizophrenia Bulletin*, 36(5), 919–934.

Batt, K. E., Shores, E. A., & Chekaluk, E. (2008). The effect of distraction on the Word Memory Test and Test of Memory Malingering in patients with a severe brain injury. *Journal of the International Neuropsychological Society*, 14(6), 1074–1080.

Blaskewitz, N., Merten, T., & Kathmann, N. (2008). Performance of children on symptom validity tests: TOMM, MSVT, and FIT. *Archives of Clinical Neuropsychology*, 23(4), 379–391.

Boone, K. B., Lu, P., Back, C., King, C., Lee, A., Philpott, L., . . . Warner-Chacon, K. (2002). Sensitivity and specificity of the Rey Dot Counting Test in patients with suspect effort and various clinical samples. *Archives of Clinical Neuropsychology*, 17(7), 625–642.

Bornstein, R. A., Podraza, A. M., Para, M. F., Whitacre, C. C., Fass, R. J., Rice, R. R., & Nasrallah, H. A. (1993). Effect of minor head injury on neuropsychological performance in asymptomatic HIV–1 infection. *Neuropsychology*, 7, 228–234.

Brockhaus, R., & Merten, T. (2004). Neuropsychologische diagnostik suboptimalen leistungsverhaltens mit dem Word Memory Test [Neuropsychological assessment of suboptimal performance: The Word Memory Test]. *Der Nervenarzt*, 75(9), 882–887.

Butterfield, L. C., Cimino, C. R., Oelke, L. E., Hauser, R. A., & Sanchez-Ramos, J. (2010). The independent influence of apathy and depression on cognitive functioning in Parkinson's disease. *Neuropsychology*, 24(6), 721–730.

Carone, D. A. (2008). Children with moderate/severe brain damage/dysfunction outperform adults with mild-to-no brain damage on the Medical Symptom Validity Test. *Brain Injury*, 22(12), 960–971.

Carone, D. A., Iverson, G. L., & Bush, S. S. (2010). A model to approaching and providing feedback to patients regarding invalid test performance in clinical neuropsychological evaluations. *The Clinical Neuropsychologist*, 24(5), 759–778.

Chafetz, M. D., Abrahams, J. P., & Kohlmaier, J. (2007). Malingering on the social security disability consultative exam: A new rating scale. *Archives of Clinical Neuropsychology*, 22(1), 1–14.

Chafetz, M. D., Prentkowski, E., & Rao, A. (2011). To work or not to work: Motivation (not low IQ) determines symptom validity test findings. *Archives of Clinical Neuropsychology*, 26(4), 306–313.

Chilovi, B. V., Conti, M., Zanetti, M., Mazzù, I., Rozzini, L., & Padovani, A. (2009). Differential impact of apathy and depression in the development of dementia in mild cognitive impairment patients. *Dementia and Geriatric Cognitive Disorders*, 27(4), 390–398.

Clarke, D. E., Ko, J. Y., Kuhl, E. A., van Reekum, R., Salvador, R., & Marin, R. S. (2011). Are the available apathy measures reliable and valid? A review of the psychometric evidence. *Journal of Psychosomatic Research*, 70(1), 73–97.

Clarke, D. E., Ko, J. Y., Lyketsos, C., Rebok, G. W., & Eaton, W. W. (2010). Apathy and cognitive and functional decline in community-dwelling older adults: Results from the Baltimore ECA longitudinal study. *International Psychogeriatrics*, 22(5), 819–829.

Constantinou, M., Bauer, L., Ashendorf, L., Fisher, J. M., & McCaffrey, R. J. (2005). Is poor performance on recognition memory effort measures indicative of generalized poor performance on neuropsychological tests? *Archives of Clinical Neuropsychology, 20*(2), 191–198.

Constantinou, M., & McCaffrey, R. J. (2003). Using the TOMM for evaluating children's effort to perform optimally on neuropsychological measures. *Child Neuropsychology, 9*(2), 81–90.

Courtney, J. C., Dinkins, J. P., Allen, L. M. III & Kuroski, K. (2003). Age related effects in children taking the Computerized Assessment of Response Bias and Word Memory Test. *Child Neuropsychology, 9*(2), 109–116.

Dawson, K. S., Batchelor, J., Meares, S., Chapman, J., & Marosszeky, J. E. (2007). Applicability of neural reserve theory in mild traumatic brain injury. *Brain Injury, 21*(9), 943–949.

Dean, A. C., Victor, T. L., Boone, K. B., Philpott, L. M., & Hess, R. A. (2009). Dementia and effort test performance. *The Clinical Neuropsychologist, 23*(1), 133–152.

Donders, J. (2005). Performance on the Test of Memory Malingering in a mixed pediatric sample. *Child Neuropsychology, 11*(2), 221–227.

Donders, J. (2011). Pediatric traumatic brain injury: Effects of questionable effort. In J. E. Morgan, I. S. Baron, & J. H. Ricker (Eds.), *Casebook of clinical neuropsychology* (pp. 183–190). New York, NY: Oxford University Press.

Donders, J., & Boonstra, T. (2007). Correlates of invalid neuropsychological test performance after traumatic brain injury. *Brain Injury, 21*(3), 319–326.

Donders, J., & Strong, C. A. H. (2011). Embedded effort indicators on the California Verbal Learning Test–Second Edition (CVLT–II): An attempted cross-validation. *The Clinical Neuropsychologist, 25*(1), 173–184.

Drane, D. L., Williamson, D. J., Stroup, E. S., Holmes, M. D., Jung, M., Koerner, E., . . . Miller, J. W. (2006). Cognitive impairment is not equal in patients with epileptic and psychogenic nonepileptic seizures. *Epilepsia, 47*(11), 1879–1886.

Duncan, A. (2005). The impact of cognitive and psychiatric impairment of psychotic disorders on the Test of Memory Malingering (TOMM). *Assessment, 12*(2), 123–129.

Egeland, J., Sundet, K., Rund, B. R., Asbjørnsen, A., Hugdahl, K., Landrø, N. I., . . . Stordal, K. I. (2003). Sensitivity and specificity of memory dysfunction in schizophrenia: A comparison with major depression. *Journal of Clinical and Experimental Neuropsychology, 25*(1), 79–93.

Etherton, J. L., Bianchini, K. J., Greve, K. W., & Ciota, M. A. (2005). Test of Memory Malingering performance is unaffected by laboratory-induced pain: Implications for clinical use. *Archives of Clinical Neuropsychology, 20*(3), 375–384.

Faust, D., Hart, K., & Guilmette, T. J. (1988). Pediatric malingering: The capacity of children to fake believable deficits on neuropsychological testing. *Journal of Consulting and Clinical Psychology, 56*(4), 578–582.

Faust, D., Hart, K. J., Guilmette, T. J., & Arkes, H. R. (1988). Neuropsychologists' capacity to detect adolescent malingerers. *Professional Psychology: Research and Practice, 19*, 508–515.

Foussias, G., & Remington, G. (2010). Negative symptoms in schizophrenia: Avolition and Occam's razor. *Schizophrenia Bulletin, 36*(2), 359–369.

Gierok, S. D., Dickson, A. L., & Cole, J. A. (2005). Performance of forensic and non-forensic adult psychiatric inpatients on the Test of Memory Malingering. *Archives of Clinical Neuropsychology, 20*(6), 755–760.

Goodrich-Hunsaker, N. J., & Hopkins, R. O. (2009). Word Memory Test performance in amnesic patients with hippocampal damage. *Neuropsychology, 23*(4), 529–534.

Gorissen, M., Sanz, J. C., & Schmand, B. (2005). Effort and cognition in schizophrenia patients. *Schizophrenia Research, 78*(2–3), 199–208.

Green, P., & Flaro, L. (2003). Word Memory Test performance in children. *Child Neuropsychology, 9*(3), 189–207.

Green, P., Montijo, J., & Brockhaus, R. (2011). High specificity of the Word Memory Test and Medical Symptom Validity Test in groups with severe verbal memory impairment. *Applied Neuropsychology, 18*(2), 86–94.

Henry, M., Merten, T., Wolf, S. A., & Harth, S. (2010). Nonverbal Medical Symptom Validity Test performance of elderly healthy adults and clinical neurology patients. *Journal of Clinical and Experimental Neuropsychology, 32*(1), 19–27.

Hilsabeck, R. C., Thompson, M. D., Irby, J. W., Adams, R. L., Scott, J. G., & Gouvier, W. D. (2003). Partial cross-validation of the Wechsler Memory Scale-Revised (WMS-R) general memory-attention/concentration malingering index in a nonlitigating sample. *Archives of Clinical Neuropsychology, 18*(1), 71–79.

Howe, L. L., Anderson, A. M., Kaufman, D. A., Sachs, B. C., & Loring, D. W. (2007). Characterization of the Medical Symptom Validity Test in evaluation of clinically referred memory disorders clinic patients. *Archives of Clinical Neuropsychology, 22*(6), 753–761.

Howe, L. S., & Loring, D. W. (2009). Classification accuracy and predictive ability of the Medical Symptom Validity Test's dementia profile and genuine memory impairment profile. *The Clinical Neuropsychologist*, 23(2), 329–342.

Kirk, J. W., Harris, B., Hutaff-Lee, C. F., Koelemay, S. W., Dinkins, J. P., & Kirkwood, M. W. (2011). Performance on the Test of Memory Malingering (TOMM) among a large clinic-referred pediatric sample. *Child Neuropsychology*, 17(3), 242–254. Advance online publication. doi: 10.1080/09297049.2010.533166

Kirkwood, M. W., & Kirk, J. W. (2010). The base rate of suboptimal effort in a pediatric mild TBI sample: Performance on the Medical Symptom Validity Test. *The Clinical Neuropsychologist*, 24(5), 860–872.

Kirkwood, M. W., Kirk, J. W., Blaha, R. Z., & Wilson, P. E. (2010). Noncredible effort during pediatric neuropsychological exam: A case series and literature review. *Child Neuropsychology*, 16(6), 604–618.

Kirkwood, M. W., Yeates, K. O., Randolph, C., & Kirk, J. W. (2011). The implications of symptom validity test failure for ability-based test performance in a pediatric sample. *Psychological Assessment*, 24(1), 36–45. Advance online publication. doi: 10.1037/a0024628

Lange, R. T., Iverson, G. L., Brooks, B. L., & Rennison, V. L. A. (2010). Influence of poor effort on self-reported symptoms and neurocognitive test performance following mild traumatic brain injury. *Journal of Clinical and Experimental Neuropsychology*, 32(9), 961–972.

Levy, M. L., Cummings, J. L., Fairbanks, L. A., Masterman, D., Miller, B. L., Craig, A. H., . . . Litvan, I. (1998). Apathy is not depression. *The Journal of Neuropsychiatry and Clinical Neurosciences*, 10(3), 314–319.

Locke, D. E., Smigielski, J. S., Powell, M. R., & Stevens, S. R. (2008). Effort issues in post-acute outpatient acquired brain injury rehabilitation seekers. *NeuroRehabilitation*, 23(3), 273–281.

Loring, D. W., Larrabee, G. J., Lee, G. P., & Meador, K. J. (2007). Victoria Symptom Validity Test performance in a heterogeneous clinical sample. *The Clinical Neuropsychologist*, 21(3), 522–531.

Loring, D. W., Marino, S. E., Drane, D. L., Parfitt, D., Finney, G. R., & Meador, K. J. (2011). Lorazepam effects on Word Memory Test performance: A randomized, double-blind, placebo-controlled, crossover trial. *The Clinical Neuropsychologist*, 25(5), 799–811.

Lu, P. H., & Boone, K. B. (2002). Suspect cognitive symptoms in a 9-year-old child: Malingering by proxy? *Clinical Neuropsychology*, 16(1), 90–96.

MacAllister, W. S., Nakhutina, L., Bender, H. A., Karantzoulis, S., & Carlson, C. (2009). Assessing effort during neuropsychological evaluation with the TOMM in children and adolescents with epilepsy. *Child Neuropsychology*, 15(6), 521–531.

Macciocchi, S. N., Seel, R. T., Alderson, A., & Godsall, R. (2006). Victoria Symptom Validity Test performance in acute severe traumatic brain injury: Implications for test interpretation. *Archives of Clinical Neuropsychology*, 21(5), 395–404.

Marshall, P., & Happe, M. (2007). The performance of individuals with mental retardation on cognitive tests assessing effort and motivation. *The Clinical Neuropsychologist*, 21(5), 826–840.

Martins, M., & Martins, I. P. (2010). Memory malingering: Evaluating WMT criteria. *Applied Neuropsychology*, 17(3), 177–182.

McCaffrey, R. J., & Lynch, J. K. (2009). Malingering following documented brain injury: Neuropsychological evaluation of children in a forensic setting. In J. E. Morgan & J. J. Sweet (Eds.), *Neuropsychology of malingering casebook* (pp. 377–385). New York, NY: Psychology Press.

Meisenzahl, E. M., Schmitt, G. J., Scheuerecker, J., & Möller, H. J. (2007). The role of dopamine for the pathophysiology of schizophrenia. *International Review of Psychiatry*, 19, 337–345.

Merten, T. M., Bossink, L., & Schmand, B. (2007). On the limits of effort testing: Symptom validity tests and severity of neurocognitive symptoms in nonlitigant patients. *Journal of Clinical and Experimental Neuropsychology*, 29(3), 308–318.

Moore, B. A., & Donders, J. (2004). Predictors of invalid neuropsychological test performance after traumatic brain injury. *Brain Injury*, 18(10), 975–984.

Mulin, E., Leone, E., Dujardin, K., Delliaux, M., Leentjens, A., Nobili, F., . . . Robert, P. H. (2011). Diagnostic criteria for apathy in clinical practice. *International Journal of Geriatric Psychiatry*, 26(2), 158–165.

O'Bryant, S. E., Finlay, C. G., & O'Jile, J. R. (2007). TOMM performances and self-reported symptoms of depression and anxiety. *Journal of Psychopathology and Behavioral Assessment*, 29(2), 111–114.

Rees, L. M., Tombaugh, T. N., & Boulay, L. (2001). Depression and the Test of Memory Malingering. *Archives of Clinical Neuropsychology*, 16(5), 501–506.

Rohling, M. L., Green, P., Allen, L. M. III & Iverson, G. L. (2002). Depressive symptoms and neurocognitive test scores in patients passing symptom validity tests. *Archives of Clinical Neuropsychology*, 17(3), 205–222.

Rudman, N., Oyebode, J. R., Jones, C. A., & Bentham, P. (2011). An investigation into the validity of effort tests in a working age dementia population. *Aging & Mental Health*, 15(1), 47–57.

Simon, J. J., Biller, A., Walther, S., Roesch-Ely, D., Stippich, C., Weisbrod, M., & Kaiser, S. (2010). Neural correlates of reward processing in schizophrenia—relationship to apathy and depression. *Schizophrenia Research*, 118(1–3), 154–161.

Singhal, A., Green, P., Ashaye, K., Shankar, K., & Gill, D. (2009). High specificity of the Medical Symptom Validity Test in patients with severe memory impairment. *Archives of Clinical Neuropsychology*, 24(8), 721–728.

Slick, D. J., Tan, J. E., Strauss, E., Mateer, C. A., Harnadek, M., & Sherman, E. M. S. (2003). Victoria symptom validity test scores of patients with profound memory impairment: Nonlitigant case studies. *The Clinical Neuropsychologist*, 17(3), 390–394.

Starkstein, S. E., Ingram, L., Garau, M. L., & Mizrahi, R. (2005). On the overlap between apathy and depression in dementia. Journal of Neurology, Neurosurgery & Psychiatry, 76(8), 1070–1074.

Stern, Y. (Ed.). (2007). *The concept of cognitive reserve: A catalyst for research*. In Cognitive reserve: Theory and applications (pp. 1–4). New York, NY: Taylor & Francis.

Suhr, J., Hammers, D., Dobbins-Buckland, K., Zimak, E., & Hughes, C. (2008). The relationship of malingering test failure to self-reported symptoms and neuropsychological findings in adults referred for ADHD evaluation. *Archives of Clinical Neuropsychology*, 23(5), 521–530.

Sullivan, B. K., May, K., & Galbally, L. (2007). Symptom exaggeration by college adults in attention-deficit hyperactivity disorder and learning disorder assessments. *Applied Neuropsychology*, 14(3), 189–207.

Teichner, G., & Wagner, M. T. (2004). The Test of Memory Malingering (TOMM): Normative data from cognitively intact, cognitively impaired, and elderly patients with dementia. *Archives of Clinical Neuropsychology*, 19(3), 455–464.

Van Hout, M. S. E., Wekking, E. M., Berg, I. J., & Deelman, B. G. (2008). Psychosocial and cognitive rehabilitation of patients with solvent-induced chronic toxic encephalopathy: A randomised controlled study. *Psychotherapy and Psychosomatics*, 77(5), 289–297.

Woods, S. P., Conover, E., Weinborn, M., Rippeth, J. D., Brill, R. M., Heaton, R. K., & Grant, I. (2003). Base rate of Hiscock Digit Memory Test failure in HIV-associated neurocognitive disorders. *The Clinical Neuropsychologist*, 17(3), 383–389.

Yanez, Y. T., Fremouw, W., Tennant, J., Strunk, J., & Coker, K. (2006). Effects of severe depression on TOMM performance among disability-seeking outpatients. *Archives of Clinical Neuropsychology*, 21(2), 161–165.

Index